CRITICAL CARE

ANESTHESIOLOGY: A PROBLEM-BASED LEARNING APPROACH

Series Editor: Magdalena Anitescu, MD

Published and Forthcoming Titles

Pain Management edited by Magdalena Anitescu

Anesthesiology edited by Tracey Straker and Shobana Rajan

Pediatric Anesthesia edited by Kirk Lalwani, Ira Todd Cohen, Ellen Y. Choi, and Vidya T. Raman

Neuroanesthesia edited by David E. Traul and Irene P. Osborn

Cardiac Anesthesia edited by Mohammed M. Minhaj

Critical Care edited by Taylor A. Johnston, Steven E. Miller, and Joseph Rumley

Perioperative Care edited by Deborah Richman and Debra Pulley

Regional Anesthesiology and Acute Pain Medicine edited by Nabil Elkassabany and Eman Nada

Obstetric Anesthesia edited by Rebecca Minehart, Jaime Daly, and Heather Nixon

Professional, Ethical, Legal, and Educational Lessons in Medicine edited by Kirk Lalwani, Ira Cohen, Ellen Choi, and Berklee Robins

CRITICAL CARE

A PROBLEM-BASED LEARNING APPROACH

EDITED BY

Taylor A. Johnston, Steven E. Miller, and Joseph Rumley

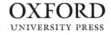

OXFORD
UNIVERSITY PRESS

OXFORD
UNIVERSITY PRESS

Oxford University Press is a department of the University of Oxford. It furthers
the University's objective of excellence in research, scholarship, and education
by publishing worldwide. Oxford is a registered trade mark of Oxford University
Press in the UK and certain other countries.

Published in the United States of America by Oxford University Press
198 Madison Avenue, New York, NY 10016, United States of America.

© Oxford University Press 2022

Library of Congress Cataloging-in-Publication Data
Names: Johnston, Taylor A., editor. | Miller, Steven E. (Anesthesiologist),
editor. | Rumley, Joseph, editor.
Title: Critical care : a problem-based learning approach / Taylor A. Johnston,
Steven E. Miller, [Joseph Rumley].
Other titles: Critical care (Johnston) | Anesthesiology (Oxford University Press)
Description: New York, NY : Oxford University Press, [2022] |
Series: Anesthesiology a problem based learning |
Includes bibliographical references and index.
Identifiers: LCCN 2020041482 (print) | LCCN 2020041483 (ebook) |
ISBN 9780190885939 (hardback) | ISBN 9780197523575 (epub) |
ISBN 9780190885946 (online)
Subjects: MESH: Critical Care—methods | Critical Illness—therapy |
Problem-Based Learning
Classification: LCC RC86.8 (print) | LCC RC86.8 (ebook) | NLM WX 18.2 |
DDC 616.02/8—dc23
LC record available at https://lccn.loc.gov/2020041482
LC ebook record available at https://lccn.loc.gov/2020041483

DOI: 10.1093/med/9780190885939.001.0001

1 3 5 7 9 8 6 4 2

Printed by Lakeside Book Company, United States of America

CONTENTS

CONTRIBUTORS

Ashish A. Ankola, MD
Fellow in Pediatric Critical Care Medicine
Department of Anesthesiology, Critical Care and Pain
Medicine
Boston Children's Hospital
Boston, MA, USA

Brent Barta
Anesthesiology Associates
Bryan Healthcare
Lincoln, Nebraska

Ayush Batra, MD
Assistant Professor
Department of Neurology & Pathology
Northwestern University Feinberg School of Medicine
Chicago, IL, USA

Suzanne Bennett, MD
Associate Professor
Department of Anesthesiology
University of Cincinnati College of Medicine-UC Health
Cincinnati, OH, USA

Payal Boss, MD
Anesthesiologist, Anesthesia Practice Consultants
Grand Rapids, MI, USA

Robert Bowen, MD, MPH
Assistant Professor
Department of Anesthesiology
Washington University in St. Louis
Saint Louis, MO, USA

Kristen Carey Rock, MD
Assistant Professor
Department of Anesthesia and Critical Care
University of Pennsylvania
Bryn Mawr, PA, USA

Manuel R. Castresana, MD, FCCM, FACA, FASA
Professor Anesthesiology, Surgery and Respiratory Tera
Department of Anesthesiology
Medical College of Georgia
Augusta, GA, USA

Floria E. Chae, MD
Assistant Professor Clinical
Department of Anesthesiology
The Ohio State University Medical Center
Columbus, OH, USA

Tarif A. Choudhury, MD
Pediatric Cardiac Intensivist
Divisions of Pediatrics Critical Care Medicine and Pediatric
Cardiology
Morgan Stanley Children's Hospital of New York at
Columbia University School of Medicine
New York, NY, USA

Matthew D. Coleman, MD
Anesthesiologist
Department of Anesthesiology
North Shore LIJ, Anesthesiology
Chappaqua, NY, US

Douglas Coursin
Pulmonary & Critical Care Staff
Clinical Science Center
Madison, WI

Justin Daniels, MD
Assistant Professor
Department of Anesthesiology and Critical Care
University of Kansas Medical Center
Overland Park, Kansas, USA

J. David Bacon, MD
Intensivist
Department of Anesthesiology, Critical Care Division
University of Kentucky
Lexington, KY, USA

Paul D. Weyker, MD
Associate Professor, Anesthesiology, Critical Care, and
Interventional Pain Medicine
Department of Clinical Science
Kaiser Permanente Bernard J. Tyson School of Medicine
San Francisco, CA, USA

Alessandro R. DeCamilli, MD
Attending Physician, Anesthesia and Critical Care
Department of Anesthesiology and Critical Care
Medicine
Memorial Sloan Kettering Cancer Center
New York, NY, USA

Ricardo Diaz Milian, MD
Associate Professor
Department of Anesthesiology and Perioperative
Medicine
Augusta University
Augusta, GA, USA

Murtaza Diwan, MD
Assistant Professor
University of Michigan
Ann Arbor, MI, USA

Eric Feduska, MD
Physician
Department of Anesthesiology
Thomas Jefferson University Hospital
Philadelphia, PA, USA

Andre F. Gosling, MD
Cardiothoracic Anesthesiology Fellow
Department of Anesthesiology
Duke University Hospital
Durham, NC, USA

Edward D. Foley, MD
Critical Care Medicine Specialist
Department of Anesthesiology
Augusta University, Medical College of Georgia
Augusta, GA, USA

Rachel Maldonado Freeman, MD
Assistant Clinical Professor
Department of Anesthesiology
University of Texas Health Science Center San Antonio
San Antonio, TX, US

Eric Fried, MD
Assistant Professor
Department of Anesthesiology, Perioperative, and Pain
Medicine
ICAHN of School of Medicine, Mount Sinai Hospital
New York, NY, USA

Haley Goucher Miranda, MD
Assistant Professor of Anesthesiology and Critical Care
Medicine
Department of Anesthesiology
The University of Kansas Health System
Lenexa, KS, USA

Erin S. Grawe, MD
Director of Perioperative Medicine
Department of Anesthesiology
University of Cincinnati
Cincinnati, OH, USA

John Hance, MD, MPH
Cardiothoracic Surgeon
East Tennessee Cardiovascular Surgery Group
Methodist Medical Center
Oak Ridge, TN, USA

Kevin W. Hatton, MD, PhD
Clinical Professor
Department of Anethesiology
University of Kentucky College of Medicine
Lexington, KY, USA

Tracey Eng, Master of Medical Science in Anesthesiology
Certified Anesthesiology Assistant
Department of Anesthesiology
Grady Memorial Hospital
Alpharetta, GA, USA

Selby B. Johnson II, MD
Cardiothoracic Anesthesiology Fellow
Department of Anesthesiology and Critical Care
Duke University Medical Center
Durham, NC, USA

Taylor A. Johnston, MD
Associate Professor of Anesthesiology at CUMC
Division of Cardiothoracic Anesthesiology
Director, Anesthesia Services for Interventional Cardiology
New York, NY, USA

Neil A. Nadkarni, MD
Fellow
Ken and Ruth Davee Department of Neurology
McGaw Northwestern Memorial Hospital
Chicago, IL, USA

Jonathan Ketzler, MD
Anesthesiologist/Intensivist
Department of Anesthesia and Critical Care
University of Wisconsin Hospital
Madison, WI, USA

Eric Leiendecker, MD
Cardiac Anesthesiologist and Intensive Care Medicine Specialist
Department of Anesthesiology
University of Wisconsin
Madison, WI, USA

Sarah Maben, MD
Anesthesiologist & Intensivist
Department of Anesthesia
Lahey Hospital & Medical Center
Burlington, MA, USA

Jennifer McDonald, MD
Residency Program Director
Teaching Faculty, Division of Critical Care
Department of Anesthesiology
Nuvance - Vassar Brothers Medical Center
Poughkeepsie, NY, USA

Connor McNamara, MD
Assistant Professor, Critical Care Anesthesiology
Department of Anesthesiology and Perioperative Medicine
University Hospitals Cleveland Medical Center
Westlake, OH, USA

Maggie Mechlin, MD
Assistant Professor of Clinical Anesthesiology
Department of Anesthesiology
University of Cincinnati College of Medicine
Montgomery, OH, USA

Steven E. Miller, MD
Assistant Professor of Anesthesiology
Department of Anesthesia
Columbia University in the City of New York
New York, NY, USA

Aaron M. Mittel, MD
Assistant Professor
Department of Anesthesiology
Columbia University Medical Center
New York, NY, USA

Joti Juneja Mucci, MD
Critical Care Medicine Specialist
Department of Anesthesiology
Cleveland Clinic
Cleveland, OH, USA

Laurence Ring, MD
Assistant Professor
Department of Anesthesiology
Columbia University
Old Tappan, NJ, USA

Oscar Roldan, MD
Critical Care Anesthesiologist
Department of Anesthesiology
Northshore University Hospital
Long Island City, NY, US

Erik Romanelli, MD, MPH
Obstetric Anesthesiologist
Department of Anesthesiology
Montefiore Medical Center/Albert Einstein College of
Medicine
New York, NY, USA

Joseph Rumley, MD
Assistant Professor
Department of Anesthesiology
Columbia University
New York, NY, USA

Jennifer A. Salant, MD
Fellow, Pediatric Critical Care
Pediatrics, Division of Critical Care and Hospital Medicine
Columbia University Medical Center
New York, NY, USA

S. Veena Satyapriya, MD
Assistant Clinical Professor
Department of Anesthesiology
The Ohio State University Wexner Medical Center
New Albany, OH, USA

Shahzad Shaefi, MD, MPH
Assistant Professor in Anaesthesia, Harvard Medical School
Department of Anesthesia, Critical Care and Pain Medicine
Beth Israel Deaconess Medical Center
Boston, MA, USA

Liang Shen, MD, MPH
Assistant Professor of Clinical Anesthesiology
Department of Anesthesiology
Weill Cornell Medicine
New York, NY, USA

Hannah Shin, DO
Resident Physician
Department of Surgery
Philadelphia College of Osteopathic Medicine
Philadelphia, PA, USA

Jared Staab, DO, MA
Critical Care Medicine Specialist
Department of Anesthesiology
University of Kansas Medical Center
Kansas City, KS, USA

James N. Sullivan, MD
Anesthesiologist, Intensivist/Associate Professor of
Anesthesiology
Department of Anesthesiology
University of Nebraska
Omaha, Nebraska, Douglas

Lauren Sutherland, MD
Assistant Professor
Department of Anesthesiology
Columbia University Irving Medical Center
New York, NY, USA

Christopher Tam, MD
Assistant Professor of Clinical Anesthesiology
Department of Anesthesiology
Weill Cornell Medical Center
Rego Park, NY, USA

Shaun L. Thompson, MD
Assistant Professor
Department of Anesthesiology
University of Nebraska Medical Center
Omaha, NE, USA

Joshua Trester, MD
Assistant Professor of Anesthesiology and Critical Care
Department of Anesthesiology
University of Cincinnati
Cincinnati, OH, USA

Katherine V. Biagas, MD
Professor and Vice Chair
Department of Pediatrics
The Renaissance School of Medicine at Stony Brook University
Stony Brook, NY, US

Emily Anne Vail, MD, MSc
Assistant Professor
Department of Anesthesiology and Critical Care
University of Pennsylvania
Philadelphia, PA, USA

Gebhard Wagener, MD
Professor
Department of Anesthesiology
Columbia University Medical Center
New York, NY, USA

Dennis Wells, MD
Congenital Cardiac Surgery Fellow
Department of Cardiothoracic Surgery
Cincinnati Children's Hospital Medical Center
Cincinnati, OH, USA

Brian Woods, MD
Director, General Anesthesia Division
Department of Anesthesiology
St Francis Hospital
Roslyn, NY, USA

Elrond Teo, MBBS
Cardiothoracic and Transplant Anesthesiologist
Department of Anesthesiology
Piedmont Atlanta Hospital
Marietta, GA, USA

Xiwen Zheng, MD
Anesthesiologist
Department of Anesthesiology
Memorial Healthcare System
Pembroke Pines, FL, USA

Nicholas C. Zimick, MD, MS
Cardiothoracic and Critical Care Anesthesiologist
Department of Anesthesia Associates of Morristown
Morristown Medical Center
Convent Station, NJ, USA

1.

REFRACTORY ASTHMA IN THE PEDIATRIC PATIENT

Jennifer A. Salant and Katherine V. Biagas

STEM CASE AND KEY QUESTIONS

A previously healthy 5-year-old male with a history of mild bronchiolitis as an infant presents with a 12-hour history of respiratory distress. His family reports that he has been experiencing cough, congestion, and rhinorrhea without fever over the prior 48 hours. His parents admonish one prior episode of wheezing in the setting of a viral illness for which he was prescribed an albuterol metered dose inhaler (MDI) with a spacer. He did not improve after an MDI dose at home. His parents brought him to the emergency department (ED) for further management. On examination he is tachypneic for age and has prolonged expiratory phase with scattered wheeze throughout both lung fields. He is unable to speak in full sentences.

WHAT ARE THE PHYSICAL FINDINGS OF ACUTE ASTHMA EXACERBATION? WHAT ARE THE INITIAL MANAGEMENT STEPS IN THE ED?

The patient is administered albuterol and ipratropium, both by nebulizer, and receives an IV dose of methylprednisone. Upon re-examination, his air entry shows minimal improvement. His saturations are starting to worsen, and he is now hypoxemic with a saturation of 86% on room air. Supplemental oxygen via nasal cannula is administered along with a bolus of normal saline, intravenous magnesium, and subcutaneous terbutaline. A repeat dose of ipratropium and continuous nebulized albuterol is started before an arterial blood gas is obtained: pH 7.49, CO_2 26, O_2 81, and HCO_3 22. His tachypnea and hypoxemia are not improved, and he is placed on continuous positive airway pressure (CPAP) respiratory support with a nasal mask interface. The ED team deems an admission to be necessary, and transfer to the pediatric intensive care unit (PICU) is arranged.

WHAT ARE THE THERAPEUTIC STRATEGIES FOR MANAGEMENT IN THE PICU, AND WHAT MEDICATIONS SHOULD BE CONSIDERED?

Once admitted to the PICU, despite CPAP support and continuous nebulized albuterol therapy, the patient is noted to have continued tachypnea and progressively decreased aeration. Another dose of intravenous terbutaline is given, an infusion is initiated, and he is escalated to biphasic positive airway pressure (BiPAP) therapy to reduce the work of breathing. Thirty minutes later, the terbutaline infusion is increased, but as time passes he becomes less responsive to verbal and tactile stimuli. Lung sounds become increasingly difficult to auscultate, and a repeat arterial blood gas reveals a worsening respiratory acidosis: pH 7.12, CO_2 72, O_2 74, and HCO_3 23. The PICU team prepares to intubate the patient.

WHAT PRECAUTIONS SHOULD BE TAKEN WHEN PREPARING TO INTUBATE THIS PATIENT? WHAT INITIAL MECHANICAL VENTILATION SETTINGS SHOULD BE CONSIDERED?

The patient's nasogastric contents are suctioned, and he undergoes induction with ketamine and rocuronium. Bag mask ventilation is performed, and the patient's trachea is successfully intubated with a 5.5-microcuff endotracheal tube. Immediately upon positive pressure ventilation, he becomes hypotensive to 76/40 and is administered a second normal saline bolus after which his blood pressure improves to 87/55. He is placed on a volume-controlled, spontaneous intermittent mechanical ventilation mode, but the ventilator begins alarming because appropriate tidal volumes are not being achieved. The patient requires high driving pressures for adequate chest rise and without elevated pressures (>40 cm H_2O) adequate tidal volumes are not being achieved. The PICU team switches him to a pressure control spontaneous intermittent mechanical ventilation mode with a rate of 10 and in inhaled time of 1.0. To achieve appropriate tidal volumes, he requires a positive end expiratory pressure (PEEP) of 7 cm H_2O and a peak inspiratory pressure of 35 cm H_2O. His fraction of inhaled oxygen is set at 1.0, and on these settings his first post-intubation arterial blood gas is pH 7.05, CO_2 80, O_2 85, and HCO_3 26.

IN THE SETTING OF WORSENING RESPIRATORY STATUS ON POSITIVE PRESSURE VENTILATION, WHAT FURTHER THERAPIES SHOULD BE CONSIDERED?

The PICU team increases the patient's steroid dose to the maximum for his weight and slowly up-titrates the terbutaline infusion. The decision is made to start a helium:oxygen gas mixture ("heliox") to allow for less turbulent gas flow while on the ventilator. Given the patient's mild hypoxemia, the team orders 70:30 helium:oxygen. Concerned for his persistent respiratory failure, the team contemplates other measures that may be taken to help this patient. The anesthesia team is called to discuss initiation of potent inhaled anesthetic therapy. The PICU team also considers initiating the patient's transfer to a center that specializes in extracorporeal membrane oxygenation (ECMO) support with a plan to initiate veno-venous ECMO cannulation.

DISCUSSION

Asthma is the most common chronic childhood disease worldwide, affecting over 24 million people in the United States and costing the healthcare system over $56 billion per year [1]. While asthma is ideally managed in the outpatient setting, there are a spectrum of clinical presentations and acute exacerbations that often require admission to the intensive care unit (ICU). The ICU provider must be prepared to treat the entire spectrum of disease manifestations. The term *status asthmaticus* refers to a severe or life-threatening manifestation of asthma in which respiratory distress and bronchospasm persists despite aggressive therapies. Status asthmaticus accounts for approximately 20% of childhood hospitalizations [2], but the prevalence of asthma is decreasing in children [3] with fewer than 10% having near-fatal events.

ETIOLOGY AND PATHOGENESIS

Asthma is a heterogeneous inflammatory lower airways disease that manifests as bronchospasm and obstruction increasing the resistance to gas entry and preventing whatever is inhaled from being exhaled. This ultimately leads to difficulties in both oxygenation and ventilation as well as hypotension secondary to severely increased intrathoracic pressure decreasing cardiac output.

HALLMARKS OF ACUTE ASTHMA
EXACERBATION
Physical Findings

The physical examination of patients suffering from an asthma exacerbation differ based on degree of severity. Tachypnea, especially with a prolonged expiratory phase and wheezes, are the hallmark symptoms of the disease. These are often accompanied by coughing, shortness of breath, and chest tightness. Mild hypoxemia, as a consequence of ventilation-perfusion mismatch, is often present. Hypercarbia, secondary to hypoventilation, coupled with somnolence, is a sign of respiratory failure and impending respiratory arrest.

Airway Response and Pathology

The lower airways are most acutely affected. Exacerbations are often due to the interaction of an environmental trigger with genetic predisposition for the disease [4]. An inflammatory cascade begins, resulting in swelling, mucus production, and bronchospasm. This leads to obstructive physiology.

MEDICAL MANAGEMENT OF
SEVERE ASTHMA

The medical management of asthma focuses largely on the use of medications that reduce airway inflammation and relax bronchospasm. Medications are depicted in Table 1.1.

Inhaled Bronchodilators: Short-Acting Beta-2 Agonists and Anticholinergics

The treatment of asthma exacerbations typically begins in the ED with rapid smooth muscle relaxation through initiation of an inhaled beta-2 agonist, either as intermittent doses or by continuous nebulization [3], which aims to relax airway obstruction. Racemic albuterol is most commonly prescribed, although the levorotatory or L-enantiomer levalbuterol and long-acting salbutamol are also prescribed agents. Inhaled anticholinergic medications, such as ipratropium, are often added to further enhance smooth muscle relaxation through antagonism of acetylcholine receptors. Ipratropium is never used as monotherapy for asthma [3] and inhaled anticholinergic agents may reduce morbidity by preventing hospital admission; there are no data to suggest their utility once the patient is admitted to the hospital [2].

It should be noted that bronchodilation may transiently increase ventilation–perfusion mismatch as some lung segments may open partially allowing for oxygenation and the resultant reversal of hypoxic pulmonary vasodilation. This transient and mild hypoxemia can be managed with supplemental oxygen via nasal cannula. Thus, a transient reduction in pulse oximetry in the setting of inhaled therapies may be an indication that the patient is responding to therapy, as opposed to a heralding sign of patient decompensation.

Long-Acting Beta-2 Agonists

While inhaled short-acting beta-2 agonists are preferred initial agents, systemic administration of long-acting beta-2 agonists (LABAs), such as terbutaline or salbutamol, should be considered for patients whose airway obstruction is so severe that inhaled therapies cannot reach distal airways. Terbutaline is a commonly prescribed LABA that can be administered as a bolus dose via a subcutaneous or intravenous route or continuously as an intravenous infusion. Evidence suggests that early initiation of a terbutaline infusion while in the ED may decrease the need for mechanical ventilation in those admitted to the PICU [5]. While not useful in the acute setting, inhaled LABAs are commonly prescribed to outpatients to improve disease control and prevent acute attacks. However, long-term use of LABAs results in downregulation of beta-receptors and decreased responsiveness to beta-agonist rescue therapies during acute exacerbations [2].

Table 1.1. COMMONLY PRESCRIBED MEDICATIONS FOR STATUS ASTHMATICUS

MEDICATION	DOSE	MECHANISM OF ACTION	SIDE EFFECT PROFILE
Albuterol (inhaled continuous)	Children <12 years: 0.5 mg/kg/hour by continuous nebulization Children >12 years: 10–15 mg/hour by continuous nebulization	Beta-2 agonist	Tachycardia, nervousness, tremors, chest pain, edema, flushing, anxiety, nausea
Corticosteroids	2 mg/kg load followed by 1 mg/kg IV every 12 hours. In severe cases, dose may be increased to 1mg/kg IV every 6 hours Maximum dose is 60 mg IV every 6 hours	Anti-inflammatory	Hyperglycemia, agitation
Terbutaline (subcutaneous)	Children <12 years: 0.01 mg/kg/dose every 20 minutes for three doses, then every 2 to 6 hours as needed >12 years: 0.25 mg/dose, may repeat three times every 20 minutes	B-receptor mediated smooth muscle dilation	Tachycardia, arrhythmia, hypotension (diastolic)
Terbutaline (intravenous)	Loading dose of 2–10 mcg/kg bolus over 20 minutes followed by a 0.08–00.4 mcg/kg/min infusion. This may be titrated up in increments of 0.1 mcg/kg/min every thirty minutes to a maximum of 10 mcg/kg/minute	As above	As above
Helium-oxygen mixture (Heliox) (continuous inhaled)	Mixtures of 70%/30% and 80%/20% helium:oxygen are available. Concentrations of helium less than 60% do not result in improvement in gas flow; accordingly, heliox should not be mixed with additional supplemental oxygen	Increased laminar flow during periods of turbulence in distal airways	
Magnesium sulfate	25 to 75 mg/kg (max 2000 mg) as a single dose over 20 to 60 minutes	Alteration of calcium flow through sarcoplasmic reticulum	Flushing, hypotension, vasodilation, acute decrease in cardiac contractility
Theophylline	Initial dosing recommendations are to achieve a serum concentration goal of 10 mcg/mL during the first 12–24-hour period. Loading dose (if no theophylline administered within previous 24 hours): 4.6 mg/kg IV (preferred) or 5 mg/kg orally followed by an infusion. Children 1 to <9 years: 0.8 mg/kg/hour Children 9 to <12 years: 0.7 mg/kg/hour Adolescents 12 to <16 years: 0.5 mg/kg/hour (0.7 mg/kg/hour in cigarette or marijuana smokers); maximum 900 mg/day Adolescents >16 years: 0.4 mg/kg/hour Those with cardiac decompensation, cor pulmonale, sepsis with multiorgan failure, or shock: 0.2 mg/kg/hour; maximum 400 mg/day	Phosphodiesterase inhibition in airway smooth muscles	Tachycardia, headache, hyperactivity, restlessness, decreased seizure threshold, tremors, nausea, emesis.
Ketamine	1 mg/kg bolus, followed by 5–20 mcg/kg/min infusion, titrating to effect	Catecholamine release with resultant bronchodilation	Sialorrhea, tachycardia, laryngospasm, agitation/ hallucinations

Corticosteroids

Systemic corticosteroids are the most important therapy for acute, severe asthma exacerbations. Corticosteroids improve asthma flare-ups through two mechanisms. Initially, corticosteroids upregulate beta-2 receptors in bronchial smooth muscle cells and allow these tissues to have an amplified response to inhaled beta-2 agonists. Overtime, corticosteroids decrease inflammation by decreasing pro-inflammatory cytokines and airway swelling [2]. While enteral prednisone/prednisolone or dexamethasone are appropriate agents for systemic therapy, many patients admitted to the ICU are unable to safely consume or absorb oral medications. Therefore, patients are prescribed IV methylprednisolone while the patient is on continuous inhaled therapy [1], until the patient is safely able to take oral therapy.

Magnesium Sulfate

Magnesium relaxes smooth muscle by antagonizing calcium flow through the sarcoplasmic reticulum. Studies have demonstrated the effectiveness of magnesium administered to children who present to the ED with moderate to severe asthma flares [2]. Magnesium is often administered after a bolus of normal saline to mitigate magnesium's side effect of hypotension. The use of nebulized magnesium is also currently being investigated [2], although its benefit remains unclear.

Methylxanthines

Methylxanthines are a class of phosphodiesterase inhibitors that include caffeine, theophylline, and aminophylline. Methylxanthines cause smooth muscle relaxation by increasing intracellular cyclic adenosine monophosphate [2] and are often administered as a continuous infusion during acute exacerbations. Side effects frequently include tachycardia, a lowered seizure threshold, and numerous drug–drug interactions involving specific isozymes of the cytochrome P450 pathway. Along with their narrow therapeutic window and need for frequent monitoring of drug levels, use of these medications has fallen out of favor.

Ketamine

Ketamine is an anesthetic with multiple mechanisms of action affecting the N-methyl-D-aspartate (NMDA), opioid, monoaminergic, and muscarinic receptors. Often it is used as a sedative in the setting of refractory status asthmaticus and is especially useful in situations of cardiopulmonary instability due to its sympathomimetic like properties (see "Intubation and Mechanical Ventilation"). As a noncompetitive NMDA receptor antagonist, ketamine is a dissociative anesthetic agent with a side effect of bronchodilation. As compared with other sedative induction agents, ketamine doesn't cause significant peripheral vasodilation that can decrease preload or reduce afterload, making it a particularly useful agent for endotracheal intubation in this setting [2]. Its bronchodilatory effects also make it an ideal agent for continuous sedative infusion once a patient is intubated. It should be noted that ketamine's side effect profile includes sialorrhea, for which anticholinergics like glycopyrrolate or atropine are often used to treat during continuous therapy or as a premedication prior to bolus administration. Additionally, ketamine can be associated with laryngospasm, which can be life-threatening, when used alone for induction of anesthesia at subtherapeutic doses.

Heliox

The use of a helium–oxygen gas mixture, also referred to as "Heliox," is useful in the setting of status asthmaticus as its use improves laminar flow and reduces turbulence in the distal airways. The use of Heliox is also thought to help deliver inhaled beta-2 agonists to distal airways by allowing for better air entry [6]. Formulations of Heliox come in two standard concentrations: 70%:30% and 80%:20% helium:oxygen ratios, respectively. Therefore, it is important to note that Heliox should not be initiated in patients with significant hypoxemic respiratory failure, as the proportion of oxygen in these mixtures may not be significant enough to support them.

Inhaled Halogenated Anesthetics

Halothane, sevoflurane, isoflurane, and desflurane are the inhaled anesthetics used to treat refractory status asthmaticus. These inhaled anesthetics are direct-acting relaxants of smooth muscle and can be used to reverse underlying bronchoconstriction. Additionally, inhaled anesthetics have a rapid onset of action and provide sedation while they are being administered. Of the inhaled agents, isoflurane is the most commonly used. It is low in cost, does not result in accumulated breakdown products, and requires the fewest reservoir refills over time [6]. It also does not have the arrhythmic side effect profile of halothane. The use of inhaled anesthetics in the ICU and outside of the operating room is institution-specific and requires conversation with anesthesiology colleagues as well as knowledge of intuition protocols.

Extracorporeal Membrane Oxygenation

In cases of refractory hypoxemia and/or hypercarbia despite medical management, support of the patient using ECMO should be considered. Veno-venous cannulation may support the patient's gas exchange until resolution of severe bronchospasm. Children placed onto ECMO for respiratory failure have an approximately 43% mortality rate, with the chances of death increasing with degree of initial hypoxemia [7]. Pediatric ECMO requires experienced providers who balance the potential benefit of survival with the ECMO risk of thrombosis, bleeding, and stroke. If ECMO cannulation is a consideration, early referral to a pediatric ECMO center is essential.

VENTILATION STRATEGIES

Noninvasive Mechanical Ventilation: High-Flow Nasal Cannula, CPAP, and BiPAP

No specific recommendations exist regarding the use of noninvasive ventilatory strategies for pediatric patients with severe asthma exacerbations, but the indications for intervention and escalation of support include persistent hypoxemia, hypercarbic respiratory failure, altered mental status, and progressive acidemia secondary to anaerobic metabolism [8]. A case series has shown that use of high-flow nasal cannula may prevent invasive ventilation in certain patients admitted to the PICU, as well as decrease recovery time and shorten length of stay [9]. However, there are no specific guidelines regarding high-flow nasal cannula for status asthmaticus, and its utility remains variable and institution-dependent.

Other noninvasive modalities may be used in these patients. Their use is intended to relieve the increased work of breathing of increased airway resistance and stent smaller airways to allow for exhalation to prevent dynamic hyperinflation. CPAP is often employed in the ED or ICU for persistent hypoxemia or signs of impending respiratory failure. If the patient does not improve despite CPAP and continuous nebulized treatments, BiPAP is sometimes used, although its use has not been shown to decrease hospital or PICU admission rates, length of stay, or recovery time [10]. There is currently no evidence to either support or negate the use of CPAP or

BiPAP in status asthmaticus [11]; however, many clinicians find it appropriate to try these therapies prior to intubation and mechanical ventilation.

Intubation and Mechanical Ventilation

In the asthmatic patient refractory to medical therapy, endotracheal intubation is indicated for persistent severe hypoxemia and hypercarbia or when metabolic acidosis persists. When preparing to intubate these patients, it is important to be aware of the cardiopulmonary interactions that may occur. The introduction of positive pressure within the thorax decreases venous return of blood, which decreases preload, and often results in predictable hypotension. This may be addressed by the administration of a bolus of crystalloid fluid prior to, or during, intubation. The choice of induction agents is also crucial. As previously discussed, ketamine has properties that counteract the pathophysiology of status asthmaticus, making it a common choice.

Ventilator settings should be chosen to promote adequate oxygenation while allowing for permissive hypercapnia and mild respiratory acidosis to help minimize air trapping and hyperinflation. Clinicians must keep in mind the dynamic pressure changes associated with the use of positive pressure ventilation in these patients and take measures to mitigate the risk of barotrauma and pneumothorax. Patients often require elevated ventilator driving pressures to maintain appropriate lung and chest wall expansion, and use of a pressure-control ventilation mode can prevent unanticipated peak pressures and decrease the risk of barotrauma. As patients have a need for prolonged expiratory phases, a lower respiratory rate with a higher inspiratory pressure and inspiratory time will result in increased tidal volumes and an inspiratory to expiratory ratio (I:E) of 1:4 or 1:5; this is a crucial maneuver to minimize air trapping. Given that patients may have varying degrees of dead space, use of end-tidal CO_2 monitor is not a reliable measure of ventilation. If patients have persistent respiratory failure despite the aforementioned ventilator adjustments, administration of neuromuscular blockade should be considered to allow the care team to take full control of respiratory mechanics. The pressure at end-expiration after a ventilatory pause allows the clinician to obtain the patients intrinsic PEEP (sometimes referred to as "auto-PEEP"). If neuromuscular blockade is needed, a lower PEEP that still allows for oxygenation should be used to minimize peak pressures and barotrauma. However, if the patient is breathing spontaneously, clinicians should attempt to "match" PEEP with intrinsic PEEP such that the patient can overcome this pressure during inspiration.

CONCLUSIONS

- The clinical syndrome of acute asthma exacerbation, or status asthmaticus, is a life-threatening condition that may require ICU admission, but fewer than 10% of patients having near-fatal events.

- Initial management focuses on treatment with inhaled bronchodilating agents and corticosteroids with the use of supplemental oxygen to overcome the resulting hypoxemia of treatment.

- For patients with unresponsive disease, the addition of inhaled anticholinergics, methylxanthines, and magnesium sulfate are additional therapeutic options.

- Patients with impending respiratory failure may require noninvasive measures of respiratory support despite not having been shown to reduce the duration of the event or the need for intubation.

- Clinicians need to be vigilant and look for signs of progressive respiratory failure that would signal the need for endotracheal intubation and mechanical ventilator support as appropriate.

- When mechanical intubation is unable to provide enough supportive care, escalating therapies for these higher risk patients can include heliox, neuromuscular blocking agents, halogenated inhaled anesthetics, and even ECMO.

REFERENCES

1. Giuliano, J.S., et al., *Corticosteroid Therapy in Critically Ill Pediatric Asthmatic Patients.* Pediatr Crit Care Med, 2013. **14**: p. 467–470.
2. Rehder, K.J., *Adjunct Therapies for Refractory Status Asthmaticus in Children.* Respir Care, 2017. **62**(6): p. 849–865.
3. Stenson, E.K., M.J. Tchou, and D.S. Wheeler, *Management of Acute Asthma Exacerbations.* Curr Opin Pediatr, 2017. **29**(3): p. 305–310.
4. Mims, J.W., *Asthma: Definitions and Pathophysiology.* Int Forum Allergy Rhinol, 2015. 5 Suppl 1: p. S2–S6.
5. Doymaz, S. and J. Schneider, *Safety of Terbutaline for Treatment of Acute Severe Pediatric Asthma.* Pediatr Emer Care, 2018. **34**: p. 299–302.
6. Carrié, S. and T.A. Anderson, *Volatile Anesthetics for Status Asthmaticus in Pediatric Patients: A Comprehensive Review and Case series.* Pediatric Anesthesia, 2015. **25**(5): p. 460–467.
7. Bailly, D.K., et al., *Development and Validation of a Score to Predict Mortality in Children Undergoing Extracorporeal Membrane Oxygenation for Respiratory Failure: Pediatric Pulmonary Rescue With Extracorporeal Membrane Oxygenation Prediction Score.* Crit Care Med, 2017. **45**(1): p. e58–e66.
8. Pardue Jones, B., et al., *Pediatric Acute Asthma Exacerbations: Evaluation and Management From Emergency Department to Intensive Care Unit.* J Asthma, 2016. **53**(6): p. 607–617.
9. Mayfield, S., J. Jauncey-Cooke, and F. Bogossian, *A Case Series of Paediatric High Flow Nasal Cannula Therapy.* Aust Crit Care, 2013. **26**(4): p. 189–192.
10. Golden, C., et al., *Clinical Outcomes After Bilevel Positive Airway Pressure Treatment for Acute Asthma Exacerbations.* JAMA Pediatr, 2015. **169**(2): p. 186–188.
11. Korang, S.K., et al., *Non-Invasive Positive Pressure Ventilation for Acute Asthma in Children.* Cochrane Database Syst Rev, 2016. 9: p. CD012067.
12. Hurfurd, W.E., *The Bronchospastic Patient.* Int Anesthesiol Clin, 2000. **38**(1): p. 77–90.
13. Maffei, F.A., et al., *Duration of Mechanical Ventilation in Life-Threatening Pediatric Asthma: Description of an Acute Asphyxial Subgroup.* Pediatrics, 2004. **114**(3): p. 762–767.
14. Sur, S., et al., *Sudden Onset Fatal asthma. A Distinct Entity With Few Eosinophils and Relatively More Neutrophils in the Airway Submucosa.* Am Rev Respir Dis, 1993. **148**: p. 713–719.

15. Morales, D.R., et al., *Adverse Respiratory Effect of Acute β-Blocker Exposure in Asthma*. Chest, 2014. **145**(4): p. 779–786.
16. Zorc, J.J. and C.B., Hall, *Bronchiolitis: Recent Evidence on Diagnosis and Management*. Pediatrics, 2010. **125**(2): p. 342–349.

REVIEW QUESTIONS

1. A 6-year-old-girl with a past medical history of recurrent, severe asthma is brought to the ED with wheezing and tachypnea. Her HR is 135, RR 45, BP 110/70 and SaO2 on 4 liters per minute of 100%FiO2 by face mask is 94%. She is treated with 5 mg of inhaled albuterol by nebulization and is given 1 mg/kg of methylprednisone intravenously. Her RR improves to 32 and her HR is 125. Her SaO2 drops to 89% and her wheezing becomes louder on auscultation. Which of the following best explains her worsened hypoxemia?

A. Poor response to the beta-agonist
B. Beta-agonist driven reduction in airways resistance
C. Beta-agonist driven reduction in hypoxic pulmonary vasoconstriction
D. Pneumothorax

Answer and Explanation: 1. C. A decrease in SaO2 is a common clinical outcome after the administration of bronchodilators. At first glance, this may be interpreted as worsening disease process; however, this patient seems to be improving clinically. Therefore, the most likely choice is that this patient is experiencing ventilation/perfusion (V/Q) mismatch in the setting of albuterol administration due to a reduction of hypoxic pulmonary vasoconstriction. Therefore answer C is correct. Answer A is incorrect, as the patient's tachypnea is improving and her wheeze is louder suggesting improved air entry. Answer B would only be correct if her saturations were improving. While a pneumothorax would result in worsening hypoxemia, answer D is far less likely as the patient is clinically improving, does not have new unilateral breath sounds, and has decreasing tachycardia and tachypnea.

2. A 7-year-old girl with history of previous PICU admissions for severe persistent asthma presents to the ED with diffuse wheezing, prolonged exhalation, and respiratory failure. She is intubated using sedatives and neuromuscular blockade. She is treated with nebulized beta-agonists, inhaled anticholinergics, intravenous magnesium sulfate, and intravenous steroids. She is admitted to the PICU where she is placed on positive pressure ventilation with pressure control mode. An expiratory pause maneuver is performed demonstrating an intrinsic PEEP of 4. Her chest radiograph shows: severe hyperinflation, a small heart, and an oral endotracheal tube in good position. Which of the following describes the patient's pulmonary vascular state?

A. The pulmonary vascular resistance is unchanged from the patient's baseline
B. The pulmonary vascular resistance is lower than the patient's baseline
C. The pulmonary vascular resistance is higher than the patient's baseline

D. Determination of the patient's direction of change in pulmonary vascular resistance requires direct measurement of pulmonary vascular pressures

Answer and Explanation: C. A severe asthma exacerbation has significant effects on a patient's cardiopulmonary interactions. Air trapping, worsening gas exchange, V/Q mismatch, and dynamic hyperinflation leading to increased pulmonary vascular resistance (PVR) are often seen in the setting of severe bronchospasm [12]. Therefore, answers A and B are incorrect. Answer D is also incorrect as one can also determine the direction of change in PVR by following other indicators of cardiopulmonary interactors, such as degree of hyperinflation on CXR, or measurements of end expiratory pressures while the patient is mechanically ventilated and paralyzed. As these markers improve, PVR also would improve, therefore direct measurement is not necessary.

3. A 10-year-old boy with an acute exacerbation of asthma presents to the ED of an outside hospital. He is intubated and transferred to a regional children's center for further care. Upon arrival to the PICU, he is noted to have the following vital signs: Temp 37.0, HR 178, RR 20 on ventilator, BP 82/45, SaO2 93% on 70% FiO2. His physical exam is remarkable for decreased air movement throughout both lung fields, no audible wheezes, and distended neck veins. What is the best, next therapeutic option for this patient?

A. Administer a dose of albuterol via metered dose inhaler
B. Administer a dose of intravenous magnesium sulfate
C. Decrease the IMV rate and inspiratory time on the ventilator
D. Administer a 20 mL/kg normal saline bolus by intravenous push

Answer and Explanation: D. The most important intervention for this patient is to provide adequate preload to establish appropriate circulation in the setting of his severe hyperinflation. Therefore, choice D is the best answer. While bronchodilators are a mainstay of asthma therapy, choice A is incorrect as continuous albuterol is preferable to a single metered-dose inhaler dose in such extreme circumstances. Answer B would also be a helpful adjuvant therapy, but would need to be administered after a normal saline bolus because of its common side effect of hypotension. While decreasing the IMV rate is appropriate for asthma, an arterial blood gas is needed to assess the degree of hypercarbia prior to making this change. Therefore, choice C is incorrect.

4. A 5-year-old boy previously healthy boy is brought to the ED by his parents after they noticed a new wheeze while playing whiffle ball in the park. While waiting in triage, he becomes acutely cyanotic and unresponsive, and is rushed to a resuscitation room. Vital signs are: Temp 37.2, HR 171, RR 62, BP 79/48, SaO2 67%. Rapid, shallow breathing is noted on exam with no appreciable air movement. He is successfully intubated and transferred to the PICU. His respiratory status improves dramatically over the next 18 hours. Which of the following is an expected clinical finding for this patient?

A. Bilateral patchy opacities on CXR with normal lung expansion
B. Neutrophilic predominance on complete blood count
C. Bilateral pneumothorax
D. Foreign body on CXR

Answer and Explanation: B. Acute asphyxial asthma is a near-fatal presentation that can be seen in both adults and children. Acute asphyxial asthma is characterized by respiratory distress followed by rapid respiratory decompensation, lack of air movement, and non-responsiveness that often improves quickly after intubation and a short period of mechanical ventilation [13]. This disease process has some distinct aspects of pathophysiology that make it unique from other presentations of asthma. There is often less mucus plugging and a neutrophilic predominance on CBC instead of the eosinophilia that is commonly seen in asthma exacerbations [14]. Therefore answer B is correct. Answer A is a common finding in acute respiratory distress syndrome (ARDS). This patient's rapid improvement is not consistent with this disease process. Pneumothorax, choice C, is also incorrect as it would not improve without evacuation. Choice D, foreign body, is also unlikely as it would be unlikely that the patient would improve without removal.

5. A 3-month-old boy with Trisomy 21 and a large VSD presents to his pediatrician for a check-up. The infant's examination is remarkable for tachypnea (RR 32) and a soft, but audible, expiratory wheeze. The parent reports also that the infant is not feeding as well as he used to and is sometimes unable to complete a 4 ounce feeding. The pediatrician notes that this infant has gained only 200 g in weight since his last visit at 7 weeks of age. Because of the wheezing, tachypnea, and failure to thrive, the pediatrician refers the child to the ED of a regional children's hospital for further evaluation. The ED physician who sees the infant 2 hours later confirms the signs and symptoms described, formulates a differential diagnosis, and performs a clinical evaluation to confirm her diagnosis. What clinical evaluation does the ED physician perform?

A. Orders 2.5 mg of inhaled albuterol to be administered to the infant
B. Orders a PA chest X-ray, EKG, echocardiogram, and 0.5 mg/kg furosemide to be administered intravenously to the infant
C. Orders lateral decubitus chest X-rays alternating the right side and left side dependent
D. Orders an upper GI and pH probe studies

Answer and Explanation: B. The differential diagnosis of wheezing in children is broad as "not everything that wheezes is asthma" and should also include cardiac and gastrointestinal causes. This patient, known to have a ventricular septal defect, has been failing to thrive and is showing signs of respiratory distress consistent with pulmonary over-circulation. The appropriate therapy for this patient is evaluation of his cardiac status with EKG and echocardiogram, a PA CXR to evaluate for cardiomegaly and lung fields, and diuretic therapy. Answer A is the appropriate therapy for asthma, but that is not consistent with this patient's disease process. Choice C is the

appropriate examination to evaluate for foreign body aspiration. Choice D is also incorrect; an upper GI and pH probe study are appropriate evaluations for reflux, which certainly can cause failure to thrive and wheezing in infants, but is less likely given this patient's cardiac physiology.

6. A 14-year-old boy has been admitted to the PICU on non-invasive positive pressure ventilation for an acute exacerbation of asthma. He is treated with steroids, continuous albuterol, and a terbutaline infusion. On PICU day 2 he is intubated in the setting of hypercarbic respiratory failure. His respiratory acidosis continues to worsen and his most recent blood gas shows a pH of 6.9 and a PCO2 of 104. His lungs remain extremely hyperinflated on exam. Which of the following is the appropriate next step in caring for this patient?

A. Placement onto high frequency oscillatory ventilation
B. Discussion of activating ECMO team or transfer to an ECMO center for venovenous cannulation
C. A dose of intravenous bicarbonate to immediately improve his acidosis
D. Deflating the cuff of the endotracheal tube to allow for passive ventilation around the tube

Answer and Explanation: B. This patient in status asthmaticus is truly refractory to the provided interventions and requires further escalation. His respiratory acidosis, if left untreated, may lead to cardiac arrest. At this point, choice B, discussion of ECMO cannulation is the appropriate next step. Use of a potent inhaled anesthetic, such as isofluorane, is also an appropriate choice if available in one's institution but this was not provided as a choice. Choice A, the use of high-frequency oscillatory ventilation, runs the risk of an acute increase in mean airway pressure that may inhibit venous return and result in cardiac arrest nor is there any robust data for the use of high frequency oscillatory ventilation in asthmatic patients. Administering bicarbonate, choice C, is also incorrect as bicarbonate is metabolized into carbon dioxide in the red blood cells and may worsen respiratory acidosis. Choice D, deflating the cuff around the endotracheal tube, is a maneuver used during high frequency oscillatory ventilation to allow for passive flow of carbon dioxide around the endotracheal tube but is inappropriate in a decompensating patient who is failing SIMV.

7. A 13-year old boy with a history of hypertension presents to the ED with severe respiratory distress. He is administered intravenous methylprednisolone and admitted to the PICU on BiPAP and continuous albuterol. His blood pressure on admission is noted to be 160/105 and he is agitated. His urine studies show no abnormalities and a renal-bladder ultrasound is normal. Of the following anti-hypertensive agents, which should be avoided in patients with asthma?

A. Esmolol
B. Hydralazine
C. Nifedipine
D. Nicardipine

Answer and Explanation: A. Esmolol, despite being a selective beta-1 receptor blocking agent, runs the risk of inhibiting beta-1 receptors as well, especially at higher doses, and might result in bronchoconstrictive properties which can exacerbate asthma symptoms. While some studies have shown that beta blockade can be safely used in certain populations [15], it is not without the significant risk of worsening bronchospasm. Choice B, hydralazine, peripherally vasodilates and relaxes smooth muscle and is not known to worsen asthma exacerbations. Similarly, nifedipine and nicardipine (choices C and D, respectively), are calcium-channel blockers that prevent calcium influx into muscular cells and therefore result in muscle relaxation and dilation. Neither of these drugs have been shown to worsen asthma exacerbations.

8. A 9-year-old patient with a history severe asthma and poor medication adherence is intubated in the ED for respiratory failure. Once connected to the ventilator, he is placed on SIMV VC with a tidal volume of 200 mL. An end tidal probe is placed at the end of his endotrachieal tube and it reads a CO_2 of 49 mmHg. An arterial blood gas drawn at the same time shows a $PaCO_2$ of 92 mmHg. Which of the following choices best explains the discrepancy between his end tidal CO_2 and his pCO_2?

A. Anatomic dead space within the patient's respiratory tract
B. Fixed dead space caused by the ventilator tubing
C. A small air bubble introduced into the arterial blood gas sample
D. Physiologic dead space within the patient's alveoli

Answer and Explanation: D. The difference between end tidal CO_2 and $PaCO_2$ is accounted for by dead space, both anatomic and physiologic. Anatomic dead space is fixed in all people, and includes areas of the respiratory system that do not participate in gas exchange from the nose to the terminal bronchioles. Physiologic dead space includes alveoli that are unable to participate in gas exchange due to pathology. In healthy people, anatomic dead space is equivalent to physiologic dead space, and is approximately 30% of tidal volume. When dead space increases, this is due to worsening physiologic dead space and therefore D is correct. A is incorrect, as anatomic dead space is fixed and therefore would not account

for such a large discrepancy in values. Choice B is also wrong as $EtCO_2$ probe is placed as close to the patient as possible and therefore should not account for such a large discrepancy in numbers. Choice C is wrong as a small air bubble would not account for increased CO_2 in a sample.

9. For the same patient above, what is the volume of dead space?

A. 20 mL
B. 47 mL
C. 93 mL
D. 175 mL

Answer and Explanation: C. Percent dead space can be calculated by the Bohr equation: Tidal volume x ($PaCO_2$ – End tidal CO_2) / $PaCO_2$. In this case, 200 mL x (92-49)/92 = 93 mL. Therefore, C is the correct answer indicating that, for this patient, dead space accounts for nearly 50% of the lung tidal volume.

10. A six-month-old ex-32-week girl arrives to the ED in severe respiratory distress. Vital signs are as follows: T 39.3, HR 170, BP 82/55, RR 52, SpO2 87%. Her exam is notable for wheezing and copious nasopharyngeal secretions. Nebulized albuterol is trialed without significant improvement. She begins grunting and head bobbing. Which is the following next best step for this patient?

A. Intramuscular epinephrine
B. Intravenous terbutaline
C. Inhaled ipratropium
D. Positive pressure ventilation and aggressive suctioning

Answer and Explanation: D. Given a lack of response to albuterol, this patient likely has bronchiolitis instead of reactive airway disease. Bronchiolitis is a common illness among infants and young children, and is most commonly attributable to the respiratory syncytial virus (RSV) [16]. The treatment for bronchiolitis is supportive care providing suctioning and positive pressure, answer D. One of the hallmarks of bronchiolitis is a lack of response to bronchodilator therapy, even when the patient exhibits wheezing, making choices A-C all incorrect.

2.

AIRWAY OBSTRUCTION, BLEEDING, AND PAIN CONTROL AFTER TONSILLECTOMY

Selby B. Johnson II and Emily Anne Vail

STEM CASE AND KEY QUESTIONS

A 4-year-old, 22-kilogram boy with enlarged tonsils and adenoids undergoes routine adenotonsillectomy (T&A) for obstructive sleep apnea (OSA).

WHAT ARE THE INDICATIONS FOR T&A? IS DIAGNOSTIC TESTING REQUIRED TO DETERMINE WHETHER A CHILD MAY BENEFIT FROM T&A?

During the immediate postoperative period, the patient recovers without apparent complication. He is discharged home with pain well controlled on oral acetaminophen and oxycodone.

WHAT ARE THIS PATIENT'S RISK FACTORS FOR POSTOPERATIVE COMPLICATIONS? HOW IS ELIGIBILITY FOR SAME-DAY DISCHARGE DETERMINED?

The patient slowly recovers from the procedure. He complains of pain when eating solid food despite regular treatment with pain medication. Oral intake of food and liquids has been insufficient. On the seventh day after surgery, the patient's mother notices blood coming from the child's mouth while brushing his teeth. She immediately takes him to the emergency department.

WHAT ARE THE RISK FACTORS FOR INCREASED POSTOPERATIVE PAIN? WHAT ARE THE ANALGESIC MODALITIES BEST USED TO TREAT POSTOPERATIVE PAIN? WHAT ARE THE RISKS OF THE USE OF OPIOIDS IN THIS POPULATION?

Upon examination in the emergency department, vital signs include

- Temperature: 36.3°C
- Pulse: 110 beats per minute
- Respiratory rate: 20 breaths per minute
- Noninvasive blood pressure: 90/68 mmHg
- SpO$_2$ 95% on room air

The patient appears in mild distress. Auscultation of the lungs does not reveal wheezing, rhonchi, or stridor. Examination of the mouth elicits exquisite pain. There is no visible bleeding or clots in the tonsillar fossae. Laboratory studies reveal a leukocyte count of $12.5 \times 10^3/\mu L$ and hematocrit of 24.7%. The patient is admitted to a pediatric ward for observation and continuous pulse oximetry. He is kept nil per os with ice chips for comfort. Lactated Ringer's solution is used to provide hydration. A single dose of intravenous dexamethasone is administered to decrease edema. The patient receives acetaminophen and oxycodone every 4 hours as needed for pain. Overnight, the patient intermittently desaturates below 90%. His mother reports that she has observed multiple apneic episodes similar to those present preoperatively.

WHAT IS SLEEP-DISORDERED BREATHING? WHAT ARE ITS RISK FACTORS IN PEDIATRIC PATIENTS? OTHER THAN SNORING, IN WHAT WAYS CAN THE CONDITION PRESENT? HOW IS IT DIAGNOSED AND TREATED?

During morning rounds, the clinical team observes unexpected inspiratory stridor characteristic of laryngeal edema. Repeat examination reveals significantly increased edema and hyperemia of the posterior oropharynx. Lung sounds remain unremarkable. The clinical team initiates supplemental oxygen therapy and administers an additional dose of dexamethasone, then transfers the patient to the pediatric intensive care unit (ICU) for close observation and further treatment.

HOW SHOULD AIRWAY OBSTRUCTION BE MANAGED IF IT DOES OCCUR? IS THERE A ROLE FOR NON-INVASIVE POSITIVE PRESSURE VENTILATION?

The boy's desaturations increase in frequency and the clinical team decides to perform endotracheal intubation to protect his airway. After anesthesia induction, direct laryngoscopy reveals bilateral white scabs in the tonsillar beds, moderate active bleeding within the oropharynx and a small clot just posterior to the glottic opening. The intubating clinician carefully suctions the oropharynx then secures the airway on the first attempt with size 5.0 mm cuffed endotracheal tube.

WHAT ARE SOME OF THE AIRWAY CHALLENGES EXPECTED IN PATIENTS WITH POST-TONSILLECTOMY HEMORRHAGE? HOW ARE PRIMARY AND SECONDARY POSTOPERATIVE BLEEDING DIFFERENT? DOES TREATMENT DIFFER FOR THE 2 CONDITIONS?

After successful intubation, the ICU team transfers the patient to the operating room for exam under anesthesia and hemostasis. The anesthesiologist administers fentanyl, acetaminophen, a third dose of dexamethasone, and dexmedetomidine. He avoids ketorolac to reduce the risk of further bleeding. The surgeon identifies an area of active bleeding, which she controls with electrocautery. Anesthetic emergence and extubation are uneventful. The patient is transferred to the postanesthesia recovery unit, breathing spontaneously with adequate oxygenation and minimal pain.

WHAT RARE INTRAPULMONARY COMPLICATION MAY OCCUR AFTER TONSILLECTOMY? WHAT IS THE POSTOPERATIVE COURSE FOR THESE PATIENTS?

The patient is admitted to the ward for overnight observation with continuous pulse oximetry. Oral pain medication and ice chips adequately control his dysphagia. His vital signs remain stable overnight without further episodes of apnea or desaturation. The patient is discharged home with his mother the next morning and makes a full recovery by the time of his routine postoperative evaluation in the surgeon's office.

DISCUSSION

T&A has been performed in children for decades. After the discovery of the role of group A beta-hemolytic streptococcal pharyngitis in the pathogenesis of rheumatic heart disease, otherwise healthy children frequently underwent prophylactic surgery. As diagnostic tools and antibiotic therapy for group A strep improved, the need for and incidence of surgery have decreased (1). At present, there are 2 indications for T&A in children; recurrent tonsillitis and sleep-disordered breathing (SDB).

INDICATIONS FOR SURGERY

Recurrent Tonsillitis

The Pittsburgh pharyngotonsillitis study reported by Paradise et al. identified children most likely to benefit from T&A (2). The Paradise criteria inform the American Academy of Pediatrics and American Academy of Otolaryngology—Head and Neck Surgery Clinical Practice Guidelines for Tonsillectomy and Adenoidectomy in children. The guidelines recommend T&A for patients with 7 or more sore throat episodes in the preceding year, 5 or more episodes in the preceding 2 years, or 3 or more episodes in each of the preceding 3 years. The guidelines also recommend surgery for children with recurrent infections complicated by peritonsillar abscess (3).

Sleep-Disordered Breathing

The most common present-day indication for surgery is SDB (1). SDB includes a range of conditions, from increased upper airway resistance syndrome to obstructive sleep apnea (OSA). Patients with upper airway resistance syndrome have daytime hypersomnolence characterized by airflow limitation without frequent respiratory disturbances or desaturation. Patients with OSA experience partial or complete obstruction of the airway during sleep (11). Resultant abnormalities in ventilation and sleep patterns, particularly in the latter condition, may profoundly affect hormonal regulation and cardiovascular physiology (3). Even with mild forms of SDB, children typically experience both daytime and nighttime symptoms. Nighttime symptoms include snoring or choking, night terrors, and sleepwalking. Daytime symptoms are generally associated with behavioral issues such as prolonged eating time and decreased appetite, changes in speech quality, and signs mimicking attention deficit disorder (3). The most common cause of SDB in children is tonsillar and adenoid hypertrophy, but hypertrophy alone does not correlate with the degree of SDB symptoms. Instead, combined tonsillar and adenoid size, presence of craniofacial abnormalities, and neuromuscular tone all determine SDB severity (3). Polysomnography is the gold standard method of diagnosis. According to the American Society of Anesthesiologists, diagnosis of moderate OSA in pediatric patients requires an apnea–hypopnea index (AHI) between 6 and 10; severe OSA requires an apnea–hypopnea index of greater than 10 (11). Children with increased upper airway resistance have a normal polysomnogram despite observed snoring and straining to breathe during sleep (1).

POSTOPERATIVE CARE

Most healthy children between 3 and 4 years of age may be safely discharged home within several hours of surgery. Younger patients frequently have difficulty with postoperative hydration and may require at least one night of admission to ensure adequate oral fluid resuscitation. Patients with insufficient oral intake, intractable vomiting or bleeding may require prolonged monitoring in the postanesthesia care unit or postoperative admission. Children with preoperative OSA may still experience obstructive apnea and desaturation after surgery. These patients typically require admission for one night of postoperative observation (8).

Postoperative complications include pain, hemorrhage, airway obstruction, dehydration, post-obstruction pulmonary edema, and Grisel's syndrome.

Pain

The primary cause of morbidity posttonsillectomy is oropharyngeal pain. This can cause dysphagia, dehydration, and weight loss. Caregiver misunderstanding or hesitation in administering analgesics at home necessitates education about effective pain control prior to hospital discharge (2). In a study conducted by Fortier et al., up to a fourth of children with severe pain after T&A received little to no analgesic medication on the first day of hospital discharge (9). Pain is especially difficult to manage in patients with SDB, who are at increased risk of both hyperalgesia requiring opioid treatment and respiratory depression from opioids. Hyperalgesia results from chronic hypoxia and intermittent sleep fragmentation, which upregulates systemic inflammation and reactive oxygen species (12). Education and clear communication can improve pain control and enhance recovery for all patients.

Analgesic medications are essential to patient satisfaction and recovery. Clinicians frequently avoid nonsteroidal anti-inflammatory drug (NSAIDs) because of historical concerns for an increased risk of bleeding; however, a recent case series comparing 6,014 patients treated with ibuprofen versus codeine failed to demonstrate a statistically significant difference in risk of post-tonsillectomy hemorrhage (6). To reduce the potential risk of renal toxicity, clinicians should instruct caregivers to withhold NSAIDs if they suspect dehydration. Nonetheless, parents should be educated on the importance of renal toxicity in the setting of dehydration when considering NSAID therapy. Acetaminophen is also a suitable option best administered on a scheduled, rather than as needed, basis (16).

Opioid medications are the most effective choice for treatment of severe pain after T&A. Although the combination of acetaminophen and codeine may be simple and effective in some patients, a US Food and Drug Administration black box warning contraindicates its use in children. Significant genetic polymorphisms in the CYP2D6 enzyme required to metabolize codeine to its active ingredient increases the risk of both under- and overdose among patients. Hydrocodone and oxycodone, which do not require synthesis of an active metabolite, are more reliably metabolized and therefore safer opioid options. Clinicians and caregivers should remember that all opioids are associated with significant side effects, including respiratory depression, nausea, vomiting, and constipation (2).

Postoperative Nausea and Vomiting

Postoperative nausea and vomiting may be severe enough to delay discharge or require overnight hospital admission for treatment and intravenous hydration. A 2003 Cochrane systematic review found that dexamethasone 0.5 mg/kg significantly reduced the incidence of emesis in the early postoperative period. Dexamethasone treatment was also associated with improved tolerance of a soft diet and a significant decrease in postoperative pain (5).

Hemorrhage

Hemorrhage may be primary or secondary. Primary hemorrhage, which occurs within 24 hours of surgery, is attributable to inadequately controlled or missed intraoperative bleeding. Risk of primary hemorrhage varies with the surgeon's approach to intraoperative hemostasis. Historically, surgeons performed tonsillectomy with cold dissection techniques, which required ligation of individual blood vessels during tissue removal (2). Newer diathermic, or "hot" surgical tools, including electrocautery, radiofrequency, and coblation, achieve more reliable hemostasis and are less likely to lead to primary hemorrhage (7).

The etiology of secondary hemorrhage is less clear and most often occurs in patients with significant pain and inadequate oral intake. It is more common in older children and adolescents. Choice of surgical technique may also be associated with risk of secondary hemorrhage (7). Loss of eschar from the tissue beds occurs 3 to 4 weeks after surgery. It does not typically cause hemorrhage unless it exposes a blood vessel. Most cases of secondary hemorrhage are minor, requiring observation and intravenous hydration without reoperation. However, patients with signs of active bleeding or observed clot in the tonsillar fossa require an immediate return to the operating room for surgical intervention (1).

Airway Obstruction

Surgical manipulation, including cautery and tissue retraction, can cause posterior oropharyngeal edema and acute airway obstruction. There are many risk factors for airway obstruction after T&A, including age less than 3 years and severe OSA. Other risk factors include underlying syndromic conditions with neurological problems, congenital heart disease, prematurity, and craniofacial abnormalities.

If clinicians suspect that postoperative airway obstruction is likely, patients require closer observation in an ICU. If airway obstruction does occur, patency may be restored by insertion of a nasal airway and administration of bronchodilators, racemic epinephrine, and heliox (8). If desaturations persist despite these measures, the patient may require noninvasive mechanical ventilatory support or even reintubation. The clinical team should prepare for a possible difficult airway scenario with different sizes of endotracheal tubes, stylets, 2 well-illuminated direct laryngoscopes, a video laryngoscope, and even an advanced airway device such as a pediatric flexible fiberoptic bronchoscope (8).

Dehydration

A required trial of oral intake before hospital discharge may prevent readmission for dehydration in some patients. Ice chips or cold drinks not only provide hydration, they also relieve throat pain. Chewing gum or gummy candies may provide additional relief by relaxing pharyngeal muscles (1). Intravenous fluids may be necessary for patients in the immediate postoperative period or, in rare cases, if patients struggle to maintain hydration after hospital discharge.

Postobstructive Pulmonary Edema

Acute postobstructive pulmonary edema is classified as Type 1 and Type 2. Type 1 develops after relief of acute airway obstruction, such as laryngospasm. Type 2 acute postobstructive pulmonary edema, which is extremely rare, develops after relief of chronic airway obstruction. During chronic airway obstruction, patients develop increased intrinsic positive end-expiratory pressure to compensate for smaller negative intrathoracic pressures generated during inspiration. When a patient is extubated immediately after surgical relief of chronic airway obstruction, intrathoracic pressures rapidly decrease, which may increase intrathoracic venous return and lead to pulmonary edema. Type 2 postobstructive pulmonary edema may develop after T&A in patients with or without comorbid disease (13). Clinical presentation usually includes hypoxemia and pink frothy sputum, with diffuse crackles and occasional wheezing present on physical exam. Chest radiographic abnormalities are nonspecific. Chest computed tomography is rarely obtained but may demonstrate central and nondependent ground glass attenuation (14). With close monitoring and temporary use of noninvasive or invasive positive pressure ventilation, pulmonary edema resolves in 2 to 3 days (14). Diuretic therapy is generally not warranted (13).

Grisel's Syndrome

Defined as nontraumatic subluxation of the atlanto-axial joint following peri-pharyngeal inflammation, Grisel's syndrome is a rare condition associated with oropharyngeal or cervical infection or surgery. If patients experience persistent neck pain and stiffness after T&A, clinicians must consider Grisel's syndrome, especially when torticollis is also present. Cervical instability from Grisel's syndrome may have devastating neurological consequences, including quadriplegia and sudden death (15).

CONCLUSIONS

- SDB is the most common present-day indication for T&A in children.

- Common complications of T&A include postoperative pain, airway obstruction, and dehydration. Patients less than 3 years of age and those with comorbid disease are more likely to suffer complications after surgery.

- Patients with craniofacial abnormalities, a history of prematurity, and severe OSA are among those at risk for postoperative airway obstruction. These patients require planned postoperative admission.

- Development of newer surgical techniques has caused a decrease in both primary and secondary hemorrhage after T&A.

- Multimodal pain control with acetaminophen, NSAIDs, and opioids is effective in treating postoperative pain in post-tonsillectomy patients. Adequate pain treatment, including education of caregivers at time of discharge, is necessary to prevent patient discomfort, dehydration, and malnutrition.

- Rare complications of T&A include Type 2 acute postobstructive pulmonary edema and Grisel's syndrome.

REFERENCES

1. Wetmore, RF. Surgical management of the tonsillectomy and adenoidectomy patient. World Journal of Otorhinolaryngology. 2017 Mar 3;3(3):176–182.
2. Paradise JL, Bluestone CD, Bachman RZ, et al. Efficacy of tonsillectomy for recurrent throat infection in severely affected children: results of parallel randomized and nonrandomized clinical trials. New England Journal of Medicine. 1984 Mar 15;310:674–683.
3. Baugh RF, Archer SM, Mitchell RB. Clinical practice guideline: Tonsillectomy in children. Otolaryngology—Head and Neck Surgery. 2011 Jan 1; 144(1 Suppl):S1–S30.
4. Marcus CL, Moore RH, Rosen CL, et al. A randomized trial of adenotonsillectomy for childhood sleep apnea. New England Journal of Medicine. 2013 Jun 20;368(25):2366–2376.
5. Steward DL, Welge JA, Myer CM. Steroids for improving recovery following tonsillectomy in children. Cochrane Database of Systematic Reviews. 2011 Aug 10;(8):CD003997. doi:10.1002/14651858.
6. Pfaff J.A., Hsu K., Chennupati S.K, et al. The use of ibuprofen in post tonsillectomy analgesia and its effect on post tonsillectomy hemorrhage rate. Otolaryngology—Head and Neck Surgery. 2016 May 16;155:508–513.
7. Mowatt G, Cook JA, Fraser C, et al. Systematic review of the safety of electrosurgery for tonsillectomy. Clinical Otolaryngology. 2006 Mar 20;31(2):95–102.
8. Cote C, Lerman Jerrold, Anderson B., eds. A Practice of Anesthesia for Infants and Children. 6th ed. Philadelphia: Elsevier; 2018.
9. Fortier MA, MacLaren JE, Martin SR, et al. Pediatric pain after ambulatory surgery: where's the medication? Pediatrics. 2009 May 29;124(4):e588–e595.
10. Spencer DJ, Jones JE, et al. Complications of adenotonsillectomy in patients younger than 3 years. Archives of Otolaryngology—Head & Neck Surgery. 2012 Apr;138(4):335–339.
11. Gross, JB, Bachenberg, KL, Benumof, JL. Practice guidelines for the perioperative management of patients with obstructive sleep apnea: a report by the American Society of Anesthesiologists Task Force on Perioperative Management of patients with obstructive sleep apnea. Anesthesiology. 2006 May;104(5):1081–1093.
12. Lam KK, Kunder S, Wong J, Doufas AG, Chung F. Obstructive sleep apnea, pain, and opioids: is the riddle solved? Current Opinion in Anesthesiology. 2016 Feb; 29(1):134–140.
13. Guffin TN, Har-El G, Sanders A, et al. Acute postobstructive pulmonary edema. Otolaryngology—Head and Neck Surgery. 1995 Feb 1;112(2):235–237.
14. Bhaskar B, Fraser JF. Negative pressure pulmonary edema revisited: pathophysiology and review of management. Saudi Journal of Anaesthesia. 2011 Sep;5(33):308–313.
15. Bocciolini C, Dall'Olio, Cunsolo E, Cavazzuti PP, Laudadio P. Grisel's syndrome: A rare complication following adenoidectomy. ACTA Otorhinolaryngologica Italica. 2005 Aug;25(4):245–249.

1. What is the recommended intraoperative pediatric dose of dexamethasone for the prevention of postoperative nausea and vomiting?

 A. 0.3 mg/kg
 B. 8 mg
 C. 0.5 mg/kg
 D. 12 mg

2. A 3-year-old boy demonstrates poor oral intake 2 days after T&A. He does not feel up to drinking anything and refuses a soft diet. Should this patient be readmitted to the hospital? Why?

 A. Yes, because he is at risk for airway obstruction
 B. No, because he has not yet developed any serious postoperative complications
 C. Yes, because he is at risk for uncontrolled pain
 D. Yes, because he is at risk for postoperative bleeding

3. What are 3 other comorbidities associated with SDB in pediatric patients?

 A. Obesity, craniofacial abnormalities, hypotonia
 B. Obesity, craniofacial abnormalities, kidney disease
 C. Obesity, seizures, asthma
 D. Asthma, kidney disease, craniofacial abnormalities

4. What was historically the most common indication for T&A?

 A. SDB
 B. Tonsillar and adenoid enlargement
 C. Group A beta-hemolytic streptococcal infections
 D. Recurrent bacterial tonsillitis

5. Which medication listed below should *not* be administered to pediatric patients?

 A. Codeine
 B. Hydrocodone
 C. Oxycodone
 D. Tylenol

6. An 8-year-old patient and her parents present several days after T&A due to shortness of breath and pink frothy sputum production. A chest radiograph demonstrates nonspecific hazy opacities. What imaging modality and findings are more specific for this condition?

 A. Magnetic resonance imaging of chest with nonspecific hyperdense areas
 B. Computed tomography chest with central and dependent ground glass attenuation
 C. Lung ultrasound with diffuse A lines
 D. Computed tomography of chest with central and nondependent ground glass attenuation

7. Which surgical technique for T&A is associated with increased risk of primary hemorrhage?

 A. Cold dissection
 B. Electrocautery
 C. Coblation
 D. Hot dissection

8. A patient with adenoid hypertrophy strains to breathe at night, but the patient's caregivers deny that the patient snores. They have not witnessed any episodes of apnea. What would a polysomnogram reveal and diagnose in this child?

 A. Abnormal polysomnogram, consistent with OSA
 B. Normal polysomnogram, not consistent with OSA
 C. Abnormal polysomnogram, consistent with upper airway resistance syndrome
 D. Normal polysomnogram, consistent with upper airway resistance syndrome

9. All of the following are daytime symptoms in a child with SDB *except*

 A. Symptoms mimicking attention deficit disorder
 B. Morning headaches
 C. Frequent urination
 D. Decreased appetite

10. All of the following are Paradise criteria for T&A for recurrent tonsillitis *except*

 A. 3 or more sore throats in the past 2 years
 B. 5 or more sore throats in the past 2 years
 C. 3 or more sore throats in the past 3 years
 D. 7 or more sore throats in the past year

ANSWERS

 1. Answer C: When administering dexamethasone to pediatric patients, the appropriate dose for the prevention of postoperative nausea and vomiting is 0.5 mg/kg. According to a 2003 Cochrane systematic review, this dose reduced the incidence of postoperative emesis within 24 hours of surgery by half (5).

 2. Answer C: Patients 3 years of age and younger are typically unable to maintain postoperative hydration due to uncontrolled pain. Young children require at least one night of postoperative admission to ensure adequate oral intake and prevent dehydration and hospital readmission (10).

 3. Answer A: Other risk factors for SDB in children include underlying neurological problems, congenital heart disease, prematurity, and craniofacial syndromes.

 4. Answer C: After group A beta-hemolytic streptococcus was discovered as the causative pathogen in rheumatic heart disease, T&As were frequently performed for treatment and prevention of the infection. With improvements in diagnosis and treatment of group A beta-hemolytic strep, T&A is now performed only for patients with recurrent tonsillitis, tonsillar abscess or SDB (1).

 5. Answer A: Although codeine may be an effective oral opioid for some patients, it carries a Food and Drug Administration black box warning for use in children. There is significant genetic variation in the CYP2D6 enzyme that metabolizes codeine to its active metabolite morphine, which increases the likelihood of both under- and overdosing.

Hydrocodone and oxycodone do not require metabolism to an active metabolite and are therefore safer and more reliable (1).

6. Answer D: Acute post-obstructive pulmonary edema Type 2 is a rare condition that occurs after relief of chronic airway obstruction. Chest radiographs may show nonspecific hazy opacities. Chest computed tomography, if obtained, may demonstrate characteristic ground glass attenuation in the central and nondependent areas of the lungs (14).

7. Answer A: Hot dissection, coblation, and electrocautery are all surgical techniques proven effective for hemostasis in T&A. All carry lower risk of primary hemorrhage than cold dissection techniques (1).

8. Answer D: Moderate-to-severe tonsillar hypertrophy alone does not correlate with the severity of SDB and is not required for its diagnosis. Polysomnography is the gold standard for diagnosis of SDB. Children with increased upper airway resistance have a normal polysomnogram despite observed snoring and straining to breathe during sleep (1, 4).

9. Answer C: Daytime symptoms are generally associated with behavioral issues such as prolonged eating time, decreased appetite, a change in speech quality and signs mimicking attention deficit disorder (1).

10. Answer A: According to the Paradise Criteria for Tonsillectomy in Pediatrics and Adolescents, surgery should be considered in patients with recurrent tonsillitis meeting one of the following criteria:

- 7 or more sore throats within 1 year
- 5 or more sore throats within 2 years
- 3 or more sore throats within 3 years

A sore throat with temperature >100.9°F, tender cervical lymphadenopathy, tonsillar exudate, or culture positive Group A beta hemolytic strep pharyngitis are also indications for T&A.

3.

THE FAILING FONTAN

Ashish A. Ankola and Tarif A. Choudhury

STEM CASE AND KEY QUESTIONS

A 10-year-old female with a history of hypoplastic left heart syndrome (HLHS) and a restrictive atrial septum now presents to the emergency department with worsening cyanosis. She had undergone a staged palliative surgery earlier in childhood, most recently involving an extracardiac fenestrated Fontan procedure at 4 years old. She has had a nonproductive cough, rhinorrhea, and a fever for the past 2 days, but she denies any chest pain or palpitations. She complains of increased shortness of breath with activity over this week as well even with simple daily activities such as walking up stairs. Her vital signs include a fever of 102.6°F, a room air oxygen saturation of 77%, a blood pressure of 73/44 mmHg, and a heart rate of 135 bpm. She appears to be in respiratory distress with tachypnea and retractions, but on exam minimal crackles are audible and a cardiac murmur is not auscultated. The liver edge is felt 3 cm below the right costal margin, and her extremities are cool but with 1+ pulses without brachio-femoral delay. An intravenous access is placed and multiple crystalloid fluid boluses are administered with minimal, transient increases in blood pressure before dwindling back to baseline. A right, femoral, central venous line is placed and reveals a central venous pressure of 21 mmHg and a norepinephrine infusion is started at 0.03 mcg/kg/min to augment the mean arterial pressure to 60 mmHg. An intensive care unit consult is called due to concern for impending cardio-respiratory failure and the patient is placed on noninvasive positive pressure ventilation (NIPPV).

WHAT IS A NORMAL ARTERIAL OXYGEN SATURATION FOR A PATIENT WITH A FONTAN WITH AND WITHOUT A FENESTRATION? WHAT WORKUP WOULD YOU PURSUE TO DETERMINE THE ETIOLOGY OF CYANOSIS HERE?

Upon discovery of the patient's cyanosis and hypotension, her mother promptly tells you that her baseline saturations are usually in the mid-90s on room air. A chest X-ray is performed (Figure 3.1) demonstrating cardiomegaly, diffuse pulmonary edema, bilateral pleural effusions, and low lung volumes.

A complete blood count returns with a hemoglobin of 13.8 g/dL and a hematocrit of 41% with a complete metabolic panel that is within normal limits except for an elevated direct bilirubin (2.2 mg/dL) and alkaline phosphatase (615 units/L).

Urine and blood cultures are sent and still pending, but a nasopharyngeal swab for influenza returns positive.

An electrocardiogram exhibits sinus rhythm and a transthoracic echocardiogram is performed showing low normal right ventricular systolic function, with an unrestrictive atrial septal defect, moderate tricuspid regurgitation, and laminar flow seen through the Fontan and Glenn anastomoses into the branch pulmonary arteries. The Fontan fenestration (Figure 3.2) is patent with right to left flow. The gradient across the fenestration is 11 mmHg. As the echocardiogram is completed, an arterial blood gas is 7.2/60/42/21 while on NIPPV.

WHAT PHYSIOLOGIC PRINCIPLES MUST YOU CONSIDER AS YOU PREPARE TO INTUBATE THIS PATIENT? WHAT SEDATION WOULD YOU USE?

Rapid sequence intubation is performed utilizing ketamine, glycopyrrolate, versed, and rocuronium with extracorporeal membrane oxygenation (ECMO) backup. The patient is mechanically ventilated and the delivery of positive pressure is titrated as close to functional residual capacity as possible. The patient's respiratory acidosis improves with serial arterial blood gas assessment. She remains intubated for 5 days and then is successfully liberated to NIPPV. In the ensuing days, the norepinephrine infusion is able to be decreased and eventually discontinued about the same time she is weaned off of

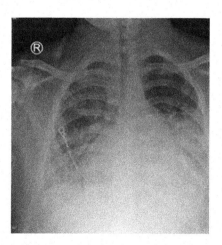

Figure 3.1 A posteroanterior chest radiograph of a 10-year-old girl with Fontan physiology presenting with shortness of breath.

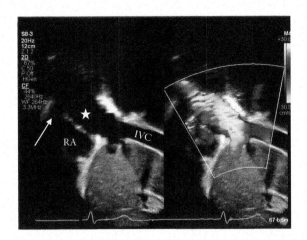

Figure 3.2 Transthoracic echocardiogram. The star denotes the fontan conduit and the arrow denotes the fenestration.

positive pressure support to nasal cannula. Despite normalization of his chest X-ray and work of breathing, she is unable to wean off supplemental oxygen via nasal cannula as her saturations remain in the low to mid-80s. Increases in flow and percent oxygen make no difference in her saturations.

WITH RESPIRATORY CAUSES OF RESIDUAL CYANOSIS NOW RULED OUT, WHAT OTHER CAUSES OF CYANOSIS NEED TO BE EXPLORED? HOW WOULD YOU DO THIS?

The patient is sent to the cardiac catheterization laboratory to further evaluate her hemodynamics. During the catheterization, her Fontan pressure is 17 mmHg with no significant gradient to the pulmonary arteries. Her pulmonary capillary wedge pressure is 9 mmHg yielding a transpulmonary gradient (TPG; Fontan pressure minus the assumed left atrial pressure derived from the pulmonary capillary wedge pressure of 9 mmHg) is 8 mmHg, and there is no gradient across the atrial septum. The right ventricular end diastolic pressure is 9 mmHg, and there is no gradient across the neo-aortic arch. A large veno-venous (VV) collateral decompressing the innominate vein and draining into the right upper pulmonary vein is found (Figure 3.3) and successfully occluded with a device.

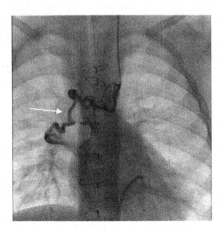

Figure 3.3 A reverse exposure posteroanterior chest radiograph. The white arrow denotes a venovenous collateral.

The Fontan pressures remains 17 mmHg after the intervention while the saturations have improved to 91% on room air. The rest of the patient's hemodynamics were unchanged after collateral closure.

WHAT MEDICAL MANAGEMENT WOULD YOU PURSUE WITH THIS INFORMATION?

The patient is started on sildenafil following the cardiac catheterization. She is subsequently weaned from oxygen support and discharged home tolerating saturations in the low 90s on room air.

DISCUSSION

Initially described by Francois Fontan in 1971 as a corrective procedure for patients with tricuspid atresia, the Fontan procedure has now become the end stage of palliation for most, if not all, patients with univentricular heart disease. The specific surgical interventions involved in each respective stage of single ventricle palliation depend on the patient's underlying anatomy; however, the principles are universally the same. As a reference lesion, HLHS requires 3 stages of surgical palliation culminating in the Fontan procedure. Patients born with HLHS have left-sided structures that are in capable of delivering a full cardiac output to the body and therefore must depend on their right ventricle to deliver blood to both the systemic and pulmonary vascular beds via a patent ductus arteriosus (Figure 3.4). Frequently the patent ductus arteriosus is kept open by means of a prostaglandin infusion started at birth and continued until the first stage of palliation.

The first stage is performed in infancy, a Norwood procedure, consisting of the creation of a "neo-aorta" utilizing the hypoplastic ascending aorta and the native pulmonary artery.

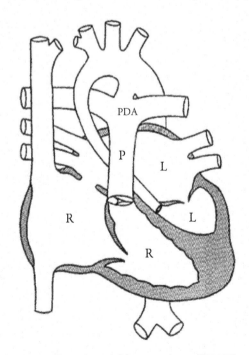

Figure 3.4 Diagram of hypoplastic left heart syndrome (HLHS).

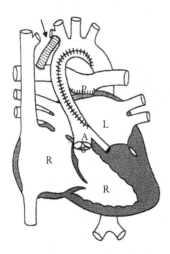

Figure 3.5 Diagram of hypoplastic left heart syndrome (HLHS) after a Norwood Procedure.

However, even together, these are usually insufficient, and a synthetic patch material is often required. An atrial septostomy is created establishing one large common atrium, and the final step is the establishment of a reliable source of pulmonary blood flow through either a right ventricle to pulmonary artery (PA) conduit or an aorto-pulmonary shunt (Figure 3.5, aorto-pulmonary shunt denoted by arrow). This circulation results in cyanosis with a resting saturation of 75% to 85% because of the complete mixing of oxygenated and deoxygenated blood in the conjoined atrium. The single systemic ventricle must now do twice the work as it provides parallel pulmonic and systemic blood flow.

Over time, these patients becomes more cyanotic as they outgrow their shunts and the second stage of palliation is undertaken. The Glenn procedure is usually performed around 4 to 6 months of age and consists of creating a superior cavopulmonary anastomosis, which connects the superior vena cava to the right PA (Figure 3.6, arrow showing Glenn connection). This converts the physiology from a single ventricle with parallel circulation back to a series circulation but still results in cyanosis due to mixing of some deoxygenated blood (from the lower body) with oxygenated blood (from the pulmonary

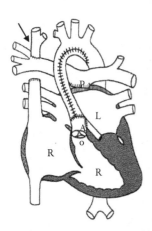

Figure 3.6 Diagram of hypoplastic left heart syndrome (HLHS) after a Glenn Procedure.

veins). In addition to the reliable source of pulmonary blood flow this circulation provides, it also allows for a decrease in volume loading to the patient's single ventricle[1] as venous blood passively flows directly into the lungs from the upper body bypassing the heart. This surgery can result in a slightly higher saturation (mid- to high 80s) compared to those after the Norwood procedure and with a more stable source of pulmonary blood flow. Children are then followed for a few years, allowing them to grow more before they embark on their third stage of palliation, the Fontan procedure.[2]

HISTORY OF THE FONTAN PROCEDURE

The original Fontan procedure, also known as the "atriopulmonary" Fontan, involved surgical connection of the right atrium to the left PA in addition to the Glenn procedure, where the superior vena cava is connected to the right pulmonary artery. The principle was to completely divert deoxygenated venous blood directly into the pulmonary circulation and entirely restore the series circulation of the pulmonary and systemic vascular beds and therefore resolve the patient's cyanosis.[3] The right atrium is used as a surrogate-pumping chamber to theoretically prevent systemic venous hypertension. This original procedure underwent multiple modifications in its early stages, and after the work of de Leval et al., the total cavopulmonary connection (TCPC) was introduced as an alternative to the atriopulmonary Fontan and is now the basis of the Fontan procedure we see in clinical practice today.[4]

The TCPC involves either the use of an intra-atrial baffle of the inferior vena cava (IVC) to the PA, also known as the lateral tunnel (LT) Fontan, or the use of an extracardiac conduit (ECC), frequently made of Gore-Tex, to baffle the IVC to the PA (Figure 3.7). This was introduced after in vitro models showed the inefficiencies of the right atrium as a subpulmonary chamber.[4] Both approaches are used and have associated risks and benefits.

The theoretical benefits of an LT Fontan (Table 3.1) include growth potential due to the use of native tissue and potentially less nidus for thrombogenesis associated with the foreign material in the ECC. The theoretical merits of the ECC Fontan lie in its avoidance of right atrial suture lines, less manipulation of the sinus node, and a decreased propensity for atrial dilation resulting in an overall decreased potential for atrial arrhythmias. The ECC Fontan can also be performed without the need for cardioplegic arrest during surgery and helps to improve preservation of myocardial function during. Despite these pros and cons, no study has consistently shown an advantage of one surgical technique over the other and practice patterns vary from center to center.[2,5,6]

The concept of a fenestration in the Fontan baffle was introduced in the early 1990s as an option for higher risk patients.[2] At the time of TCPC, a connection is made between the medial wall of the Fontan baffle and the right atrium to serve as a right to left shunt. Physiologically, this serves to preserve cardiac output in patients with impaired passive forward flow in the Fontan circulation by allowing deoxygenated blood to escape into the systemic circulation and preserve cardiac output. This is not without sacrifices as an increase in certain comorbidities including desaturation (usually into the low

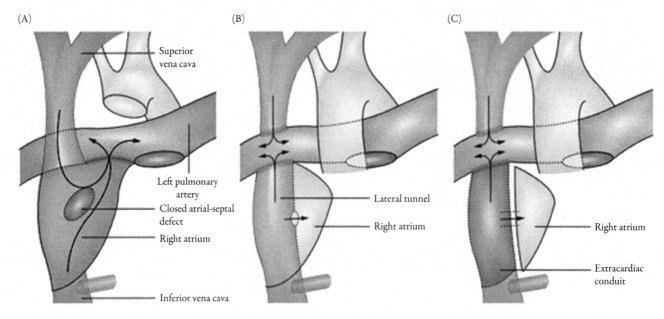

(A)   (B)   (C)

Superior
vena cava

Left pulmonary
artery
Closed atrial-septal
defect
Right atrium

Inferior vena cava

Lateral tunnel

Right atrium

Right atrium

Extracardiac
conduit

Figure 3.7 Diagrams of types of total cavopulmonary connection (TCPC). (A) Atriopulmonary connection. (B) Intracardiac total cavopulmonary connection (lateral tunnel). (C) Extracardiac total cavopulmonary connection.
Original by deLeval MR, The Fontan circulation: a challenge to William Harvey? Nat Clin Pract Cardiovasc Med. 2005;2(4):202–208.

90s percent range), risk of systemic thromboembolism, and possible need for fenestration closure in the future. Fontan fenestration has been shown to decrease postoperative length of stay, duration of chest tube output, and need for early reintervention[7–9] and patency of fenestration has not been shown to have significant deleterious effects long term. Currently, a fenestration is placed on a patient specific basis and is center and surgeon dependent. Patients with borderline pre-Fontan hemodynamics secondary to significant residual lesions that could not be optimized further such as significant systemic ventricular dysfunction, atrioventricular valve dysfunction, elevated pulmonary vascular resistance (PVR), or evidence of obstruction across the pulmonary vascular bed usually undergo fenestration at the time of Fontan completion.

The Fontan procedure is usually performed anywhere from 2 to 5 years of age depending on center preference and patient symptomatology. With advances in surgical technique and peri- and postoperative care, short-term survival is >95% and long-term survival ranges from 70% to 90%.[2]

FONTAN PHYSIOLOGY

The Fontan procedure completes a process of separation of the systemic and pulmonary circulations in children with univentricular hearts. Venous, deoxygenated blood is directly routed to the lungs in a passive manner without a subpulmonary pump. Oxygenated blood enters the heart via the pulmonary veins, traverses a common atrium to the single ventricle with minimal to no restriction, and is pumped to the body. The pulmonary and systemic circulations remain in series but with minimal intracardiac mixing, such as in the Glenn circulation, and this should result in a near fully saturated patient unless a fenestration is placed.

This circulation requires a number of different anatomic and physiologic parameters to be met in order to be successful:

1. The Fontan pathway must have unobstructed systemic venous drainage into the pulmonary arteries via the Fontan conduit.

2. The pressure in this system must be higher than atrial pressure to help drive forward flow into the lungs.

3. The pulmonary arteries need to be adequately sized and unobstructed.

4. The PVR must be low and ideally less than 2 to 3 WU/m^2.

5. The pulmonary veins must be unobstructed in their drainage into the left atrium.

6. Once inside the heart, if there is only a single right ventricle, there needs to be unobstructed flow between the native atria.

Table 3.1 COMPARISON OF FONTAN TYPES

TYPE OF FONTAN	RISK OF ARRHYTHMIAS	GROWTH POTENTIAL	POTENTIAL AVOIDANCE OF CARDIOPLEGIC ARREST	FOREIGN MATERIAL
Lateral tunnel	X	X		
Extracardiac			X	X

7. The atrioventricular valve should be functioning well, without stenosis or regurgitation.[10,11]

8. The single ventricle should have good systolic and diastolic function, and there should be no obstruction of flow through the aorta.

These tenets of Fontan physiology originally described by Fontan himself are now termed the "Commandments of Fontan Physiology" and are used to guide practitioners regarding appropriateness for Fontan candidacy.[2,3]

This three-step process is not without its caveats. The single ventricle remained volume overloaded through the course of the first two stages of palliation undoubtedly resulting in alterations in ventricular systolic and diastolic function through remodeling over time. In keeping the pulmonary and systemic circulations in series, oxygen saturation is improved and ventricular load is diminished, but the lack of a subpulmonary pump and the reliance of passive flow from the systemic veins into the lungs predisposes patients to systemic venous hypertension and chronic low cardiac output. The hydraulic activity of the subpulmonary ventricle provides suction to systemic venous flow and its absence in the Fontan patient attenuates the patient's ability to compensate for flow restriction.[12] The heart's ability to augment cardiac output and alter the degree of systemic venous congestion is significantly impaired. This decrease in cardiac output further causes

systemic arterial vasoconstriction resulting in increased ventricular afterload and can add to ventricular diastolic dysfunction with time and further complicate the long term success of this physiology.[2,10,11]

CAUSES OF ELEVATED FONTAN PRESSURES

Fontan patients with signs and symptoms of congestive heart failure are frequently found to have elevated pressures in the Fontan circuit. Knowledge of whether or not a patient has a fenestration and their baseline oxygen saturations is crucial to diagnosing issues as they arise. In a patient with a fenestration, impedance to flow through the Fontan circulation can manifest in cyanosis due to the nature of this right to left shunt in maintaining cardiac output.[1,10] However, in a patient without a fenestration, signs of elevated Fontan pressures may manifest without cyanosis and may be similar to signs and symptoms seen in congestive heart failure with a decrease in exercise tolerance, an increase in shortness of breath especially with exercise, and swollen lower extremities.

In a biventricular cardiac system, the TPG is the difference between the mean PA pressure and systemic atrial pressure and normal TPGs are typically <10. Normal pressures in the Fontan circuit are 10–15 mmHg and the TPG is usually less than 3 to 5 mmHg. A good diagnostic approach to the failing Fontan is to create a differential diagnosis separated into those with a normal versus elevated TPG (Table 3.2).

Table 3.2 DIFFERENTIAL DIAGNOSIS OF THE FAILING FONTAN WITH ELEVATED FONTAN PRESSURES

CAUSE OF FONTAN FAILURE	TREATMENT
Elevated transpulmonary gradient	
1. Increased pulmonary vascular resistance	
a. Pulmonary arterial hypertension	a. Pulmonary vasodilators (ie, inhaled nitric oxide, sildenafil, bosentan, prostacylclin analogues)
b. Pulmonary causes	
1. Atelectasis	1. Chest physiotherapy, suctioning
2. Pleural effusion	2. Diuretics
3. Pneumothorax	3. Chest tube placement
4. Pneumonia	4. Antibiotics
2. Mechanical obstruction in Fontan circuit	
a. Pulmonary artery/vein stenosis	a. Transcatheter or surgical intervention
b. Clot in Fontan pathway	b. Anticoagulation or thrombolytic therapy
Normal transpulmonary gradient	
1. Ventricular dysfunction	
a. Systolic ventricular dysfunction	a. Inotropes, diuretics
b. Diastolic dysfunction	b. Diuretics, milirinone
2. Atrioventricular valve regurgitation/stenosis	a. Diuretics, milrinone, surgical intervention
3. Atrial septal restriction	a. Balloon atrial septostomy
	b. Surgical intervention
4. Dysrhythmias	
a. Sinus node dysfunction	a. Pacemaker
b. AV dyssynchrony	b. Pacemaker, antiarrhythmic therapy
1. Complete heart block	
2. Junctional ectopic tachycardia	
3. Ventricular tachycardia	
4. Atrial flutter	

The intimate relationship between the pulmonary and cardiovascular system is highlighted in the Fontan patient. While maintenance of adequate pulmonary mechanics and gas exchange is essential to preserve normal cardiac output, the use of positive pressure ventilation in these patients can have a paradoxical effect. By increasing intrathoracic pressure with mechanical ventilation, passive venous return to the lungs is reduced and cardiac output can be decreased. In patients with a fenestration, this increase in venous pressures can result in an increase in right-to-left shunting causing a worsening of oxygen saturations. As such, positive pressure ventilation should be employed only when absolutely necessary.

Although different modes of ventilation exist, the hallmark approach to ventilating a Fontan patient is to maintain functional residual capacity (FRC) while using the lowest mean airway pressure possible. At FRC (Figure 3.8), atelectasis is minimized and alveolar gas exchange is optimized thus maximizing the relationship of ventilation to perfusion. Both under- and overinflation of the lungs is known to cause resultant pulmonary vasoconstriction and increase PVR.[13] Vigilant surveillance by CXR to identify pulmonary causes of ventilation to perfusion mismatch such as atelectasis, pneumothorax, pleural effusions, and pneumonia are necessary. Chest physiotherapy, diuresis, chest tube placement, antibiotics, and judicious use of positive pressure ventilation may be necessary to treat the underlying processes.

Elevated TPG may also occur as a result of endothelial changes and subsequent precapillary pulmonary hypertension. Certain cardiac anatomic risk factors predispose the Fontan patient to the development of pulmonary hypertension including pulmonary vein stenosis, atrioventricular valve dysfunction, systolic dysfunction, diastolic dysfunction, and a history of intact atrial septum. In addition, the lack of pulsatile pulmonary blood flow in the Fontan circulation predisposes these patients to endothelial dysfunction in the pulmonary vascular bed. Pulsatile blood flow normally

induces shear force-induced release of nitric oxide from the vascular endothelium, causing vasodilation.[14] This phenomenon is diminished in Fontan patients. Additionally, Fontan patients have been shown to have increased levels of endothelin-1, a pulmonary vasoconstrictor, which further contributes to the elevation in PVR.[15] Diagnosis of pulmonary arterial hypertension is confirmed with cardiac catheterization and pulmonary vasodilators such as oxygen, sildenafil, bosentan, prostacyclin analogues, and inhaled nitric oxide can be used to treat patients with elevated PVR. In addition to maintaining a normal acid base status the minimization agitation, and in some cases using sedation +/− neuromuscular blockade, can be used to discourage the worsening pulmonary hypertension.

ELEVATED TRANSPULMONARY GRADIENT: MECHANICAL OBSTRUCTION IN FONTAN PATHWAY

Anatomic obstruction can occur at any point along the Fontan pathway from the systemic veins to the pulmonary veins. Obstruction can be secondary to stenosis that develops at anastomotic sites or unaddressed residual lesions from prior palliations that progress to clinical significance and can include PA or vein stenoses. Diagnosis can be suggested by echocardiography and Doppler interrogation of these areas can provide an estimation of the degree of obstruction across the region of interest.[2] Doppler interrogation can also quantify the gradient across a Fontan fenestration, which, if elevated, can suggest an elevated TPG. Echocardiography can be a useful screening tool for structural abnormalities; however, it has its limitations in the ability to accurately identify and delineate residual lesions.[16,17] Confirmation of diagnosis can be achieved with cardiac catheterization or advanced imaging such as cardiac computed tomography or magnetic resonance imaging. Treatment includes catheter interventions, such as balloon angioplasty or stent placement, as well as surgical relief of mechanical obstructions. Another form of mechanical obstruction includes thrombosis at any point along the Fontan pathway, and treatment would consist of anticoagulation or possibly even thrombolytic therapy in severe or acute cases.

NORMAL TRANSPULMONARY GRADIENT

Atrial hypertension is another mode of impedance achieved by transmitting intracardiac pressures to the Fontan circuit by increasing pulmonary venous congestion. Mechanisms of atrial hypertension include systolic and diastolic dysfunction, atrioventricular valve regurgitation or stenosis, and atrial septostomy restriction. Diagnosis can be made with echocardiography and, in some cases, necessitates cardiac catheterization, particularly when diagnosing diastolic dysfunction. Reversible causes of systolic dysfunction such as systemic outflow tract obstruction should be sought out and often requires a combination of echocardiogram and cardiac catheterization to solidify this diagnosis.

Dysrhythmias that result in atrioventricular dyssynchrony, such as junctional rhythm, junctional ectopic tachycardia, atrial flutter/fibrillation, complete heart block, and ventricular

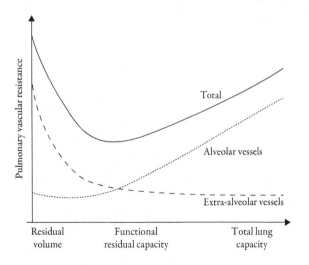

Figure 3.8 Pulmonary vascular resistance as it relates to lung volume, demonstrating that at FRC, atelectasis is minimized and alveolar gas exchange is optimized.

tachycardia will also result in elevated Fontan pressures due to atrial hypertension. Initial recognition by telemetry and central venous pressure waveform analysis (if the patient has a central line) should be followed by formal electrocardiography. Treatment should be targeted to address the underlying dysrhythmia, and in the case of junctional rhythms (not junctional tachycardia), where sinus node dysfunction is implied, pacemaker implantation should be considered to provide atrioventricular synchrony.

Temporizing measures while concomitantly seeking definitive treatment (where possible) includes judicious use of diuretics; vasoactive medications; and, when refractory to these therapies, minimization of metabolic demand. In the case of a restrictive atrial septum, catheterization or surgical relief of obstruction should be employed early rather than late.

Vasoactives employed for systolic dysfunction include inotropic agents such as epinephrine, dobutamine, and milrinone. Milrinone can also be utilized in patients with diastolic dysfunction due to its theoretical ability to enhance lusitropy. If faced with refractory Fontan failure despite medical therapies, especially in the face of severe ventricular dysfunction, ECMO can be utilized but its use is not without challenges. Cannulation strategies for Fontan patients can be difficult, and survival following ECMO remains very poor in this patient population.[18]

OTHER MECHANISMS OF CYANOSIS IN THE FONTAN PATIENT

In addition to the cyanosis that can result from right to left shunting at the fenestration level, there are other mechanisms of cyanosis that should be considered. One cause of cyanosis finds its origins back at the time of Glenn circulation. As a result of IVC blood never reaching the pulmonary arteries, there is a lack of hepatic blood flow to the lungs after the Glenn operation and a resultant deficiency of an "hepatic factor"[19] involved in mediating angiogenesis through anti angio genic factors. This usually manifests in patients who have their Fontan operations later in life, and the end result is right to left shunting within the lungs secondary to pulmonary arteriovenous malformations (AVMs). Depending on the number of AVMs, patient phenotypes may range from being asymptomatic to progressive cyanosis despite completing the TCPC.[16]

Diagnosis can be suggested by contrast echocardiography utilizing agitated saline, with visualization of late bubbles on the systemic side, but is more commonly confirmed with cardiac catheterization and angiography. Pulmonary AVMs have been shown to regress following heart transplantation and after Fontan completion.[20] In patients with clinically significant pulmonary AVMs, treatment can be considered through transcatheter embolism or surgical resection.[19] Currently, the lack of understanding of the molecular etiology of pulmonary AVMs and their expected natural history has made medical therapy very challenging.[19]

Elevations in Fontan pressure can also cause the opening or creation of VV collateral vessels, like in our previously discussed patient. These vessels, some of which were channels that were patent earlier in embryologic development, can reopen

and drain into the left atrium, pulmonary veins, or coronary sinus and effectively result in a right to left shunt.[21] Diagnosis can be made by cardiac catheterization and treatment involves device closure of collaterals as long closing these channels do not result in clinically significant increases in Fontan pressures that would compromise cardiac output.

MANAGEMENT OF RESPIRATORY FAILURE IN THE FAILING FONTAN

Given the limitations in augmenting cardiac output that are inherent in Fontan circulation, anesthetic considerations and cardiopulmonary interactions regarding Fontan physiology requires a critical understanding of the variables that dictate venous return. Guyton et al demonstrated the gradient between mean systemic filling pressure (MSFP) and right atrial pressure are what drives venous return.[22] Venous capacitance and fluid status contribute to the makeup of MSFP.[23] Krishnan et al. described the decreased venous capacitance and resultant increase venous tone at baseline in Fontan patients when compared to normal patients.[24] This principle needs to be preserved to maintain cardiac output and therefore the choice of induction anesthetic should be in concert with this philosophy. Drugs such as propofol that are potent peripheral vasodilators should be used with caution as they increase venous capacitance[25] and therefore may compromise venous return and resultant cardiac output in the Fontan patient. As opposed to ketamine, which liberates endogenous catecholamines thus increasing total peripheral resistance,[26] decreasing pulmonary resistance has minimal myocardial depressant effects. An alternative approach would be high dose fentanyl or etomidate in combination with small to moderate dose fentanyl. Despite etomidate's favorable hemodynamic profile, it should be used with caution in patients with sepsis due to risks of adrenal insufficiency.[27,28] This point should be further highlighted in a Fontan patent who is unable to generate the supranormal cardiac index necessary to combat the vasodilatory shock state of adrenal insufficiency or septic shock. Induction should be coupled with liberal volume resuscitation as the cardiopulmonary effects of positive thoracic pressure induced by bag mask and later by mechanical ventilation are exaggerated due to the absence of a subpulmonary ventricle.

Following intubation, the variables that manipulate venous return (venous return = MSFP – right atrial pressure) require meticulous control. The exception in the Fontan circulation is the pulmonary arteries are the first downstream resistor of the systemic venous return as opposed to the right atrium in normal patients with biventricular circulation. As a result, you must substitute mean pulmonary pressure for right atrial pressure (venous return = MSFP – mean PA pressure) and must manipulate PVR to augment venous return. Ventilating to FRC with the least amount of mean airway pressure is desired to generate the lowest PA pressure. Ideally, a mode of ventilation that allows for patient triggered breaths, or even totally spontaneous breaths with assistance, will promote more venous return as compared to unsynchronized positive pressure breaths. The beneficial effects of negative pressure breathing, including the incorporation of using a Cuirass (external negative pressure ventilation vest) to facilitate ventilation, have been described as a method of augmenting Fontan flow.[29] This strategy of negative pressure breathing should be used with caution in Fontan patients with moderate to severe systolic ventricular dysfunction since the negative intrathoracic pressure will increase afterload in a ventricle that is unlikely to acutely tolerate this new loading condition.

CONCLUSIONS

- A thorough knowledge of single ventricle physiology, and each patient's unique baseline hemodynamics, will increase chances for success when caring for the patient with a failing Fontan circulation.

- Multimodality evaluation of the cardiovascular system is necessary in evaluating the failing Fontan patient.

- Meticulous manipulation of cardiopulmonary interactions are necessary in the failing Fontan patient.

- If cyanosis is refractory to maneuvers that optimize pulmonary mechanics, noninvasive and invasive cardiovascular imaging may help elucidate and manage cardiac causes of cyanosis.

- Medical, interventional, and surgical therapies exist to optimize Fontan hemodynamics and should be considered on a case-by-case basis depending on underlying hemodynamic assessments.

REFERENCES

1. Margossian R, Zak V, Shillingford AJ, et al. The effect of the superior cavopulmonary anastomosis on ventricular remodeling in infants with single ventricle. *J Am Soc Echocardiogr.* 2017;30(7):699–707.e1. doi:10.1016/j.echo.2017.03.005.
2. Feinstein JA, Benson DW, Dubin AM, et al. Hypoplastic left heart syndrome: current considerations and expectations. *J Am Coll Cardiol.* 2012;59(1 Suppl):S1–S42. doi:10.1016/j.jacc.2011.09.022.
3. Fontan F, Baudet E. Surgical repair of tricuspid atresia. *Thorax.* 1971:240–248. doi:10.1136/thx.26.3.240.
4. De Leval MR, Deanfield JE. Four decades of Fontan palliation. *Nat Rev Cardiol.* 2010;7(9):520–527. doi:10.1038/nrcardio.2010.99.
5. Robbers-Visser D, Miedema M, Nijveld A, et al. Results of staged total cavopulmonary connection for functionally univentricular hearts; comparison of intra-atrial lateral tunnel and extracardiac conduit. *Eur J Cardio-thoracic Surg.* 2010;37(4):934–941. doi:10.1016/j.ejcts.2009.10.016.
6. Kumar SP, Rubinstein CS, Simsic JM, et al. Lateral tunnel versus extracardiac conduit Fontan procedure: a concurrent comparison. *Ann Thorac Surg.* 2003;76(5):1389–1397. doi:10.1016/S0003-4975(03)01010-5.
7. Lemler MS. Fenestration improves clinical outcome of the Fontan procedure: a prospective, randomized study. *Circulation.* 2002;105(2):207–212. doi:10.1161/hc0202.102237.
8. Atz AM, Travison TG, McCrindle BW, et al. Late status of Fontan patients with persistent surgical fenestration. *J Am Coll Cardiol.* 2011;57(24):2437–2443. doi:10.1016/j.jacc.2011.01.031.
9. Salazar JD, Zafar F, Siddiqui K, et al. Fenestration during Fontan palliation: now the exception instead of the rule. *J Thorac Cardiovasc Surg.* 2010;140(1):129–136. doi:10.1016/j.jtcvs.2010.03.013.
10. Gewillig M. The Fontan circulation. *Heart.* 2005;91(6):839–846. doi:10.1136/hrt.2004.051789.
11. Gewillig M, Brown SC. The Fontan circulation after 45 years: update in physiology. *Heart.* 2016;102(14):1081–1086. doi:10.1136/heartjnl-2015-307467.
12. La Gerche A, Gewillig M. What limits cardiac performance during exercise in normal subjects and in healthy Fontan patients? *Int J Pediatr.* 2010;2010:1–8. doi:10.1155/2010/791291.
13. Simmons DH, Linde LM, Miller JH, O'Reilly RJ. Relation between lung volume and pulmonary vascular resistance. *Circ Res.* 1961;9(2):465–471. doi:10.1161/01.RES.9.2.465.
14. Goldberg DJ, French B, McBride MG, et al. Impact of oral sildenafil on exercise performance in children and young adults after the Fontan operation: a randomized, double-blind, placebo-controlled, crossover trial. *Circulation.* 2011;123(11):1185–1193. doi:10.1161/CIRCULATIONAHA.110.981746.
15. Mahle WT, Todd K, Fyfe DA. Endothelial function following the Fontan operation. *Am J Cardiol.* 2003;91(10):1286–1288. doi:10.1016/S0002-9149(03)00289-3.
16. Kutty S, Rathod RH, Danford DA, Celermajer DS. Role of imaging in the evaluation of single ventricle with the Fontan palliation. *Heart.* 2016;102(3):174–183. doi:10.1136/heartjnl-2015-308298.
17. Margossian R, Schwartz ML, Prakash A, et al. Comparison of echocardiographic and cardiac magnetic resonance imaging measurements of functional single ventricular volumes, mass, and ejection fraction (from the Pediatric Heart Network Fontan Cross-Sectional Study). *Am J Cardiol.* 2009;104(3):419–428. doi:10.1016/j.amjcard.2009.03.058.
18. Rood KL, Teele SA, Barrett CS, et al. Extracorporeal membrane oxygenation support after the Fontan operation. *J Thorac Cardiovasc Surg.* 2011;142(3):504–510. doi:10.1016/j.jtcvs.2010.11.050.
19. Kavarana MN, Jones JA, Stroud RE, Bradley SM, Ikonomidis JS, Mukherjee R. Pulmonary arteriovenous malformations after the superior cavopulmonary shunt: mechanisms and clinical implications. *Expert Rev Cardiovasc Ther.* 2014;12(6):703–713. doi:10.1586/14779072.2014.912132.
20. Lamour JM, Hsu DT, Kichuk MR, Galantowicz ME, Quaegebeur JM, Addonizio LJ. Regression of pulmonary arteriovenous malformations following heart transplantation. *Pediatr Transplant.* 2000;4(4). doi:10.1034/j.1399-3046.2000.00126.x.
21. Magee AG, McCrindle BW, Mawson J, Benson LN, Williams WG, Freedom RM. Systemic venous collateral development after the bidirectional cavopulmonary anastomosis: prevalence and predictors. *J Am Coll Cardiol.* 1998;32(2):502–508. doi:10.1016/S0735-1097(98)00246-0.
22. Guyton AC, Lindsey AW, Abernathy B, Richardson T. Venous return at various right atrial pressures and the normal venous return curve. *Am J Physiol—Leg Content.* 1957;189(3):609–615. doi:10.1152/ajplegacy.1957.189.3.609.
23. Guyton AC, Polizo D, Armstrong G. Mean circulatory filling pressure measured immediately after cessation of heart pumping. *Am J Physiol.* 1954;179(2):261–267. doi:10.1152/ajplegacy.1954.179.2.261.
24. Krishnan US, Taneja I, Gewitz M, Young R, Stewart J. Peripheral vascular adaptation and orthostatic tolerance in Fontan physiology. *Circulation.* 2009;120(18):1775–1783. doi:10.1161/CIRCULATIONAHA.109.854331.
25. Hoka S, Yamaura K, Takenaka T, Takahashi S. Propofol-induced increase in vascular capacitance is due to inhibition of sympathetic vasoconstrictive activity. *Anesthesiology.* 1998;89(6):1495–1500. doi:10.1097/00000542-199812000-00028.
26. Tweed WA, Minuck M, Mymin D. Circulatory responses to ketamine anesthesia. *Anesthesiology.* 1972;37(6):613–619. doi:10.1097/00000542-197212000-00008.
27. Schenarts CL, Burton JH, Riker RR. Adrenocortical dysfunction following etomidate induction in emergency department patients. *Acad Emerg Med.* 2001;8(1):1–7. doi:10.1111/j.1553-2712.2001.tb00537.x.
28. Bruder EA, Ball IM, Ridi S, Pickett W, Hohl C. Single induction dose of etomidate versus other induction agents for endotracheal

intubation in critically ill patients. *Cochrane Database Syst Rev.* 2015;2017(6). doi:10.1002/14651858.CD010225.pub2.
29. Shekerdemian LS, Bush A, Shore DF, Lincoln C, Redington AN. Cardiopulmonary interactions after Fontan operations: augmentation of cardiac output using negative pressure ventilation. *Circulation.* 1997;96(11):3934–3942. doi:10.1161/01.CIR.96.11.3934.

REVIEW QUESTIONS

1. A 4-year-old patient with hypoplastic left heart syndrome returns from the operating room after undergoing an extracardiac Fontan procedure. His surgeon mentions to you that his Fontan is fenestrated. The patient is on nasal cannula postoperatively and you are aiming to wean this off. What saturation goal should be expected for this patient in room air?

   A. 100%
   B. 90%
   C. 80%
   D. 70%

Answer and Explanation: The correct answer is B. An expected minimum room air saturation for a patient with a fenestrated Fontan is roughly 90%. Normally, a Fontan patient should be fully saturated as the pulmonary and systemic circulations are placed in series without any residual shunts. When a Fontan is fenestrated, a connection is made between the medial wall of the Fontan baffle and the right atrium which can then serve as a right to left shunt. Physiologically, this serves to preserve cardiac output in patients with impaired passive forward flow in the Fontan circulation. This is done at the expense of desaturation, usually into the low 90% range.

2. Which of the following is FALSE regarding Fontan physiology?

   A. The pulmonary and systemic circulations are in series.
   B. Pulmonary blood flow is passive.
   C. PVR should be high.
   D. Pulmonary venous return serves as preload for the single ventricle.

Answer and Explanation: The correct answer is C. The Fontan circulation requires that the patient's PVR be *low*, not high. The Fontan circulation requires a number of different anatomic and physiologic parameters to be met to be successful. The systemic veins drain passively into the pulmonary arteries, placing the pulmonary and systemic circulations in series. These connections must be unobstructed both into and out of the lung vasculature. The PVR must be low and ideally less than 2 to 3 WU×m² to allow for effective forward flow into the lungs. Pulmonary venous return comes back to the common atrium, ultimately serving as preload to the single ventricle. While this physiology allows patients with single ventricle physiology to survive with relatively normal saturations, this ultimately predisposes them to chronic systemic venous hypertension and low cardiac output.

3. Which of the following is a theoretical advantage of the lateral tunnel Fontan over the extracardiac Fontan?

   A. Decreased potential for arrhythmias
   B. Growth potential over time

   C. Decreased atrial dilation
   D. Potential avoidance of cardioplegic arrest

Answer and Explanation: The correct answer is B. The lateral tunnel Fontan involves the creation of an intra-atrial baffle of the IVC to the pulmonary artery, utilizing native tissue. This theoretically allows for growth potential over time. Its downsides include manipulation of the atrium with multiple suture lines, creating a nidus for atrial arrhythmias, and atrial dilation due to its use of the atrium as a filling chamber. The extracardiac Fontan is performed utilizing a conduit of foreign material, such as Gore-Tex, that is placed just to the side of the atrium. This approach avoids manipulation and suturing of the atrium, minimizing the risk of atrial arrhythmias. The extracardiac Fontan can also potentially be performed without the need of cardioplegic arrest given its predominant extracardiac location and lack of intracardiac manipulation.

4. A 4-year-old patient 3 days post-op from an extracardiac fenestrated Fontan operation remains intubated and on a milrinone infusion. You are unable to wean his ventilator due to persistent hypercarbia and hypoxemia. His echocardiogram reveals no obvious Fontan pathway obstruction and shows good single ventricular function. You determine that his lack of progression is due to Fontan failure in the presence of an elevated TPG. Which of the following is a potential cause of this type of Fontan failure?

   A. Ventricular dysfunction
   B. Junctional tachycardia
   C. Atrioventricular valve regurgitation
   D. Pleural effusions

Answer and Explanation: The correct answer is D. Failure of the Fontan circulation has multiple different causes. The easiest way to work through the differential diagnosis of Fontan failure is by separating causes into those with elevated or normal TPGs, the difference between the mean PA pressure and atrial pressure (should be <5 mmHg). Two major groups of diagnoses that increase the TPG are pathologic elements that increase PVR and causes of mechanical obstruction in the Fontan pathway. In this patient, an echocardiogram has ruled out obvious mechanical obstruction from the Fontan baffle to the pulmonary veins; therefore, causes of increased PVR remain the most likely diagnosis. PVR can be increased by any pulmonary derangement that deviates lung volume from functional residual capacity, such as pleural effusion, atelectasis, pneumothorax, or pneumonia. Identification and treatment of this could then potentially result in improvement in the patient's trajectory.

5. A 10-year-old patient post-Fontan is admitted to the intensive care unit with hypoxemic and hypercarbic respiratory failure. He continues to decline despite noninvasive ventilation and is becoming progressively hypotensive, and you are faced with intubating him. Which of the following is the most appropriate induction anesthetic agent for this patient's intubation?

   A. Propofol
   B. High-dose fentanyl + midazolam

C. Ketamine

D. Thiopental

Answer and Explanation: The correct answer is C. Ketamine would be the most appropriate induction agent for this patient given the underlying principles that govern Fontan physiology. Patients post-Fontan preload rely on systemic venous return passively flowing into the pulmonary arteries, and therefore agents that decrease vascular tone such as propofol or midazolam may be a detrimental to maintain cardiac output. Additionally, this patient's progressive hypotension will also necessitate avoidance of agents that can cause myocardial depression such as thiopental. Ketamine increases vascular tone and, in the presence of preserved catecholamine stores, does not cause myocardial depression. These are both desirable characteristics in an induction agent for a Fontan patient.

6. Causes of Fontan failure can be broken down into those that have a normal or increased TPG. Which of the following is *not* a cause of Fontan failure with a normal TPG?

A. Systolic dysfunction

B. Atrioventricular valve regurgitation

C. Atrial septal restriction

D. Pulmonary vein stenosis

Answer and Explanation: The correct answer is D. The easiest way to work through the differential diagnosis for Fontan failure is by separating causes into those with elevated or normal TPGs, the difference between the mean PA pressure and atrial pressure (should be <5 mmHg). All pathologic entities that result in Fontan failure with a normal TPG cause atrial hypertension. Working backwards from the single ventricle—systolic and diastolic dysfunction can raise ventricular end diastolic pressure, thereby raising atrial pressure. The atrioventricular valve can be either stenotic or regurgitant, resulting in atrial hypertension. In some anatomic forms, restriction at the atrial level by means of a small atrial communication can result in atrial hypertension. Arrhythmias that result in atrioventricular dyssynchrony, such as ventricular or junctional tachycardia or complete heart block, can also result in a normal TPG. Pulmonary vein stenosis, while a potentially important cause of Fontan failure, results in an increased TPG by increased mean PA pressure without an increase in atrial pressure.

7. You have just intubated a 6-year-old female who is post-Fontan and presented with respiratory failure. Which of the following are consequences of excessive positive pressure ventilation in this patient?

A. Increased ventricular afterload

B. Increased pulmonary blood flow

C. Decreased pulmonary blood flow

D. Decreased ventricular preload

E. C and D

Answer and Explanation: The correct answer is E. Fontan patients are devoid of a subpulmonary ventricle as systemic venous return flows passively into the pulmonary vascular bed. Positive pressure ventilation can decrease both pulmonary blood flow and, as a result, single ventricular preload in this patient population. Positive pressure ventilation results in increased pleural pressure which is then transmitted to the pulmonary vascular bed. In a Fontan patient, this results in the potential for impedance to passive pulmonary blood flow due to this increase in pulmonary arterial pressure. This can result in decreased pulmonary venous return to the single ventricle, its only source of preload in this physiologic state. Unlike its effects on the pulmonary circulation, positive pressure ventilation results in decreased ventricular afterload and can be beneficial in Fontan patients with ventricular dysfunction when used judiciously.

8. You admit a 6-year-old female who underwent Fontan completion without fenestration 2 years ago who now presents with persistent hypoxemia. She is placed on high-flow nasal cannula and her SpO_2 is 85% despite 100% FiO_2 by blender and the addition of inhaled nitric oxide. Her echocardiogram shows laminar flow in the Fontan baffle, trivial atrioventricular valve regurgitation, and normal ventricular function. Her chest X-ray shows normal lung expansion without focal infiltrates or pleural effusions. She is scheduled for cardiac catheterization to evaluate her hypoxemia. Which of the following are possible causes of her persistent hypoxemia?

A. Pulmonary vein stenosis

B. VV collateral formation

C. Elevated PVR

D. Aortopulmonary collateral formation

Answer and Explanation: The correct answer is B. The formation of VV collaterals is the most likely cause of persistent hypoxemia despite maximal medical therapy in this patient with a nonfenestrated Fontan and no obvious pulmonary disease. VV collaterals tend to form in patients with elevated Fontan pressures as a means of pressure "pop-off" and can drain to a variety of locations. When these collaterals drain to the atrium, bypassing the lungs, they result in a right to left shunt and can cause persistent hypoxemia depending on their number and size. These collaterals can be identified using angiography in the catheterization lab and can be occluded if clinically appropriate. Pulmonary vein stenosis and elevated PVR are all potential causes of hypoxemia in a Fontan patient who has a patent fenestration. In this patient, significant Fontan obstruction or increased PVR would result in hypotension, not hypoxemia, given the patient's lack of fenestration. Aortopulmonary collaterals can also form in patients after Fontan completion who have inadequate pulmonary blood flow. These collaterals increase pulmonary blood flow resulting in increased saturation at the potential expense of worsening ventricular end diastolic pressure secondary to supranormal pulmonary venous return.

4.

THE ACUTE RESPIRATORY DISTRESS SYNDROME

Sarah Maben, Andre F. Gosling, and Shahzad Shaefi

STEM CASE AND KEY QUESTIONS

A 27-year-old male with no prior medical history presents to an outside hospital with 1 day of severe epigastric abdominal pain, nausea, and bilious vomiting. This is the first episode, and he has no sick contacts. He has no allergies and takes no medications on a regular basis. On physical exam, temperature is 102.3°F, blood pressure is 89/52, heart rate is 110, and respiratory rate is 20. His white blood cell count is 16.3 K/μL, creatinine 2.3 mg/dL, and serum lactate is 2.8 mmol/L. Liver enzymes, calcium, and coagulation profile are normal. Blood drawn is reported as grossly lipemic, and because of this finding, the patient's triglycerides level is checked and reveals a massively elevated level of 1850 mg/dL. Treatment with intravenous fluids at 10mL/kg is started immediately. In the emergency department, an abdominal computed tomography (CT) scan shows peripancreatic fat stranding consistent with a diagnosis of acute hypertriglyceridemic pancreatitis. Further discussion with the patient reveals a family history of hypertriglyceridemia, although this patient has not been on treatment. Less than 24 hours in the hospital, the patient develops progressive shortness of breath, somnolence, and hypoxia. He is intubated and sedated with propofol and fentanyl infusions prior to transferring him to a tertiary care center.

WHAT IS THE DEFINITION OF ARDS? HOW IS IT DIFFERENT FROM RESPIRATORY FAILURE ALONE?

In the intensive care unit (ICU), an arterial blood gas shows a PaO_2 of 73 mmHg with an FiO_2 of 1 (100% inspired oxygen) and a chest X-ray shows bilateral pulmonary infiltrates. He is started on broad spectrum antibiotics including mereopenem for possible necrotizing pancreatitis. He is ventilated with volume control at a tidal volume of 5mL/kg predicted body weight and positive end-expiratory pressure (PEEP) of 12 cm H_2O. Over the next several hours, he becomes increasingly difficult to ventilate. The $PaCO_2$ starts to rise, and ventilator plateau pressures are >30 mmHg. Bladder pressure is measured at 21 mmHg, requiring emergent surgical abdominal decompression at the bedside. Postoperatively, he remains hypoxemic and hypercarbic but plateau pressures are <30 mmHg.

WHAT ARE THE DIFFERENT TREATMENT MODALITIES FOR ARDS?

Supportive care for the patient's acute pancreatitis continues with aggressive fluid hydration at 10 mL/kg/h. Despite this, urine output drops to <0.5 mL/kg/h, and he develops uremia with anasarca. He is started on continuous veno-venous (VV) dialysis with ultrafiltration, and aggressive fluid therapy is terminated. A chest X-ray continues to show bilateral pulmonary infiltrates that are worsening. A transthoracic echocardiogram reveals a normal ejection fraction of 60% and normal cardiac valve structure. Frequent arterial blood gases show decreasing PaO_2 levels despite 100% FiO_2 and escalating PEEP and plateau pressures have risen over 30 mmHg despite his abdominal fascia remaining open. Sedation is deepened and a Cisatracurium infusion for neuromuscular blockade is started prior to turning the patient prone. After 12 hours of prone ventilation, his hypoxemia and hypercarbia have remained unchanged. The cardiac surgical team is consulted for possible extra-corporeal membrane oxygenation (ECMO).

HOW HIGH IS THE MORTALITY RATE FOR ARDS?

Cardiac surgeons cannulate the patient for VV ECMO. Over the next 2 days, despite improvement in PaO_2 and $PaCO_2$ levels, the patient develops worsening hypotension requiring infusions of norepinephrine, vasopressin, and epinephrine. His arterial blood gas shows a pH of 7.02, pO_2 52 mmHg, pCO_2 45 mmHg, sodium bicarbonate level of 10 mEq/L, and lactate level of 12.5 mmol/L. A sodium bicarbonate infusion is started, but his bicarbonate level remains unchanged. Given the overall poor prognosis, the patient's code status is changed to DNR. Overnight his cardiac rhythm changes to pulseless electrical activity, and he passes away with family at bedside.

DISCUSSION

First described by Ashbaugh and colleagues in 1967, ARDS continues to cause significant morbidity and mortality in the ICU. In a 2016 study involving 29,144 patients, 10% of all ICU patients and 23% of all mechanically ventilated patients met criteria for ARDS. There was a 46% mortality rate for patients with severe ARDS. While survivors of ARDS have not been extensively studied, they are at risk for skeletal muscle, neurological, psychological, and pulmonary complications.

Diagnostically, the cardinal features of lung permeability, inflammation, and edema have transformed over the years into quantitative criteria including onset of signs after an inciting event, the severity of hypoxemia, and lung imaging modalities to evaluate pulmonary infiltrates.

ETIOLOGY AND PATHOGENESIS

ARDS is triggered by an initial insult leading to systemic inflammation. Aspiration, pneumonia, chest trauma, intra-abdominal sepsis, and acute pancreatitis are common inciting factors. The lungs are particularly vulnerable, perhaps in part due to sensitivity from the repetitive mechanical stress of positive pressure ventilation. The pulmonary response to trauma is divided into three phases: the exudative phase, proliferative phase, and fibrotic phase. The exudative phase involves injury to the bronchial epithelium, which triggers apoptosis and the release of inflammatory mediators within the lung. This, in turn, causes excessive neutrophil activation, damage to basement membrane integrity, and loss of barrier function and progresses to accumulation of a protein-rich fluid in the lungs. Surfactant is inactivated and lung compliance is markedly reduced. Tumor necrosis factor mediated tissue factor (TF) activation causes microvascular changes and microthrombi, leading to hyaline membrane formation. The flooded, noncompliant alveoli collapse, significantly reducing gas diffusion leading to a profound shunt and resultant hypoxemia.

The proliferative phase of ARDS is required for patient survival. The lung has survived a massive inflammatory insult and now must repair the damage. Activated fibroblasts and alveolar epithelial cells repair the basement membrane, begin surfactant production, and establish ion and aquaporin channels to shift intra-alveolar fluid out of the lungs. Barrier function is restored, pulmonary compliance increases, and gas diffusion approaches equilibrium.

The fibrotic phase does not occur in all patients but, if present, is a harbinger for increased morbidity and mortality, specifically prolonged mechanical ventilation. The pathophysiology is poorly understood, but the extent of lung parenchymal damage and resiliency of the activated immune system are critical determinants of the patient's ability to restore lung function.

CLINICAL MANIFESTATIONS AND DIAGNOSIS

ARDS can mimic several other common disease processes, including congestive heart failure, interstitial lung disease, severe pneumonia, and alveolar hemorrhage. Hypoxic respiratory failure is seen in all of these diagnoses, but ARDS is unique in that it develops as a response to an *initial* pulmonary insult; therefore, the time course of development is especially important to the ARDS definition. The Berlin definition of ARDS (Table 4.1), so named from the multidisciplinary panel that met in Berlin in 2011, has multiple criteria for an ARDS diagnosis.

Table 4.1 **BERLIN CRITERIA OF ARDS**

ARDS SEVERITY	PAO$_2$/FIO$_2$	MORTALITY (%)
Mild	200–300	27
Moderate	100–200	32
Severe	<100	45

1. Timing within 1 week of known clinical insult or worsening respiratory symptoms.

2. Bilateral pulmonary opacities on chest imaging not fully explained by congestive heart failure

3. PaO$_2$/FIO$_2$ (P/F ratio) of <300

1. Onset. Onset within 7 days of known clinical injury, but most patients who go on to develop ARDS will do so within 72 hours of the initial injury.

2. *Bilateral pulmonary infiltrates*: Bilateral pulmonary infiltrates, consistent with pulmonary edema; the diagnosis may be made using chest X-ray or chest CT.

3. Respiratory failure of a noncardiac etiology by objective assessment (ie, echocardiography or pulmonary capillary wedge pressure). Patients with known congestive heart failure or high pulmonary capillary wedge pressures may still be diagnosed with ARDS. However, for ARDS diagnosis, the pulmonary infiltrates cannot be fully explained by cardiogenic pulmonary edema alone.

4. *P/F Ratio:* The P/F ratio determines ARDS severity, which is correlated with mortality.

TREATMENTS OF ARDS

Treatment of ARDS (Figure 4.1) revolves around both identifying and treating the underlying etiology (e.g., aspiration pneumonia, pancreatitis, etc.) and mitigating the pulmonary inflammatory response and ventilator-associated lung injury. Volume and pressure-limited ventilation strategies along with increased levels of PEEP have been the primary therapy since the late 1990s, with dramatic reduction in mortality. Since then, the use of neuromuscular blockade, prone positioning, high-frequency oscillation ventilation (HFOV), ECMO, and inhaled NO have all been studied as part of a multimodality treatment strategy for ARDS. All except HFOV and NO have proven effective in reducing hypoxemia in certain patient populations, but more studies are needed to determine which therapies successfully reduce mortality.

PEEP and Low Tidal Volume Ventilation

A lung-protective ventilation strategy is thought to improve pulmonary compliance and alveolar oxygenation. An injured, inflamed lung has reduced alveolar aeration, thus conventional tidal volumes (10–12 mL/kg) are likely to overdistend remaining alveoli causing volutrauma. Studies done in the late 1990s showed a dramatic reduction in 28-day mortality when low tidal volumes of 6 mL/kg were used in patients with severe hypoxemic respiratory failure. Ventilation is a function of tidal volume and respiratory rate, and by reducing tidal volumes, ventilation decreases, causing hypercapnia. Using a low tidal volume ventilation strategy, the clinician accepts a level of permissible hypercapnia to achieve the desired tidal volume in the ARDS patient.

The distal alveoli are subject to repeated opening and collapse, which is termed "atelectrauma." Atelectrauma causes epithelial injury, inflammation, surfactant breakdown, and

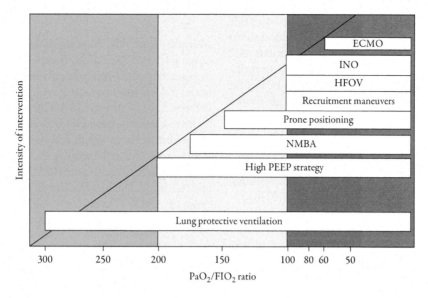

Figure 4.1 Escalating intervention versus severity of ARDS by P/F ratio.

subsequent reduced surface area for gas diffusion. Positive pressure ventilation contributes to this repeated stress on alveoli by using a high driving pressure to push a lung unit open, immediately followed by negative pressure expiration causing rapid collapse. Increased PEEP mitigates the rapid negative pressure collapse of distal alveoli by adding positive pressure to exhalation, keeping those alveoli open and available for gas exchange. This improves overall lung compliance and oxygenation. However, multiple randomized controlled trials have not shown a statistically significant reduction in overall *mortality* from this strategy. Subgroup analyses have shown that patients with moderate to severe ARDS (PaO_2/FiO_2 [P/F] < 200) may see a mortality benefit, but further diagnostic strategies are needed to identify patients who are likely to benefit from increased levels of PEEP.

There is also no clearly demonstrated optimal PEEP level. Using oxygenation as an endpoint to guide PEEP settings has not been shown to decrease overall mortality in ARDS. Patients with obesity or high intra-abdominal pressures (such as in abdominal compartment syndrome) have reduced chest wall compliance, which subsequently changes the transpulmonary pressures and may require elevated PEEP levels compared to other patients. The use of transpulmonary pressure measurements obtained using esophageal manometry has been shown to significantly increase oxygenation but again has failed to show improved mortality.

Neuromuscular Blockade

The use of neuromuscular blocking drugs such as Cisatracurium has a number of theoretical benefits in the ICU. Muscle paralysis could prevent ventilator dysynchrony, allowing intensivists to precisely control ventilation. The cumulative data have shown that the early use (within 48 hours) of Cisatracurium infusions in patients with severe ARDS is associated with a reduced overall hospital mortality rate. The use of other neuromuscular blocking drugs has not been extensively studied, but

Cisatracurium's metabolism by Hoffman elimination makes it unique. Unlike all other neuromuscular blocking drugs, its clearance is unaffected by both renal and hepatic dysfunction, both of which are common in patients with ARDS. The optimum duration of paralysis is not delineated. Use of neuromuscular blockade is also not without risk; there is concern for an increased incidence of polyneuropathy and myopathy in ICU patients treated with muscle relaxants, although further investigation is necessary to quantitate this risk.

Prone Positioning

Prone positioning has the hypothetical benefit of increased chest wall compliance and better ventilation:perfusion matching. Implementing a prone positioning study protocol has been challenging for a multitude of reasons: Variable duration of prone position, use of concurrent neuromuscular blockade, degree of ARDS severity, and treatment group crossover has plagued several randomized controlled trials on the subject. However, a 2013 randomized controlled trial showed that for patients with severe ARDS, early prone positioning for 16 hours per day along with lung protective ventilation strategies was associated with a statistically significant decrease in both 28-day and 90-day mortality rate. Previous studies used high tidal volume ventilation (10 mL/kg), had an erratic duration of time spent prone, and were conducted in centers that did not necessarily have the experience required to effectively carry out treatment of prone patients. At best, patients with severe ARDS *may* benefit from early prone positioning with concurrent use of neuromuscular blockade and low tidal volume ventilation but more definitive studies are needed.

Extracorporeal Membrane Oxygenation

Despite the promising premise, studies have failed to show a robust benefit for ECMO in ARDS. VV ECMO is an invasive method to clear carbon dioxide and oxygenate blood while bypassing injured lungs. If a patient also has heart failure, veno-arterial ECMO can return oxygenated blood to the arterial system, bypassing the heart. In theory, a patient with ARDS could benefit from VV ECMO, maintaining ventilation and oxygenation while allowing the lungs to heal. One of the major studies of ECMO in severe ARDS did show a benefit in 6-month mortality among patients transferred to ECMO centers for treatment, but results are tempered by the lack of standardization in the control group. As of this writing, there is a larger trial of early VV ECMO in patients with severe ARDS compared to a lung-protective ventilation strategy (EOLIA study: ClinicalTrials.gov NCT01470703).

Inhaled Nitrous Oxide

NO is highly lipophilic and diffuses into the pulmonary vasculature, causing localized vasodilation. Its effects could combat the ventilation:perfusion mismatch associated with hypoxic vasoconstriction. When NO comes into contact with hemoglobin in red blood cells, it produces methemoglobin, which inactivates NO. This restricts the vasodilatory effect to the pulmonary vasculature, without causing a serious drop in blood pressure from decreased systemic resistance. Multiple studies have been conducted using NO as a treatment for ARDS, but the data are lacking for a 28-day mortality benefit. Furthermore, there was evidence of harm in a significant increase of renal failure among patients treated with NO. Therefore, the use of nitric oxide is not recommended in the treatment of ARDS.

High-Frequency Oscillatory Ventilation

High-frequency oscillatory ventilation can be thought of as the ultimate low-tidal volume ventilation strategy. Patients are ventilated using small tidal volumes at high respiratory rates—up to 900 breaths per minute! Two randomized controlled trials compared HFOV to lung protective ventilation strategies, but while one trial failed to show a difference in 30-day mortality, one trial was stopped early due to an *increased* mortality rate in the HFOV group. Consequently, the use of HFOV in adult patients with ARDS is not recommended, even as a rescue strategy.

Pharmacologic Therapy

As we begin to understand the underlying pathophysiological mechanism of ARDS, there is intense research looking at potential pharmacological treatments. Many small trials show some initial benefits, but larger, randomized control trials haven't delivered on theoretical promises. Glucocorticoids, surfactant replacement, neutrophil elastase inhibitors, statins, nonsteroidal anti-inflammatory drugs, prostaglandin analogues, *N*-acetylcysteine, albuterol, recombinant activated protein C (Xigris˚), and anticoagulation have not been proven effective treatments for ARDS. Research is still ongoing looking for the holy grail of pharmacologic intervention that will provide definitive morbidity and mortality benefit for these patients.

PROGNOSIS

Mortality from ARDS increases with severity of the P/F ratio, ranging from 27% to 45%. There is significant interest in finding specific patient-related or disease-related factors that could better help predict outcomes. Among patient-related factors, increased age is correlated with increased mortality. Obesity is another patient-related factor that is currently under investigation, but without a clear correlation. Disease-related factors leading to increased mortality include severity of hypoxemia, coexisting infection, higher APACHE II (Acute Physiologic and Chronic Health Evaluation) score, and nontraumatic cause of ARDS. There is no single laboratory test that predicts severity, but there is ongoing research showing there may be genetic polymorphisms in certain patients susceptible to ARDS and who have a higher risk of death.

For patients who survive ARDS, there remains considerable physical, psychological, and cognitive morbidity on the road to recovery. The traumatic experience of hospitalization in an ICU can lead to anxiety, depression, and posttraumatic stress disorder among survivors. Muscle weakness and reduced lung function has also been noted in several studies which followed ARDS survivors for 5 years posthospital discharge. Physical and cognitive rehabilitation are common. Surviving ARDS is simply the first step in a long road to recovery.

CONCLUSIONS

- ARDS is characterized pathologically by the cardinal features of pulmonary inflammation, increased epithelial permeability, and edema.

- Diagnosis of ARDS requires 3 signs: The onset of acute hypoxemic respiratory failure within 7 days of the initial injury, bilateral pulmonary infiltrates not fully explained by cardiogenic pulmonary edema, and a P/F ratio <300. The lower the P/F is, the higher the mortality rate is.

- Low tidal volume ventilation is the mainstay of therapy. There are data to support high PEEP levels, neuromuscular blockade, prone positioning, and ECMO in select patients with severe ARDS.

- There are no strong data to support the use of inhaled NO, and HFOV may actually cause harm in the form of renal failure.

- More randomized controlled trials are needed to better elucidate patient factors that may influence response to a particular therapy.

REFERENCES

Ashbaugh DG, Bigelow DB, Petty TL, Levine BE. Acute Respiratory Distress In Adults. *Lancet*. 1967; 2(7511):319–323.

Amato MBP et al. Effect of a Protective Ventilation Strategy on Mortality in the Acute Respiratory Distress Syndrome. *New England Journal of Medicine*. 1998; 338(6): 347–354.

Anzueto A. Surfactant supplementation in the lung. Respiratory Care Clinics of North America 2002;8(2):211–236.

Bernard GR. Potential of N-acetylcysteine as treatment for the adult respiratory distress syndrome. European Respiratory Journal Supplement 1990;11:496s-8s.

Bernard GR. N-acetylcysteine in experimental and clinical acute lung injury. American Journal of Medicine 1991;91(3C):54S–9S.

Bernard GR, Artigas A, Brigham KL, Carlet J, Falke K, Hudson L, et al. Report of the American-European consensus conference on ARDS: definitions, mechanisms, relevant outcomes and clinical trial coordination. The Consensus Committee. Intensive Care Medicine 1994;20(3):225–232.

Bone RC, Slotman G, Maunder R, Silverman H, Hyers TM, Kerstein MD, et al. Randomized double-blind, multicenter study of prostaglandin E1 in patients with the adult respiratory distress syndrome. Prostaglandin E1 Study Group. Chest 1989;96(1):114–119.

Brochard L, Roudot-Thoraval F, Roupie E, Delclaux C, Chastre J, Fernandez-Mondejar E, et al. Tidal volume reduction for prevention of ventilator-induced lung injury in acute respiratory distress syndrome. The Multicenter Trial Group on Tidal Volume reduction in ARDS. American Journal of Respiratory and Critical Care Medicine 1998;158(6):1831–1838.

Brower RG, Shanholtz CB, Fessler HE, Shade DM, White P, Jr, Wiener CM, et al. Prospective, randomized, controlled clinical trial comparing traditional versus reduced tidal volume ventilation in acute respiratory distress syndrome patients. Critical Care Medicine 1999;27–8):1492–1498.

Brower RG, Ware LB, Berthiaume Y, Matthay MA. Treatment of ARDS. Chest 2001;120(4):1347–1367.

Chadda K, Annane D. The use of corticosteroids in severe sepsis and acute respiratory distress syndrome. Annals of Medicine 2002;34(7-8):582–589.

Cranshaw J, Griffiths MJ, Evans TW. The pulmonary physician in critical care - part 9: non-ventilatory strategies in ARDS. Thorax 2002;57(9):823–829.

Ferguson ND, Fan E, Camporota L, et al. The Berlin Definition of ARDS: An Expanded Rationale, Justification, and Supplementary Material. Intensive Care Med. 2012; 38:1573–1582.

Gattinoni L, Tognoni G, Pesenti A, et al. Effect of Prone Positioning on the Survival of Patients with Acute Respiratory Failure. New England Journal of Medicine. 2001; 345: 568–573.

Griffiths MJ, Evans TW. Inhaled Nitric Oxide Therapy in Adults. New England Journal of Medicine. 2005; 353:2683–2695.

Conner BD, Bernard GR. Acute respiratory distress syndrome. Potential pharmacologic interventions. Clinics in Chest Medicine 2000;21(3):563–587.

Dos Santos CC, Chant C, Slutsky AS. Pharmacotherapy of acute respiratory distress syndrome. Expert Opinion in Pharmacotherapy 2002;3(7):875–888.

Fan E, Brodie D, Slutsky A. Acute Respiratory Distress Syndrome: Advances in Diagnosis and Treatment. JAMA. 2018; 319(7):698–710.

Herridge MS, Cheung AM, Tansey CM, Matte-Martyn A, Diaz-Granados N, Al Saidi F, et al Canadian Critical Care Trials Group. One-year outcomes in survivors of the acute respiratory distress syndrome. New England Journal of Medicine 2003;348(8):683–693.

Herridge MS, Tansey CM, Matté A, et al. Functional Disability 5 Years After Acute Respiratory Distress Syndrome. New England Journal of Medicine. 2011; 364:1293–1304.

Hite RD, Morris PE. Acute respiratory distress syndrome: Pharmacological treatment options in development. Drugs 2001;61(7):897–907.

Holcroft JW, Vassar MJ, Weber CJ. Prostaglandin E1 and survival in patients with the adult respiratory distress syndrome. A prospective trial. Seminars in Respiratory Medicine 1986;7(5):40–47.

Laterre PF, Wittebole X, Dhainaut JF. Anticoagulant therapy in acute lung injury. Critical Care Medicine 2003;31(4 Suppl.):S329-36.

Lewis JF, Brackenbury A. Role of exogenous surfactant in acute lung injury. Critical Care Medicine 2003;31(4 Suppl):S324-8.

Lovat R, Preiser J-C. Antioxidant therapy in intensive care. Current Opinion in Critical Care 2003;9(4):266–270.

Luce JM. Acute lung injury and the acute respiratory distress syndrome. Critical Care Medicine 1998;26(2):369–376.

Marras T, Herridge M, Mehta S. Corticosteroid therapy in acute respiratory distress syndrome. Intensive Care Medicine 1999;25(10):1191–1193.

McIntyre RC, Pulido EJ, Bensard DD, Shames BD, Abraham E. Thirty years of clinical trials in acute respiratory distress syndrome. Critical Care Medicine 2000;28(9):3314–3331.

Peek GJ et al. Efficacy and Economic Assesment of Conventional Ventilatory Support Versus Extracorporeal Membrane Oxygenation for Severe Adult Respiratory Failure (CESAR): a Multicentre Randomised Controlled Trial. Lancet. 2009; 374: 1351–1363.

Que LG, Huang Y-C. Pharmacologic adjuncts during mechanical ventilation. Seminars in Respiratory and Critical Care Medicine 2000;21(3):223–232.

Shoemaker WC. Effectiveness of prostaglandin E1 in adult respiratory distress syndrome. Progress in Clinical and Biological Research 1987;236A:361–368.

Slotman GJ, Kerstein MD, Bone RC, Silverman H, Maunder R, Hyers TM, et al. The effects of prostaglandin E1 on non-pulmonary organ function during clinical acute respiratory failure. The Prostaglandin E1 Study Group. Journal of Trauma 1992;32(4):480–488.

Sokol J, Jacobs SE, Bohn D. Inhaled nitric oxide for acute hypoxemic respiratory failure in children and adults (C. Cochrane Database of Systematic Reviews 2002, Issue 4.

Spragg RG. Surfactant replacement therapy. Clinics in Chest Medicine 2000;21(3):531–541.

Spragg RG. The future of surfactant therapy for patients with acute lung injury - new requirements and new surfactants. Biology of the Neonate 2002;81(Suppl. 1):20–24.

Tasaka S, Hasegawa N, Ishizaka A. Pharmacology of acute lung injury. Pulmonary Pharmacology and Therapeutics 2002;15(2):83–95.

Thompson BT. Glucocorticoids and acute lung injury. Critical Care Medicine 2003;31(4 Suppl):S253-7.

Thompson BT et al. Acute Respiratory Distress Syndrome. New England Journal of Medicine. 2017; 377:562–572.

Whitehead J, Stratton I. Group sequential clinical trials with triangular continuation regions. Biometrics 1983;39(1):227–236.

Wiedemann H, Baughman R, DeBoisblanc B, Schuster D, Caldwell E, Weg J, et al. A multicenter trial in human sepsis-induced ARDS of an aerosolized synthetic surfactant (Exosurf). American Review of Respiratory Disease 1992;145(4 part 2):A184.

Wiedemann HP, Arroliga AC, Komara JJ, Jr. Emerging systemic pharmocologic approaches in acute respiratory distress syndrome. Respiratory Care Clinics of North America 2003;9(4):419–435.

REVIEW QUESTIONS

1. A 30-year-old male, with known history of opioid use disorder is brought to the hospital by emergency medical services. The patient was intubated in the field after being found down. The paramedics report that he vomited during intubation, and thick secretions were suctioned from the endotracheal tube. On hospital day 1, his arterial blood gas shows a PaO_2 of 65 mmHg on a FiO_2 of 0.8 and PEEP of 10 cmH2O. You suspect that the patient has acute respiratory distress syndrome (ARDS). All of the following are required for the diagnosis of ARDS, except

A. Onset within 7 days after a known clinical insult or new or worsening respiratory symptoms.

B. PaO2:FiO2 ratio equal or less than 300 mmHg.

C. Pulmonary Artery Wedge Pressure equal or less than 18 mmHg.

D. Presence of bilateral opacities on chest radiograph or computed tomography.

2. A 68 year-old female, with history of diabetes mellitus type 2, obesity, and hyperlipidemia presents to the emergency department with a 24-hour history of abdominal pain in the left lower quadrant. Her body temperature is 101.3 degrees F, heart rate 115 beats per minute, and blood pressure 85x60 mmHg. A CT scan of the abdomen shows diverticulitis with pneumoperitoneum and fecal contamination. She is taken to the operating room for emergent surgical exploration. On post-operative day 1, she remains intubated with worsening hypoxemia and you become concerned that she could be developing ARDS. All of the following are risk factors for the development of ARDS, *except*

   A. Pneumonia.
   B. Aspiration of gastric contents.
   C. Congestive Heart Failure.
   D. Sepsis.
   E. Pulmonary contusion.

3. A 35 year-old female, with history of morbid obesity and poorly controlled diabetes mellitus type 2 presents to the hospital complaining of weakness, dizziness, and right groin pain. She reports that her symptoms began three days ago after the appearance of an ingrown hair, which expanded very quickly. On examination, she has an area of purple skin discoloration extending from the right groin to the perineal area and mid-thigh. Palpation of the affected area reveals crepitus. Her temperature is 102 degrees F, and WBC count 23,000. She is started on broad-spectrum antibiotics and undergoes extensive surgical debridement. On post-operative day 2, her chest x-ray reveals bilateral opacities and her PaO_2:FiO_2 ratio is 123 mmHg and she is diagnosed with ARDS. What are pathological findings of ARDS?

   A. Intra-alveolar fibrin deposition and associated organizing pneumonia, without hyaline membranes.
   B. Discrete aggregates of epithelioid histiocytes and T lymphocytes, with varying numbers of multinucleated Langhans-type giant cells.
   C. Dense diffuse interstitial infiltrate of lymphocytes, plasma cells, and histiocytes, with the presence of germinal centers and multinucleated giant cells.
   D. Interstitial and alveolar edema, type II cell hyperplasia, and hyaline membrane formation, consistent with diffuse alveolar damage.

4. An 86 year-old male, with history of dementia and multiple myeloma is brought to the hospital by EMS after a fall from 10 stairs, without loss of consciousness. He is found to have fractures on right ribs 2-10 and left ribs 3-5. The patient undergoes placement of an epidural catheter for pain management and is placed on high-flow nasal oxygen. On hospital day 1, his PaO2 is found to be 52 mmHg on 60 L/min and FiO2 of 1.0. The patient is then intubated. Which of the following is a predictor of better prognosis in this patient with ARDS?

   A. Trauma-related ARDS.
   B. Age > 85 years old.
   C. PaO2:FiO2 ratio of less than 100 mmHg.
   D. Treatment with glucocorticoids.
   E. Compliance of less than 20 ml/cmH2O.

5. A 74 year-old male, with longstanding history of smoking (80 pack-years) and COPD presents to the hospital complaining of shortness of breath and chills. On exam, he is noted to have increased work of breathing and accessory muscle use. His SpO_2 on arrival was 82%. The patient is initially placed on bilevel positive airway pressure (BiPAP), but continues to be hypoxemic and 3 hours later is intubated. A CT scan of the chest is performed and demonstrates widespread patchy airspace opacities more apparent in the dependent lung zones, consistent with ARDS. What fluid management strategy is associated with better outcomes in patients with ARDS?

   A. Liberal fluid balance strategy aiming for a positive fluid balance of 500 ml to 1 L daily.
   B. Goal-directed therapy targeting a central venous pressure of more or equal than 10 mmHg.
   C. Goal-directed therapy targeting a pulmonary artery wedge pressure of more or equal than 15 mmHg.
   D. Conservative fluid balance strategy with diuresis, as tolerated.

6. A 19 year-old male, with no significant past medical history is brought to the hospital after a work-related accident. The patient fell from scaffolding from a height of approximately 35 feet. He remembers the accident and denies having lost consciousness. He is found to have multiple bilateral rib fractures, pulmonary contusions, right femoral midshaft fracture, and L2 and L3 compression fractures. On hospital day 1, the patient is noted to have increased work of breathing and worsening hypoxia, requiring endotracheal intubation. A medical student rotating in the ICU suggests that the patient is started on glucocorticoid. Which of the following better describes the effect of steroids in ARDS?

   A. Glucocorticoids are first-line agents in the treatment of ARDS and should be considered in most patients.
   B. Steroids consist of effective rescue-therapy for ARDS and should be considered in severe cases.
   C. Steroids reduce the risk of neuromuscular weakness in ARDS patients.
   D. Initiating steroids more than 14 days after ARDS onset is associated with increased mortality.

7. A 47 year-old female, with history of morbid obesity presents to the hospital with severe abdominal pain in the periumbilical region, associated with nausea and vomiting. On examination, she is found to have a periumbilical mass tender to palpation. CT scan demonstrates an incarcerated umbilical hernia and intra peritoneal fluid. The patient is emergently taken to the operating room for exploration. Intra-operatively, a segment of 30 cm of small bowel is noted to be necrotic and resection is performed. The patient is taken to the ICU intubated following the operation. She arrives in the ICU sedated, on norepinephrine and vasopressin, a blood pressure of 95x60 mmHg, heart rate of 115 beats per minute. Her chest x-ray demonstrates bilateral opacities and arterial blood gas shows a PaO2 of 67 mmHg on FiO2 of 1.0. All of the following are associated with improved survival in severe ARDS, *except*

   A. Lung-protective ventilation with tidal volumes of 6 ml/kg and plateau pressures less than 30 cmH2O.

B. Inhaled pulmonary vasodilators.

C. Prone positioning.

D. Decreases in driving pressure owing to changes in ventilator settings.

8. A 45 year-old female, with history of hypertriglyceridemia is admitted with severe epigastric pain, nausea, and vomiting. Her labs show a lipase level of 3,234 U/L, and an amylase level of 1,492 U/L. Over the next 3 days, she develops respiratory failure, requiring endotracheal intubation, with worsening hypoxemia. This morning, her arterial blood gas shows a PaO_2 of 73 mmHg on a FiO_2 of 0.8. A nurse asks if there is a benefit in paralyzing the patient. Which of the following is true regarding the use of neuromuscular blockade in ARDS?

A. Paralysis has a clear mortality benefit and should be considered in all cases of moderate or severe ARDS.

B. The benefit of paralysis is currently unclear, but it should be considered in patients with severe ARDS and ventilator dyssynchrony or intra-abdominal hypertension with increased peak pressures.

C. Vecuronium is the preferred agent as it was used in the 2 biggest trials that studied the effect of neuromuscular blockers in ARDS.

D. The benefit of paralysis has only been shown when maintained for more than 48 hours.

9. A 15-year-old female, with no previous medical history is admitted to the hospital after having developed sore throat, rhinorrhea, fever, and chills. Her symptoms progressed over 2 days, and by the time of presentation she complained of severe dyspnea. Pulse oximetry demonstrates an oxygen saturation of 90% on room air. Her workup reveals an influenza infection. The patient is admitted and started on oseltamivir but continues to worsen and develops ARDS. On hospital day 3, after institution of a lung-protective ventilation strategy, prone positioning, and neuromuscular blockade, the patient remains hypoxic with a PaO_2:FiO_2 ratio of 73 mmHg and SpO_2 of 87%. The ECMO team is consulted to evaluate the patient for VV ECMO. Which of the following is true about the use of ECMO in severe ARDS:

A. ECMO should be considered after 7 days of symptoms and failure to respond to conventional therapies.

B. Mortality is higher in patients who develop ARDS after an influenza infection.

C. Potential candidates for ECMO should be referred early to an ECMO center.

D. After ECMO is instituted, there is no need for a lung-protective strategy, and the patient should be ventilated with higher tidal volumes (8 mL/kg or more).

10. A 38-year-old male with no previous medical history is brought to the hospital after being rescued in a house fire. The patient was found down inside the house by firefighters. Despite not suffering thermal injuries, his workup reveals a carboxyhemoglobin level of 44%. He was intubated in the field due to concern for inhalational injury. Bronchoscopy reveals severe inflammation and copious carbonaceous deposits. On hospital day 2, the patient develops ARDS secondary to inhalational injury. His family members are concerned and ask about his long-term prognosis if he survives. Which of the following is true regarding functional disability after ARDS?

A. Duration of mechanical ventilation and lowest static thoracic compliance during the acute illness correlate with persistent symptoms after recovery.

B. Patients are expected to return to their baseline weight within 6 months after discharge from the ICU.

C. Psychiatric illnesses affect less than 20% of survivors from ARDS.

D. Less than 50% of survivors are expected to return to work 5 years after ARDS.

ANSWERS

1. C
2. C
3. D
4. A
5. D
6. D
7. B
8. B
9. C
10. A

5.

PULMONARY HYPERTENSION AND HEMORRHAGE REQUIRING LUNG ISOLATION

Hannah Shin, Tracey Eng, and Elrond Teo

STEM CASE AND KEY QUESTIONS

A 48-year-old female with a history of heart failure with preserved ejection fraction, obstructive sleep apnea noncompliant with home continuous positive airway pressure, and pulmonary hypertension presented to the pulmonology clinic concerning her worsening dyspnea. At that time, the initial workup consisted of a chest radiograph, electrocardiogram, and transthoracic echocardiogram (TTE) (Box 5.1). As a result, the patient is scheduled for right heart catheterization the next day for pulmonary hypertension evaluation. The data acquired from the right heart catheterization are shown in Table 5.1.

WHAT IS THE WHO CLASSIFICATION FOR PULMONARY HYPERTENSION? HOW IS PULMONARY VASCULAR RESISTANCE CALCULATED? WHAT IS THE SIGNIFICANCE OF THE LACK OF DIASTOLIC DYSFUNCTION IN THIS PATIENT?

The patient is subsequently admitted to the medical intensive care unit (ICU) for the treatment of pulmonary hypertension. Intravenous epoprostenol is initiated along with diuresis using a furosemide infusion. The patient remains hypoxic despite therapy, and in an attempt to improve cardiac output, intravenous milrinone is started. Systemic hypotension develops, and the patient requires a norepinephrine infusion. Vasopressin is added as a secondary vasopressor agent as norepinephrine levels rise quickly.

Box 5.1 TRANSTHORACIC ECHOCARDIOGRAPHY RESULTS

LV: Hyperdynamic, no regional wall motion abnormalities
RV: Severely dilated, hypertrophic, globally hypokinetic
LA: Normal
RA: Severe enlargement
RVSP: Estimated to be >145 mmHg by tricuspid regurgitation jet
RAP: Estimated to be >20 mmHg by intrahepatic inferior vena cava dilation and nonvariation
Valves:
Aortic: normal; mitral: normal; tricuspid: severe regurgitation; V_{max}, 5.79 m/s; pulmonic: mild regurgitation
Incidental: bilateral pleural effusions

Despite adequate prophylaxis, the patient becomes acutely short of breath and the clinicians feel she is too unstable to transfer for a computed tomography pulmonary angiography. Instead, a critical care ultrasound is performed with attention to deep venous thrombosis screening. A thrombus in the right common femoral vein is found, and a heparin drip is initiated. A standard set of labs is ordered, and a rise in serum creatinine alerts the team to the possibility of acute kidney injury.

The next day, the patient is noted to have a cough, which worsens throughout the day. With leukocytosis and evidence of an infiltrative pattern seen in the right lower lobe on chest radiography, broad spectrum antibiotics are started for pneumonia. Her oxygen saturation has dropped now to 90% on 8 L nasal cannula. An arterial-blood gas test shows a PaO_2 of 52 with a $PaCO_2$ of 58, consistent with both worsening hypoxemia and respiratory acidosis. A bedside lung ultrasound reveals hepatization of the right lower lobe with a large right pleural effusion that appears increased compared to the TTE just a day prior. Bilevel positive airway pressure is initiated in an attempt to improve oxygenation and ventilation and stave off intubation.

HOW CAN OXYGENATION AND VENTILATION BE OPTIMIZED IN THIS PATIENT?

The patient develops hemoptysis, and the heparin drip is stopped for 2 hours. The team is hoping that the hemoptysis will stop on its own, but continued hypoxemia forces their decision-making process. Re-expansion of the right lung is attempted with by increasing the positive airway pressure via bilevel positive airway pressure and removal of the pleural effusion via thoracentesis at the eighth intercostal space. Even though 800 mL of straw-colored fluid is successfully evacuated from the pleural space, the procedure was complicated by pneumomediastinum and massive hemoptysis.

WHAT NONSURGICAL APPROACHES ARE AVAILABLE TO CONTROL PULMONARY HEMORRHAGE?

The patient is emergently intubated and prepared for diagnostic bronchoscopy. The clinicians are able to localize the source

Table 5.1 RIGHT HEART CATHETERIZATION RESULTS

CO: 4.4 L/min	RVP: 92/15 mmHg	PAP: 92/28	Sats: PA 55% RA 65% FA 89%	CVP: 12
CI: 1.7 L/min/m2	RAP: 23mmHg	PCWP: 26 mmHg	PVR 5 WU	MAP: 61

of bleeding to the right lower lobe but find it cannot be controlled with iced saline lavage or topical epinephrine.

The patient's peak pressures continue to rise, and mechanical ventilation is becoming harder as her oxygenation worsens. Her mean pulmonary arterial pressure is now 130% of her systemic pressure. A repeat lung ultrasound on the side the thoracentesis had been performed is significant for a re-accumulation of fluid that is concerning for blood. A right chest tube is inserted emergently and 900 mL of blood return is immediately elicited. Given the worsening gas exchange, the patient is emergently cannulated for femoral-femoral (fem-fem) extracorporeal membrane oxygenation (ECMO). The cardiothoracic surgery service is consulted for surgical options as blood from the endotracheal tube (ETT) continues to worsen.

WHEN SHOULD LUNG ISOLATION BE UTILIZED? WHAT ARE THE DIFFERENT METHODS OF ONE-LUNG VENTILATION?

Emergent bronchoscopy is performed again, revealing bright red blood coming from the right lower lobe with evidence of spillage across into the left lung. Bronchoscopic attempts to stem the bleeding fail again, likely due to the massive volume of blood seen in her airways. In an effort to tamponade the bleed, an endobronchial blocker is introduced under fiberoptic guidance into the bronchus intermedius and inflated, isolating the right lower and middle lobes from the rest of the lung. This appears to impede the flow of blood out of the right lower lobe and after a quick suctioning by bronchoscopy, the rest of the airways appear to be preserved.

The patient is transported to interventional radiology for assessment and possible embolization to help address the high chest tube output. An area with radiographic blush is seen at the eighth intercostal artery and is successfully embolized. The patient is transferred back to the ICU with a markedly decreased chest tube output.

Not long after embolization, the patient becomes hypotensive with recurrent hemoptysis, and multiple units of packed red blood cells, fresh frozen plasma, and platelets are transfused. Multiple attempts at therapeutic bronchoscopy are attempted and topical epinephrine is administered into the right lower lobe and the endobronchial blocker reinflated. A large clot is removed from the left mainstem via use of a cryoprobe, but smaller clots in the lower airways are more tenacious and cannot be extracted.

Despite these efforts to mitigate the bleeding, oxygen saturation continues to diminish to the low 70s, and the patient is now unable to be manually ventilated. After a lengthy discussion, the patient's family declines advanced surgical options,

and care was redirected toward comfort. Shortly thereafter, the patient expires in the ICU with her family present at bedside.

DISCUSSION

Massive hemoptysis management is multifaceted. The speed at which a patient can deteriorate is rapid and potentially predictable. The induction of anesthesia and control of the airway is paramount. It is recommended to intubate the trachea with the largest ETT possible to facilitate bronchoscopy, which should be initiated early, as it can be both diagnostic and therapeutic in the unstable patient [1]. Rapid identification of the etiology and laterality of the hemoptysis source will provide prognostic information and guide patient management. It is usually appropriate to lavage any affected airways with iced saline mixed with epinephrine (100 mcg/mL). Some systemic absorption of epinephrine is to be expected and is oftentimes useful but also has the potential to induce cardiac arrythmias [1-3]. Antifibrinolytics, such as tranexamic acid, can be considered and administered into the gastrointestinal tract or intravenously to reduce hemoptysis or act as a bridge to more definitive interventions [4]. Bronchoscopic electrocautery may be useful depending on the etiology of the bleed. See Box 5.2 for other useful adjuncts.

It is not uncommon for patients who are in hemoptysis to develop further coagulopathy. Identification and management of coagulopathy through clinical suspicion and coagulation labs (international normalized ratio, partial thromboplastin time, thromboelastography, and fibrinogen) can guide prompt transfusions of blood products such as fresh frozen plasma, platelets, and cryoprecipitate. If worsening volume

Box 5.2 BRONCHOSCOPIC ADJUNCTS AS A NON-SURGICAL APPROACH TO MANAGING PULMONARY HEMORRHAGE

Strategy
Ice-cold saline
Topical vasoconstrictors
Balloon tamponade
Endobronchial stent placement
Endobronchial spigot
Oxidized regenerated cellulose
Cyanoacrylate glue
Electrocautery
Laser photocoagulation
Argon plasma coagulation

Adapted from Sakr L, Dutau H, Massive hemoptysis: an update on the role of bronchoscopy in diagnosis and management. *Respiration.* 2010;80(1):38–58.

overload, or the suspicion that coagulopathy reversal may precipitate volume overload, factor concentrate products should be considered as part of a balanced resuscitation. Attention to clot generation over the course of the bronchoscopy can also provide advantageous clinical information in determining the need for blood products. Specialty consultation with interventional pulmonology can secure tools to remove clot that has formed casts within the airway, such as a cryoprobe [1,5].

If bleeding is unilateral and constant, the practitioner is encouraged to assess feasibility and patient stability for endotracheal extubation and double lumen tube (DLT) reintubation. Factors to consider are current gas exchange, hemodynamic stability, ease of reintubation, and confidence of the practitioner. It is recommended that the practitioner wear full personal protective equipment and consider administration a neuromuscular blocking drug to improve first pass success. Video laryngoscopy is likely to be useful. Use of airway exchange catheters may be used but use caution and integrate bronchoscopic data (e.g., distance of the ETT to the carina) to judge the depth of catheter insertion as to not cause or exacerbate any endobronchial trauma.

If the patient is too unstable for tube exchange, the goal of care is to optimize the nonbleeding lung through lung isolation with intrabronchial balloon tamponade. This intervention requires modifying the patient's position into a lateral decubitus position with the affected lung down towards the bed [1,6]. For example, position the patient in right lateral decubitus for bleeding from right lung and left lateral decubitus for bleeding from the left lung. Intrabronchial tamponade can only be achieved by clamping the endotracheal tube followed by delayed fiberoptic, rigid bronchoscopy or surgical resection.

The strategy for lung isolation will depend on the bronchoscopic data obtained earlier. This will help balance the loss of functional lung volume with ventilation/perfusion matching. See Table 5.2 for endobronchial balloon and endotracheal tube management strategies related to bleeding location. Insertion of a DLT is not recommended as first-line airway management because the suction port of the bronchoscope that fits within the DLT lumen is often too small and thus ineffective for high volume hemoptysis, clot extraction, or endobronchial intervention through cryotherapy or electrocautery [1,3]. However, it should be considered as a second line option if other options to isolate bleeding fail.

Often times, the patient has already been intubated by a separate team or institution and the ETT in situ is small. If deemed safe to do so, it is appropriate to upsize the ETT. The smallest choice for therapeutic bronchoscopy is a 7.5, and thus it has been nicknamed "the universal tube." Preferably one would upsize to an 8.0 ETT or larger as it allows for easier and safer mechanical ventilation during prolonged bronchoscopy. If it is unsafe to manipulate the airway, it is appropriate to attempt endoscopic balloon placement to protect the nonbleeding lung and to provide intrabronchial tamponade. If this is difficult, the practitioner can take advantage of the smaller endotracheal tube. For example, if the ETT is too small and the bleed is originating from the right upper lobe, one can advance the ETT into the left mainstem to protect the left lung. Use of an ETT with subglottic suctioning will be useful to continue to measure the hemorrhage from the nonisolated lung. If space is available around the vocal cords and within the proximal trachea, a flexible bronchoscopy can passed alongside the ETT to assist in stopping the bleeding.

Assuming lung isolation has been achieved, finding a means to stop the hemorrhage is the next step in management. Endobronchoscopic data are incredibly useful for identifying laterality of bleeding and consultation with interventional radiology to identify a source for potential bronchial artery embolization may be useful as well.

In some cases of unilateral bleeding, all the previously measures may not help. At this point, the practitioner may consider whether or not the patient is a viable surgical candidate

Table 5.2 ISOLATED LOBAR BLEEDING AND ENDOTRACHEAL TUBE AND ENDOBRONCHIAL TUBE MANAGEMENT STRATEGIES

SITE OF BLEEDING	TECHNIQUE	LIKELIHOOD OF SUCCESS	RISK
RUL	Balloon to proximal right mainstem	Fair	Balloon may move
RUL	ETT to left mainstem intubation	Good	Neuromuscular blockade required ETT are usually too short Nasal Ring–Adair–Elwyn may be useful
RLL	Balloon to bronchus intermedius	Good Gas exchange to RUL is preserved	Balloon may move Neuromuscular blockade required
LLL	Balloon to LLL takeoff	Fair	Balloon may move
LUL	Balloon to LUL takeoff	Poor	Balloon frequently becomes malpositioned
LLL/LUL	Balloon to left mainstem	Good	Minimal
LLL/LUL	ETT right mainstem intubation	Fair	ETT Murphy eye may not align with the RUL takeoff so loss of the RUL functional capacity can occur

Abbreviations: ETT, endotracheal tube; RUL, right upper lobe; RLL, right lower lobe; LUL, left upper lobe; LLL, left lower lobe.

for a lobectomy or pneumonectomy. Of note, the morbidity and mortality in such patients are extremely high, upwards of 27% if performed during active bleeding, and survival is only possible with integration of VV ECMO [7,8].

Bleeding from both lungs poses a serious problem as the capacity for efficient gas exchange will deteriorate rapidly. In cases of bilateral pulmonary hemorrhage having failed other procedures, early veno-venous EMCO (VV ECMO) consultation is recommended [9]. There is growing evidence that patients can be fully supported on ECMO in a veno-venous, veno-arterial, or veno-arterio-venous configuration so that the patient can survive having their ETT clamped and disconnected from the ventilator entirely [8,10]. If possible, the separate ECMO team can wire or cannulate both femoral sites and facilitate the speed of ECMO initiation. One important caveat to veno-arterial ECMO is the need for anticoagulation; therefore, extreme caution is emphasized if it is to be considered. VV ECMO does not necessarily require anticoagulation or, in an emergency, can tolerate much lower levels of anticoagulation, especially if ECMO flows are high enough.

CONCLUSION

Pulmonary hypertension presents an added layer of complexity not only in its disease process but also in the array of complications that may arise from relatively minor procedures. For example, in our previously outlines case, a needle thoracostomy to drain a pleural effusion resulted in massive hemoptysis and hemorrhagic pleural effusion in a patient with suprasystemic pulmonary arterial hypertension. In managing such patients, one should be cognizant of the ratio between the systemic and pulmonic circulatory pressures. It should be considered that if the pulmonic to systemic pressure ratio is greater than 2:3, intraparenchymal pulmonary bleeding will act like uncontrolled noncompressible bleeding. Much like the difficult airway algorithm, heroic efforts are often required to oxygenate the patient either with either their native lungs or ECMO. Identification of localized bleeding versus diffuse bleeding should be diagnosed quickly to direct the strategies for source control (e.g., interventional radiology or surgical control).

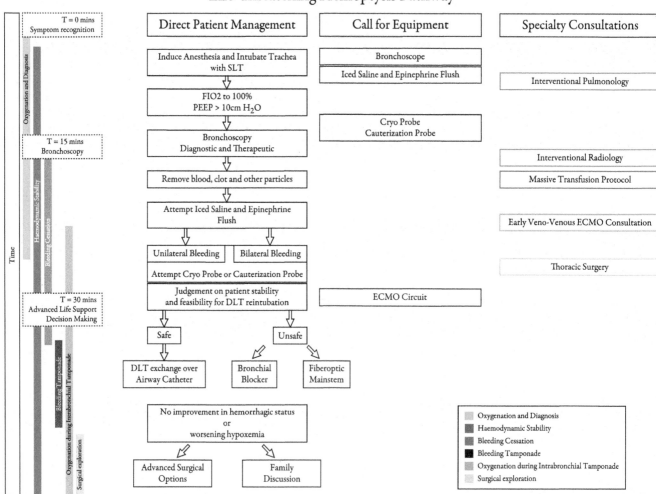

Figure 5.1 Treatment algorithm for pulmonary hemorrhage requiring lung isolation.

REFERENCES

1. Davidson K, Shojaee S, Managing massive hemoptysis, *Chest.* 2020;157(1):77–88. doi.10.1016/j.chest.2019.07.012.
2. Kalyanaraman M, Carpenter RL, McGlew MJ, et al. Cardiopulmonary compromise after use of topical and submucosal α-agonists: possible adding complication by the use of β-blocker therapy. *Otolaryngol Head Neck Surg* 1997;117:56–61.
3. Radchenko C, Alraiyes AH, Shojaee S. A systematic approach to the management of massive hemoptysis. *J Thorac Dis.* 2017;9(Suppl 10):S1069–S1086. doi:10.21037/jtd.2017.06.41.
4. Bellam BL, Dhibar DP, Suri V, et al. Efficacy of tranexamic acid in haemoptysis: a randomized, controlled pilot study. *Pulm Pharmacol Ther.* 2016;40:80–83. doi:10.1016/j.pupt.2016.07.006
5. Sehgal IS, Dhooria S, Agarwal R, Behera D. Use of a flexible cryoprobe for removal of tracheobronchial blood clots. *Respir Care.* 2015;60(7):e128–e131.
6. Sakr L, Dutau H. Massive hemoptysis: an update on the role of bronchoscopy in diagnosis and management. *Respiration.* 2010;80(1):38–58. doi:10.1159/000274492.
7. Andrejak C, Parrot A, Bazelly B, et al. Surgery for hemoptysis in patients with benign lung disease. *J Thoracic Dis.* 2018;10(6):3532–3538.
8. Nunez D, Rao R, Gray BW, et al. Massive hemoptysis from pulmonary histoplasmosis requiring emergency lung resection and extracorporeal membrane oxygenation. *J Pediatr Surg Case Rep.* 2019;48:101260. doi:10.1016/j.epsc.2019.101260
9. Endicott-Yazdani, TR, Wood C, Trinh AD, et al. Massive hemoptysis managed by rescue extracorporeal membrane oxygenation. *Baylor Univ Med Cent Proc.* 2018;31(4):479–481. doi:10.1080/08998280.2018.1487693
10. Lee CF, Huang CT, Ruan SY. Endotracheal tube clamping and extracorporeal membrane oxygenation to resuscitate massive pulmonary haemorrhage. *Respirol Case Rep.* 2018;6(5):e00321. doi:10.1002/rcr2.321

REVIEW QUESTIONS

1. Diagnostic elective right heart catheterization was performed for suspected PH and revealed the following measurements:

CO: 4.4L/min
CI 1.7L/min/m²
RA 23
RV 92/15
PAP 92/28
PCWP 26
MAP 61

What is the calculated transpulmonary gradient?

A. 3 mmHg
B. 8 mmHg
C. 23 mmHg
D. 66 mmHg

Answer: C

The transpulmonary gradient represents the pressure change that occurs as blood flow meets resistance through the pulmonary circulation. It can be calculated as MPAP – LAP with MPAP representing precapillary pressures and LAP, which can be approximated using PCWP, signifying postcapillary pressures.

2. Using the same data set above, what is the calculated PVR (dyn·s/cm5)?

A. 120 dyn·s/cm5
B. 418 dyn·s/cm5
C. Calculated SVR
D. Unable to calculate using the information given.

Answer: B
By applying Ohm's law to pulmonary hemodynamics, pulmonary vascular resistance can be calculated as
PVR = (MPAP – PCWP)/Cardiac Output × 80 (dynes)
= 23/4.4 × 80
= 418 dynes

3. No fiberoptic guidance is available. Breath sounds present in both lungs when either the tracheal or endobronchial lumens are occluded. Where is the DLT positioned?

A. Left mainstem
B. Esophageal
C. Right mainstem
D. Too proximally

Answer: D
Breath sounds heard in both lungs signify ventilation in both lungs. The only location of both lumens despite the cuffs being inflated is the trachea. This is too proximal for lung isolation.

4. Breath sounds are only audible in the left lung when either the tracheal or endobronchial is occluded. Where is the DLT positioned?

A. Left mainstem
B. Esophageal
C. Right mainstem
D. Too proximally

Answer: A
If both lumen are within the left mainstem with both cuffs inflated, breath sounds will be heard only on the left side as ventilation has not occurred on the right.

5. Using a left DLT, the tracheal and endobronchial cuffs are inflated. Breath sounds are present on the right when the bronchial lumen is ventilated. When the tracheal lumen is ventilated, there are no breath sounds on the left.

A. Left mainstem
B. Esophageal
C. Right mainstem
D. Too proximally

Answer: C
Here the endobronchial lumen is inside the bronchus intermedius. The tracheal cuff is likely occluding the right mainstem takeoff.

6. The following image is seen during fiberoptic bronchoscopy through the endobronchial lumen. What is the best next step to achieve appropriate lung isolation?

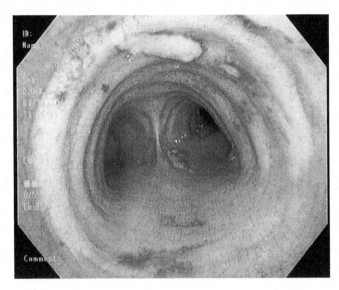

A. Inflate both tracheal and endobronchial cuffs
B. Withdraw the DLT
C. Advance the DLT
D. Deflate the endobronchial cuff

Answer: C

The image shows the bifurcation of the trachea. The tracheal rings are seen anteriorly and the striae of the membranous trachea are seen.

7. The following image is seen during fiberoptic bronchoscopy through the endobronchial lumen. What is the best next step to achieve appropriate lung isolation?

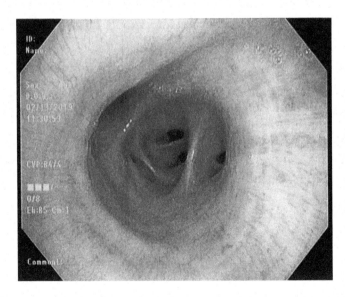

A. Inflate both tracheal and endobronchial cuffs
B. Withdraw the DLT
C. Advance the DLT
D. Deflate the endobronchial cuff

Answer: B

The bronchoscope is within the bronchus intermedius past the right upper lobe takeoff.

8. The second carina is seen

A. In the bronchus intermedius
B. At the right upper lobe takeoff
C. Right middle lobe takeoff
D. Left mainstem

Answer: D

9. Label the letters in the bronchus intermedius

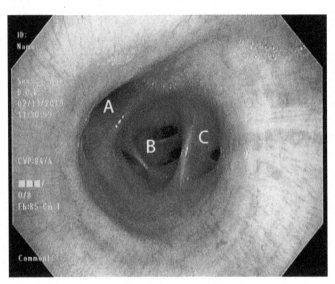

Answers: A: right middle lobe; B: right lower lobe; C: superior segment, right lower lobe

10. Label the letters in the left mainstem.

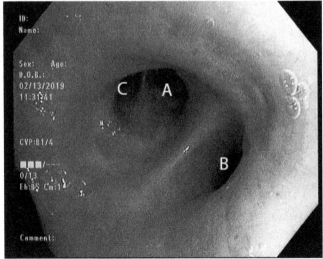

Answers: A: lingula, B: left lower lobe, C: left upper lobe

6.

VENTILATOR AND CHEST TUBE MANAGEMENT FOR PNEUMOTHORAX IN A PATIENT WITH BULLOUS EMPHYSEMA

Shaun L. Thompson and James N. Sullivan

STEM CASE AND KEY QUESTIONS

A 66-year-old male with a history of chronic obstructive pulmonary disease (COPD) presents from home to the emergency department due to increased shortness of breath. His symptoms began earlier in the week and has progressively worsened over the past couple of days. He notes increased effort to breath, coughing, and the amount of productive cough that he has had compared to his baseline. Vital signs reveal an oxygen saturation of 86%, a pulse of 102 bpm, a blood pressure of 155/92, a respiratory rate of 28 breaths per minute, and a temperature of 37°C. An initial supine chest X-ray reveals hyperinflated lungs consistent with the patient's COPD. A large air space opacity in the area of the right upper lobe and diffuse infiltrates in the left and right lower lobes are present. The patient continues to have increased work of breathing. An arterial blood gas reveals the following values: 7.31/63/54 on 10 L/min of oxygen therapy delivered by nasal cannula. In an attempt to reduce the patient's work of breathing, noninvasive ventilation is attempted without significant improvement. Inhaled bronchodilators, systemic corticosteroids, and antibiotics are started per guideline recommendations for a potential COPD exacerbation [1–3]. Despite this, the patient continues to decline and has worsening hypoxia and signs of significant fatigue requiring endotracheal intubation. Following intubation, the patient's oxygen saturation declines further and hemodynamic compromise also occurs. Physical examination subsequently reveals diminished breath sounds on the left side and no breath sounds on the right side. A pneumothorax is feared, and rapid diagnosis is desired. Because of its high sensitivity and specificity, 95% and 94%, respectively, bedside lung ultrasound is performed and demonstrates a large right pneumothorax [4].

WHAT OTHER CAUSES OF HYPOXIA SHOULD BE INCLUDED IN THE DIFFERENTIAL DIAGNOSIS?

There are many life-threatening conditions that can cause acute hypoxia and a timely diagnosis must be made. In addition to pneumothorax, the differential diagnosis for acute hypoxia in this patient includes COPD exacerbation, mucus plugging of the airways, pulmonary embolism, pulmonary edema, acute heart failure, and pneumonia. A brief medical history and good physical exam can quickly differentiate these conditions allowing for rapid treatment decisions to be made. In this situation, the diagnosis of pneumothorax was aided by bedside ultrasonography of the thorax.

WHAT IS THE NEXT INTERVENTION THAT SHOULD BE PERFORMED?

Due to the patient's deteriorating condition and diagnosis of pneumothorax, emergent decompression of the chest with tube thoracostomy should be performed. In the event that a tube thoracostomy cannot be rapidly performed, needle decompression can be used emergently until definitive treatment can be performed. Needle decompression is performed by placing a large bore intravenous catheter, typically 14 gauge or 16 gauge, into the second intercostal space in the midclavicular line. In this case, a pigtail catheter was introduced in the mid-axillary line in the 4th intercostal space with a rush of air noted after placement. The chest tube was then placed on wall suction for continued evacuation of the pneumothorax. The patient's oxygen saturation subsequently improved, and he was transferred to the intensive care unit for further management.

WHAT OTHER DIAGNOSTIC TESTING SHOULD BE PERFORMED ON THIS PATIENT?

Following treatment of the patient's acute hypoxic episode, additional causes of respiratory failure should be investigated and ruled out. Given the patient's history of bullous emphysema a computer tomography (CT) scan of the chest was performed to evaluate the lung parenchyma and confirm proper positioning of the chest tube. A contrast study to evaluate for pulmonary embolism was deemed not necessary due to the significant improvement in the patient's clinical status following the placement of the chest tube. The noncontrast scan revealed a small pneumothorax in the right hemi-thorax along with findings of severe bullous emphysema bilaterally. The CT examination also revealed thickened bronchial walls that suggested acute COPD exacerbation as the primary underlying cause for the patient's initial hypoxia and hypercarbia upon initial presentation [5]. Blood and urine cultures were obtained, along with a rapid viral panel and urine tests for streptococcus pneumonia and legionella to further evaluate for infection as a trigger for the patient's acute COPD exacerbation.

WHAT SETTINGS SHOULD BE USED FOR POSITIVE PRESSURE MECHANICAL VENTILATION IN THIS PATIENT?

In a patient with a secondary spontaneous pneumothorax (SSP), likely due to a ruptured bleb from bullous emphysema, it is essential to prevent further lung injury from positive pressure ventilation. A lung protective strategy includes lower tidal volumes based on predicted body weight of 4-8 ml/kg, higher levels of positive end-expiratory pressure (PEEP) [6], plateau pressures less than 30 mmHg, and driving pressures of less than 17 mmHg [7, 8]. PEEP can still be used in this patient despite the pneumothorax because of the presence of the chest tube that is under continuous suction for evacuation. However, PEEP should be reduced if a pneumothorax continues to persist despite chest tube evacuation.

DISCUSSION

DEFINITION AND DIAGNOSIS OF BULLOUS EMPHYSEMA

A bulla is defined as an air-filled space, 1 cm or larger in size, that develops within lung parenchyma associated with emphysematous changes [9]. The disease develops from destruction of elastic tissue in the lung by proteolysis, typically elastase [6, 10]. This in turn leads to a loss of elastic recoil within the lung. The bullae are thought to increase in size over time as air becomes trapped in the air pockets and is unable to escape due to medium airway obstruction from the emphysematous changes [10, 11]. Risk factors for the development of bullous emphysema include cigarette smoking, marijuana smoking, crack/cocaine abuse, alpha-1-antitrypsin disease, sarcoidosis and other connective tissue diseases [6].

Typically bullae are identified with plain chest radiography (chest X-ray) [6]. If bullous disease is discovered, then further evaluation with chest tomography is recommended to evaluate the size of the bullae and architecture of the underlying lung tissue [6, 9]. If the lung parenchyma shows changes consistent with emphysema, the diagnosis of bullous emphysema is made. Giant bullous emphysema is a rare subtype of bullous emphysema defined by a bulla that comprises 30% of the lung volume by itself [6].

DEFINITION AND TREATMENT OF COPD EXACERBATION

Acute exacerbation of COPD (AECOPD) is a major health problem and has been steadily increasing in incidence over the past 20 years [1–3, 12]. An acute exacerbation by definition according to the Global Initiative for Chronic Obstructive Lung Disease (GOLD) is "an event in the natural course of the disease characterized by a change in the patient's baseline dyspnea, cough, and/or sputum that is beyond normal day-to-day variations, is acute in onset, and may warrant a change in regular medication in a patient with underlying COPD" [3, p. 786]. When these events occur, they produce not only short-term worsening of symptoms for patients but also portend to long-term outcome and survival. In patients with an acute exacerbation that requires hospitalization, studies have shown that 5-year mortality is around 50% [2]. Because of this, it is important to diagnose this problem quickly and begin therapy to reduce further decompensation.

Diagnosis of AECOPD is typically made based upon symptoms and patient history. The most common complaints that patients present with during AECOPD are dyspnea, increased sputum production, and increased cough from baseline [1–3]. AECOPD are multifactorial events typically triggered by infectious causes by viral or bacterial sources [1–3, 12]. Typical viruses that are found in patients with AECOPD include rhinovirus, coronavirus, and adenovirus [3]. Bacterial organisms associated with AECOPD include streptococcus pneumoniae, haemophilus influenza, and pseudomonas aeruginosa [3]. Other triggers can be environmental in form of allergens, cigarette smoke, industrial exposures, and even extremes in temperature [1–3, 12]. These triggers typically cause a large inflammatory response in the host affecting the pulmonary function causing the previously described symptoms [1–3, 12]. Patients with severe underlying disease will have greater degree of physiological stress applied when an exacerbation occurs leading to a higher likelihood of respiratory failure necessitating non-invasive ventilation or even invasive mechanical ventilation [3]. Severity of the exacerbation can be graded based upon symptoms, extent of treatment, and need for hospitalization (Table 6.1). If CT is performed, typical findings associated with AECOPD include bronchial wall thickening and lymphadenopathy in the mediastinal or hilar lymph nodes [5].

Treatment for AECOPD has been well studied, and guidelines exists to manage these events when they do occur. The mainstay of therapy for AECOPD consists of systemic corticosteroids, inhaled bronchodilators, and empiric antibiotic

Table 6.1 **GOLD CLASSIFICATION OF SEVERITY OF ACUTE EXACERBATION OF COPD [5].**

GOLD EXACERBATION CLASSIFICATION	TREATMENT
Mild	Short acting bronchodilators
Moderate	Short acting bronchodilators + antibiotics +/− systemic corticosteroids
Severe	Admission to hospital + systemic corticosteroids + short acting bronchodilators + antibiotics +/− non-invasive ventilation

therapy [1–3, 12]. All of these modalities have been reviewed an in a meta-analysis has been shown to decrease the severity of the exacerbation and also shorten the time the patient may need to be hospitalized [1, 2]. Initial treatment with short-acting bronchodilators such as beta-agonists and anticholinergics is recommended for dyspnea and correction of bronchospasm [1–3]. Initiation of long-acting beta-agonists should be started as soon as possible as well if the patient is not already on them [1–3]. Systemic corticosteroids in either oral or intravenous form should be given to all patients suffering an AECOPD. Multiple studies have shown that they decrease the length of symptoms and has been shown to be the most beneficial treatment provided in these situations [1–3]. Initial therapy with steroids should not be done via the inhaled route as benefit was shown to be more pronounced with systemic administration over inhaled therapy [1–3]. Systemic therapy is usually continued for a duration of 1 week and then weaned off. Inhaled corticosteroids used in combination with long acting beta agonists have been shown to be beneficial for long-term treatment of COPD patients and helps with prevention of exacerbations as well [2, 3].

Antibiotic therapy is the last arm of guideline recommended treatment for AECOPD. Since infectious causes are felt to be a major precipitant of exacerbations, it makes sense that empiric antibiotic therapy is a recommended treatment. The clinical finding that suggests that a patient may benefit greatly from antibiotic treatment is the presence of purulent sputum [2, 3]. It has been shown to decrease symptoms in patients but not to the extent that systemic corticosteroids provide [1]. It is recommended that antibiotic choice be determined by local antibiograms and patient history of previous infections [2]. Antibiotic treatment should be delivered for a duration of 5 to 7 days dependent upon clinical response [2].

Respiratory distress with AECOPD is not an uncommon occurrence and may require assistance to prevent morbidity and mortality. First line treatment for respiratory failure in AECOPD is noninvasive ventilation. It has been shown to improve outcomes and reduces the rates of intubation and need of invasive mechanical ventilation [1, 2]. If noninvasive ventilation fails to improve the patient's condition, then invasive mechanical ventilation is indicated.

DEFINITION AND DIAGNOSIS OF PNEUMOTHORAX

A pneumothorax is an abnormal collection of air between the visceral and parietal pleura that causes collapse of the lung on that side. There are many causes of pneumothorax including iatrogenic, traumatic, and infection by gas producing organisms (i.e., Pneumocystis jiroveci or tuberculosis) [13]. The most common causes of iatrogenic pneumothorax are placement of central venous catheters, transbronchial biopsy, thoracentesis, and positive pressure ventilation [13, 14].

A pneumothorax is classified by size, which is determined from a CT scan or chest X-ray. A pneumothorax with a ring of air greater than 2 cm around the lung tissue is termed a large pneumothorax [15]. Management will not differ between small and large pneumothoraces and treatment decisions should be based on the clinical situation of the patient and not simply size [15].

Pneumothoraces can occur spontaneously in patients and are termed either primary or secondary. A primary spontaneous pneumothorax (PSP) is one which occurs in a patient without underlying lung disease. A secondary SP or SSP is one that occurs in a patient with underlying lung disease such as COPD, cystic lung disease, or pulmonary fibrosis [13]. The likelihood of an SSP occurring increases when a patient with underlying lung disease is placed on mechanical ventilation [16, 17]. The pathophysiology for both PSP and SSP is poorly understood but as previously stated, is multifactorial in nature [18]. In our previous example, this patient would fit the diagnosis of an SSP due to his bullous emphysema with pneumonia.

Diagnosis of pneumothorax can generally be made from a patient's history and physical exam. Symptoms of a pneumothorax may include acute shortness of breath, air hunger, chest tightness, and chest or shoulder pain. Physical signs include tachypnea, tachycardia, hypoxia, and absent or reduced lung sounds on one side of the chest. Tracheal deviation can also be a sign of pneumothorax, but it is generally a late finding. In situations where a tension pneumothorax exists, life-threatening hypotension may also be present from reduced cardiac filling due to elevated pressures in the affected hemithorax. If tension pneumothorax is suspected, emergent needle decompression is indicated and should be performed immediately without further diagnostic testing.

Absent lung sounds on one side of the chest can be a sign of pneumothorax. Tracheal deviation can also be a sign of pneumothorax but it is generally a late finding. The gold standard of diagnosis for pneumothorax is plain chest tomography [13]. Recently, ultrasonography has been shown to be both sensitive and specific for determining the presence of a pneumothorax and is becoming increasingly utilized [4, 19]. When employing bedside ultrasound to diagnose a pneumothorax, it is important to examine multiple quadrants of the lung to be certain that a pneumothorax isn't present in any area of the thorax [4, 13, 19]. Ultrasonography of the lung and pleural space for diagnosis of a pneumothorax is typically performed with a high-frequency transducer such as a linear or phased array transducer (Figure 6.1). Emitting a frequency between 5 and 10 megahertz (mHz) these probes allow for optimal imaging of more superficial structures such as the pleura. The size of these probes also allow for optimal scanning as the footprints of these transducers are small and allow them to fit into the intercostal spaces more readily. The depth of the probe is typically set as shallow as possible to obtain optimal imaging of the superficial pleural line. This depth is typically around 5 cm but can vary from patient to patient. The probe is oriented in a longitudinal orientation with the indicator of the probe directed toward the patient's head. Again, multiple views should be undertaken to rule out pneumothorax in all areas of the hemithorax being investigated.

"Lung sliding" is the clinical sign on ultrasound that represents the apposition of the visceral and parietal pleura. It

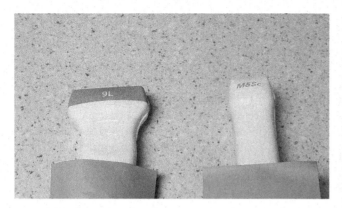

Figure 6.1 Example of linear transducer (left) and phased array transducer (right). Both can be utilized for lung ultrasonography.

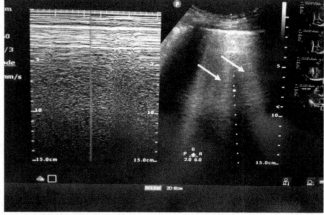

Figure 6.2 Ultrasound image showing M-mode on the left and live image on the right. Note the "seashore" sign on M-mode on the left. B-lines are noted in the live image and noted by the arrow.

appears as a "shimmer" of the pleural line on ultrasound. In the absence of lung sliding, a pneumothorax is most likely present [4, 13, 19, 20]. The presence of "B-lines" on ultrasound are also a clinical finding that will rule out pneumothorax in the area that is being studied with the ultrasound probe [4, 13, 19, 20]. B-lines represent "lung interstitial syndrome" and result from air and fluid interfaces in lung parenchyma that appear in disease entities such as interstitial pneumonia [20].

The advantage of ultrasonography for diagnosis of pneumothorax includes it can be performed rapidly at the bedside and has been shown to have high diagnostic capabilities when compared to chest X-ray and chest CT [4, 19]. Lichtenstein found that ultrasound had an accuracy around 92% when compared to CT [4]. Since many critically ill patients with pneumothoraces are in the supine position, plain chest radiography can miss pneumothoraces if the air rises to the anterior portion of the chest. In this situation, ultrasound is an optimal imaging modality as this anterior air pocket can be rapidly found with ultrasound [13]. If ultrasound images are questionable or there is still uncertainty about the presence of a pneumothorax then chest X-ray or chest CT is indicated to identify and quantify a pneumothorax [13, 15].

Lastly, M-mode ultrasound can be used to confirm a pneumothorax if the diagnosis is in doubt. The M-mode transducer can be placed on a rib space so that the ultrasound beam crosses the lung tissue. If a pneumothorax is present, then the "bar code sign" can be seen as there is no movement and the lung tissue will appear similar to the subcutaneous tissue. If there is movement of the visceral and parietal pleura, then the "seashore sign" will be present as movement of the lung tissue will appear different from the lack of movement of superficial subcutaneous tissue (see Figure 6.2). In some instances, the "lung point" can be found, which describes the area where a pneumothorax is present next to normally aerated lung tissue. This is an extremely sensitive and specific finding for pneumothorax on ultrasound (see Figure 6.3) [19]. The limiting factor of the lung point is that it can be difficult to find in patients, particularly in patients with a large pneumothorax as there are few areas where parietal and visceral pleura will be in contact with one another. However, when it is present, it is pathognomonic for the presence of a pneumothorax and carries a specificity of 100% [13].

TREATMENT OF PNEUMOTHORAX

Patients with SSP typically have a decreased pulmonary reserve and will present sooner and with more severe symptoms than someone with PSP [18]. They also have higher morbidity and mortality than patients with PSP [10, 15]. As such these patients require rapid treatment. The primary goal when

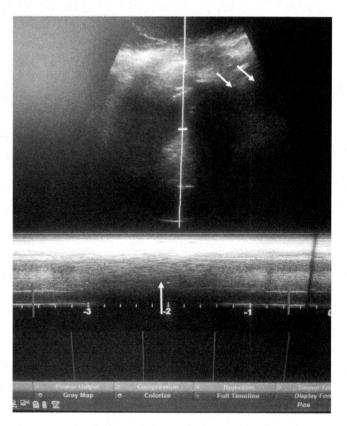

Figure 6.3 Ultrasound image of lung point. Note in the M-mode area below the image of both the "seashore sign" (white arrow) and the "barcode sign" (red arrows). With both present and intermittent lung sliding, this signifies the lung point and is specific for pneumothorax.

treating a pneumothorax is to remove the air pocket thus allowing apposition of the visceral and parietal pleural tissues and creating lung contact with the chest wall [13]. This contact permits healing of the defect and over time will result in resolution of the pneumothorax. Historically, the use of large bore chest tubes, 24 to 28 French in size, were utilized for management of a spontaneous pneumothorax in mechanically ventilated patients [21, 22]. Currently, there is growing evidence to suggest that the use of small bore, pigtail chest tubes are just as effective [15, 17, 21–24]. The advantage of using pigtail chest tubes include easier placement, fewer complications, and less patient pain and discomfort when compared to large bore chest tubes [17, 21, 23–25]. There is also some evidence to suggest that small bore pigtail catheters are associated with decreased intubation times, shorter dwell times for the chest tube, and shorter hospitalization times as well [13, 21, 24, 25].

Risks associated with placement of a percutaneous pigtail thoracostomy tube are few and very infrequent [25, 26]. Complications such as hemothorax were found to be as low as 4% with negligible rates of infection and misplacement noted in a case series by Cantin et al. [26]. One disadvantage of the pigtail catheter is that it may become obstructed more frequently than large bore chest tubes and may not adequately drain more complex effusions such as hemothorax or empyema [13, 17, 24, 25, 27]. Due to the minimal viscosity of air, small bore chest tubes are effective treatment of the spontaneous uncomplicated pneumothorax and as such are recommended based by the British Thoracic Society as first line treatment [15, 21]. The chest tube should remain in place until there is minimal drainage and resolution of the pneumothorax with minimal to no air leak. If an air leak persists or there is a persistent pneumothorax, then a large bore chest tube should be placed and surgical drainage with pleurodesis considered.

MECHANICAL VENTILATION FOR PNEUMOTHORAX

Preventing further lung damage and preventing an increased air leak while maintaining adequate patient oxygenation and ventilation are the goals of ventilator strategy in a patient with a pneumothorax on mechanical ventilation. There are currently no consensus guidelines for mechanical ventilation in a patient with a pneumothorax. Some studies suggest that elevated pulmonary pressures alone are not sufficient to cause a pneumothorax, but that high tidal volumes are related to the incidence and size of pneumothoraces [16, 28]. Given this evidence, the aim should be to reduce the amount of mechanical strain on bullae should they be present.

There have been a number of studies that have examined how large tidal volumes may induce further lung damage due to overdistention and excess strain from mechanical forces [7, 8, 29]. They have demonstrated that TV on the higher side of the physiologic range (8 mL/kg or greater) may lead to increased distention of alveoli, exacerbate barotrauma, and increases the potential for alveolar rupture/pneumothorax in patients with underlying lung disease such as COPD [15, 16, 18, 22, 23]. It has also been found that the driving pressure, which is found by the difference of plateau pressure minus the PEEP, may be the most predictive factor in determining worsening lung function and patient outcomes [7, 8]. In our patient, multiple factors predispose him to develop not only an SSP but also an iatrogenic pneumothorax from inappropriate positive pressure ventilation with high tidal volumes. Given the evidence of improved outcomes in patients with acute respiratory distress syndrome [11], there has been an increase in the utilization of low TV and high PEEP for all patients in the modern critical care unit [8, 30]. Low tidal volume ventilation is often defined as 4 to 6 mL/kg of predicted body weight (PBW).

In the setting of pneumothorax, it can be inferred that reduction of mechanical strain on airspaces will reduce the occurrence of pneumothorax and prevent the exacerbation of any underlying lung disease. Limiting the driving pressure to a value under 15 has a positive correlation with reduced incidence of acute respiratory distress syndrome and decreased morbidity and mortality [7, 8]. Positive pressure ventilation may be utilized in the presence of a pneumothorax when a chest tube thoracostomy is present to allow drainage of excess air. The level of PEEP should be titrated to reduce the amount of air leak and permit the resolution of the pneumothorax. Extubation with return of spontaneous negative pressure ventilation should be performed as soon as the patient's condition permits. Limiting the amount of time on positive pressure ventilation will hasten the resolution of the pneumothorax.

If an air leak persists despite optimal ventilator settings and chest tube thoracostomy drainage, then surgical treatment options should be considered as previously mentioned [9, 15, 24, 25, 27]. In extreme situations where ventilation and oxygenation are severely impaired due to persistent air leak, veno-venous extracorporeal membrane oxygenation can be initiated to allow low tidal volumes (4–6 mL/kg PBW) promoting closure of the defect while maintaining oxygenation and ventilation [31, 32].

CONCLUSIONS

Secondary spontaneous pneumothorax is a potentially life-threatening disease process that requires rapid detection and treatment. Due to these patients' underlying lung disease, they generally do not tolerate this change in lung dynamics well and will likely require urgent treatment. With ever improving ultrasound technology, and increasing utilization by intensivists, bedside ultrasonography can be used in situations where rapid diagnosis is required. This can be very advantageous in patients who are in acute distress and require emergent intervention, in this case for a tension pneumothorax. While chest X-ray is the gold standard for diagnosis for pneumothorax, lung ultrasonography can be a highly sensitive and specific imaging modality that can be utilized rapidly to make a diagnosis that can be life-saving [4, 15, 19, 20]. The gold standard of treatment for pneumothorax is chest tube thoracostomy drainage. Currently, there is increasing use of small bore pigtail catheters for evacuation of pneumothoraces over large bore chest tubes [15, 17, 21, 24, 25]. This change is due to the decreased morbidity and also improved outcomes that have been associated with the use of small bore chest tubes in comparison to large bore chest tubes [13, 17, 21, 24, 25].

Mechanical ventilation may be necessary in patients with SSP due to their likely intolerance of acute changes in lung dynamics and reduced pulmonary reserve. The appropriate setting of tidal volumes and PEEP can help to optimize ventilation and oxygenation and also reduce the development of further lung damage. Positive pressure ventilation can still be utilized in patients with pneumothorax with a chest tube in place to evacuate air that may still be escaping from damaged airways. Treatment of persistent air leaks despite optimal chest tube drainage and mechanical ventilation may require surgical evaluation and intervention.

REFERENCES

1. Quon, B.S., W.Q. Gan, and D.D. Sin, *Contemporary management of acute exacerbations of COPD: a systematic review and metaanalysis.* Chest, 2008. **133**(3): p. 756–766.
2. Vogelmeier, C.F., et al., *Global strategy for the diagnosis, management, and prevention of chronic obstructive lung disease 2017 report: GOLD executive summary.* Am J Respir Crit Care Med, 2017. **195**(5): p. 557–582.
3. Wedzicha, J.A., and T.A. Seemungal, *COPD exacerbations: defining their cause and prevention.* Lancet, 2007. **370**(9589): p. 786–796.
4. Lichtenstein, D., *Lung ultrasound in the critically ill.* Curr Opin Crit Care, 2014. **20**(3): p. 315–322.
5. Hackx, M., et al., *Severe COPD exacerbation: CT features.* COPD, 2015. **12**(1): p. 38–45.
6. Ghattas, C., T.J. Barreiro, and D.J. Gemmel, *Giant bullae emphysema.* Lung, 2013. **191**: p. 573–574.
7. Fuller, B.M., et al., *Pulmonary mechanics and mortality in mechanically ventilated patients without acute respiratory distress syndrome: a cohort study.* Shock, 2018. **49**(3): p. 311–316.
8. Amato, M.B., et al., *Driving pressure and survival in the acute respiratory distress syndrome.* N Engl J Med, 2015. **372**(8): p. 747–755.
9. van Berkel, V., E. Kuo, and B.F. Meyers, *Pneumothorax, bullous disease, and emphysema.* Surg Clin North Am, 2010. **90**(5): p. 935–953.
10. Chesnutt, M.S., and T.J. Prendergast, Pulmonary Disease, in Pathophysiology of Disease: An Introduction to Clinical Medicine, 7e, G.D. Hammer and S.J. McPhee, Editors. 2013, McGraw-Hill Education: New York, NY.
11. Morgan, M.D.L., C.W. Edwards, J. Morris, and H.R. Matthews, *Origin and behaviour of emphysematous bullae.* Thorax, 1989. **44**(7): p. 533–538.
12. O'Donnell, D.E., and C.M. Parker, *COPD exacerbations. 3: Pathophysiology.* Thorax, 2006. **61**(4): p. 354–361.
13. Yarmus, L., and D. Feller-Kopman, *Pneumothorax in the critically ill patient.* Chest, 2012. **141**(4): p. 1098–1105.
14. Baumann, M.H., and M. Noppen, *Pneumothorax.* Respirology, 2004. **9**(2): p. 157–164.
15. MacDuff, A., et al., *Management of spontaneous pneumothorax: British Thoracic Society pleural disease guideline 2010.* Thorax, 2010. **65** Suppl 2: p. ii18–31.
16. Hsu, C.W., and S.F. Sun, *Iatrogenic pneumothorax related to mechanical ventilation.* World J Crit Care Med, 2014. **3**(1): p. 8–14.
17. Tsai, W.K., et al., *Pigtail catheters vs large-bore chest tubes for management of secondary spontaneous pneumothoraces in adults.* Am J Emerg Med, 2006. **24**(7): p. 795–800.
18. Tschopp, J.M., et al., *Management of spontaneous pneumothorax: state of the art.* Eur Respir J, 2006. **28**(3): p. 637–650.
19. Lichtenstein, D., et al., *The "lung point": an ultrasound sign specific to pneumothorax.* Intens Care Med, 2014. **26**(10): p. 1434–1440.
20. Lichtenstein, D.A., and G.A. Meziere, *Relevance of lung ultrasound in the diagnosis of acute respiratory failure: the BLUE protocol.* Chest, 2008. **134**(1): p. 117–125.

21. Lin, Y.C., et al., *Pigtail catheter for the management of pneumothorax in mechanically ventilated patients.* Am J Emerg Med, 2010. **28**(4): p. 466–471.
22. Baumann, M.H., et al., *Management of Spontaneous Pneumothorax: An American Collge of Chest Physicians Delphi Consensus Statement.* Chest, 2001. **119**: p. 590–602.
23. Chen, C.H., et al., *Secondary spontaneous pneumothorax: which associated conditions benefit from pigtail catheter treatment?* Am J Emerg Med, 2012. **30**(1): p. 45–50.
24. Iepsen, U.W., and T. Ringback, *Small-bore chest tubes seem to perform better than larger tubes in treatment of spontaneous pneumothorax.* Dan Med J, 2013. **60**(6): p. A4644.
25. Chang, S.H., et al., *A systematic review and meta-analysis comparing pigtail catheter and chest tube as the initial treatment for pneumothorax.* Chest, 2018. **153**: p. 1201–1212.
26. Cantin, L., et al., *Chest tube drainage under radiological guidance for pleural effusion and pneumothorax in a tertiary care university teaching hospital: review of 51 cases.* Can Respir J, 2005. **12**(1): p. 29–33.
27. Schipper, P.H., et al., *Outcomes after resection of giant emphysematous bullae.* Ann Thorac Surg, 2004. **78**(3): p. 976–982; discussion p. 976–982.
28. Steier M, N. Ching, E.B. Roberts, and T.F. Nealon Jr., *Pneumothorax complicating continuous ventilatory support.* J Thorac Cardiovasc Surg, 1974. **67**(1): p. 17–23.
29. Davies, J.D., M.H. Senussi, and E. Mireles-Cabodevila, *Should a tidal volume of 6 mL/kg be used in all patients?* Respir Care, 2016. **61**(6): p. 774–790.
30. Talmor, D., et al., *Mechanical ventilation guided by esophageal pressure in acute lung injury.* N Engl J Med, 2008. **359**(20): p. 2095–2104.
31. Marek, S., et al., *Extracorporeal membrane oxygenation in the management of post-pneumonectomy air leak and adult respiratory distress syndrome of the non-operated lung.* Perfusion, 2017. **32**(5): p. 416–418.
32. Slade, M., *Management of pneumothorax and prolonged air leak.* Semin Respir Crit Care Med, 2014. **35**(6): p. 706–714.

REVIEW QUESTIONS

1. A 72-year-old male presents to the emergency department with acute hypoxia, tachycardia, and shortness of breath. Chest X-ray reveals a pneumothorax of the right side. The patient has a history of moderate COPD with bullous changes noted on previous CT scans. What is the classification of this pneumothorax?

   A. Iatrogenic pneumothorax
   B. Secondary spontaneous pneumothorax
   C. Primary spontaneous pneumothorax
   D. Traumatic pneumothorax

2. A patient is diagnosed with an SSP due to the rupture of a bleb in the left lung. There is a space of 3 cm surrounding the left lung and the patient is symptomatic with pulse oximetry reading 89% on non-rebreather mask. What is the next best course of action for treatment of this patients' pneumothorax?

   A. Placement of a large bore chest tube in the left hemithorax in the midaxillary line at the fourth rib space.
   B. Observation as the patient is maintaining adequate oxygen saturation for a patient with COPD.
   C. Immediate intubation due to hypoxia
   D. Placement of small bore, pigtail chest tube in the midaxillary line at the 4th rib space.

3. An elderly male patient who suffered from a spontaneous pneumothorax is intubated due to respiratory distress and severe hypoxia. What are the ideal settings for mechanical ventilation for this patient. Patient is 5'9" in height and 75 kg.

A. Volume control, TV of 800 mL, PEEP 8 mmHg, RR 16 breaths per minute
B. Pressure control, PIP of 48 mmHg, PEEP 5, RR of 14 breaths per minute
C. Volume control, TV of 500 mL, PEEP 5 mmHg, RR of 14 breaths per minute
D. Volume control, TV of 1000 mL, PEEP 14, RR of 20 breaths per minute

4. A patient is diagnosed with a spontaneous pneumothorax with tension component due to hypotension. Chest tube decompression is indicated but the kit is not readily accessible and must be delivered and will take a few minutes to arrive. What is the next best step in management of this patient?

A. Needle decompression with a 14-gauge catheter in the midclavicular line in the second intercostal space
B. Observation and supportive care until chest tube kit arrives
C. Emergent intubation and placement of central venous catheter for vasopressors
D. Needle decompression with a 14 gauge catheter in the midaxillary line in the fifth intercostal space

5. Despite placement of a pigtail chest tube, a patient has a persistent pneumothorax after one week of treatment. What is the next best step in treatment?

A. Continued observation
B. Thoracic surgery consultation
C. Replacement of the pigtail chest tube
D. Placement of a second pigtail chest tube

6. What ventilatory parameter has been associated with improved outcomes in patients on mechanical ventilation with lung injury?

A. Plateau pressures of 40 mmHg
B. Driving pressure of less than 17 mmHg
C. Tidal volumes of 10 to 12 mL/kg of predicted body weight
D. Avoidance of use of positive end-expiratory pressure

7. What parameter is most closely associated with the development of pneumothorax in patients requiring mechanical ventilation?

A. Plateau pressure
B. Peak inspiratory pressure
C. Low tidal volumes (6–8 ml/kg PBW)
D. High tidal volumes (10–12 ml/kg PBW)

8. A 22-year-old male with Marfan syndrome presents with acute shortness of breath. A 1 cm ring of air is noted surrounding his left lung. He has no previous history of lung disease. What classification does his pneumothorax fit?

A. Iatrogenic pneumothorax

B. Primary spontaneous pneumothorax
C. Secondary spontaneous pneumothorax
D. Traumatic pneumothorax

9. When should a pigtail catheter be upgraded to a large bore chest tube for management of a pneumothorax?

A. Persistent air leak
B. Due to patient body habitus
C. To place on wall suction
D. For minimal pleural effusion

10. A patient presents with tachycardia, acute shortness of breath, hypotension, and tachypnea. Ultrasound of the lungs is performed at the bedside while awaiting the arrival of the portable chest X-ray machine. What findings on ultrasound are consistent with the presence of a pneumothorax?

A. Presence of A-lines
B. Presence of B-lines
C. Absence of lung sliding
D. "Seashore sign" with M-mode

ANSWERS

1. B—Spontaneous pneumothorax can be either termed primary or secondary based upon pre-existing lung disease. This patient has bullous lung disease as shown on previous CT examination so therefore has an SSP. A PSP is a situation where the patient has no previously documented lung disease.

2. D—Treatment of an SSP typically requires placement of a chest tube for evacuation of air in the pleural space. Historically, large bore chest tubes were placed for this purpose. There is growing evidence to suggest that the use of small bore, pigtail chest tubes are just as effective [3, 17, 21–24]. The advantage of using pigtail chest tubes include easier placement, fewer complications, and less patient pain and discomfort when compared to large bore chest tubes [17, 21, 23–25]. There is also some evidence to suggest that small bore pigtail catheters are associated with decreased intubation times, shorter dwell times for the chest tube, and shorter hospitalization times as well [1, 21, 24, 25].

3. C—There are currently no consensus guidelines for mechanical ventilation in a patient with a pneumothorax. Some studies suggest that elevated pulmonary pressures alone are not sufficient to cause a pneumothorax, but that high tidal volumes are related to the incidence and size of pneumothoraces [16, 28]. Given this evidence, the aim should be to reduce the amount of mechanical strain on bullae should they be present. Lung protective ventilation with low tidal volumes should be utilized in this situation to limit strain on the lungs. The level of PEEP should be titrated to reduce the amount of air leak and permit the resolution of the pneumothorax. Extubation with return of spontaneous negative pressure ventilation should be performed as soon as the patient's condition permits.

4. A—Due to the acute decompensation and hypotension that this patient is suffering from, emergent needle

decompression of the pneumothorax is indicated. This is performed by using a 14-gauge catheter and placing it in the second intercostal space in the midclavicular line. Once air is evacuated from the chest, hemodynamics should improve. Further studies to rule out hemothorax should be performed as well. Once a chest tube kit arrives, then chest tube thoracostomy should be performed for definitive treatment.

5. B—If an air leak persists despite optimal ventilator settings and chest tube thoracostomy drainage, then surgical treatment options should be considered [2, 3, 24, 25, 27]. Surgical options include pleurodesis, direct evacuation of air and debris from the chest wall, and possible placement of one-way valves to help with correction of bronchopleural fistula.

6. B—In the setting of pneumothorax, it can be inferred that reduction of mechanical strain on airspaces will reduce the occurrence of pneumothorax and prevent the exacerbation of any underlying lung disease. Limiting the driving pressure to a value under 15 has a positive correlation with reduced incidence of acute respiratory distress syndrome and decreased morbidity and mortality [10, 11].

7. D—There have been a number of studies that have examined how large tidal volumes may induce further lung damage due to overdistention and excess strain from mechanical forces [10, 11, 29]. They have demonstrated that TV on the higher side of the physiologic range (8 mL/kg or greater) may lead to increased distention of alveoli, exacerbate barotrauma, and increase the potential for alveolar rupture/pneumothorax in patients with underlying lung disease such as COPD [3, 16, 18, 22, 23].

8. B—This type of spontaneous pneumothorax fits into the designation of PSP due to the lack of previous lung disease in this patient. Treatment can be conservative at first with observation and supplemental oxygen in patients with PSP. However, if the patient's clinical condition deteriorates, then chest tube thoracostomy is indicated in a similar manner to that of SSP.

9. A—Due to the minimal viscosity of air, small bore chest tubes are effective treatment of the spontaneous uncomplicated pneumothorax and as such are recommended based by the British Thoracic Society as first-line treatment [3, 21]. The chest tube should remain in place until there is minimal drainage and resolution of the pneumothorax with minimal to no air leak. If an air leak persists or there is a persistent pneumothorax, then a large bore chest tube should be placed and surgical drainage with pleurodesis considered.

10. C—While chest X-ray is the gold standard for diagnosis for pneumothorax, lung ultrasonography can be a highly sensitive and specific imaging modality that can be utilized rapidly to make a diagnosis that can be life-saving [3, 7, 19, 20]. "Lung sliding" is the clinical sign on ultrasound that represents the apposition of the visceral and parietal pleura. It appears as a "shimmer" of the pleural line on ultrasound. In the absence of lung sliding, a pneumothorax is most likely present [1, 7, 19, 20]. The advantage of ultrasonography for diagnosis of pneumothorax includes it can be performed rapidly at the bedside and has been shown to have high diagnostic capabilities when compared to chest X-ray and chest CT [7, 19].

7.

RUPTURED ESOPHAGEAL VARICES AND COMPLICATIONS OF MASSIVE BLOOD TRANSFUSION

Joti Juneja Mucci and Connor McNamara

STEM CASE AND KEY QUESTIONS

A 55-year-old man with a past medical history of alcoholism presents from home with massive hematemesis and syncope. He is now lethargic and only oriented to person. He is tachycardic and hypotensive.

WHAT ARE THE INITIAL PRIORITIES FOR MANAGING THIS PATIENT? IS THERE ANY INDICATION FOR BLOOD WORK OR TESTS/ CONSULTS?

The patient was considered to need both volume resuscitation and a secure airway. Large bore peripheral intravenous (IV) access was obtained, and intravascular volume resuscitation was commenced initially with crystalloid and un-crossmatched O-negative blood, while crossmatched blood was being obtained from the blood bank. Concurrently, a rapid sequence induction was performed and the patient intubated for airway protection. Laboratory tests for complete blood count (CBC), coagulation studies, liver function, and a basic metabolic panel were sent. After these initial steps, central venous access and invasive arterial monitors were placed. The gastroenterology and interventional radiology teams were alerted to the ongoing massive hemorrhage.

WHAT IS THE DEFINITION OF A MASSIVE TRANSFUSION? WHAT IS THE ROLE OF BLOOD IN OXYGEN DELIVERY? HOW CAN COAGULOPATHY DEVELOP IN THIS SETTING?

Four units of blood were transfused as quickly as possible, and the institutional massive transfusion protocol was initiated. Resuscitation continued, transfusing packed red blood cells (pRBCs):fresh frozen plasma (FFP) in a 1:1 ratio, with platelets and cryoprecipitate administered approximately each 4 U aliquot of pRBCs and FFP. An octreotide bolus of 100 mcg was given, and an infusion of 25 mcg/hr commenced. Norepinephrine infusion was started, targeting mean arterial pressure 65 mmHg. Admission laboratory values showed Hb 8, platelets 67, arterial lactate 12, partial thromboplastin time >180, international normalized ratio >18. Core body temperature was 35°C. Diffuse oozing was noted for venipuncture and line insertion sites. At this time the patient was maintaining adequate blood pressure with volume resuscitation and vasopressors, and the gastroenterologists wished to perform an esophagogastroduodenoscopy in the intensive care unit (ICU) setting. The patient was transferred to the medical ICU.

WHAT ARE THE POTENTIAL COMPLICATIONS OF A MASSIVE BLOOD TRANSFUSION?

Upon arrival to the medical ICU, the patient required ongoing resuscitation with blood products. A blood warmer was used to continue volume resuscitation, and forced air warming instituted to warm the patient peripherally. Norepinephrine requirement began to increase. Of note, Hb was 8 g/dL, lactate 8 mmol/L, Ca2+ 0.7 mmol/L, core temperature 35.5°C. Electrocardiogram (ECG) is shown in Figure 7.1.

One gram calcium chloride was administered. The gastrointestinal (GI) department performs an esophagogastroduodenoscopy (EGD) and discovers ruptured esophageal varices that were banded. The patient stabilizes and massive transfusion is stopped. He is maintained sedated and intubated. Several hours after arriving the patient becomes febrile, tachypneic, and has increasing oxygen requirement on the vent.

WHAT IS TRALI? WHAT IS TACO?

The patient's chest radiograph (CXR) shows bilateral pulmonary opacities, and bedside transthoracic echocardiogram shows normal ejection fraction and valves, with no obvious fluid overload. Central venous oxygen saturation is 63%. Ventilation parameters are altered to utilize low tidal volume lung ventilation and elevated positive end-expiratory pressure. After a period of hemodynamic stability and no evidence of further bleeding, furosemide was used to gently diurese the patient. Over the next 48 hours, the ventilatory support requirements decreased, and the patient was weaned to successful extubation. He was able to be discharged to the floor hospital day 4.

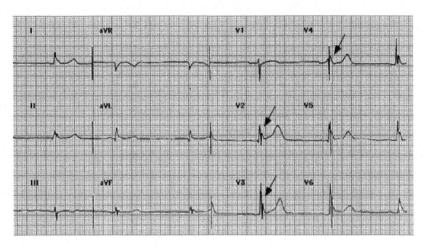

Figure 7.1 Electrocardiogram in a patient with severe hypothermia. The arrow indicates Osborn or J-waves.

DISCUSSION

INITIAL MANAGEMENT

The main priority should be stabilizing the patient. Two large bore (18 G or larger) IVs should be placed. Central access is not required unless vasopressor support is necessary. Two large short peripheral IVs are superior for resuscitation to the most typically placed central venous catheter. Poiseuille's Law can explain this:

where Q is flow rate, P is pressure, r is radius, n is fluid viscosity, and l is length of tubing. It can be seen that doubling the radius of an IV will increase the flow rate 16 fold, and increasing the length decreases the flow rate.

In addition to obtaining IV access, intubation and mechanical ventilation may be necessary due to hematemesis and altered mental status.

A type and cross match should be sent for blood as quickly as possible in addition standard labs (CBC, comprehensive metabolic panel, coagulation studies) and a lactate. Un-crossmatched O-negative or type-specific blood can be used in place of fully crossmatched blood if necessary.

Gastroenterology should be consulted for emergent EGD and potential banding. In addition, Interventional Radiology may be needed for transjugular intrahepatic portosystemic shunt/embolization if gastroenterology is unable to stop the bleeding.

MASSIVE TRANSFUSION

Several definitions exist. Massive blood transfusion is defined as loss of >1 blood volume within a 24-hour period. Average blood volume for an adult is 70cc/kg. Thus, for an average 70 kg male, blood volume would be approximately 4.9 L. Other definitions include transfusion of >10 units of pRBCs in 24 hours [1].

A dilutional coagulopathy can develop if coagulation factors and platelets are not replaced during the period of transfusion. In a massive transfusion situation, red blood cells (RBCs) are typically transfused in a 1:1 or 1:2 ratio with FFP to prevent further coagulopathy. Platelets should also be given as indicated.

Transfusing cold blood products can exacerbate coagulopathy and causes other cardiac abnormalities. In a massive transfusion situation, every attempt should be made to warm blood prior to transfusion. Delaying transfusion however should be avoided if a patient is rapidly exsanguinating.

The most common complications seen with massive blood transfusion includes:

- Volume overload
- Coagulopathy
- Hypocalcemia
- Metabolic alkalosis/citrate toxicity
- Hyperkalemia
- Hypothermia
- Transfusion-related acute lung injury (TRALI)
- Transfusion-associated circulatory overload (TACO)

VOLUME OVERLOAD

Any large amount of fluids has the potential to expand intravascular volume and can lead to pulmonary edema. This is more of a concern in patients with decreased cardiac or renal function.

COAGULOPATHY

Transfused RBCs dilute the pools of platelets and coagulation factors and therefore clotting factors and platelets should be transfused as well.

Disseminated intravascular coagulation (DIC) may occur because of injured/under perfused tissues. Adequate volume resuscitation and tissue perfusion may prevent the propagation of DIC by acidosis or tissue hypoxia.

HYPOCALCEMIA

Significant hypocalcemia can occur because calcium forms complexes with citrate. This change can lead to paresthesias and/or cardiac arrhythmias in some patients [2]. Citrate is used as a preservative in blood and also prevents clotting. Transfusion of large amounts of blood products has the potential to decrease calcium significantly. In an emergency, calcium chloride should be administered (vs. calcium gluconate) as calcium chloride has 3× more elemental calcium versus calcium gluconate.

IV calcium gluconate is preferred over IV calcium chloride in nonemergency settings due to the potential for extravasation and tissue necrosis with calcium chloride. Calcium chloride should only be given centrally.

One gram of calcium gluconate salt is equal to 93 mg of elemental calcium.

One gram of calcium chloride salt is equal to 270 mg of elemental calcium.

METABOLIC ALKALOSIS/ CITRATE TOXICITY

This may occur as citrate is metabolized to bicarbonate in the liver. The metabolism of each mmol of citrate generates 3 mEq of bicarbonate (approximately 23 meq of bicarbonate in each unit of blood). As a result, metabolic alkalosis can occur if the renal ischemia or underlying renal disease prevents the excess bicarbonate from being excreted in the urine. Hypokalemia is possible as potassium moves into cells in exchange for hydrogen ions that move out of the cells to minimize the degree of extracellular alkalosis [3, 4].

However, metabolic acidosis is more frequently encountered due to poor tissue perfusion.

HYPERKALEMIA

The amount of potassium increases with duration of storage of the RBCs as the cells lyse. Stored RBCs at day 7 contain ~12 mEq of potassium and approximately 40 mEq at day 21 [2].

HYPOTHERMIA

Hypothermia reduces the enzymatic activity of plasma coagulation factors and also prevents the activation of platelets via traction on the glycoprotein Ib/IX/V complex by von Willebrand factor [5].

Hypothermia causes characteristic ECG changes because of slowed impulse conduction through potassium channels. This results in prolongation of all the ECG intervals, including RR, PR, QRS, and QT. There may also be elevation of the J point (only if the ST segment is unaltered), producing a characteristic J or Osborn wave that represents distortion of the earliest phase of membrane repolarization (Figure 7.1). The height of the Osborn wave is roughly proportional to the degree of hypothermia [6, 7].

TRALI, TACO, AND ACUTE LUNG INJURY

TRALI is a phenomenon of rapidly occurring lung injury temporally related to blood product transfusion. It is probably underdiagnosed because its symptomatology is similar to other disease presentations such as acute respiratory distress syndrome (ARDS).

The National Heart, Lung, and Blood Institute use the following working definition of ARDS [8]:

Development of ALI (acute lung injury) as defined as

- Acute onset

- Hypoxemia (PaO_2/FiO_2 ratio ≤300 mmHg)

- Bilateral pulmonary opacities on frontal CXR

- Absence of left atrial hypertension (pulmonary artery occlusion pressure ≤18 if measured)

In patients without other ALI risk factors:

- New onset of ALI during or within 6 hours after transfusion of plasma-containing blood product.

In patients with other ALI risk factors:

- New onset of ALI during or within 6 hours after the end of transfusion of a plasma-containing blood products

- Clinical course suggestive of TRALI—the ALI is not attributable to the ALI risk factor and the patient was clinically stable before transfusion.

HOW DOES TRALI OCCUR?

The exact mechanism of action of TRALI is not fully known. There are several theories. The first revolves around antibodies from stored blood products activating leukocytes in the recipient leading to inflammation and damage to the pulmonary capillary endothelium [9]. Specific HLA antigens seem to be at fault.

A second theory involves a two hit hypothesis. A patient has specific risk factors that "prime" neutrophils prior to transfusion. Subsequent transfusion releases lipids/cytokines from stored blood products activating the neutrophils and causing damage [9].

WHAT ARE THE RISK FACTORS?

There are transfusion related risk factors and patient specific risk factors.

Transfusion related [8, 10]:

- Plasma containing blood products (FFP, platelets, whole blood, cryoprecipitate), particularly from multiparous female donors

- Specific antibodies present in plasma blood products (Anti HLA-2, Anti-HNA)

Patient-specific risk factors:

- Higher interleukin-8 level
- Shock (of all types)
- Liver surgery (mainly transplantation)
- Chronic alcohol abuse
- Positive fluid balance
- Peak Airway pressure >30 if on a ventilator prior to TRALI development
- Current smoking

ARE THERE ANY OTHER SYMPTOMS THAT PATIENTS PRESENT WITH?

Unfortunately the very nonspecific symptoms likely contribute to TRALI being underreported. Other than hypoxemia typical of lung injury, patients may also have fever, tachycardia, tachypnea, and hypotension to the point of needing vasopressor support [11].

WHAT ARE OTHER CAUSES OF ALI?

Specific things to consider in your differential are TACO, an anaphylactic type transfusion reaction, bacterial contaminated blood products, or ARDS from underlying medical condition [10]. Sepsis, burns, and trauma are other causes of ALI not associated with blood transfusions.

TACO is lung injury associated with increased osmotic pressure within capillaries leading to fluid leak, as opposed to TRALI that causes pulmonary edema by capillary endothelial damage and fluid leak.

It is defined as symptoms and signs of acute pulmonary edema within 6 hours of blood transfusion with signs/symptoms of left atrial hypertension or volume overload [12]. Diuretics should help in this situation.

These signs and symptoms include acute respiratory distress, hypertension, hypoxemia, and signs of acute congestive heart failure [12].

WHAT IS THE DIFFERENCE BETWEEN TRALI AND TACO?

TRALI typically presents as a more severe form of ARDS, with PaO_2/FiO_2 (P/F) ratios <200. Furthermore, TRALI is an inflammatory pulmonary edema and thus diuretics may not be useful. However, TACO often coexists with TRALI in cases of massive transfusion and can thus complicate the clinical picture.

TACO is typically less severe with P/F ratios between 200 and 300. TACO by itself should respond to diuretic therapy or fluid removal in patients requiring dialysis.

IF THE PATIENT MEETS THE CRITERIA FOR TRALI, WHAT CAN BE DONE?

- If recognized during a blood transfusion, stop the transfusion and send it to the blood bank. They can test the product for antibodies/bacteria, etc. and may quarantine additional blood products from that donor.
- Order any studies that may help differentiate TRALI from your other differentials:
  o CBC (WBC may decrease in TRALI) [13]
  o B-type natriuretic peptide
  o CXR
  o Echocardiogram or bedside ultrasound
  o Tryptase (to r/o anaphylaxis)

Otherwise treatment is supportive. Patients may require mechanical ventilation and vasopressor support. Extreme cases may require extracorporeal life support. If required, mechanical ventilation should follow ARDSnet protocol to decrease the risk of further lung injury. Judicious use of further blood products if necessary as additional transfusions can worsen outcome [14].

WHAT IS THE MORBIDITY AND MORTALITY ASSOCIATED WITH TRALI?

Mortality from TRALI varies widely depending on the study, and has been reported as low as 5% to as high as 35% [11]. Misdiagnosis and likely underreporting of TRALI makes it difficult to define true morbidity or mortality data. In patients who had additional risk factors for ALI their mechanical ventilation days, ICU length of stay, hospital length of stay, and mortality were significantly higher [11].

CONCLUSIONS

- Ruptured esophageal varices can present with massive hematemesis and hemodynamic instability requiring massive blood transfusion.
- Airway protection may be necessary in addition to large bore IV access.
- In the setting of ongoing bleeding associated with hemodynamic instability, transfusion should not be delayed while awaiting crossmatched blood products; it may be necessary to give un-crossmatched O-negative blood.
- The clinician should also anticipate the potential complications of massive blood transfusion and have a plan to prevent them. This may include
  o Warming of blood products prior to transfusion.
  o Having calcium preparations readily available to treat hypocalcemia.

o Replacing clotting factors and platelets to prevent dilutional coagulopathy.

o Monitoring for cardiac arrhythmias.

- Hypoxia can occur due to volume overload or TRALI may occur and require supportive care ± diuresis.

REFERENCES

1. Savage, S.A., et al., The new metric to define large-volume hemorrhage: results of a prospective study of the critical administration threshold. J Trauma Acute Care Surg, 2015. 78(2): p. 224–229; discussion 229-30.
2. Smith, H.M., et al., Cardiac arrests associated with hyperkalemia during red blood cell transfusion: a case series. Anesth Analg, 2008. 106(4): p. 1062–1069.
3. Lier, H., et al., Preconditions of hemostasis in trauma: a review: the influence of acidosis, hypocalcemia, anemia, and hypothermia on functional hemostasis in trauma. J Trauma, 2008. 65(4): p. 951–960.
4. Bruining, H.A., R.U. Boelhouwer, and G.K. Ong, Unexpected hypopotassemia after multiple blood transfusions during an operation. Neth J Surg, 1986. 38(2): p. 48–51.
5. Holcomb, J.B., et al., Damage control resuscitation: directly addressing the early coagulopathy of trauma. J Trauma, 2007. 62(2): p. 307–310.
6. Mattu, A., W.J. Brady, and A.D. Perron, Electrocardiographic manifestations of hypothermia. Am J Emerg Med, 2002. 20(4): p. 314–326.
7. Aslam, A.F., et al., Hypothermia: evaluation, electrocardiographic manifestations, and management. Am J Med, 2006. 119(4): p. 297–301.
8. Sayah, D.M., M.R. Looney, and P. Toy, Transfusion reactions: newer concepts on the pathophysiology, incidence, treatment, and prevention of transfusion-related acute lung injury. Crit Care Clin, 2012. 28(3): p. 363–372.
9. Toy, P., and C. Lowell, TRALI—definition, mechanisms, incidence and clinical relevance. Best Pract Res Clin Anaesthesiol, 2007. 21(2): p. 183–193.
10. Benson, A.B., M. Moss, and C.C. Silliman, Transfusion-related acute lung injury (TRALI): a clinical review with emphasis on the critically ill. Br J Haematol, 2009. 147(4): p. 431–443.
11. Looney, M.R., et al., Prospective study on the clinical course and outcomes in transfusion-related acute lung injury. Crit Care Med, 2014. 42(7): p. 1676–1687.
12. Roubinian, N. and E.L. Murphy, Transfusion-associated circulatory overload (TACO): prevention, management, and patient outcomes. Int J Clin Transfusion Med, 2015. 2015–3): p. 17–28.
13. Toy, P., et al., Transfusion-related acute lung injury: incidence and risk factors. Blood, 2012. 119(7): p. 1757–1767.
14. Gong, M.N., et al., Clinical predictors of and mortality in acute respiratory distress syndrome: potential role of red cell transfusion. Crit Care Med, 2005. 33(6): p. 1191–1198.

QUESTIONS

1. A 57-year-old male is admitted for hematemesis. He undergoes an EGD and is found to have a bleeding gastric ulcer. The bleeding could not be controlled with clipping nor epinephrine injection. The decision is made to send the patient to interventional radiology for coiling of bleeding vessel. During an 8 hour time period, he is transfused 12 RBCs, 6 FFP, and three 5-pack platelets. Which of the following would not be considered a complication of massive blood transfusion?

A. Coagulopathy
B. Citrate toxicity
C. Hypocalemia
D. Hypokalemia

Answer: D

A dilutional coagulopathy can result if blood is not transfused along with clotting factors in the setting of massive transfusion. Citrate toxicity can occur as citrate is used as a preservative in blood products. This can result in a metabolic alkalosis and/or hypocalcemia as citrate binds calcium. Hyperkalemia would be more common due to hemolysis of older red cells.

2. A 63-year-old female with history of end-stage liver disease secondary to alcoholic cirrhosis presented to the emergency department with massive hematemesis due to bleeding esophageal varices. She is intubated prior to an EGD for worsening hypoxia and airway protection. Over the course of several hours, she is transfused red cells, platelets, and FFP. Her oxygenation continues to worsen and her CXR shows bilateral pulmonary edema. She requires positive end-expiratory pressure 12, 80% FiO_2 to maintain SpO_2 in the low 90s. What are the significant findings in TRALI?

A. Severe hypoxemia, manifested by P/F ratio <200
B. Less responsive to diuretics
C. Acute onset
D. All of the above

Answer: D

TRALI typically presents as a more severe form of ARDS, with P/F ratios <200. Furthermore, TRALI is an inflammatory pulmonary edema and thus diuretics may not be useful. However, TACO often coexists with TRALI in cases of massive transfusion and can thus complicate the clinical picture.

3. A 33-year-old female undergoes emergency hysterectomy after standard vaginal delivery due to ongoing bleeding from retained products of conception. After 8 units of red blood cell transfusions, bleeding is well controlled and labs are resent. Ionized calcium was noted to be 0.86, hemoglobin 10.5, international normalized ratio 1.3, platelets, 102. Which of the following are not signs and symptoms of hypocalcemia?

A. Paresthesias
B. Hypertension
C. Hypotension
D. Cardiac arrhythmias

Answer: B

Significant hypocalcemia can occur because calcium forms complexes with citrate. This change can lead to paresthesias and/or cardiac arrhythmias in some patients [2]. Citrate is used as a preservative in blood and also prevents clotting. Transfusion of large amounts of blood products has the potential to decrease calcium significantly. Hypotension is often seen with low levels of ionized calcium.

4. What is the definition of massive blood transfusion?

A. Loss of one blood volume
B. Transfusion of 10 or more units in 24 hours

C. Transfusion of 2 units within 1 hour

D. Both A and B

Answer: D

Several definitions exist. Massive blood transfusion is defined as loss of >1 blood volume within a 24-hour period. Average blood volume for an adult is 70 cc/kg. Thus, for an average 70 kg male, blood volume would be approximately 4.9 L. Other definitions include transfusion of >10 units of pRBCs in 24 hours.

6. In the setting of hypocalcemia related to massive blood transfusion, why is calcium chloride preferred?

A. Less concern for tissue necrosis

B. Can be given peripherally or centrally

C. Three times more potent than calcium gluconate

D. Less likely to cause hypertension

Answer: C

In an emergency, calcium chloride should be administered (versus calcium gluconate) as calcium chloride has 3× more elemental calcium versus calcium gluconate. IV calcium gluconate is preferred over IV calcium chloride in nonemergency settings due to the potential for extravasation and tissue necrosis with calcium chloride. Calcium chloride should only be given centrally.

6. A 45-year-old male with a history of alcoholism and recent admission for pneumonia and bacteremia presents with hematemesis and shock. He is diagnosed with massive GI bleed from unknown source. GI is being consulted for emergent EGD. Which of the following is the most appropriate access for massive transfusion?

A. In-situ single lumen peripheral inserted central catheter (PICC) line

B. Triple lumen central venous catheter

C. Multiple large bore peripheral IVs (18 g or larger)

D. PICC line and 22-gauge IV

Answer: C

Based on Poiseuille's law, the larger the diameter catheter and smaller the length the higher the flow rate. Given this knowledge, 2 "large bore" IVs, typically defined as 18 G or larger is the best choice. The typical triple lumen catheter does have at least 1 port that is 18 G and 16 G, however its length (smallest 16 mm) vs a 18 G IV (4 cm) make the triple lumen catheter far inferior for massive resuscitation. PICC lines have even smaller gauges (20 cm) and can be more than double the length of a central line, leading to very slow flow rates.

7. A 50-year-old man had hemorrhagic shock for a bleeding gastric ulcer. This was subsequently banded. During his resuscitation he received 5 L crystalloid and 10u of warmed pRBC for approximately 4 L of blood loss. During this event his lactate was never above normal limits. He is noted now to have noted oozing from around his IV sites. Coagulation studies are sent. What is the most likely cause of his coagulopathy?

A. DIC

B. Dilutional coagulopathy

C. Acute liver failure

D. Hypothermia

Answer: B

When large amount of blood is lost, the best resuscitation method is equal resuscitation, meaning for every 1 unit of pRBC transfused, 1 U of FFP and 1 unit of platelets should also be given (unit of platelets are usually "packed," so that 1 transfusion is usually multiple packed platelets 4/5). Resuscitation as in the question above likely resulted in dilutional coagulopathy given crystalloid and only pRBC resuscitation. The other answers can all cause coagulopathy but are less likely given the context of the question.

8. What is the most likely reason for developing metabolic alkalosis shortly after a massive transfusion for acute GI bleed?

A. Citrate toxicity

B. Contraction alkalosis

C. Diarrhea

D. Both B and C

Answer: A

pRBC are usually stored with citrate to help prevent clotting while waiting to be transfused by chelating calcium. When large volumes of pRBC are transfused, this also leads to large volume of citrate. Citrate is then metabolized into bicarbonate in the liver that can at times overwhelm the bodies buffering system and the kidneys ability to filter the excess bicarbonate. This is especially true when massive hemorrhage leads to end organ dysfunction such as acute kidney injury/acute tubular necrosis, further impairing the kidneys ability to filter bicarbonate. Renal replacement therapy is sometimes needed to reverse the metabolic alkalosis.

9. Which of the following blood products has the lowest risk of causing TRALI?

A. FFP

B. Cryoprecipitate

C. Whole blood

D. pRBC

Answer: D

FFP and other products containing similar blood factors (cryoprecipitate and whole blood) lead to the highest risk of TRALI following a transfusion. This is particularly true if from multiparous female donors, whose donated blood is often excluded from these products. TRALI following pRBC transfusion can occur, but is much less common. As stated above the mechanism for TRALI has not been fully elucidated.

10. A 45-year-old male with a history of hepatitis C underwent emergent transjugular intrahepatic portosystemic shunt procedure after esophageal banding by EGD failed to stop an upper GI bleed requiring massive transfusion. He has now been weaned off vasopressors, but remains on mechanical ventilation. His current vitals are temperature, 34.3°C; blood pressure, 90/60, heart rate, 60; respiratory rate, 18 (not

overbreathing the vent); oxygenation saturation, 99%. His 12-lead ECG is shown in the following figure.

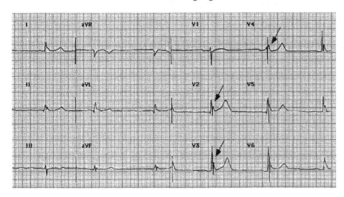

What is the cause of the ECG feature indicated by the arrow in this clinical setting?

A. Hypokalemia
B. Hypocalcemia
C. Hypothermia
D. Ischemia

Answer: C.

In severe hypothermia, Osborn waves/J point can be identified on ECG, as identified of the ECG as shown. Hypothermia causes slowing of impulse conduction through potassium channels, leading to prolongation of all ECG intervals. The J point/Osborn waves represent the earliest phase of membrane repolarization.

8.

TREATMENT FOR HEMORRHAGIC CVA/ANEURYSM WITH CEREBRAL ARTERIAL VASOSPASM

Matthew D. Coleman and Oscar Roldan

STEM CASE AND KEY QUESTIONS

A 51-year-old woman with a history of poorly controlled hypertension presents with a sudden onset of bifrontal headache, described to her spouse as "the worst headache of my life." After her family notices she is becoming confused and has started to vomit, they activate emergency medical services, and she is rushed to the hospital. On arrival to the emergency department, it is apparent she is becoming increasingly somnolent and is showing signs of right hemiparesis. In the emergency department she opens eyes to painful stimulation only, is unable to make comprehensible sounds, and localizes to pain. Brain stem reflexes are intact. Her vitals are heart rate 106, blood pressure 200/100, SpO_2 98% on 2 L NC O_2, and temperature 99.3°F.

WHAT IS THE PRESENTING GLASGOW COMA SCALE SCORE FOR THIS PATIENT? WHAT COULD ACCOUNT FOR HER RAPID DECLINE IN NEUROLOGIC FUNCTION? AT WHAT POINT SHOULD SHE BE INTUBATED TO SECURE HER AIRWAY?

With a Glasgow Coma Scale (GCS) score of 9, the decision is made to intubate at this time (opens her eyes to painful stimulation for 2 points, she makes incomprehensible sounds for 2 points, and localizes to pain for 5 points). Given emergency medical services' description of her "thunderclap headache," the emergency medicine physician orders a STAT noncontrast head CT (NC-HCT).

WHAT DRUGS SHOULD BE USED IN SECURING HER AIRWAY? SUPPOSING THE HEAD COMPUTED TOMOGRAM IS NEGATIVE, WHAT WOULD YOUR DIFFERENTIAL DIAGNOSIS INCLUDE?

Due to her rapidly declining mental state, she is intubated for airway protection. A modified rapid sequence intubation by a skilled practitioner is performed using propofol and rocuronium, and the patient is maintained on a propofol infusion. A NC-HCT is obtained. It shows acute subarachnoid hemorrhage (SAH) with blood in the basal cisterns,

thick clot in the bilateral sylvian fissures, and intraventricular hemorrhage.

WHAT GRADE OF SUBARACHNOID HEMORRHAGE DOES THIS PATIENT HAVE? WHAT CLINICAL PRESENTATION AND FINDINGS ON COMPUTED TOMOGRAM WOULD LEAD YOU TO CONSULT NEUROSURGERY?

A neurosurgical consultation is obtained and an emergent external ventricular drain (EVD) is placed. Angiography is performed revealing an anterior communicating artery aneurysm. The aneurysm is secured with coils, and she is transferred to the intensive care unit (ICU).

WHAT IS THE OPTIMAL BLOOD PRESSURE MANAGEMENT FOR THIS PATIENT? AFTER COILING, IS THERE STILL A RISK THAT THE PATIENT WOULD REBLEED?

On presentation, the patient has elevated blood pressures and was treated with intravenous (IV) labetalol with some improvement, but after the computed tomography (CT) scan she continues to have elevated systolic blood pressures (SBPs) greater than 180 mmHg. Nicardipine infusion is initiated and her SBP is lowered to approximately 140 mmHg and nimidopine 60 mg Q4 hours is started to reduce the incidence of cerebral vasospasm. By the time she arrives in the neuro ICU, the nicardipine has been uptitrated to 10 mg/hour.

WHAT IS CEREBRAL SALT WASTING, AND HOW DOES IT DIFFER FROM THE SYNDROME OF INAPPROPRIATE ANTIDIURETIC HORMONE? HOW SHOULD HYPONATREMIA BE TREATED IN THESE PATIENTS?

On post bleed day 2, she develops polyuria and her serum sodium concentration decreases to 129 meq/L. With a controlled SBP, she is no longer receiving nicardipine but despite aggressive volume replacement, she remains volume negative for the day. She is started on a 2% sodium chloride infusion at 50 mL/hour in addition to isotonic maintenance fluids. Free water is also eliminated as much as possible from her medication infusions. Over the following 2 days her sodium increases slowly to 135 meq/L

WHAT IS THE RISK OF CEREBRAL VASOSPASM? ON WHAT DAY POST BLEED DOES THE RISK OF VASOSPASM BEGIN, AND WHEN DOES THE RISK PEAK? WHAT IS DELAYED CEREBRAL ISCHEMIA, AND HOW IS IT MANAGED?

On post bleed day 3, a transcranial doppler (TCD) is performed with a velocity in the M1 branch of the ipsilateral middle cerebral artery of 120 m/s. She appears stable from a cardiopulmonary standpoint and the decision is made to discontinue her sedation. She emerges from sedation, is able to follow commands appropriately, and is successfully liberated from mechanical ventilation. By morning rounds on post bleed day 7, she is noted to be more lethargic and by the afternoon is noted to have a new right hemiparesis.

WHAT ROLE DOES TRANSCRANIAL DOPPLER PLAY IN DIAGNOSING CEREBRAL VASOSPASM? ARE THERE OTHER DIAGNOSTIC MODALITIES AVAILABLE TO DIAGNOSE VASOSPASM?

A TCD is obtained emergently demonstrating a velocity in the middle cerebral artery of 220 m/s indicating early signs of cerebral vasospasm. Coupled with her new onset hemiplegia, she is taken to cerebral angiogram that confirms vasospasm. Balloon angioplasty is performed and post dilatation and IV verapamil is injecting injected. Her symptoms improve over the next several days, and by day 12 she is transferred from the ICU.

WHAT IS THE PROGNOSIS FOR PATIENTS WITH ASAH?

After discharge from the hospital, she spent several months in an extended care facility receiving extensive physical and occupational rehabilitation. One year after her aneurysm bleed, she has made considerable progress but continues to have significant disability.

DISCUSSION

EPIDEMIOLOGY AND RISK FACTORS

Intracranial aneurysms exist in about 1-2% of the general population. SAH from spontaneous rupture of intracranial aneurysms accounts for 5% to 10% of strokes annually in the United States. The exact numbers may be higher due to the high prehospital mortality associated with these events. The incidence varies throughout the world with the highest incidence in Finland. As a subset of stroke, patients with a spontaneous rupture of an aneurysm resulting in subarachnoid hemorrhage(aSAH) tend to be much younger in age and occur more commonly in women than men. The peak age of rupture appears to be in the 50s [1].

Risk factors associated with aSAH include hypertension, family history of SAH or aneurysms (first-degree relative with an intracranial aneurysm), and prior history of SAH regardless of the presence of untreated aneurysms. The behavioral risk factors for aSAH include alcohol, tobacco, and cocaine use. Genetic diseases such as autosomal dominant polycystic kidney disease and type IV Elhers-Danlos syndrome also increase the risk substantially.

PATHOGENESIS

Intracranial aneurysms occur most commonly at bifurcation points in the cerebral vasculature. Connective tissue diseases causing weakness of the vasculature walls, such as with Ehlers-Danlos syndrome, increase the likelihood of developing aneurysms. However, the majority of intracranial aneurysms occur in individuals with no known genetic predisposition. Bifurcations result in increased turbulent blood flow, and it is theorized the resultant increase in wall tension causes weakening, and eventual outpouching, of the vessel wall over time. As the size of the aneurysm increases, the wall weakens further, and the likelihood of rupture sharply increases. This can be illustrated by Laplace's relationship of the radius of a vessel on the wall tension: $T = (P \cdot R)/2$, where T is tension, P is the pressure, and R is the radius of the vessel. Even with the pressure held constant, as the radius of the aneurysm increases the wall tension of the aneurysm continues to increase the risk of rupture.

DIAGNOSIS

The telltale sign of SAH is the sudden, thunderclap, headache. It is typically bifrontal in nature and is described as the worst headache of one's life. The headache occurs almost immediately following the rupture and reaches maximum severity in seconds, hence the term "thunderclap." In 10% of cases, the headache is frequently preceded by a less severe headache week to months prior, known as the sentinel headache. This may represent a leak or enlargement with subsequent irritation of the tissue surrounding the aneurysm and is often misdiagnosed as a migraine or tension headache [2]. In addition to the pathognomonic headache, patients can present with nausea, vomiting, nuchal rigidity, cranial nerve palsies, aphasias, and even hemiparesis. Altered mental status can be assessed by the GCS, one of the most widely used and studied scales in medicine (Table 8.1).

While it has become the standard or care to intubate head trauma patients with a GCS of 8 or less, this datum is not as robust for other forms of altered mental state. At this time, there is no cutoff recommendation for GCS scores in SAH hemorrhage patients that correlates to a need for intubation. However, lower scores, rapidity of progression of symptoms, and need for procedural airway control are often factors that influence the decision to intubate.

NC-HCT is the initial diagnostic test performed to identify aSAH. In the first hours to days following hemorrhage, NC-HCT has a very high sensitivity but in a low-grade SAH, CT may be negative. CT angiography is very sensitive in

Table 8.1 GLASGOW COMA SCALE

CATEGORY	SCORE
Eyes opening	
Spontaneous	4
To speech	3
To pain	2
None	1
Verbal response	
Oriented to time, place, and person	5
Confused	4
Inappropriate words	3
Incomprehensible sounds	2
None	1
Motor response	
Obeys commands	6
Localizes to pain	5
Withdrawals to pain, flexion	4
Abnormal flexion	3
Abnormal extension	2
None	1

Table 8.2 HUNT AND HESS SCALE

GRADE	PRESENTATION
I	Asymptomatic, or mild headache and slight nuchal rigidity
II	Moderate to severe headache, nuchal rigidity, no neurologic deficit other than cranial nerve palsy
III	Drowsiness, confusion, or mild focal deficit
IV	Stupor, moderate to severe hemiparesis, early decerebrate rigidity, vegetative disturbances
V	Deep Coma, decerebrate rigidity

survive, 8% to 20% will suffer long-term disability. The highest mortality occurs during the initial bleeding event, and the second highest rate occurs during recurrent bleeding events. Clinically significant cerebral vasospasm attributes to a third wave of mortality.

The two most commonly used scales for grading SAH and for determining prognosis are the Hunt and Hess Grading Scale and the World Federation of Neurosurgical Societies scale (see Tables 8.2 and 8.3). Both scales focus on the severity of presenting neurologic symptoms [5, 6].

The Fisher Scale (Table 8.4) grades the SAH by the amount and location of blood on the computer tomography scan [7]. A more recent modified Fisher Scale (Table 8.5) was developed by Claassen el al that takes into account some of the limitations of the original Fisher Scale in predicting cerebral vasospasm [8]. The Fisher scales are used for risk stratification for development of cerebral vasospasm and delayed cerebral ischemia.

INITIAL MANAGEMENT OF SUBARACHNOID HEMORRHAGE

Following a diagnosis by clinical presentation and confirmation by NC-HCT, the initial management of a patient with aneurysmal SAH, as with any critically ill patient, is to stabilize the cardiopulmonary systems. For the patient that is rapidly deteriorating, airway management is critical. Once the decision to intubate is made, the goals surrounding intubation should be considered. The patient should be considered a full stomach and treated as such during intubation. She should

identifying and characterizing aneurysms >3 mm but sensitive decreases rapidly with aneurysm size. If the clinical suspicion is high, a lumbar puncture (LP) can be performed. Lumbar puncture will detect blood or xanthochromia in the cerebrospinal fluid (CSF) if SAH is present. However, as trauma from the puncture itself can also result in blood in the CSF, several tubes of CSF should be obtained, tested, and compared. If the amount of blood decreases with each subsequent tube, the likelihood of SAH is decreased and local trauma is more likely the cause. When other modalities yield equivocal results, specific magnetic resonance imaging modalities that utilize fluid-attenuated inversion recovery, proton density, diffusion-weighted imaging, and gradient echo sequences are also sensitive in identifying blood in the subarachnoid space and can help establish a diagnosis of SAH. However, these scans require patients to lie flat for an extended period of time and are not feasible for those patients with significantly increased intracranial pressures (ICPs) or rapidly worsening mental status.

PROGNOSIS

Spontaneous SAH carries a very high morbidity and mortality. Upwards of 12% will not survive the initial bleed and 25% will die within the first 24 hours [3]. Thirty-day mortality in the United States is in the range of 30% to 60%. Of those who

Table 8.3 WORLD FEDERATION OF NEUROSURGICAL SOCIETIES SCALE

GRADE	CRITERIA
I	GSC 15 without focal deficit
II	GSC13–14 without focal deficit
III	GSC 13–14 with focal deficit
IV	GCS 7–12 with or without focal deficit
V	GSC 3–6 with or without focal deficit

Table 8.4 FISHER SCALE

GROUP	BLOOD PATTERN ON NC-HCT
1	No detectable SAH
2	Diffuse SAH, no localized clot >3 mm or vertical layers > 1 mm thick
3	Localized clot > 5 × 3 mm thick in subarachnoid space, or vertical layers >1 mm in thickness
4	Intraparenchymal or intraventricular hemorrhage with either absent or minimal SAH

also be suspected of having an elevated ICP, and appropriate drugs should be chosen so as to avoid further spikes in ICP. Pain management is critical and will further stabilize the blood pressure to avoid ongoing hemorrhage or rebleeding. Care should also be taken when deciding what drugs to use to intubate and sedate. Close neurologic exams will be necessary to guide further treatment.

With the airway under control and cardiopulmonary stability achieved, the focus should be on identifying and treating acute hydrocephalus and elevated ICP. An urgent neurosurgical consult should be obtained and a systematic approach to treating elevated ICP should be employed. A patient with signs of acute obstructing hydrocephalus on CT, or a high-grade SAH should have an external ventriculostomy drain placed. This will aid in draining CSF, thus treating elevated ICP, and will allow continuous monitoring of the ICP waveform. In high-grade SAH, the placement of a ventriculostomy drain is an emergent, life-saving procedure.

In addition to placing an EVD and draining CSF, multiple steps should be considered to further reduce ICP. Pain management is often a first step in treating elevated ICP in SAH. Intravenous opioids and deep sedatives, like propofol, can be administered as long as the hemodynamics are maintained. It is important to keep in mind that close monitoring of the neurological exam can be helpful in clinical decision-making

Table 8.5 THE MODIFIED FISHER SCALE

CT FINDINGS	IVH	MODIFIED FISHER SCALE
Diffuse thick SAH	Present	4
	Absent	3
Localized thick SAH	Present	4
	Absent	3
Diffuse thin SAH	Present	2
	Absent	1
Localized thin SAH	Present	2
	Absent	1
No SAH	Present	2
	Absent	0

and short-acting sedatives at the lowest clinically effective dose are preferred. Hyperventilation, in the acute setting, will rapidly decrease ICP by causing cerebral vasoconstriction thus decreasing the flow of blood into the skull. However, too much hyperventilation could result in cerebral ischemia if used for longer periods of time. The body will respond to prolonged hyperventilation with a metabolic acidosis to counteract the respiratory alkalosis, thus reducing the effects.

Osmotic diuretics can also be administered to reduce the ICP. Mannitol 1 to 1.5 gram/kg infused over 15 to 30 minutes will result in a decrease in cerebral spinal fluid. Hypovolemia can result sometimes after excess diuresis and hemodynamics should be carefully monitored. As an alternative to mannitol, hypertonic saline boluses of 23.4% will decrease ICP for several hours. Hypertonic saline should be administered through a central line, can be complicated by fluid overload and may result in acute kidney injury. Both treatments can result in electrolyte abnormalities.

In severe cases of refractory elevated ICP, a barbiturate coma or hypothermia may be necessary. Both will reduce oxygen consumption thereby protecting the patient's brain when cerebral perfusion pressure is low. Cerebral perfusion pressure can be calculated as the difference between mean arterial pressure and either ICP or central venous pressure, whichever is higher. In the case of SAH, the ICP is pathologically high and the barrier to proper cerebral oxygenation.

After protecting the patient from elevated ICP, the focus should now be directed on reducing the chances of rebleeding. Reversal of anticoagulation, antifibrinolytic therapy, definitive coiling or clipping, and blood pressure management will all reduce this risk. There is a growing body of data, suggesting a role for antifibrolytic therapy to reduce bleeding. Transexamic acid is being given as part of experimental protocols of early response to SAH as part of a catheter-based or open surgical intervention for control of the aneurysm thought to be responsible for the SAH. The data seem to imply a reduction in mortality as well as a reduction in rebleeding rates with the use of transexamic acid protocols without an increase in vasospasm or vascular thrombosis.

For patients being anticoagulated, steps should be taken to reverse the coagulopathy if possible given that the rate or morbidity and mortality from SAH while anticoagulated is incredibly high. Patients on coumadin should receive both phytonadione (Vitamin K) as well as coagulation factors. Classically, coumadin reversal is performed using fresh frozen plasma but more recently 3-factor and 4-factor prothrombin complex concentrates have been used with a faster time to reversal of anticoagulation and only a slightly increased risk of thrombosis.[14]

BLOOD PRESSURE MANAGEMENT IN ASAH

aSAH patients will commonly present with elevated blood pressures both as a cause for the initial rupture and as a physiologic compensation of increased ICP. The primary focus after initial diagnosis and stabilization of the patient is to prevent rebleeding: 4% of unsecured aneurysms rebled within 24 hours, and 27% rebled within 14 days. The majority of rebleeding events (>50%) occur within the first 6 hours after the initial event, and this correlates to the subset of patients with the highest mortality [1]. Therefore, early treatment of uncontrolled hypertension to prevent rebleeding is crucial. The hypertension is a physiologic response to reduced cerebral blood flow and may be further compounded by pain and agitation. Pain and agitation should be addressed with short-acting agents to facilitate frequent neurologic assessments and if hypertension persists, IV medications should be administered. The goal SBP should be between 140 and 160 mmHg as the reduction in SBP is associated with a reduction in the risk of rebleeding. If the blood pressure is reduced too much, cerebral blood flow may be altered and ischemia can result. Labetalol is a primary alpha-1 antagonist, with some lesser beta-1 and beta-2 antagonistic effects as well, that results in arterial vasodilation thus lowering systemic blood pressure. It has a quick onset of action and can be given by IV bolus, IV infusion, and orally. It is an excellent first line treatment for mild to moderate hypertension in low grade SAH but keeping in mind that it does have a relatively long half-life and is not easily titratable. Nicardipine is a primary arterial vasodilator that is quick onset, short-acting, and easily titratable and does not increase ICP.[9] It should be considered as the drug of choice in high-grade SAH and in severe hypertensive cases. There is no role for nitroglycerin or sodium nitroprusside as these medications have been shown to cause cerebral venous dilation and could worsen intracranial hypertension.

ENDOVASCULAR TREATMENT AND CLIPPING OF ANEURYSMS AFTER SAH

Early securing of the aneurysm is also of paramount importance. Both endovascular and open clipping are suitable ways to secure aneurysms thus reducing the risk of rebleeding substantially. The decision to secure the aneurysm through microsurgical versus endovascular technique is beyond the scope of this discussion. The issues that determine one approach versus the other are the severity of the SAH, the patient comorbidities, the location and geometry of the aneurysm, and the timing. In low grade, World Neurologic Federation Scores (WNFS) 1–3, SAH, endovascular treatment is preferable when possible. In Higher grade, WNFS 4–6, it is less clear whether endovascular or surgical treatment is preferable.[10] Certainly, surgical clipping is more invasive and poses a greater risk to patients with significant medical comorbidities; however, the inherent risk of death or long-term disability is so high in this subgroup that both treatments pose a similar risk profile. Comparing both approaches, surgical clipping is the most secure way to prevent rebleeding when done without complication, as there is a greater risk of rebleeding with coiled aneurysms that still contain filling defects. However, as endovascular technologies continue to evolve, studies are finding reductions in morbidity and mortality from rebleeding as well as improvement in vasospasm outcomes. In most centers, endovascular treatment is becoming the first-line therapy for acute aSAH treatment.

CEREBRAL SALT WASTING AND SYNDROME OF INAPPROPRIATE ANTIDIURETIC HORMONE

Cerebral salt wasting is often seen in SAH. Sodium and free water losses occur in the form of polyuria and may be due to decreases in the concentration of natriuretic peptides. These losses ultimately lead to dehydration and severe hyponatremia and can occur for days following SAH. It is important to not misdiagnose cerebral salt wasting (CSW) for syndrome of inappropriate antidiuretic hormone (SIADH) and treat the intravascular volume depleted patient with fluid restriction. CSW should be treated with isotonic fluid administration in mild cases and with hypertonic, 2% or 3% sodium chloride or sodium acetate solutions in refractory cases.

SIADH can occur after traumatic brain injury, postoperative craniotomy, and in patients after SAH. SIADH results in hyponatremia with euvolemia or volume overload. Despite the difference in volume status of the classic SIADH patient as compared to the CSW patient, it is often difficult to make the diagnostic distinction. In SIADH, the urine osmolality is >100 mOsm/kg and urine sodium >40 mmol/L. The treatment for SIADH involves free water restriction, and if severe enough, treating with vasopressin receptor antagonist such as conivaptan or tolvaptan which cause diuresis with sodium retention. In SAH patients in which the differentiation between CSW and SIADH is unclear, hyponatremia should be assumed to be CSW and the patient treated with isotonic or hypertonic saline given that intravascular volume depletion may increase the risk for, and worsen outcomes of, cerebral vasospasm.

CEREBRAL VASOSPASM AND DELAYED CEREBRAL ISCHEMIA

Cerebral vasospasm is one of the most common and most serious complications following spontaneous SAH. In severe hemorrhage, Fisher 3 or modified Fisher 3–4, had the highest incidence of vasospasm with demonstrable angiographic evidence in 70% of patients [11]. The cause of cerebral vasospasm is not totally understood, but it seems clear that the greater the amount of heme in the subarachnoid space, the higher the incidence of vasospasm. The likelihood of vasospasm starts in increase between post bleed days 3 and 5, peaking on day 7, and diminishing by day 10. It can, however, be seen up to 21 days after SAH. The neurologic exam will often be the first clue to the presence of vasospasm. Patients often become lethargic and may develop specific symptoms related to the location of the spasm. If the spasm is severe enough to cause ischemia for a prolonged period of time, infarction can occur. Symptomatic vasospasm occurs in 20% to 30% of the patients after spontaneous SAH and is termed "delayed cerebral ischemia" (DCI). If not treated aggressively, DCI can result in long-term disability or death.

While the gold standard for diagnosis of cerebral vasospasm is cerebral angiography, detecting vasospasm is best done using frequent neurologic exams and serial TCD measurements during the time period in which the patient is at greatest risk, between post bleed day 3 to 10. Due to the risks and logistics involved in performing cerebral angiography (transporting critically ill patients, contrast nephropathy, bleeding, groin hematoma, etc.), TCD is the more frequently used for screening purposes and angiography for confirmation and treatment of a spastic vessel.

Treatment of SAH induced cerebral vasospasm includes hemodynamic alterations, vasodilatory drugs, and balloon angioplasty. Nimidopine given orally 60 mg Q4 hours from time of presentation will decrease the incidence and duration of vasospasm [12]. In the past, triple H therapy had been advocated and consisted of hypervolemia, hemodilution, and hypertension. The idea was to increase the cerebral blood flow to the ischemic brain tissue by giving large amounts of fluid in the form of crystalloids or colloids and increasing the delivery pressure with inotropic or vasopressor medications, elevating the SBP to 160 to 220. This often resulted in fluid overload and had significant cardiac, pulmonary, and renal complications. More recent data has suggested a more conservative, goal-directed approach of augmenting cardiac output, measuring and optimizing cerebral perfusion pressure, and cerebral oxygenation be employed [13]. Cardiac output monitoring, cerebral tissue oxygen content, and jugular bulb oxygen tension monitoring has improved the ability of the intensivist to achieve these goals without blindly giving large amounts of fluid.

CONCLUSIONS

- Spontaneous aneurysmal SAH carries a high morbidity and mortality. Timely diagnosis and treatment greatly improve outcomes.

- After diagnosis, and stabilization, preventing early rebleeding is the most important goal.

  - Treat pain and agitation

  - Treat hypertension

  - Optimize cerebral perfusion

  - Aggressively treat elevated ICP

  - Reverse anticoagulation if present and consider antifibrinolytic therapy if a delay in securing the aneurysm is expected

  - Rapid mobilization of the teams necessary to quickly treat the patient

- In high-grade SAH or evidence of obstructive hydrocephalus on imaging, urgent neurosurgical placement of an EVD could be life-saving.

- Securing the aneurysm, once the patient is stable, will sharply decrease rebleeding risk.

- If hyponatremia in SAH develops CSW or SIADH are possible. Avoid hypovolemia and treat severe hyponatremia with hypertonic saline.

- Have a high clinical suspicion for cerebral vasospasm after SAH especially from post bleed days 3 to 10. Use serial neurological examination to detect clinical vasospasm. TCD is noninvasive and useful in detecting cerebral vasospasm.

- Cerebral vasospasm should be treated aggressively to prevent DCI with

  - oral nimodipine 60 mg every 4 hours.

  - Induced hypertension SBPs 160 to 220 .

  - Goal-directed treatment with volume and hemoglobin optimization, cardiac output augmentation, and cerebral perfusion pressure optimization.

  - Endovascular treatment including balloon angioplasty and intraarterial vasodilator injections.

REFERENCES

1. Connolly ES, Rabinstein AA, Carhuapoma JR, et al. Guidelines for the Management of Aneurysmal Subarachnoid Hemorrhage: a guideline for healthcare professionals from the American Heart Association/ American Stroke Association. Stroke. 2012;43:1711–1737.
2. Kowalski RG, Claassen J, Kreiter KT et al. Initial misdiagnosis and outcome after subarachnoid hemorrhage. JAMA. 2004;291(7):866–869.
3. Schievink WI, Wijdicks EF, Parisi JE, Peipgras DG, Whisnant JP. Sudden Death from aneurysmal subarachnoid hemorrhage. Neurology. 1995;45:871–874.
4. Suarez JI, Tarr RW, Selman WR. Aneurysmal subarachnoid hemorrhage. N Engl J Med. 2006;354:387–396.
5. Hunt WE, Hess RM. Surgical risk as related to time of intervention in the repair of intracranial aneurysms. J Neurosurg. 1968;28:14–20.
6. Drake C. Report of World Federation of Neurological Surgeons Committee on a Universal Subarachnoid Hemorrhage Grading Scale. J Neurosurg. 1988;68:985–986.
7. Fisher CM, Kristler JP, Davis JM. Relation of cerebral vasospasm to subarachnoid hemorrhage visualized by computerized tomographic scanning. Neurosurgery 1980;6:1–9.
8. Classen J, Bernardini GL, Kreiter KT et al. Effect of cisternal and ventricular blood on risk of delayed cerebral ischemia after subarachnoid hemorrhage: the Fisher Scale revisited. Stroke 2001;32:2012–2020.
9. Narotam PK, Puri V, Roberts JM, Taylon C, Vora Y, Nathoo N. Management of hypertensive emergencies in acute brain disease: evaluation of the treatment effects of intravenous nicardipine on cerebral oxygenation. J Neurosurg. 2008;109:1065–1074.
10. Molyneux Y, Kerr RS, Yu LM et al. International Subarachnoid Aneurysm Trial (ISAT) of neurosurgical clipping versus endovascular coiling in 2143 patients with ruptured intracranial aneurysms: a randomized comparison of effects on survival, dependency, seizures, rebleeding, subgroups, and aneurysm occlusion. Lancet 2005;366:809–817.
11. Millikan CH. Cerebral vasospasm and ruptured intracranial aneurysm. Arch Neurol. 1975;32:433–449.
12. Pickard JD, Murray GD, Illingworth R, Shaw MDM, Teasdale GM, Foy PM, Humphrey PRD, Lang DA, Nelson R, Richards P, Sinar J, Nailey S, Skene A. Effect of oral nimodipine on cerebral infarction and outcome after subarachnoid haemorrhage: British Aneurysm Nimodipine trial. Br Med J. 1989;298:636–642.
13. Francoeur CL, Mayer SA. Management of delayed cerebral ischemia after subarachnoid hemorrhage. Critical Care. 2016;20:277.

14. Sarode R, Milling T Jr, Refaai M, Mangione A, Schneider A, Durn B, and Goldstein J. Efficacy and safety of a 4-Factor prothrombin complex concentrate in patients on vitamin K antagonists presenting with major bleeding. Circulation. 2013;128:1234–1243.

REVIEW QUESTIONS

1. Which of the following statements on strict glucose control in SAH patients is false?

   A. Increased incidence of hypoglycemic events with strict glucose control.
   B. Decreased rates of cerebral vasospasm with controlled glucose levels.
   C. Strict glucose control protocols lead to a decrease in hospital mortality.
   D. There is no defined range of glucose levels which correlate with optimal glucose control.

Correct answer: C
Latorre JG, Chou SH, Nogueira RG et al. Effective glycemic control with aggressive hyperglycemia management is associated with improved outcome in aneurysmal subarachnoid hemorrhage. Stroke. 2009;40(5),1644–1652.
The effect of intensive insulin therapy on infection rate, vasospasm, neurologic outcome, and mortality in neuro ICU after intracranial aneurysm clipping in patients with acute subarachnoid hemorrhage: a randomized prospective pilot trial.
Bilotta F, Spinelli A, Giovannini F, Doronzio A, Delfini R, Rosa G. J Neurosurg Anesthesiol. 2007 Jul;19(3):156–160.
Strict glucose control does not affect mortality after aneurysmal subarachnoid hemorrhage.
Thiele RH, Pouratian N, Zuo Z, Scalzo DC, Dobbs HA, Dumont AS, Kassell NF, Nemergut EC. Anesthesiology. 2009 Mar;110(3):603–610. doi:10.1097/ALN.0b013e318198006a.

2. A 63-year-old male with a past medical history of hyperlipidemia presents to the emergency department for confusion. NC-HCT revealed a subarachnoid hemorrhage, which was successfully embolized in the angiography suite. On postoperative day 2, the patient became dyspneic and desaturated which resulted in an emergent intubation. Chest radiography revealed pulmonary edema and vascular congestion. All of the following are characteristics of Takatsubo's Cardiomyopathy in Subarachnoid Hemorrhage *except*

   A. New onset ECG abnormalities such as ST elevations or T wave inversions.
   B. Irreversible echocardiographic changes in ejection fraction and/or wall motion abnormalities.
   C. Severe reduction in ejection fraction secondary to left ventricular mid and apical segments.
   D. Higher incidence with a greater Hunt and Hess score.

Correct answer: B
Abd TT, Hayek, SS, Cheng JW. Incidence and clinical characteristics of Takotsubo's cardiomyopathy among patients with aneurysmal subarachnoid hemorrhage: retrospective analysis of 2,276 patients. Journal of the American College of Cardiology Mar 2013;61(10 Suppl):e562; doi:10.1016/S0735-1097(13)60562-8.
Abd TT, Hayek S, Cheng JW, Samuels W, Lerakis S. Takotsubo's cardiomyopathy is associated with severe subarachnoid hemorrhage: retrospective analysis of 1,251 patients. Circulation. 2012;126(Suppl 21):Abstract 13973.

3. A 71-year-old female with a past medical history of congestive heart failure, hypertension, Type II diabetes mellitus, and chronic kidney disease is diagnosed with vasospasm following a subarachnoid hemorrhage. Which of the following is the greatest concern regarding the use of "triple H therapy" in this patient?

   A. Anemia
   B. Hypertensive crisis
   C. Worsening renal failure
   D. Pulmonary edema

Correct answer: D
Hoff RG, Rinkel GJ, Verweij BH, Algra A, Kalkman CJ. Pulmonary edema and blood volume after aneurysmal subarachnoid hemorrhage: a prospective observational study. Crit Care. 2010;14(2):R43. doi:10.1186/cc8930

4. A 75-year-old female is 2 days status post cerebral angiography and coiling for a SAH. You are notified by your intern of "odd" changes within the patients ECG. A 12-lead ECG is ordered, what do you most expect to see?

   A. Widened QRS, Prolonged QT interval, Peak T waves
   B. ST segment depressions, U waves, T wave abnormalities
   C. Prolonged PR interval, absent T waves with decreased Ejection fraction on ECHO
   D. Third-degree AV block

Correct answer: B
Chatterjee S. ECG changes in subarachnoid haemorrhage: a synopsis. Neth Heart J. 2011;19(1):31–34. doi:10.1007/s12471-010-0049-1

5. An 81-year-old patient develops hyponatremia following a craniotomy for a subdural hematoma. Urine electrolytes and urine osmolality are increased, and serum sodium and serum osmolality are decreased. At the bedside, you find the patient to be hypovolemic. What treatment modality is best?

   A. Fluid restriction
   B. Salt tablets
   C. DDAVP
   D. Normal saline

Correct answer: D
Sorkhi H, Salehi Omran MR, Barari Savadkoohi R, Baghdadi F, Nakhjavani N, Bijani A. CSWS versus SIADH as the probable causes of hyponatremia in children with acute cns disorders. Iran J Child Neurol. 2013;7(3):34–39.

6. Oral Nimodipine is a Class 1, Level A recommendation for the management of SAH, which of the following is the only other class 1, level A recommendation for SAH?

   A. Cerebral angiography with endovascular coiling

B. Treatment of high blood pressure with antihypertensives
C. NC-HCT for initial diagnosis of SAH
D. Use of hypertonic IV fluids

Correct answer: B

Diringer MN. Management of aneurysmal subarachnoid hemorrhage. Crit Care Med. 2009;37(2):432–440. doi:10.1097/CCM.0b013e318195865a

7. Which of the following strategies for a rapid sequence intubation in a patient with increased ICP is least favorable?

A. Pretreatment with fentanyl, induction with propofol and succinylcholine followed by direct laryngoscopy in a hypertensive patient
B. Induction with remifentanil, etomidate, and high dose rocuronium followed by video assisted laryngoscopy in a normotensive patient
C. Induction with etomidate, and succinylcholine followed by video assisted laryngoscopy in a hypotensive patient
D. Ketamine induction followed by fiberoptic guided intubation in a normotensive patient

Correct answer: D

Kramer N, Lebowitz D, Walsh M, Ganti L. Rapid sequence intubation in traumatic brain-injured adults. Cureus. 2018;10(4):e2530. doi:10.7759/cureus.2530

Jung JY. Airway management of patients with traumatic brain injury/C-spine injury. Korean J Anesthesiol. 2015;68(3):213–219. doi:10.4097/kjae.2015.68.3.213

8. Which of the following grading scales is used to predict and/or correlate risk of vasospasm?

A. Hunt and Hess Scale
B. World Federation of Neurological Surgeons
C. Fischer Radiological Scale
D. Ogilvy and Carter Combination Scale

Correct answer: C

Rosen, DS, Macdonald RL. Subarachnoid hemorrhage grading scales. Neurocri Care 2005;2(2):110–118.

9. Delayed cerebral ischemia is better predicted with which of the following modalities?

A. Cerebral angiography
B. MRI head
C. CT head
D. Transcranial Doppler

Correct answer: D

Kumar G, Shahripour RB, Harrigan MR. Vasospasm on transcranial Doppler is predictive of delayed cerebral ischemia in aneurysmal subarachnoid hemorrhage: a systematic review and meta-analysis. J Neurosurg. 2016 May;124(5):1257–1264. doi:10.3171/2015.4.JNS15428

10. Which of the following is the gold standard for the diagnosis of vasospasm following subarachnoid hemorrhage?

A. Transcranial doppler
B. Magnetic resonance angiography
C. Cerebral angiography
D. Jugular venous bulb oximetry

Correct answer: C

Mascia L, Del Sorbo L. Diagnosis and management of vasospasm. F1000 Med Rep. 2009;1:33. doi:10.3410/M1-33

9.

MOTOR VEHICLE ACCIDENT WITH SKULL FRACTURE AND C-SPINE COMPROMISE, ELEVATED ICP, AND SPINAL SHOCK—A CASE PRESENTATION

Eric Fried and Nicholas C. Zimick

STEM CASE AND KEY QUESTION

A 43-year-old restrained male driver struck a highway barrier at an estimated 70 miles per hour. Emergency services arrived, extricated the driver from the overturned vehicle, and placed him on an immobilizer board with a cervical collar. Initial assessment reveals an unresponsive patient with facial lacerations, periorbital ecchymoses, a weak pulse, and tachypnea with labored breathing. He grimaces and withdraws his upper extremities to pain, but he does not move spontaneously, open his eyes, or follow commands. Pupils are noted to be equal, 3 mm in diameter, and reactive to light. Initial vital signs are blood pressure 85/40 mmHg, heart rate 140, respiratory rate 30, and oxygen saturation 86% on room air.

WHAT IS THIS PATIENT'S GLASGOW COMA SCALE SCORE?

Large bore intravenous (IV) access is obtained, 2 liters of 0.9% normal saline is administered for hypotension, and supplemental oxygen via a non-rebreather face mask is given for hypoxemia. The patient is then transported to the nearest trauma center approximately 15 minutes away. On arrival his blood pressure is 143/85, his heart rate is 120 bpm, respiratory rate is 30 per minute, oxygen saturation is 90% on 100% non-rebreather face mask, and his temperature is 36.5°C. A neurologic examination remains the same, with a Glasgow Coma Scale (GCS) of 6 (E1cV1M4).

SHOULD THIS PATIENT HAVE AN ENDOTRACHEAL TUBE PLACED?

Given the patient's hypoxemia, GCS of 6, and inability to protect his airway the medical team decides to perform endotracheal intubation. He is given succinylcholine (1 mg/kg), etomidate (0.3 mg/kg), and intubated in the emergency department during the primary survey. The procedure is performed with manual in-line stabilization and following tube placement bilateral chest rise, condensation, and continuous end-tidal carbon dioxide are used to confirm proper tube position. An oral-gastric sump tube is placed to empty the stomach. The patient is then sedated with dexmedetomidine.

NOW THAT THE PRIMARY SURVEY HAS BEEN COMPLETED AND THE AIRWAY SECURED, WHAT ARE THE COMPONENTS OF THE SECONDARY SURVEY?

The secondary survey is remarkable for a step off in the left temporal bone, concerning for a skull fracture. There are also decreased breath sounds over the left hemithorax. Focused Assessment with Sonography for Trauma (FAST) exam is subsequently performed and reveals a left pleural effusion, hyperdynamic cardiac function, and no free fluid in the abdomen. A left-sided chest tube is placed and drains 300 cc of bright red blood. Following this the patient's oxygen saturation rises to 100% on an FiO_2 of 100%. A urinary catheter is placed and the patient is taken the computed tomography (CT) scanner for a CT of his head, neck, chest, abdomen, and pelvis.

CT of the head and neck reveals a left temporal bone fracture and concomitant epidural hemorrhage with a 3 mm midline shift and effacement of the lateral ventricles.

CT of the chest demonstrates a C7 fracture with dislocation and spinal cord impingement, as well as a fracture of the left sixth and seventh ribs, with well-positioned chest and endotracheal tubes. CT of the abdomen and pelvis are unremarkable.

WHAT SYNDROMES SHOULD BE EXPECTED IN THIS PATIENT? IS THERE A ROLE FOR STEROID TREATMENT? IS THERE A ROLE FOR HYPOTHERMIA?

Neurosurgery is consulted for the C7 fracture with spinal cord impingement complicated by spinal shock and epidural hemorrhage with intracranial hypertension. Neurologic exam now evidences anisocoria with a 3 mm responsive pupil on the right, and a 6 mm minimally responsive pupil on the left. He does not open his eyes to pain or move spontaneously. Although he continues to withdraw his upper extremities to pain, his lower extremities are no longer responsive, and he has developed priapism. At this time, the patient's blood pressure is 80/40 mmHg and his heart rate is 54 bpm. His respiratory rate is 30 and dyssynchronous with the ventilator. His oxygen saturation remains 99% on 100% FiO_2 and his body temperature is 35.5°C.

WITH THIS COMPLICATED CLINICAL PICTURE, WHAT IS YOUR DIFFERENTIAL DIAGNOSIS FOR THE PATIENT'S WORSENING NEUROLOGIC STATUS? WHAT IS SPINAL SHOCK? WHAT IS INTRACRANIAL HYPERTENSION? HOW WOULD YOU MANAGE EACH SCENARIO SEPARATELY, AND HOW WOULD YOU MANAGE THEM TOGETHER AS IN THIS CASE?

The patient is further resuscitated with 250 cc hypertonic saline and 2 liters of lactated Ringer's solution. A subclavian central line is placed, and he is started on a norepinephrine infusion, with an increase in blood pressure to a goal of 90 mmHg mean arterial pressure. After hemodynamic stabilization, he is taken emergently to the operating room for a decompressive craniotomy, epidural hematoma evacuation, and a cervical–spinal decompression and spinal fusion.

SHOULD THIS PATIENT HAVE HAD AN EXTERNAL VENTRICULAR DRAIN PLACED INSTEAD OF A CRANIOTOMY?

The operative course is uncomplicated. The bleeding epidural vessel is found and cauterized with an estimated blood loss of 1 L. Neuromonitoring is attempted intraoperatively, but there are no baseline motor evoked potentials elicited, and somatosensory evoked potentials are low amplitude and high latency.

Postoperatively, the patient's epidural bleeding resolves and he regains consciousness. Unfortunately, his C7 fracture with spinal cord impingement results in paralysis from C7 caudad. He is transferred from the hospital on postoperative day 21 to a long-term care facility, wheelchair bound.

DISCUSSION

Spinal shock and intracranial hypertension are 2 common and serious sequelae of trauma, which frequently occur after high-speed motor vehicle accident.[1] We will start this discussion with spinal shock and then continue our discussion with intracranial hypertension.

SPINAL SHOCK

Spinal shock is the initial period after spinal cord injury where all spinal cord function may be lost caudal to the level of injury with resultant loss of bladder and bowel control, reflex activity, flaccid paralysis, and anesthesia. In males with a high spinal cord lesion, priapism may also develop. These patients may also develop hypotension and bradycardia due to spinal cord injury causing vasoplegia and loss of cardiac

accelerator fibers (levels T1–T4). These signs and symptoms may last from several hours to several weeks and are often referred to as "spinal shock."[2]

Pathophysiology

The initial loss of function in spinal shock may be due to potassium loss from within the injured cord cells and its accumulation in the extracellular space, reducing axonal transmission. Once potassium levels normalize and equilibrate between the intracellular and extracellular spaces, spinal shock fades and spastic paresis replaces flaccid paralysis. Complete recovery after transient paralysis is often seen in younger patients who sustain athletic injuries.[3]

Assessment

Caring for patients with spinal shock requires a primary assessment, since the level of spinal cord injury can result in hemodynamic instability and respiratory impairment.
  Primary assessment:

A Airway (establish/secure and/or open airway, when necessary)

B Breathing

C Circulation (pulse check, heart rate, blood pressure)

D Disability (neurologic status, Glasgow Coma Scale, sensory motor exam, digital rectal examination)

E Exposure (remove clothing, check for environmental exposures)

Generally, any patient with a head injury, loss of consciousness, confusion, or complaints of weakness, spinal pain, and/or loss of sensation, should be evaluated for spinal cord injury. Great care must be taken to avoid aggravating the injury by minimizing spine movement. After placement of a rigid cervical collar, other modalities include log-roll movements for turns and patient transfer with a stiff backboard.[3]
  The Glasgow Coma Scale was first described in 1974 and is a commonly used tool for assessing neurologic status in patients, especially after trauma. It has three components: eye opening, motor exam, and verbal expressions. Each is assigned a score, the best of which is recorded: eyes (4), verbs (5), and motors (6). The lowest GCS possible is 3, and the highest is 15. When a patient is intubated, a "T" is placed next to the numerical sum to indicate such, for example, 8T; when the eyes are closed, a "c" is placed next to the eye score. This scale allows for graphical representation of each best score daily for the duration of coma, so any provider will have an idea of the progression of disease.[8,9]

Management

Nearly a third of patients with cervical spinal cord injuries require intubation within the first 24 hours for both hypoxic respiratory failure and airway protection. Hypoxia can adversely affect neurologic outcome, and so it is particularly important to avoid hypoxia whenever possible. The intubation technique for these patients must minimize motion of the cervical spine to prevent any extension of the injury. Elective intubation should be performed with a flexible fiberoptic laryngoscope, while emergent intubation should be performed with rapid sequence induction and in-line cervical spinal immobilization. Immobilization of the neck and body should be maintained until spinal injury has been ruled out.[5] This can be performed with a c-collar or the two-provider method. Neurogenic shock after spinal cord injury can result in hypotension due to blood pooling in the extremities that have lost sympathetic tone. Neurologic examination of mental status and cranial nerve function should always be performed, as head injury often accompanies spinal cord injury. Bladder tone must be evaluated, and a urinary catheter should be placed as soon as possible to avoid harm from overdistention.[3]

At the minimum, a head CT should be performed in trauma patients regardless of suspected spinal cord injury, to evaluate for occult pathology. The bones of the spine can be imaged with plain radiographs (static or dynamic films), or CT, while soft tissue evaluation can be made with magnetic resonance imaging (MR), as long as the spine is stabilized prior to the study.[3]

Complications

Cardiovascular. The major cardiovascular complications of acute spinal cord injury typically include hypotension and bradycardia, although frequently seen together, they depend upon the level of injury as well as concurrent comorbid disease, including hypovolemia due to bleeding, which frequently occurs during traumatic injuries. Hypotension with bradycardia may result from disruption of autonomic pathways leading to a decrease in vascular resistance and an inability to accelerate heart rate to compensate for cardiac output. In order to ensure adequate cord perfusion and minimize ischemic injury, guidelines recommend maintaining a mean arterial blood pressure (MAP) of at least 85 to 90 mmHg, targeting spinal cord perfusion pressure (SCPP) of at least 60 mmHg, using IV fluids, blood product transfusion, and vasopressors. For high cervical lesions, bradycardia due to unbalanced vagal tone can be seen any time in the first two weeks after injury and may require external pacing or atropine. Later autonomic dysreflexia may occur with episodic paroxysmal hypertension with bradycardia, flushing, sweating, and headache.[3]

Pulmonary. Respiratory failure, pulmonary edema, and pneumonia, are the most frequent pulmonary complications leading to early morbidity and mortality in patients with spinal cord damage.[4] Weakness of the diaphragm and chest wall muscles impairs clearance of secretions, which in turn leads to respiratory infection, atelectasis and hypoventilation.[3]

Hematological. Venous thromboembolism and pulmonary embolism are also common complications in patients with spinal injuries due to their immobilization after injury, with an incidence of 50% to 100% in untreated patients. Most of these occur between 72 hours and 14 days following the injury.[5]

Pain. Patients typically require pain relief after spinal injuries. In addition to surgical intervention for stabilization, opiates are frequently used, but their benefits must be weighed against their sedating and respiratory depressive side effects, especially in light of neurologic examinations which will be performed by the team throughout their ICU stay. Other modalities may include non-steroidal anti-inflammatory drugs (NSAIDs), acetaminophen, clonidine, ketamine, and local anesthetics; the specifics of these are beyond the scope of this chapter.[3]

INTRACRANIAL HYPERTENSION

Normally, the brain, spinal cord, blood, and cerebrospinal fluid (CSF) are contained within skull and the vertebral canal, with a minimal amount of compliance provided by the intra-cerebral ventricles, intervertebral spaces. Intracranial hypertension in the adult patient is defined by an intracranial pressure (ICP) greater than 5 to 15 mmHg. Any significant increase in volume will result in a large increase in pressure within this enclosed space. ICP greater than 20 mmHg generally requires treatment, while an ICP of greater than 40 mmHg is life-threatening intracranial hypertension. The Monro–Kellie hypothesis states: "that the sum of the intracranial volumes of CSF, brain, blood and other components is constant, and any increase in one volume must be offset by a decrease in another, or else the pressure increases."[2]

Pathophysiology

To understand intracranial hypertension and its management, we must first describe cerebral perfusion. The cerebral perfusion pressure (CPP) is equal to the MAP minus the greater of either ICP or central venous pressure (CVP). MAP is defined as one third the systolic blood pressure (SBP) added to two thirds the diastolic blood pressure (DBP):
As the cranium is a fixed volume, MAP and ICP are thus inversely related. Increasing MAP or decreasing ICP will increase the CPP, and *vice versa*. Generally, the brain is thought able to autoregulate cerebral blood flow across a wide range of CPPs (50–150 mmHg), however, this protective mechanism may be altered or absent following injury.[2]

Intracranial hypertension can be caused by processes that occur intracranially, extracranially, or postoperatively.

Assessment

All patients with suspected intracranial hypertension should have close ICP monitoring, which can range from serial physical exams to direct measurement, and frequently includes standard ASA monitors, temperature, blood glucose, and fluid balance. A urinary catheter is often necessary for accurate urine measurement, and point-of-care ultrasound or a central venous catheter may be used to evaluate intravascular volume status.[2]

Ventriculostomy catheters are the standard for invasive ICP monitoring. An intraventricular catheter (ICP "bolt") is placed by a surgeon and connected to a dry pressure transducer. It can be used for therapeutic drainage of CSF and ICP monitoring, and it is relatively inexpensive; however, the transducer height and a continuous fluid column are crucial for accurate repeated measurement. Some form of ICP monitoring should be performed in all traumatic brain injury (TBI) patients with an abnormal head CT and a GCS of 8 or less after resuscitation, patients with a normal head CT and at least two of the following: age > 40 years, motor posturing, or systolic blood pressure < 90 mmHg.[2] Patients who can follow commands are generally considered low risk for developing intracranial hypertension (ICH) and can be followed with serial neurologic examinations.[2]

Management

To maintain CPP in the desired range, ICP and MAP must be optimized and aggravating factors limited. One goal is maintaining ICP less than 20–25 mmHg, while concurrently ensuring CPP is greater than 60 mmHg.[2] To reduce ICP, venous outflow resistance should be minimized and CSF displacement from the intracranial department to the spinal compartment should be enhanced. This can be accomplished by elevating the head of the bed at minimum 20 degrees and keeping the head in a neutral position to prevent obstruction of the jugular veins. Cables and wires must not be draped across the patient's neck as this could further restrict venous outflow. Other obstructions to cerebral venous drainage include indwelling internal jugular catheters and elevated intra-thoracic and intra-abdominal pressure (such as pneumothorax or abdominal compartment syndrome). Central venous catheters are often placed in the subclavian vein to facilitate cerebral venous drainage.[2]

Hypoxia and hypercapnia are common in patients with intracranial hypertension, especially in head trauma patients, and can increase ICP dramatically. Close monitoring and optimization of ventilation are crucial to control ICP. Mechanical positive-pressure ventilation, although often necessary to treat respiratory insufficiency, may elevate ICP. Positive end-expiratory pressure (PEEP) can increase ICP by decreasing venous return thereby increasing cerebral venous pressure and ICP. Hyperventilation can temporarily decrease ICP until compensation occurs. A decrease in $PaCO_2$ causes constriction of cerebral arteries by increasing the pH of the CSF. This results in a reduction of cerebral blood volume and ICP. This reduction of ICP lasts only 11 to 20 hours due to the rapid equilibration between the CSF pH and the arterial CO_2 level. Although hyperventilation is useful as a bridge to other therapies that reduce ICP, it can also have a detrimental effect by reducing global cerebral blood flow and risking tissue hypoperfusion/ischemia. Hyperventilation should thus be reserved only for patients with elevated ICP, not all TBI patients.[2]

Fever may induce dilation of cerebral, an increase in cerebral blood flow and thus a resultant increase in ICP. It is therefore essential to control fever with antipyretics and cooling blankets, as well as treating any suspected infection with antibiotic therapy, when appropriate. Hypothermia may also be an adjunct therapy to reduce ICP, although studies haven't shown any improvement in neurologic outcome.

Seizures after TBI are related to the severity of the injury and will increase the cerebral metabolic oxygen demand and increase the ICP, resulting in decreased CPP and cerebral oxygen delivery establishing a deteriorating cycle of ischemic tissue damage. Phenytoin has been shown to reduce the incidence of seizures during the first week after trauma, and it is recommended for seizure prophylaxis in patients with TBI for 7 days following injury.[6] Continued seizure prophylaxis beyond 7 days is reserved for patients with active seizures.[2]

Adequate sedation and analgesia are important in the patient with TBI to prevent elevated blood pressure and ICP. Short-acting sedatives and analgesics are preferred to long-acting agents, in order to permit neurologic examination. Over-sedation may confound accurate assessment of the patient's neurologic status. Patients with refractory intracranial hypertension may be treated with a "barbiturate coma," where deep barbiturate sedation is titrated to burst suppression on electroencephalogram. This therapy can increase the likelihood of controlling ICP at the cost of the inability to perform a neurologic examination for days. In addition to deep sedation, paralysis with neuromuscular blockers may be used, but their use should be limited to (i) allow assessment of neurologic status and (ii) decrease the incidence of myopathy and polyneuropathy, which may accompany prolonged neuromuscular blocker use.[2]

Hyperosmolar therapy with mannitol or hypertonic saline is commonly used to acutely reduce ICP. Intravenous administration of mannitol will reduce ICP in 1 to 5 minutes with a peak effect in 20 to 60 minutes, and may last 1.5 to 6 hours. Increasing the osmotic gradient between the CSF compartment and the vascular compartment will induce a redistribution of volume from the former to the latter. Hyperosmolar therapy is contraindicated in patients with heart failure where the rapid intravascular volume increase may precipitate pulmonary edema or exacerbate cardiac volume overload. Following the volume redistribution, hyperosmolar therapy results in diuresis, thus close monitoring of urinary output and IV fluid administration is necessary.[2]

Steroids are commonly used to reduce vasogenic cerebral edema for primary and metastatic brain tumors. Improvement in a patient's neurologic signs and mental status may be evident within hours of steroid administration due to the reduction in cerebral edema and ICP, which may continue to decrease for several days. However, steroids have not be shown to be beneficial in other neurosurgical disorders including TBI or spontaneous intracerebral hemorrhage. They may in fact have a detrimental effect.[2]

CONCLUSION

This 43-year-old patient presented with decreased mental status after a motor vehicle accident. His initial GCS was 6 (E1cV1M4), he was intubated during the primary survey and resuscitated with IV fluids. Primary and secondary surveys were completed, following the A/B/C/D/E protocol of Advanced Trauma Life Support, and a FAST displayed no free fluid in the abdomen. A CT was performed which showed a skull fracture and an unstable cervical fracture with cord compression. Emergent surgical intervention allowed for patient improvement, with persistent paraplegia below the level of the injury. Our discussion focused on the pathophysiology, assessment, management, and complications of 2 major conditions exhibited by our patient: spinal shock and intracranial hypertension. Major teaching points include:

- The Monro–Kellie hypothesis states that the sum of the intracranial volumes of CSF, brain, blood and other components is constant, and any increase in one volume must be offset by a decrease in another, or else the pressure increases.

- It is essential to maintain the mean arterial pressure to achieve adequate cerebral and spinal perfusion pressure

- Treatment goals should include Maintenance of ICP less than 20 to 25 mmHg.

- Maintenance of CPP greater than 60 mmHg with adequate MAP

Efforts should be focused on limiting factors that aggravate or precipitate elevated ICP.[2]

Although the patient was not able to make a full recovery, a strong understanding of these conditions is paramount to tailor management strategies for patients who present with multiple comorbid conditions involving the central nervous system.

REFERENCES

1. Hasler RM, Exadaktylos AK, Bouamra O, et al. Epidemiology and predictors of cervical spine injury in adult major trauma patients: a multicenter cohort study. J Trauma Acute Care Surg 2012;72:975–981.
2. Rangel-Castilla L, Gopinath S, Robertson CS. Management of intracranial hypertension. Neurol Clin. 2008;26(2):521–541.
3. Hansebout RR, Kachur E. Acute traumatic spinal cord injury. Post TW, ed. UpToDate Inc. https://www.uptodate.com. Accessed on March 2, 2019.
4. Stevens RD, Bhardwaj A, Kirsch JR, Mirski MA. Critical care and perioperative management in traumatic spinal cord injury. J Neurosurg Anesthesiol. 2003; 15(3):215–229.
5. Merlij GJ, Crabbe S, Paluzzi RG, Fritz D. Etiology, incidence, and prevention of deep vein thrombosis in acute spinal cord injury. Arch Phys Med Rehabil. 1993;74(11):1199–1205.
6. Hadley MN, Walters BC, Grabb PA, et al. Cervical spine immobilization before admission to the hospital. Neurosurgery 2002;50:S7–S17.
7. "The Brain Trauma Foundation. The American Association of Neurological Surgeons. Joint Section NeuroTrauma and Critical Care. Role of Antiseizure prophylaxis following Head Injury. Journal of Neurotrauma. 2000;17(6–7):549–553. http://doi.org/10.1089/neu.2000.17.549
8. Health, Myburgh J, Cooper DJ, Finfer S, et al.; SAFE Study Investigators; Australia and New Zealand Intensive Care Society Clinical Trials Group; Australian Red Cross Blood Service; George Institute for International Health. Saline or albumin for fluid resuscitation in patients with traumatic brain injury. N Engl J Med. 2007;357(9):874–884.
9. Institute of Neurological Sciences, Glasgow. What is the Glasgow Coma Scale? https://www.glasgowcomascale.org/what-is-gcs/. Accessed February 25, 2019.
10. Teasdale G, Jennett B. Assessment of coma and impaired consciousness: a practical scale. Lancet 1974;2:81–84. https://doi.org/10.1016/S0140-6736(74)91639-0.

REVIEW QUESTIONS

1. Steroids are indicated for the treatment of which of the following:

   A. TBI
   B. Vasogenic edema
   C. Acute spinal cord injury
   D. Epidural hematoma with midline shift

2. All of the following are determinants of spinal cord perfusion pressure, *except*

   A. SBP
   B. peak airway pressure
   C. ICP
   D. MAP

3. Which of the following neuromuscular blocking drugs may increase ICP?

   A. Neostigmine
   B. Atracurium
   C. Succinylcholine
   D. Rocuronium

4. The ICP treatment goals include all of the following *except*

   A. Maintenance of ICP less than 25 mmHg.
   B. Targeting CVP of 8–10mmHg.
   C. Maintenance of CPP greater than 60 mmHg.
   D. Limiting factors that aggravate elevated ICP

5. Which of the following is *least* likely to increase ICP?

   A. Use of PEEP at 5mmHg
   B. Bronchospasm
   C. Ventilator dyssynchrony
   D. $EtCO_2 = 45$mmHg

6. Which of the following is *not* a component of Cushing's triad?

   A. Hypertension
   B. Altered mental status
   C. Bradycardia
   D. Irregular breathing

7. Which of the following medications will cross a normal (intact) blood–brain barrier?

   A. Glycopyrrolate
   B. Mannitol
   C. Albumin
   D. Atropine

8. What test is the gold standard for ruling out elevated ICP?

   A. Lumbar puncture with opening pressure
   B. Absence of papilledema on fundoscopic examination
   C. Computed tomography
   D. Pupillary diameter on pupillometry

9. A low CSF pressure headache has all of the following characteristics, *except*

   A. Supine amelioration
   B. Photophobia
   C. Typically self-resolves
   D. Torticollis

10. Which of the following results from a rupture of bridging veins within the cranium?

   A. Subdural hematoma
   B. Subarachnoid hemorrhage
   C. Epidural hematoma
   D. Intraparenchymal hemorrhage

11. You go to see a patient who, upon evaluation, speaks in full sentences but is confused, localizes to painful stimuli, and opens eyes only in response to voice. What is this patient's Glasgow Coma Scale?

   A. 11
   B. 12
   C. 13
   D. 14

12. What is the sodium concentration (mEq/L) of 0.9% normal saline?

   A. 135
   B. 140
   C. 145
   D. 154

13. Which of the following drugs has been shown to decrease the incidence of seizures for the first 7 days after TBI and is recommended for seizure prophylaxis?

   A. Phenytoin
   B. Pentobarbital
   C. Propofol
   D. Oxcarbazepine

14. Which of the following is an absolute contraindication to 1.5 Tesla MRI of the brain after intracranial hemorrhage?

   A. Sternal closure wires from prior cardiac surgery
   B. Retained epicardial pacing wires from prior cardiac surgery
   C. Inferior vena cava filter
   D. CRT-D implanted cardiac defibrillator placed 12 weeks ago

15. Which of the following is the correct equation for mean arterial pressure?

   A. ⅓*(SBP) + ⅔*(DBP)
   B. (SBP +DBP)/2
   C. (SBP – CVP)*2 – DBP
   D. 2*(SBP – DBP)/3*(DBP)

16. When does the peak effect of mannitol occur to decrease intracerebral pressure?

   A. 0.1–0.3 hours
   B. 1.0–1.5 hours
   C. 0.3–1.0 hours
   D. 1.5–6 hours

17. Which of the following is *true* regarding cerebral autoregulation?

   A. It is rarely impaired, even in the setting of TBI.
   B. There is little change in cerebral blood flow between 50 mmHg to 150 mmHg.
   C. It is a vasodilatory response to high mean arterial pressure.
   D. It operates independent of partial pressure of CO_2.

18. What name is given regarding constant sum of intracranial volumes?

   A. Monroe Doctrine
   B. Pythagorean theorem
   C. Galen's theory
   D. Monro–Kellie hypothesis

19. Which levels of the sympathetic nervous system carry the cardiac accelerator fibers?

   A. T5–T12
   B. C7–C8
   C. T1–T4
   D. C3–C5

ANSWERS

1. B. Vasogenic edema. Steroids are commonly used to reduce vasogenic cerebral edema for primary and metastatic brain tumors. Steroids have not be shown to be beneficial in other neurosurgical disorders like TBI or spontaneous intracerebral hemorrhage, and in fact may have a detrimental effect.

2. B. Peak airway pressure. Although peak airway pressure may increase intrathoracic pressure, the equation for CPP, and thus, spinal cord perfusion pressure is CPP = MAP–ICP. MAP is determined by ⅓ SBP + ⅔ DBP.)

3. C. Succinylcholine. Succinylcholine is the only depolarizing neuromuscular blocking drug which will result in muscular contraction prior to inhibition of neuromuscular transmission. These "fasciculations" run the risk of elevating ICP. All of the other medications do not cause depolarization

by exerting their mechanism of action, and thus are least likely to increase ICP.

4. B. Targeting CVP = 8–10 mmHg. ICP treatment goals are A, C, and D, as listed in the discussion. There is no specific CVP target for management of ICP.

5. A. Use of PEEP at 5 mmHg. A low/physiologic dose of positive end expiratory pressure of 5 mmHg will merely overcome the resistance of the airway circuit and will have a negligible effect on venous drainage, and therefore will not significantly increase ICP. Bronchospasm and ventilator dyssynchrony will both result in much larger elevations in intrathoracic pressure, inhibiting cerebral venous drainage, thereby increasing ICP.

6. B. Altered mental status. Cushing's triad is a sign of impending cerebral herniation and encompasses three physical examination findings: hypertension (A), bradycardia (C), and irregular breathing patterns (D). Although altered mental status is frequently seen in these patients, it is not a part of the triad.

7. D. Atropine. Atropine (D) is the only substance listed, which will cross a physiologically normal (i.e., intact) blood–brain barrier, thus resulting in central anticholinergic effect of sedation. Glycopyrrolate (A) is a charged molecule at physiologic pH and therefore does not cross the blood–brain barrier. Mannitol (B) is a large molecule which does not cross the blood–brain barrier. Albumin (C) is a large, electrically negative protein, which also does not cross normal endothelium.

8. C. CT. Head CT (C) is the gold standard for ruling out elevations in ICP, as it is both sensitive and specific and should be performed prior to lumbar puncture in patients who may have elevated ICP. Lumbar puncture with opening pressure (A) allows the measurement of ICP, however, should not be used to rule out elevations, as cerebral herniation may occur if performed in patients with high ICP. Papilledema (B) is a physical exam finding that is indicative of elevated ICP but is not sensitive enough to effectively rule out the presence of elevated ICP. Pupillary diameter (D) does not reliably change with changes in ICP, however, loss of pupillary reflexes may indicated changes in ICP, often preceding herniation.

9. D. Torticollis (torticollis, or stiff-neck, is a part of the constellation of physical exam findings called "meningeal signs" and is not typically seen in low CSF pressure headaches. These headaches are usually self-resolving (C) and are characterized by exacerbation in upright position, amelioration in supine position (A), frontal in nature, and photophobia (B) commonly co-exists.

10. A. Subdural hematoma. Rupture of bridging veins results in a subdural hematoma, whereas arterial rupture, commonly of the middle meningeal artery, results in Epidural hematoma (C). Subarachnoid (B) and intraparynchymal (D) hemorrhages typically result from rupture of cerebral aneurysms or hemorrhagic cerebrovascular accidents.

11. B. 12. This patient's score is: E3M5V4 = 12.

12. D. 154 mEq/L. The sodium content of 0.9% normal saline is 154 mEq/L (D). The extracellular content of plasma is typically 140 mEq/L (B). The content of lactated Ringer's is approximately 135 mEq/L (A). The choice 145 mEq/L (C) is the upper limit of normal for extracellular plasma sodium concentration.

13. A. Phenytoin. Only phenytoin (A) has been shown to decrease the incidence of seizures in the first 7 days after TBI (see previous discussion). Although all answer choices will raise seizure threshold and decrease cerebral metabolic demand, phenytoin is the correct answer.

14. B. Retained epicardial pacing wires from prior cardiac surgery. Epicardial pacing wires are frequently cut after cardiac surgery and abandoned in situ. In this case, the patient will never be able to have an MRI (B). The other choices: inferior vena cava filter (C), CRT-D automated implantable cardioverter defibrillator placed more than 6 weeks ago (after 1996; D), and sternal closure wires (A) are all safe to undergo MRI at 1.5 Tesla. If the patient needs a 3 Tesla examination, each specific device should be checked with the manufacturer prior to the study.

15. A. ⅓*(SBP) + ⅔*(DBP). Choice A is the correct formula for mean arterial pressure; see previous discussion.

16. C. 0.3 to 1.0 hours. The time to peak effect of mannitol to reduce ICP is 0.3 to 1.0 hour, or 20 to 60 minutes (C). The duration of effect is 1.5 to 6 hours (D). A and B are incorrect.

17. B. There is little change in cerebral blood flow between 50 mmHg and 150 mmHg. Choice A is incorrect because TBI frequently results in loss of cerebral autoregulation. Autoregulation results in a vasoconstrictive response to high mean arterial pressure (C, incorrect), and a vasodilatory response to low MAP, both to regulate cerebral blood flow. The partial pressure of CO_2 (D) does indeed affect cerebral autoregulation, which is the rationale for moderate hyperventilation to a pCO_2 of 25 to 30 mmHg to decrease cerebral blood flow.

18. D. Monro–Kellie hypothesis. The Monro–Kellie hypothesis (D) states that the sum of the intracranial volumes of CSF, brain, blood, and other components is constant, and any increase in one volume must be offset by a decrease in another, or else the pressure increases. The Monroe Doctrine (A) is a U.S. policy of opposing European colonialism in the Americas beginning in 1823. The Pythagorean theorem (B) states the relationship between the squares of the three sides of triangle, $A^2 + B^2 = C^2$. Galen's theory (C) expresses that illness is caused by an imbalance of the four humors: blood, phlegm, black bile, and yellow bile.

19. C. T1–T4. The cardiac accelerator fibers are carried along the left sympathetic chain, typically at levels T1–T4 (C); see discussion. Choice A is incorrect as it is low thoracic (T5–12), which innervates the intercostals and adrenal glands but plays no direct role in cardiac innervation. There is little to no cervical innervation to the heart, and C3–C5 give rise to the phrenic nerve, which innervates the diaphragm (B and D).)

10.

ANTI-NMDA RECEPTOR ENCEPHALITIS

Jennifer McDonald and Steven E. Miller

An 18-year-old girl presents to the emergency department with a severe headache and facial twitching that started earlier this morning. When asked, she acknowledges that she has had recurrent headaches recently along with fevers and myalgias. While awaiting further testing in the emergency department, her condition worsens, and she begins to drool uncontrollably with increased facial and mouth twitching. An emergency computed tomography (CT) scan is ordered, but before it can be done she starts to exhibit tonic–clonic upper and lower extremity movements, and she is no longer responsive.

WHAT IS THE DIFFERENTIAL DIAGNOSIS FOR NEW ONSET SEIZURES IN THIS PATIENT?

She is given intravenous lorazepam and the seizure movements stop. Fosphenytoin is loaded at a dose of 15 mg/Kg over 15 minutes. She is transferred to the neurology stepdown unit for observation with stable vital signs but remains lethargic. After a few hours, she appears to be more energetic but is no longer making sense with her words and is progressively getting more agitated and confused. Another seizure occurs, but this time it takes lorazepam 2 mg and then another 4 mg before her movements stop again. Despite supplemental oxygen by mask, her saturations remain in the upper 80s. The decision is made to intubate her for respiratory support and airway protection; Propofol 2 mg/Kg and Rocuronium 0.5 mg/Kg is administered, and the intubation occurs without incidence.

WHAT IS THE NEXT STEP IN THE DIAGNOSTIC WORKUP FOR THIS PATIENT?

Before a sedative infusion can be started, she is wracked by another seizure. A loading dose of levetiracetam 1000 mg (15 mg/Kg) is loaded and her tonic–clonic movements cease again. She is started on 50 mcg/Kg/min of propofol for sedation with the adjuvant side effect that it might help shut down her seizures for a time. A full viral panel is sent, pancultures are taken, and a lumbar puncture is performed looking for an infectious etiology. A CT is finally done but reveals no bleeding or space occupying lesions of any kind. She is ordered for an magnetic resonance image (MRI), but she breaks through

her antiepileptic drugs into a tonic–clonic seizure again. The decision is made to institute a benzodiazepine coma and midazolam 0.5 mg/Kg is loaded and an infusion of 0.5 mg/Kg/hour is stated. The seizure doesn't break this time, and the midazolam is reloaded and the infusion increased to 1 mg/Kg/hour. The movements stop, but there is concern for nonconvulsive status epilepticus (NCSE) as she remains tachycardic and hypertensive despite the sedative infusions. Bedside electroencephalography (EEG) is applied and confirms NCSE; 1 mg/Kg of midazolam is given intravenously and then repeated until she achieves EEG silence. Her infusion rises to 3 mg/Kg, and her heart rate finally decreases but with it her blood pressure drops precipitously and she is started on a norepinephrine infusion.

IS MRI STILL APPROPRIATE GIVEN HER INSTABILITY? IS THERE A ROLE FOR BRAIN BIOPSY IF THERE IS ANYTHING ABNORMAL?

An MRI of her head with single-photon emission computed tomography (SPECT) and fluid attenuated inversion recovery (FLAIR) is performed with significant signs of bilateral hyperintensity on the FLAIR studies, right greater than left, in the temporal and hippocampal regions. To a lesser degree the parietal lobes, parasagittal frontal lobes, and sulci particularly towards the vertex all have increased FLAIR signals. Radiology reads the study as possible viral or bacterial meningitis, but things like vector-borne or herpes encephalitis could also present in this fashion. While awaiting cultures, she is started on broad-spectrum antibiotics and antivirals. An HIV Ab and viral load as well as HSV-1/2 Ab are added to the original labs sent. After 3 days, all the infectious markers have come back negative. The decision is made not to proceed to open brain biopsy in the face of overwhelmingly negative tests so far. She remains on midazolam infusion at very high doses as there are still signs of abnormal EEG bursts intermittently without NCSE.

WHAT IS THE TREATMENT REGIMEN FOR POSSIBLE AUTOIMMUNE ENCEPHALITIS? IS THERE ANY ROLE FOR FULL BODY IMAGING?

The decision is made to start high-dose steroids to treat possible autoimmune encephalitis, methylprednisolone 125 mg intravenous (IV) q8h and then to continue 50 mg IV q12. After 3 days, a repeat MRI reveals a significant improvement in FLAIR signal. Her midazolam infusion is stopped and 6 hours later she suffers another tonic–clonic seizure. The sedatives are restarted but now only 1.5 mg/Kg/hour is needed to obtain a near silent EEG. After some success with steroid therapy, the decision is made to try IV immunoglobulin (IVIg) 2 G/kg for 5 days. By the third day she has tolerated a reduction in midazolam infusion to 1 mg/Kg/hour but she breaks into urticarial and some expiratory wheezes are noted by the respiratory therapy team. Diphenhydramine and nebulizers are used to stabilize her allergic reaction, but she suffers a breakthrough seizure again and a midazolam bolus is given, and her infusion is raised back to its previous level.

The decision is made to send her for a full body CT scan with contrast looking for a source for her current syndrome. The CT scan discovers 2 cm masses in each of her ovaries, cystic in nature, and her right ovarian mass has an ossified center. Given its appearance there is a high suspicion for bilateral ovarian teratomas. In discussion with her family, her parents prefer not to remove her ovaries at this time.

CAN CONTROL OF AUTOIMMUNE ENCEPHALITIS BE ACHIEVED WITHOUT REMOVAL OF HER TERATOMAS?

She is instead started on weekly rituximab 375 mg/m² along with cyclophosphamide 750 mg/m² monthly. By her fifth week of therapy, she has been given a tracheostomy and percutaneous feeding tube as she is still suffering from an altered cognitive state. She has tolerated the withdrawal of her benzodiazepine infusion, but she remains on high doses of three different antiepileptic drugs and still has breakthrough seizures requiring IV benzodiazepines at times. Given her slow progression, her parents decide to go ahead with the bilateral oophorectomies. The laparoscopic surgery proceeds without complications and pathology confirms the masses were fully matured ovarian teratomas and the right mass even included a tooth. Over the next several weeks, she continues to improve more rapidly and is able to interact with physical and occupational therapy. A full year later, after much rehabilitation, she is able to return to high school to get her diploma.

DISCUSSION

NMDAR PRESENTATION

Unlike other types of paraneoplastic encephalidities, anti-NMDAR encephalitis presents predominantly in young women (4:1 female:male predominance), with a characteristic constellation of neuro-cognitive, dystonic and psychiatric symptoms, is highly responsive to treatment, and results in few long-term sequelae in patients who recover from the initial acute illness.[1-3] Monosymptomatic syndrome presentations are rare and occur in less than 5% of cases.[1,4]

Prodrome

Prior to presentation with acute neurologic or psychologic symptoms, many patients with anti-NMDAR encephalitis experience a non-specific viral prodrome, consisting of low-grade fever, headache, nausea, vomiting, diarrhea or upper respiratory tract symptoms.[1,5] It is unclear if the prodrome is an initial immune activation or an unrelated non-specific viral illness is unknown.[3]

Psychiatric Symptoms

Initial psychiatric symptoms can include emotional disturbances (such as apathy, anxiety or depression, fear, and/or loneliness)[3] and may progress to more severe symptoms such as impaired impulse control, inappropriate or bizarre behaviors, hypersexuality, hyperreligiosity, paranoia, or social withdrawal.[1,6] In children, behavioral changes may manifest as temper tantrums, hyperactivity, or irritability.[1]

Acute psychiatric symptoms displayed by patients included personality or behavioral changes bizarre behaviors, delusional or paranoid thoughts, and hallucinations[7] that may progress to confusion, restlessness, anxiety or agitation, slurring of words or echolalia,[3] and disintegration of language[1] Progressive symptoms included inappropriate smiling, mutism, unresponsiveness to verbal commands.[2]

Due to these symptoms, patients often present initially to psychiatrists or diagnosed with psychiatric disorder.[2-5]

Neurologic Symptoms

Neuro-psychological symptoms attributable to NMDAR Encephalitis may include abnormal movements (ataxia, ocular deviation or disconjugation, choreoathetosis, dystonia, opisthotonis posturing, catatonia) as well as characteristic oro-facio-lingual movements, which include lip-smacking or licking, chewing movements, jaw opening, grimacing.[5] Some patients experience cognitive decline prior to more severe neurologic symptoms, such as decreased attention, impaired working memory, and executive function resulting in confusion and/or inability to perform previously simple tasks.[2,6] Progression of disease often includes development of generalized or partial complex seizures, decreased level of consciousness (including catatonic-like episodes) and dissociative responses similar to the states induced by NMDAR antagonists such as phencyclidine or ketamine.[1,5] Advanced neurologic signs include central hypoventilation requiring mechanical ventilation, and a late-state neurological manifestation of NMDAR encephalitis is autonomic instability, which can include tachycardia, diaphoresis, tachypnea, hypertension, or labile blood pressures.[2,3] Severe autonomic dysfunction can manifest as autonomic "storms" causing fluctuation from tachycardia to bradycardia with cardiac pauses.[1] For patients with psychiatric symptoms treated with antipsychotics, the progression to rigidity and autonomic instability may mimic symptoms of neuroleptic malignant syndrome.[1]

DIFFERENTIAL DIAGNOSIS

- Viral encephalitides such as Herpes (HSV, HHV-6, VZV), arbovirus (West Nile, EEE, WEE), Rhabdovirus (rabies)

- Autoimmune disorders including systemic lupus erythematosus cerebritis, Sjögren's syndrome

- Intracranial tumor—primary mass or metastasis

- Cerebral infection such as toxoplasmosis, tuberculosis, HIV

- Toxic ingestion

- Neuroleptic malignant syndrome or serotonin syndrome

- Acute psychotic episode or schizophrenia

- Malingering

Cognitive decline without delirium may be a useful sign for consideration of autoimmune encephalitis.[6] Due to the prevalence of psychiatric symptoms seen in anti-NMDAR encephalitis, testing for antibodies to the NR1 subunit of the NMDA receptor should be considered in any patient (especially women under 50 years old) demonstrating new-onset psychosis, particularly if accompanied by neurologic symptoms (dyskinesias, speech disorders, memory deficit, seizures, or autonomic dysfunction).[1,7,8]

DIAGNOSTIC MODALITIES AND RELEVANT CLINICAL STUDIES

CSF

Initial cerebral spinal fluid (CSF) evaluation may demonstrate lymphocytic pleocytosis often with increased protein concentration and normal glucose, oftentimes with oligoclonal bands.[1,5] A sine qua non of NMDAR encephalitis is the presence of antibodies to the NMDA receptor.[5] Gresa Arribas et al. found that the presence of NMDAR Antibodies in the CSF is 100% sensitive for patients with disease (as compared to 85% sensitivity in serum) and 100% specific.[9] The severity of patient symptoms and/or recovery correlates to CSF NMDAR antibody titers.[3,5] Serial CSF antibody titers that decreased earlier and to a greater extent appear to prognosticate a good outcome, although, interestingly, most patients ultimately have a decrease in both serum and CSF titers regardless of outcome.[9]

Serum

Serum antibodies to the NR1/NR2B heteromer of the NMDAR were found in a majority of patients,[2] which, like antibody titers in the CSF, usually decrease or are not found during the recovery and rehabilitation phase.[2,3] Serum testing alone may miss >10% diagnoses of NMDAR encephalitis, but is more likely correlated to presence of teratoma. Serum titers are higher in patients with teratoma, and those without teratoma who have a poor outcome.[9] However, post recovery,

patients may still have persistently high serum titers without detectable titers in the CSF, suggestive of an immune process that was initially triggered systemically by a tumor.[1]

MRI and SPECT

MRI is abnormal in 50% of patients (abnormalities consisted of FLAIR sequences involving hippocampi, cerebral, and cerebellar cortex),[1] while SPECT may show nonspecific variable multifocal cortical and subcortical abnormalities.

Electroencephalography

EEG can show nonspecific, slow or disorganized activity consistent with diffuse cerebral dysfunction, and slow, rhythmic activity in the delta–theta range that predominates in the catatonic-like state.[10]

Brain biopsy does not aid in the diagnosis of NMDAR encephalitis.[1]

Tumor Screening

Ovarian teratoma is found in more than half of patients who present with anti-NMDAR encephalitis.[3] Black women are more likely to have a tumor when compared to other ethnic groups.[1] Tumors are detected in only 5% of male patients.[1] MRI, CT, and ultrasound (pelvic and transvaginal) scans are useful screening tools for tumor. Other serological tumor markers are frequently negative.[1]

In some patients, tumors are only identified after exploratory laparoscopies.

MECHANISM OF NMDAR ENCEPHALITIS

The NMDA receptor is composed of 2 subunits: the NR1 (glycine-binding) subunit and the NR2 (glutamate-binding) subunit. Expression of the NR1/NR2B heteromer of the NMDAR is found preferentially in the prefrontal cortex, amygdala, and hypothalamus and is essential in neuronal plasticity, learning, and memory. Density of expression of the NR2B subunit-containing NMDAR correlates with the increased reactivity with the anti-NMDAR antibodies in the hippocampus and forebrain and plays a role in executive function and memory.[11] Decreased NMDAR activity is associated with schizophrenia and NMDAR-binding drugs can cause hallucinations, paranoia, and dyskinesias.[8,12] The decreased NMDAR function associated with dysregulated glutamate release and increased corticomotor excitability[13] can account for the behavioral deficits in patients with the disease.[14]

At autopsy, immunoglobulin G (IgG) deposits were discovered in the hippocampus and amygdala without evidence of complement deposits.[15] The lack of complement and cytotoxic T-cell deposits in brain tissue, as well as the reversibility of NMDAR dysfunction with disease resolution, suggest a *functional* disruption of NMDARs, rather than irreversible, T-cell-mediated damage.[15] Dalmau et al. demonstrated a concentration-dependent decrease in cell-surface fraction of synaptic NMDAR in rat hippocampal samples when exposed to patients' IgG, which was later reversed when IgG exposure was removed,[3] suggesting selective antibody-mediated capping and internalization of surface NMDARs in a titer-dependent fashion, as the structural integrity of the neurons and synapses was not affected.[14] Other GABA-ergic receptors, such as AMPA receptors, are not affected by anti-NMDAR antibodies.[14]

Development of anti-NMDAR encephalitis may be triggered by an infectious process, as suggested by evidence of concurrent infection or, in rare cases, recent vaccination or booster vaccination.[1] Tumors removed from patients with NMDAR encephalitis often contained neural tissue with expression of NMDARs.[3,5] Most patients (80%)[1] have intrathecal production of antibodies: Dalmau et al. demonstrated intact blood–brain barriers in 53 of 58 patients, suggesting intrathecal synthesis of antibodies, as well as higher CSF antibody titers when compared to serum titers.[3] Furthermore, CSF titers were slower to decrease than serum titers. Dalmau et al. suggest that, similar to lupus models, infection or hypertension may make the blood–brain barrier more susceptible to antibody penetration into the central nervous system.[5]

TREATMENT

Initial Treatment

First-line immunotherapy

- Corticosteroids
- IVIg
- Plasma exchange or plasmapheresis[16]

According to Dalmau's unpublished data, only 48% of patients without tumor have improvement to first-line immunotherapy.[1] All 3 initial treatment modalities have an inability to cross the blood–brain barrier, and given that most patients have intrathecal synthesis of antibodies, it explains why many patients do not improve with initial first-line immunotherapy.[8]

Second-Line Immunotherapy

Patients who did not respond to initial immunomodulatory therapy showed improvement when given rituximab (an anti-CD20 monoclonal antibody that targets B cells)[1,15,17] and also appear to benefit from cyclophosphamide, which crosses the blood–brain barrier.[3,16] Furthermore, second-line immunotherapy may decrease the risk of recurrence.[8]

Other proposed immunotherapies include alemtuzumab, an anti-CD52 monoclonal antibody affecting memory B and T cells has (given concurrently with intrathecal methotrexate administration)[18] and bortezomib (when combined with rituximab), which eliminates plasma cells, but does not cross the blood–brain barrier, both of which have demonstrated benefit.[8]

Surgical Resection of Ovarian Teratoma

Identification of teratoma is considered a good prognostic factor.[3] While tumor removal decreases the severity and duration

of symptoms, spontaneous recovery without tumor removal has been identified.[2]

Special Patient Populations

Dalmau et al. report 3 pregnant patients who were treated safely with first-line immunotherapy, and recovery improved after delivery or termination of pregnancy.[1]

Supportive Treatment

Administration of anti-epileptic medications to decrease seizure frequency and incidence of abnormal movements can be attempted. However, seizure-like activity attributable to anti-NMDAR encephalitis is not typically amenable to anti-epileptic drugs, and some severe cases of status epilepticus have required phenobarbital-induced coma.[1] Initial treatments aimed at alleviating persistent dyskinesias such as anti-epileptics (phenytoin, phenobarbital, valproate) or antipsychotics (quetiapine, haloperidol) can be given, but are often insufficient to treat dyskinesias, and anesthetics such as propofol and/or midazolam infusions have been used with good effect. In rare cases, despite adequate sedation, dyskinesias can be severe enough to necessitate a short period of non-depolarizing neuro-muscular junction antagonists to prevent injury (Dalmau, unpublished data). Patients with severe movement disorders requiring prolonged sedation are at risk for propofol infusion syndrome, especially considering they are often treated concomitantly with steroids (which is an independent risk factor for propofol infusion syndrome).[1]

Intensive care unit level care is typically required for patients with autonomic instability. Continuous cardiac and hemodynamic monitoring may be required for patients with hyper- or hypotension or blood pressure lability, and temporary pacing may be necessary for patients with prolonged cardiac pauses or asystole.[19,20] Prolonged mechanical ventilation may be required for patients with severe hypoventilation.[2]

PROGNOSIS AND RECOVERY

The reversible nature of the internalization of the NMDAR (as opposed to a cytotoxic effect) can account for the dramatic and rapid recovery of patients with anti-NMDAR encephalitis when compared to permanent dysfunction seen in other paraneoplastic encephalidities. Approximately 75% of patients with NMDAR encephalitis have a favorable outcome (full recovery or mild sequelae), but the remainder of patients have severe, persistent disability or die.[1] Mortality is estimated at 4%, with death occurring, on average, of 3.5 months from disease onset. Causes of death included sepsis, sudden cardiac arrest, acute respiratory distress or failure, refractory *status epilepticus*, or tumor progression.[1]

Initial

While recovery is generally takes weeks to months before significant clinical improvement (median of 12 weeks),[7] patients with early identification and resection of tumor (within the first 4 months since onset) show more rapid recovery (8 weeks vs. 10–11 weeks) with fewer severe deficits compared to patients with unrecognized tumor or no tumor.[3]

Long-Term Recovery and Sequelae

Although initial response to treatment may be rapid (as compared to other encephalidities), full recovery can be protracted, lasting up to 3 years. Many patients require prolonged hospitalization (at least 3–4 months).[1] Recovery occurs gradually as a multistage process in reverse order of symptom presentation, with delayed or incomplete restoration of pre-illness social behavior and/or executive function.[1] Even patients who show full recovery or recovery with only mild deficits continue to have evidence of frontal lobe dysfunction (including poor inhibition and/or impulse control, poor attention, and/or deficits of executive function and memory).[3,21] Short-term memory testing can reveal more subtle deficits in attention, working memory, executive functions, and general intellectual abilities that affect daily activities persisting for several years after resolution of acute disease.[18] Better cognitive outcome occurred in patients with early immunotherapy as compared to delayed immunotherapy.[18]

Relapses

Relapses occur in 20% to 25% of patients,[1,22] and are seen more commonly in patients with unrecognized tumor or no tumor or patients for whom immunotherapy was delayed.[19] Relapses may present with partial aspects of the syndrome, with speech disorder, psychiatric symptoms, conscious-attention disturbance, and/or seizures as the most common manifestations. Relapses presenting as typical NMDAR encephalitis were comparatively rare.[19] Periodic screening for teratomas is recommended for at least 2 years following recovery.[1]

FUTURE DIRECTION

At the time of writing, a small study is underway to evaluate the efficacy of transcranial direct current stimulation on cognitive dysfunction due to decreased cortical plasticity,[23] and recruitment has not yet begun for a trial examining immunoadsorption therapy with short- and long-term follow-up.[24]

CONCLUSION

- Reversible neuro-psychiatric condition
- Increased index of suspicion
- Early immunological and tumor excision (if appropriate)
- Supportive care, including intensive care unit management, as needed
- Second-line treatment for refractory cases
- Appropriate counseling of patient and family
- Rehabilitation and follow-up care.

RECOMMENDED READING

Graus F, Titulaer MJ, Balu R, et al. A clinical approach to diagnosis of autoimmune encephalitis. *Lancet Neurol* 2016;15:391–404.
Dalmau J, Lancaster E, Martinez-Hernandez E, et al. Clinical experience and laboratory investigations in patients with anti-NMDAR encephalitis. *Lancet Neurol* 2011;10:63–74.

REFERENCES

1. Dalmau J, Lancaster E, Martinez-Hernandez E, et al. Clinical experience and laboratory investigations in patients with anti-NMDAR encephalitis. *Lancet Neurol* 2011;10:63–74.
2. Iizuka I, Sakai F, Ide T, et al. Anti-NMDA receptor encephalitis in Japan: long-term outcome without tumor removal. *Neurology* 2008;70:504–511.
3. Dalmau J, Gleichman AJ, Hughes EG, et al. Anti-NMDA-receptor encephalitis: case series and analysis of the effects of antibodies. *Lancet Neurol* 2008;7:1091–1098.
4. Panzer JA, Lynch DR. Treatment of anti-NMDA receptor encephalitis—time to be bold? *Nat Rev Neurol* 2013;9:187–189.
5. Dalmau J, Tüzün E, Wu H, et al. Paraneoplastic anti-N-methyl-D-aspartate Receptor encephalitis associated with ovarian teratoma. *Ann Neurol* 2007;61:25–36.
6. Vahter L, Kannel K, Sorro U, et al. Cognitive dysfunction during anti-NMDA-receptor encephalitis is present in early phase of the disease. *Oxford Medical Case Reports* 2014; 4:74–76.
7. Vitaliani R, Mason W, Ances B, et al. Paraneoplastic encephalitis, psychiatric symptoms, and hypoventilation in ovarian teratoma. *Ann Neurol* 2005;58(4):594–604.
8. Titulaer MJ, Kayser MS, Dalmau J. Prevalence and treatment of anti-NMDA receptor encephalitis—author's reply. *Lancet Neurol* 2013;12:424–426.
9. Gresa-Arribas N, Titulaer MJ, Torrents A, et al. Antibody titres at diagnosis and during follow-up of anti-NMDA receptor encephalitis: a retrospective study. *Lancet Neurol* 2014;13:167–177.
10. Florence NR, Davis RL, Lam C, et al. Anti-N-methyl-D-aspartate receptor (NMDAR) encephalitis in children and adolescents. *Ann Neurol* 2009;66:11–18.
11. Morris RG, Anderson E, Lynch GS, et al. Selective impairment of learning and blockade of long-term potentiation by an N-methyl-D-aspartate receptor agonist AP5. *Nature* 1986;319:774–776.
12. Lynch DR, Guttmann RP. Excitotoxicity: perspectives based on N-methyl-D-aspartate receptor subtypes. *J Pharmacol Exp Ther* 2002;300:717–723.
13. Manto M, Dalmau J, Didelot A, et al. Afferent facilitation of corticomotor responses is increased by IgGs of patients with NMDA-receptor antibodies. *J Neurol* 201; 258:27–33.
14. Hughes EG, Peng X, Gleichman AJ, et al. Cellular and synaptic mechanisms of anti-NMDA receptor encephalitis. *J Neurosci* 2010;30(17):5866–5875.
15. Lancaster E, Dalmau J. Neuronal autoantegens—pathogenesis, associated disorders and antibody testing. *Nat Rev Neurol* 2012;8(7):380–390.
16. Bartolini L. How do you treat anti-NMDA receptor encephalitis? *Neurol Clin Pract* 2016;6:69–72.
17. Ishiura H, Matsuda S, Higashihara M, et al. Response of anti-NMDA receptor encephalitis without tumor to immunotherapy including rituximab. *Neurology* 2008;71:1921–1923.
18. Liba Z, Seronova V, Komarel V, et al. Prevalence and treatment of anti-NMDA receptor encephalitis—correspondence. *Lancet Neurol* 2013;12:424–425.
19. Nazif TM, Vázquez J, Honig LS, et al. Anti-N-methyl-D-aspartate receptor encephalitis: an emerging cause of centrally mediated sinus node dysfunction. *Europace* 2012;14:1188–1194.
20. Mehr SR, Neeley RC, Wiley M, et al. Profound autonomic instability complicated by multiple episodes of cardiac asystole and refractory

bradycardia in a patient with anti-NMDR encephalitis. *Case Rep Neurol Med* 2016;2016:7967526.

21. Finke C, Kopp UA, Prüss H, et al. Cognitive deficits following anti-NMDA receptor encephalitis. *J Neurol Neurosurg Psychiatry* 2012;83(2):195–198. doi:10.1136/jnnp-2011-300411.

22. Gabilondo I, Saiz A, Galán L, et al. Analysis of relapses in anti-NMDAR encephalitis. *Neurology* 2001;77:996–999.

23. Transcranial direct current stimulation on cortical plasticity in patients with anti-NMDA receptor encephalitis. ClinicalTrials.gov: NCT01865578.

24. Prospective assessment of efficacy of immunoadsorption therapy in managing childhood NMDA-receptor (NMDAR) antibodies encephalitis. ClinicalTrials.gov: NCT03274375.

SUPPLEMENTAL CHARTS AND IMAGES

IMMUNOMODULATORY PROTOCOL

First Line
IVIg 0.4 g/kg/day × 5 days
Methylprednisolone 1 g/day × 5 days
With clinical evaluation after 10 to 15 days

Second Line
Rituximab 375 mg/m^2/week × 4 weeks
Cyclophosphamide 750 mg/m^2/month × 4–6 months
Ongoing Treatment for Patients Without Tumor
Mycophenolate mofetil or azathioprine × 1 year
Comprehensive Immunotherapy
Rituximab
Plasmapheresis (6 treatments over 10 days)
IVIg
Methylprednisolone
Source: Dalmau[1] and Bartolini[16]

CHAPTER REVIEW QUESTIONS

1. For patients diagnosed with NMDAR Encephalitis, anticipated recovery would be expected to be

   A. immediate, with no or minimal residual dysfunction.
   B. gradual (over many weeks to months), but with no residual dysfunction or only mild deficits.
   C. initially a fast recovery, but with persistent residual dysfunction.
   D. gradual improvement with persistent residual dysfunction.

Answer: B. Initial recovery can take weeks to months, but 75% of patients have a favorable outcome (full-recovery or mild sequelae).

2. Initial (first-line) treatment of NMDAR encephalitis should include (choose all that apply)

   A. IVIg
   B. Steroids
   C. Rituximab
   D. Cyclophosphamide

Answer: A and B. IVIg, corticosteroids and plasma exchange are considered first-line therapy for Anti-NMDAR Encephalitis. Rituximab and cyclophosphamide are considered second-line treatments.

3. Good prognostic indicators include (choose all that apply)

   A. Decrease in anti-NMDAR titers in CSF after initial treatment
   B. Presence of a teratoma
   C. Female sex

Answer: A and B. Although teratoma is only present in 5% of male patients, male sex is not considered to be an independent risk factor for poor prognosis.

4. The most sensitive and specific diagnostic test for NMDAR encephalitis is

   A. anti-NMDAR serum titers
   B. anti-NMDAR CSF titers
   C. EEG
   D. MRI

Answer: B. Presence of Anti-NMDAR Antibodies in CSF titers is both highly sensitive and highly specific for Anti-NMDAR Encephalitis. Serum titers are less sensitive than CSF titers but tend to correlate with presence of a teratoma. EEG, MRI, and SPECT are nonspecific for anti-NMDAR encephalitis.

5. After confirmation of diagnosis of Anti-NMDAR Encephalitis, subsequent diagnostic testing should include

_____.

Answer: MRI, CT, or ultrasound tumor screening for teratoma.

6. True or false: Most patients respond to initial (first-line) treatment of anti-NMDAR encephalitis.

Answer: False. Fewer than 50% of patients respond to initial treatments, as most patients have intrathecal synthesis of anti-NMDAR antibodies and these modalities do not cross the blood–brain barrier.

7. In addition to psychiatric illness, which of the following should prompt a higher index of suspicion for anti-NMDAR encephalitis?

   A. Long-standing history of psychiatric disease.
   B. Age >50.
   C. Neuro-psychologic symptoms, such as abnormal oro-facio-lingual movements.
   D. Male sex

Answer: C. Psychiatric symptoms of anti-NMDAR encephalitis are typically sudden-onset without long-standing history of prior disease. Anti-NMDAR encephalitis is more prevalent in young women.

11.

MANAGEMENT OF ACUTE ISCHEMIC STROKE WITH INTERVENTIONAL CLOT RETRIEVAL

Neil A. Nadkarni and Ayush Batra

STEM CASE AND KEY QUESTIONS

A 63-year-old right-handed woman with a prior medical history of hypertension and hyperlipidemia presented to a hospital emergency room 2½ hours after developing weakness on the right side with marked difficulty in communication witnessed by her daughter. Her blood glucose was normal. Vital signs are notable for an irregularly irregular pulse and blood pressure of 190/110 mmHg. Neurology is immediately consulted and an National Institutes of Health Stroke Scale (NIHSS) was performed that revealed a stroke scale of 14 for alteration of consciousness, inability to follow commands, left gaze preference, right hemianopia, right facial paresis, right hemiparesis (arm greater than leg), and a moderate global aphasia. She is rushed to radiology for a noncontrast computed tomography (CT) scan of her head. The radiologist reads the CT scan as "no sign of acute stroke is seen."

THE CT BRAIN SHOWS NO EVIDENCE OF HEMORRHAGE OR INFARCTION. DOES THE PATIENT HAVE A STROKE? WHAT SYNDROME DOES THIS PATIENT HAVE? WHAT IS THE IMMEDIATE NEXT DIAGNOSTIC TESTING REQUIRED?

Neurology is called and a diagnosis of left middle cerebral artery (MCA) acute stroke syndrome is made given the constellation of symptoms (cortical signs present on neurological examination including aphasia, hemianopia, and gaze preference toward side of lesion in combination with a contralateral hemiparesis of face and arm greater than leg). A second CT is ordered, this time including angiography with perfusion imaging of the head and neck, and it confirms a left MCA and left internal carotid artery (ICA) occlusion with a hyperdensity within the region of the left MCA territory. (See Figures 11.1 and 11.2.)

WHAT ARE THE NEXT STEPS IN WORKUP AND/OR TREATMENT?

Labetalol is given intravenously and her blood pressure decreases to 175/95 mmHg. The decision is made to deliver

alteplase for thrombolysis, and blood pressure monitoring frequency is increased. However, there is no apparent improvement in symptoms.

A normal CT excludes intracranial hemorrhage (ICH) but does not have the sensitivity to diagnose an acute ischemic stroke (AIS) (1). Early ischemic signs include hyperdense MCA sign, early hypodensity in the lenticular nucleus, loss of the insular ribbon, hemispheric sulcal effacement, and loss of the gray–white matter interface (2). There is no evidence of early hypodensity within the suspected ischemic territory on the CT brain, although there is evidence of a hyperdensity within the left MCA proximal territory. The decision is made to take her immediately to interventional radiology for

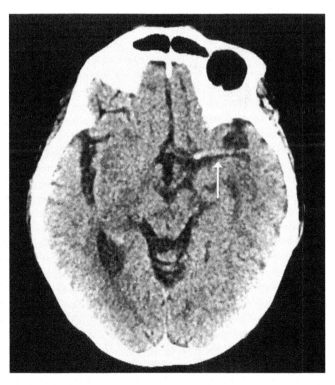

Figure 11.1 Noncontrast CT brain in acute ischemic stroke with suspected large vessel occlusion. A stat CT brain image reveals no hemorrhage and no clear hypodensity indicative of stroke. Of note, there is a hyperdensity in the left MCA (arrow) suggestive of clot (hyperdense left MCA sign).

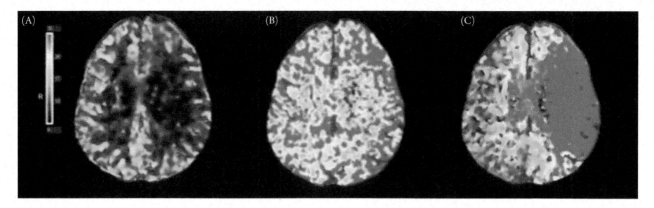

Figure 11.2 CT perfusion of the brain in acute ischemic stroke with large vessel occlusion. Perfusion based CT imaging reveals no change in flow for (A) cerebral blood flow with delays in the left hemisphere for both (B) mean transit time and (C) time to peak.

mechanical thrombectomy for large vessel occlusion (LVO), and the anesthesia team is activated for support.

WHAT KIND OF ANESTHESIA SUPPORT MUST BE GIVEN AS THE PATIENT GOES TO THE ANGIOGRAPHY SUITE?

As she is not agitated nor combative, the decision is made to attempt the procedure using monitored anesthesia care at the start. Minimal doses of propofol are used to facilitate the patient's comfort, and the anesthesia gives the go-ahead to continue.

WHAT HAPPENS DURING A MECHANICAL THROMBECTOMY? HOW IS REPERFUSION ACHIEVED AND CONFIRMED?

After appropriate vascular access is established (either through the femoral artery or less commonly the brachial or radial arteries), angiography of the left ICA demonstrates a partially occlusive thrombus at the nexus of the posterior cavernous segment of the left ICA and proximal MCA. Aspiration thrombectomy based on the ADAPT technique (9) is initially used after which repeat angiography demonstrates recanalization of the left ICA cavernous segment but propagation of a smaller thrombus in the left MCA inferior division. Thus, the recanalization of the left ICA vessel did not lead to reperfusion of the MCA at this point. Subsequently, a microcatheter was advanced distally to the clot after which a stent retriever was deployed with aspiration thrombectomy of the left MCA segment. A final repeat angiography of the left ICA and common carotid artery is performed and demonstrates complete recanalization of the left MCA territory, graded TICI-3, and the patient's hemiparesis on the right side immediately improves. The systemic blood pressure is immediately reduced, typically below a systolic blood pressure of 160 mmHg, to minimize risk of subsequent reperfusion injury. The right femoral artery access site in the groin is sealed off with a vascular closure device, and pressure is maintained on the site prior to transferring the patient to the neurocritical care intensive care unit. (See Figure 11.3.)

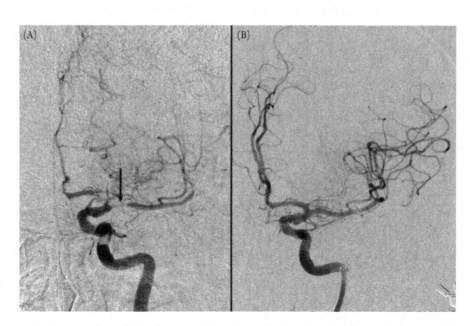

Figure 11.3 Cerebral angiography during mechanical thrombectomy. (A) Occlusive clot (arrow) at the left MCA bifurcation. (B) TICI 3 recanalization is achieved postprocedurally.

She is placed on telemetry, an echocardiogram is ordered, as well as a full lipid panel and hemoglobin A1C. She starts physical and occupational therapy and is showing significant improvement and is successfully discharged to subacute rehabilitation.

DISCUSSION

Stroke is the leading cause of disability worldwide and the fifth leading cause of death in the United States with 795,000 cases a year, 87% of which are ischemic strokes (11). AIS signifies actionable stroke syndromes for which therapy can be offered to salvage brain tissue and limit degree of disability. LVOs—which involve sudden thrombosis or embolus of vertebral, basilar, carotid terminus, and middle and anterior cerebral arteries—comprise 46% of stroke syndromes (12). LVOs also portend a worse outcome than strokes resulting from small vessel disease. Notably, 13% of LVOs can actually present as transient ischemic attacks (TIAs) or stroke with NIHSS <6, thus underscoring the importance of obtaining vessel imaging for symptoms of AIS (12).

DIFFERENTIAL DIAGNOSIS

The broad differential diagnosis for this condition includes other seizure/postictal phenomena; underlying mass lesion or tumor; and infectious etiologies such as meningitis, hypertensive encephalopathy, and migraine but the most likely in this scenario is an AIS with LVO. CT imaging of the brain is required to help differentiate the causes and exclude emergent life-threatening issues such as ICH.

ETIOLOGY/PATHOGENESIS OF ARTERIAL ISCHEMIC STROKE/LVO

Stroke is in fact a syndrome and not a cause of disease per se. AIS is due to either thrombus or embolus, but the mechanisms by which these occur are manifold. Determining the etiology is critical for secondary prevention. Atrial fibrillation/arrhythmia is a major risk factor for stroke by embolic mechanism, with patients having a 3- to 5-fold higher risk after adjustment for risk factors and warrants lifelong anticoagulation. Extracranial atherosclerotic disease is another common cause with predominant artery-to-artery embolism from this location causing stroke syndromes and warranting investigation for carotid endarterectomy. Intracranial atherosclerotic disease is varied in its mechanism of stroke, including artery-to-artery embolism, in situ thrombo-occlusion, and local branch occlusion. Younger patients and those who are subject to trauma have higher rates of carotid/vertebral

dissection. Patients with long-bone fractures can be vulnerable to fat embolism. Small-vessel ischemic disease is often by in-situ thrombosis and a sequelae of chronic hypertension and hyperlipidemia. Although there are many more causes of stroke, these are among the most common and should guide decision-making on next steps in secondary prevention with appropriate neurology evaluation.

CLINICAL MANIFESTATION/DIFFERENTIAL DIAGNOSIS OF AIS/LVO

The clinical key for determining AIS/LVO at the bedside is to assess for cortical signs. Cortex is the gray matter on the surface of the brain that includes the frontal, temporal, parietal, and occipital lobes. Subcortical structures include everything else such as cerebellum, brainstem, thalamus, hypothalamus, basal ganglia, and all white matter. Cortical deficits encompass a range of higher-order functions as well as specific patterns of weakness different from subcortical lesions. Examples of cortical deficits include aphasia, neglect, gaze preference, hemianopia, and disproportionate weakness between the face and arm compared to the leg. Subcortical deficits include extraocular movement impairments, nausea, vertigo, nystagmus and diplopia, ataxia, and equal loss in sensation/strength in the face, arm and leg. Although basilar artery occlusions/thromboses can present with subcortical signs as TIAs or small emboli, further workup with vessel imaging is necessary to determine if there is an actionable LVO as this condition carries a high morbidity.

DIAGNOSTIC TESTS FOR AIS/LVO

CT Brain

Early features of ischemic stroke on noncontrast head CT can include hyperdense vessels, loss of gray–white matter differentiation, and hypoattenuation of deep nuclei. The Alberta Stroke Program Early CT Score (ASPECTS) is a 10-point quantitative score that provides reliable and reproducible detection of early (<3 hours from symptom onset) ischemic changes in patients suspected of having an acute LVO that measures various points on the caudate, lentiform nucleus, insula, and internal capsule. A point is subtracted from 10 for each of the prespecified areas with evidence of hypodensity. Scores greater than 6 were required for the thrombectomy trials and higher scores predicted the ability for better outcome (16).

CT Angiography

The administration of a contrast bolus through a large-bore intravenous (IV) needle allows for visualization of the filling defect, as well as structural evaluation of the vessels for dissection or atherosclerosis. Contrast enhanced vessel imaging also helps differentiate neurologic stroke mimics such as seizure or migraine. Furthermore, this test has proved useful in assisting interventional planning by not only localizing the suspected clot but also informing the operator of variant vascular anatomy of the aortic arch or intracranial circulation.

CT Perfusion

CT perfusion findings have good agreement with diffusion weight imaging (DWI) and perfusion magnetic resonance imaging (17). There are 3 major regions of the brain for interest in consideration for salvage therapy. Ischemic core is defined as an irreversible area of infarction. Penumbra is severely hypoperfused and nonfunctional, but still viable brain tissue, which surrounds the core. Benign oligemia is tissue area that is ischemic but will recover spontaneously.

CT perfusion involves the recursive scanning of a selected area of brain as contrast passes through an area. Several metrics in CT perfusion are used in parallel to help delineate areas for salvage therapy by measuring cerebral blood perfusion (18). These include (i) cerebral blood volume (CBV), (ii) cerebral blood flow (CBF), (iii) mean transit time (MTT), and (iv) time to peak (TTP). Collectively, these parameters (Table 11.1) will help decide if there is a mismatch in specific parts of the brain thereby amenable to intervention.

Broadly, penumbra can be estimated by delayed MTT/TTP/time to maximum plasma concentration (TMax) but compensated CBF/CBV while infarct core can be defined by delayed MTT/TTP/TMax and insufficient CBV/CBF (19). Every scanning system has its own characteristic color-coded bars, so careful interpretation is required. The length of time that the penumbra can compensate depends upon vasodilation and increase in total blood volume as well as appropriate collateral. The point at which this cannot occur anymore results in reduced CBV and subsequent ischemic core.

Magnetic Resonance Imaging

Although MRI is in fact the gold standard for stroke diagnosis, extensive costs, accessibility, and problems with workflow have limited its broad adoption in AIS therapy. DWI, a function of the rate of movement of water in tissue, demonstrates increased signal within minutes of ischemia when combined with decreased signal in the apparent diffusion coefficient. Changes in fluid attenuated inversion recovery sequences typically occur after 6 to 12 hours. A recent study has co-opted this natural timing to study the effect on alteplase in wake-up strokes—a population which previously had a prolonged last-known normal and therefore was ineligible for systemic thrombolysis. The study demonstrated a benefit for those patients who had a DWI+/fluid attenuated inversion recovery mismatch and suggest a possibility for re-introducing emergent MRI for this specific population (20).

Angiography

Recanalization and reperfusion, although often loosely interchanged in discussion, are different standards by which the success of procedure is measured (21). Recanalization measures the direct action of therapeutic intervention on treatment-related improvement in blood flow. It allows for anterograde reperfusion but doesn't necessitate it, as there can be distal emboli or completed infarcts further downstream. Reperfusion, the salvage of the penumbra tissue, is thus the ultimate goal and is often mediated by recanalization. The most commonly used primary outcome measure for recanalization/reperfusion in current clinical trials is the modified Thrombolysis in Cerebral Infarction (mTICI) (22). Estimating this scale is predicated on visually estimating how much of the target downstream territory section is re-perfused with grade 0 signifying a failed reperfusion and grade 3 signifying the best possible reperfusion. The full grading scale is shown in Table 11.2.

Current guidelines recommend TICI 2B and TICI 3 reperfusion to determine adequate reperfusion, as this was the bench mark in all the recent trials. Much of the inability for earlier trials to show significance in mechanical thrombectomy for LVO was largely attributed to inability to achieve this outcome in addition to other factors. Further investigation into gradating the difference between TICI2B and TICI3 has already been underway (aka TICI2C) and suggests improved outcome when compared to TICI2B as of preliminary studies (23).

Access is achieved through a transfemoral arterial approach with a large (8 Fr) guide catheter within which is a 5 to 6 Fr catheter directed to the circle of Willis and a microcatheter, which should be navigated to the clot over a guidewire. An alternative vascular access point is either via the brachial artery or radial artery for patients with aortoilial-femoral disease.

SYSTEMIC THROMBOLYSIS USING ALTEPLASE (RECOMBINANT TISSUE PLASMINOGEN ACTIVATOR)

The administration of alteplase requires a last known normal of less than 4.5 hours (24). Less than 10% of AIS patients meet current criteria for thrombolysis in < 4.5 hours. To complicate matters, BP must be < 185/110 pre-thrombolysis, due to higher rates of spontaneous hemorrhagic transformation afterwards (25). Blood pressure control is typically done using

Table 11.1 **CT PERFUSION PARAMETERS**

CT PERFUSION METRIC	UNITS OF MEASUREMENT	WHAT IS MEASURED?
CBV	mL of blood/100 g of brain	Total volume of flowing blood in a given volume of brain
MTT	seconds	Average time for blood transiting through the given brain region
CBF	mL of blood/100 g of brain/minute	Volume of blood passing through given volume of brain per unit of time
TTP/Tmax	Seconds	Time at which maximal enhancement of contrast occurs

Table 11.2 MTICI GRADING SCALE FOR VESSEL RECANALIZATION/REPERFUSION

mTICI 0	No perfusion
mTICI 1	Antegrade perfusion past the initial occlusion but limited distal branch filling with little or slow distal reperfusion
mTICI 2 A	Antegrade reperfusion of less than half of the occluded target artery's previously ischemic territory
mTICI 2 B	Antegrade reperfusion of more than half of the previously occluded target artery's previously ischemic territory
mTICI 3	Complete antegrade reperfusion of more than half of the previously occluded target artery ischemic territory, with absence of visualized occlusion in all distal branches

intravenous medications such as labetalol or nicardipine. The placement of nasogastric tubes, indwelling bladder catheters and intra-arterial pressure catheters should be delayed if able. If the patient were to develop acute hypertension, severe headache, nausea or vomiting, a concern for hemorrhagic conversion should be a priori and infusion should be stopped with pursuit of a stat head CT. Alteplase activates tissue plasminogen activator (tPA), which degrades fibrinogen and thus causes clot lysis. Any symptomatic hemorrhage that results following thrombolysis with alteplase should be treated with therapies that also restore fibrinogen. Lastly, if the patient were to develop orolingual angioedema—a known allergic complication tPA—airway management optimally requires awake fiberoptic intubation. Nasal-tracheal intubations are less preferred given concern for post-alteplase epistaxis. This would be done in concert with typical management of anaphylaxis (cessation of medication, steroids, diphenhydramine, epinephrine).

If alteplase eligibility is determined, thrombolysis should be offered at a dose of 0.9 mg/kg (maximum 90 mg) over 60 minutes with 10% of the dose given as a bolus over 1 minute (3). Alteplase administration requires frequent monitoring of blood pressure and neurological examinations every 15 minutes during infusion, and every 2 hours following infusion, which requires intensive care unit (ICU) or stroke unit level of care for the first 24 hours. In addition to providing thrombolytic therapy, the use of additional CT angiography (CTA) and CT perfusion to evaluate for residual LVO. In the event of thrombolysis failure, transfer to facilities capable of performing mechanical thrombectomy is now considered standard of care (4). Acute perfusion weighted imaging, either through the use of CT perfusion or in some centers perfusion MRI, helps to determine those patients eligible for mechanical thrombectomy by differentiating the proportion of brain parenchyma that is irreversibly ischemic core and which areas of the brain parenchyma is potentially salvageable with reperfusion therapy, often referred to as the penumbra (5). Of key note, perfusion imaging requires peripheral IV access for contrast bolus injection (iodinated contrast for CT-perfusion studies; gadolinium contrast for perfusion MRI studies). Though CT perfusion remains the most readily available and performed perfusion study, recent studies suggest perfusion MRI can be performed within a similar timeframe with superior imaging data (6).

Recanalization by systemic intravenous alteplase in LVO varies by location but occurs in 4% to 18% of ICA occlusions and 22% to 32% of proximal MCA occlusions (7). Given the importance of recanalization in clinical outcome (8), systemic thrombolysis is not enough in the current era. Evidence of (ii) NIHSS >6, (ii) mismatch between delayed MTT/TTP and insufficient CBV/CBF suggesting a marked "penumbra" or salvageable tissue, (iii) an ASPECTS >6 (see discussion), or (iv) a last known normal within 24 hours of presentation suggests that endovascular treatment, such as mechanical thrombectomy, is rapidly becoming the gold standard.

ANESTHESIA AND ENDOVASCULAR NEUROINTERVENTIONS

The coordination of anesthesia care is critical for the successful completion of mechanical thrombectomy in ischemic stroke. A key metric used in trials involved door-to-groin puncture times and groin puncture-to-reperfusion time for which minimization of pain and agitation is paramount. Patients with severe dominant hemisphere lesions may become very agitated necessitating general anesthesia (13). Blood pressure goals are often dictated by the interventionalist, with current American Heart Association stroke guidelines suggesting blood pressure <180/105 mmHg during the procedure (14).

There is currently no consensus on whether general anesthesia or conscious sedation is superior in acute stroke cases requiring mechanical thrombectomy. Two thrombectomy trials (ESCAPE, SWIFT PRIME) used conscious sedation predominantly with no clear impact on outcome, while one trial, MR-CLEAN, showed a decrease in treatment effect of general anesthesia compared to conscious sedation. Original retrospective studies showed superior neurologic outcomes with conscious sedation compared with general anesthesia, although prospective studies have failed to show such an association. Most of the decisions regarding method of anesthesia were predicated on NIHSS scale, baseline demographic data, and ASPECTS score. Unfortunately, retrospective studies were often clouded by variation in LVO location, endovascular intervention, and differences in baseline scores (15). As such, either method of procedural sedation has been deemed reasonable by the current American Heart Association stroke guidelines, and the appropriate approach for each patient should be determined by the treatment team. Pain control with local anesthetics to the site of entry for the catheter is imperative as well as monitoring for the uncooperative/agitated patient. For patients who exhibit signs of oropharyngeal weakness (excessive drooling, dysphagia, inability to clear secretions) or decreased arousal, practitioners should have a low threshold for intubation to ensure airway protection.

MECHANICAL THROMBECTOMY

In 2015, the results of 5 separate randomized, prospective, multicenter trials have resulted in Class I evidence for mechanical thrombectomy offering superior 90 day outcome for previously independent individuals, no change in hemorrhagic stroke, and no change in mortality as compared to intravenous thrombolysis alone (26). These trials (MR-CLEAN, EXTEND-IA, REVASCAT, ESCAPE, SWIFT-PRIME) revolutionized the stroke field by increasing the window for intervention from 4.5 hours up to 12 hours, in addition to demonstrating that the failure of earlier studies could largely be attributed to inappropriate patient selection, incomplete revascularization, and inexperienced operators (27–31). Further studies which resulted in 2018 examined patients with intracranial ICA or proximal MCA and mismatch between clinical deficit and infarct volume demonstrated better 90-day functional outcome when offered thrombectomy even between 6 to 24 hours after last known normal (32, 33). This also had no significant difference between symptomatic ICH and 90-day mortality. The emergence of mechanical thrombectomy has proved a watershed moment in the care of patients with stroke and current training for neurology, anesthesia, critical care, radiology, and neurosurgery has appropriately focused on optimizing the care of those with AIS/emergent large vessel occlusion.

The complication rate for the mechanical thrombectomy procedure has decreased with both improvement of technology and the restriction of trials to expert neuro-interventionalists at high-volume centers. A recent meta-analysis revealed "the risk of complications from mechanical thrombectomy to be about 15% (4% access-site related, 6% from artery rupture causing subarachnoid hemorrhage, intraventricular hemorrhage, additional symptomatic intracerebral hemorrhage, extracranial bleeding and perforation, and 5% from distal or new arterial territory embolization)" (10). As such, complications from the procedure mostly revolve around physical trauma introduced by the catheter, and particular care must be paid to those patients who also receive systemic thrombolysis. The most feared complication remains symptomatic ICH as a result of reperfusion injury and subsequent hemorrhagic transformation.

FOLLOW-UP AFTER STROKE

The standard workup for cerebrovascular disease is that for any patient with advanced atherosclerotic disease and should include electrocardiogram, echocardiogram, lipid panel, and hemoglobin A1C. Care involves optimizing the patient's risk factors and to determine if there is any evidence of structural

heart disease/cardiac arrhythmia. Additionally, patients should be monitored on telemetry to evaluate for paroxysmal atrial fibrillation as the occlusive cerebrovascular accident might have been embolic from a thrombus in the left atrial appendage. This patient would warrant lifelong anticoagulation if confirmed to have atrial fibrillation, based on her recurrent stroke risk. The timing of initiation of anticoagulation in this setting should be balanced with the risk of possible hemorrhagic transformation depending on the final infarct size and location.

STROKE COMPLICATION

Patients with ischemic stroke should be closely monitored for fever, pneumonia, urinary tract infection, and venous thromboembolism (34). These are often a result of systemic inflammation combined with structural deficits (oropharyngeal weakness, hemiparesis) that subsequently increase the risk for each of these conditions. As such, there should be a low threshold for workup of these morbidities in the setting of fever—which independently predicts poor outcome (35)—and/or other signs and symptoms.

Greater than 65% of patients will develop some degree of difficulty swallowing, or dysphagia, following ischemic stroke. This may warrant nasogastric feeding tube placement in the short-term and in severe cases gastrostomy tube placement (36). Recurrent aspiration, or inability to protect the airway necessitates intubation in severe stroke cases, or in posterior circulation strokes where arousal is severely impacted. Patients may also warrant tracheostomy placement due to failure to wean from the ventilator or to allow appropriate recovery of ability to protect the airway (37).

After 72 hours, patients with hemispheric stroke are at higher risk for malignant syndromes manifested with cerebral edema and sometimes hyperosmolar therapy and/or decompressive surgery. Further long-term consequences include depression, sleep-disordered breathing, cognitive impairment, poststroke epilepsy, development of contracture, increased risk for future cardiovascular events, and even caregiver fatigue and psychosocial stress (38).

CONCLUSIONS

- Aphasia, contralateral arm > leg hemiparesis, ipsilateral gaze deviation, and neglect are examples of cortical signs at the bedside that can be used to predict a LVO AIS.

- Noncontrast CT brain can exclude ICH but not AIS.

- Alteplase (tPA) can be given within 4.5 hours if all exclusion/inclusion criteria are met and blood pressure <185/110 at time of administration with the use of antihypertensives if needed.

- MRI remains the gold standard for diagnosing stroke, however CT perfusion and CTA are more readily available and should be obtained in the acute setting to assess eligibility for mechanical thrombectomy.

- Though MTT of contrast and time to maximal contrast enhancement are delayed in all ischemic areas, CBF/CBV is spared in the ischemic penumbra and compromised in irreversible core infarct.

- Mechanical thrombectomy can potentially re-perfuse tissue at risk for irreversible infarction, known as the ischemic penumbra. Patients may be eligible for mechanical thrombectomy up to 24 hours from symptom onset without increased risk for hemorrhagic transformation or reperfusion injury.

- TICI2B/TICI3 is the optimal recanalization standard to predict successful outcome.

REFERENCES

1. Chalela JA, Kidwell CS, Nentwich LM, et al. Magnetic resonance imaging and computed tomography in emergency assessment of patients with suspected acute stroke: a prospective comparison. Lancet. 2007;369(9558):293–298. doi:10.1016/S0140-6736(07)60151-2

2. Merino JG, Warach S. Imaging of acute stroke. Nat Rev Neurol. 2010;6(10):560–571. doi:10.1038/nrneurol.2010.129

3. Demaerschalk BM, Kleindorfer DO, Adeoye OM, et al. Scientific rationale for the inclusion and exclusion criteria for intravenous alteplase in acute ischemic stroke: a statement for healthcare professionals from the American Heart Association/American Stroke Association. Stroke. 2016;47(2):581–641. doi:10.1161/STR.0000000000000086

4. Barlinn J, Gerber J, Barlinn K, et al. Acute endovascular treatment delivery to ischemic stroke patients transferred within a telestroke network: a retrospective observational study. Int J Stroke. 2017;12(5):502–509. doi:10.1177/1747493016681018

5. Schaefer PW, Barak ER, Kamalian S, et al. Quantitative assessment of core/penumbra mismatch in acute stroke: CT and MR perfusion imaging are strongly correlated when sufficient brain volume is imaged. Stroke. 2008;39(11):2986–2992. doi:10.1161/STROKEAHA.107.513358

6. Simonsen CZ, Yoo AJ, Rasmussen M, et al. Magnetic resonance imaging selection for endovascular stroke therapy: workflow in the GOLIATH Trial. Stroke. 2018;49(6):1402–1406. doi:10.1161/STROKEAHA.118.021038

7. Tsivgoulis G, Katsanos AH, Schellinger PD, et al. Successful reperfusion with intravenous thrombolysis preceding mechanical thrombectomy in large-vessel occlusions. Stroke. 2018;49(1):232–235. doi:10.1161/STROKEAHA.117.019261

8. Rha J-H, Saver JL. The impact of recanalization on ischemic stroke outcome: a meta-analysis. Stroke. 2007;38(3):967–973. doi:10.1161/01.STR.0000258112.14918.24

9. Turk AS, Spiotta A, Frei D, et al. Initial clinical experience with the ADAPT technique: a direct aspiration first pass technique for stroke thrombectomy. J Neurointerv Surg. 2014;6(3):231–237. doi:10.1136/neurintsurg-2013-010713

10. Balami JS, White PM, McMeekin PJ, Ford GA, Buchan AM. Complications of endovascular treatment for acute ischemic stroke: Prevention and management. Int J Stroke. 2018;13(4):348–361. doi:10.1177/1747493017743051

11. Mozaffarian D, Benjamin EJ, et al.; Writing Group Members. Heart disease and stroke statistics—2016 update: a report from the American Heart Association. Circulation. 2016;133(4):e38–360. doi:10.1161/CIR.0000000000000350

12. Smith WS, Lev MH, English JD, et al. Significance of large vessel intracranial occlusion causing acute ischemic stroke and TIA. Stroke. 2009;40(12):3834–3840. doi:10.1161/STROKEAHA.109.561787

13. Evans MRB, White P, Cowley P, Werring DJ. Revolution in acute ischaemic stroke care: a practical guide to mechanical thrombectomy. Pract Neurol. 2017;17(4):252–265. doi:10.1136/practneurol-2017-001685

14. Powers WJ, Rabinstein AA, Ackerson T, et al. 2018 Guidelines for the early management of patients with acute ischemic stroke: a guideline for healthcare professionals from the American Heart Association/American Stroke Association. Stroke. 2018;49(3):e46–e110. doi:10.1161/STR.0000000000000158

15. Ilyas A, Chen C-J, Ding D, et al. Endovascular mechanical thrombectomy for acute ischemic stroke under general anesthesia versus conscious sedation: a systematic review and meta-analysis. World Neurosurg. 2018;112:e355–e367. doi:10.1016/j.wneu.2018.01.049

16. Barber PA, Demchuk AM, Zhang J, Buchan AM. Validity and reliability of a quantitative computed tomography score in predicting outcome of hyperacute stroke before thrombolytic therapy. ASPECTS Study Group. Alberta Stroke Programme Early CT Score. Lancet. 2000;355(9216):1670–1674

17. Campbell BCV, Christensen S, Levi CR, et al. Comparison of computed tomography perfusion and magnetic resonance imaging perfusion-diffusion mismatch in ischemic stroke. Stroke. 2012;43(10):2648–2653. doi:10.1161/STROKEAHA.112.660548

18. Lui YW, Tang ER, Allmendinger AM, Spektor V. Evaluation of CT perfusion in the setting of cerebral ischemia: patterns and pitfalls. AJNR Am J Neuroradiol. 2010;31(9):1552–1563. doi:10.3174/ajnr.A2026

19. Lin L, Bivard A, Parsons MW. Perfusion patterns of ischemic stroke on computed tomography perfusion. J Stroke. 2013;15(3):164–173. doi:10.5853/jos.2013.15.3.164

20. Thomalla G, Simonsen CZ, Boutitie F, et al. MRI-guided thrombolysis for stroke with unknown time of onset. N Engl J Med. 2018;379:611–622. doi:10.1056/NEJMoa1804355

21. Barlinn J, Gerber J, Barlinn K, et al. Acute endovascular treatment delivery to ischemic stroke patients transferred within a telestroke network: a retrospective observational study. Int J Stroke. 2017;12(5):502–509. doi:10.1177/1747493016681018

22. Zaidat OO, Yoo AJ, Khatri P, et al. Recommendations on angiographic revascularization grading standards for acute ischemic stroke: a consensus statement. Stroke. 2013;44(9):2650–2663. doi:10.1161/STROKEAHA.113.001972

23. Tung EL, McTaggart RA, Baird GL, et al. Rethinking thrombolysis in cerebral infarction 2b: which thrombolysis in cerebral infarction scales best define near complete recanalization in the modern thrombectomy era? Stroke. 2017;48(9):2488–2493. doi:10.1161/STROKEAHA.117.017182

24. Hacke W, Kaste M, Bluhmki E, et al. Thrombolysis with alteplase 3 to 4.5 hours after acute ischemic stroke. N Engl J Med. 2008;359(13):1317–1329. doi:10.1056/NEJMoa0804656

25. Bowry R, Navalkele DD, Gonzales NR. Blood pressure management in stroke: Five new things. Neurol Clin Pract. 2014;4(5):419–426. doi:10.1212/CPJ.0000000000000085

26. Lambrinos A, Schaink AK, Dhalla I, et al. Mechanical thrombectomy in acute ischemic stroke: a systematic review. Can J Neurol Sci. 2016;43(4):455–460. doi:10.1017/cjn.2016.30

27. Berkhemer OA, Fransen PSS, Beumer D, et al. A randomized trial of intraarterial treatment for acute ischemic stroke. N Engl J Med. 2015;372(1):11–20. doi:10.1056/NEJMoa1411587

28. Campbell BCV, Mitchell PJ, Kleinig TJ, et al. Endovascular therapy for ischemic stroke with perfusion-imaging selection. N Engl J Med. 2015;372(11):1009–1018. doi:10.1056/NEJMoa1414792

29. Jovin TG, Chamorro A, Cobo E, et al. Thrombectomy within 8 hours after symptom onset in ischemic stroke. N Engl J Med. 2015;372(24):2296–2306. doi:10.1056/NEJMoa1503780

30. Goyal M, Demchuk AM, Menon BK, et al. Randomized assessment of rapid endovascular treatment of ischemic stroke. N Engl J Med. 2015;372(11):1019–1030. doi:10.1056/NEJMoa1414905

31. Saver JL, Goyal M, Bonafe A, et al. Stent-retriever thrombectomy after intravenous t-PA vs. t-PA alone in stroke. N Engl J Med. 2015;372(24):2285–2295. doi:10.1056/NEJMoa1415061

32. Nogueira RG, Jadhav AP, Haussen DC, et al. Thrombectomy 6 to 24 hours after stroke with a mismatch between deficit and infarct. N Engl J Med. 2018;378(1):11–21. doi:10.1056/NEJMoa1706442

33. Albers GW, Marks MP, Kemp S, et al. Thrombectomy for stroke at 6 to 16 hours with selection by perfusion imaging. N Engl J Med. 2018;378(8):708–718. doi:10.1056/NEJMoa1713973

34. Kappelle LJ, Van Der Worp HB. Treatment or prevention of complications of acute ischemic stroke. Curr Neurol Neurosci Rep. 2004;4(1):36–41.

35. Azzimondi G, Bassein L, Nonino F, et al. Fever in acute stroke worsens prognosis: a prospective study. Stroke. 1995;26(11):2040–2043.

36. Martino R, Foley N, Bhogal S, Diamant N, Speechley M, Teasell R. Dysphagia after stroke: incidence, diagnosis, and pulmonary complications. Stroke. 2005;36(12):2756–2763. doi:10.1161/01.STR.0000190056.76543.eb

37. Bösel J. Use and timing of tracheostomy after severe stroke. Stroke. 2017;48(9):2638–2643. doi:10.1161/STROKEAHA.117.017794

38. Powers WJ, Derdeyn CP, Biller J, et al. 2015 American Heart Association/American Stroke Association focused update of the 2013 guidelines for the early management of patients with acute ischemic stroke regarding endovascular treatment: a guideline for healthcare professionals from the American Heart Association/American Stroke Association. Stroke. 2015;46(10):3020–3035. doi:10.1161/STR.0000000000000074

39. Frontera JA, Lewin JJ, Rabinstein AA, et al. Guideline for reversal of antithrombotics in intracranial hemorrhage: a statement for healthcare professionals from the Neurocritical Care Society and Society of Critical Care Medicine. Neurocrit Care. 2016;24(1):6-46. doi:10.1007/s12028-015-0222-x

40. Shaikh N. Emergency management of fat embolism syndrome. J Emerg Trauma Shock. 2009;2(1):29–33. doi:10.4103/0974-2700.44680

41. Fugate JE, Kalimullah EA, Wijdicks EFM. Angioedema after tPA: what neurointensivists should know. Neurocrit Care. 2012;16(3):440–443. doi:10.1007/s12028-012-9678-0

REVIEW QUESTIONS

1. A 44-year-old man with a history of hypertension, hyperlipidemia, and tobacco abuse present with acute onset right face, arm, and leg weakness beginning approximately 1 hour prior. His initial CT scan shows no evidence of hemorrhage, and he meets all other tPA inclusion criteria. He receives IV tPA; however, half an hour into the infusion he complains of severe headache and now has worse weakness on the right side. A repeat CT scan shows a small hemorrhage in the internal capsule. What should be done next?

   A. Continue IV tPA infusion, but monitor exam closely and repeat CT scan at end of infusion.

   B. Stop IV tPA infusion and give Vitamin K IV.

   C. Stop IV tPA infusion, monitor blood pressure closely, and give cryoprecipitate or fibrinogen concentrate.

   D. Continue tPA infusion, and give cryoprecipitate or fibrinogen concentrate.

2. A 56-year-old man with history of coronary artery disease, hypertension, and hyperlipidemia is post-operative day 0 from an uncomplicated sternotomy and 4-vessel coronary artery bypass grafting. Upon extubation, he is noted to not be moving the right side and unable to follow any commands. What are the immediate next steps?

   A. Perform emergent head CT to evaluate for hemorrhage, and if negative administer IV tPA at 0.9 mg/kg (maximums dose 90 mg) over 60 minutes with 10% of the dose given as a bolus over 1 minute.

   B. Maintain blood pressure >140/90 to ensure adequate perfusion pressure

   C. Administer IV tPA at 0.9 mg/kg (maximums dose 90 mg) over 60 minutes with 10% of the dose given as a bolus over 1 minute.

   D. Perform emergent head CT and CTA of the head to evaluate for hemorrhage or LVO.

3. A 65-year-old diabetic hypertensive woman presents to the emergency department with aphasia, right-sided facial droop, and right hemiparesis. She was last seen well the night before, approximately 12 hours ago. She undergoes an emergent head CT, which shows a hyperdense left MCA sign, and no evidence of blood or significant territorial infarction. What treatments should she undergo, if any?

   A. She is not eligible for any treatments given she is outside of the 4.5 hour window

   B. Systemic thrombolysis therapy with IV tPA

   C. Emergent thrombectomy if she has a LVO with perfusion deficit

   D. She should undergo emergent left carotid endarterectomy for suspected carotid plaque rupture

4. A 23-year-old man was recently rear-ended in a motor vehicle collision with no loss of consciousness. He presents with a full left MCA syndrome with onset 8 hours prior and on CTA is found to have a left carotid dissection with left MCA thrombus. While being taken emergently to the angiography suite for mechanical thrombectomy, he becomes increasingly agitated. What anesthesia management strategy should be used at this point?

   A. Rapid sequence induction and intubation with rocuronium for neuromuscular blockade to ensure airway protection

   B. IV Haldol, followed by fentanyl and/or versed for conscious sedation

   C. Avoid any narcotics or sedating anesthetic agents as this may drop blood pressure and worsen outcome

   D. The appropriate strategy should be determined in conjunction with the interventionalist and anesthesiologist to assess the safest and most expedient method for performing thrombectomy.

5. A 37-year-old woman is 6 weeks postpartum and develops new onset aphasia and hemiparesis. CT showed no hemorrhage, and CTA with no evidence of LVO. She was given IV tPA in the emergency department and transferred to the ICU with the remaining tPA infusion for close monitoring. While in the ICU 30 minutes later her examination improves, and she is speaking clearly with no residual hemiparesis; however, her blood pressure climbs to 210/110. What should be done next, if anything?

   A. Continue tPA infusion and allowing for permissive hypertension given improved exam.

   B. Continue tPA infusion with aggressive control of blood pressure to less than 180/105 with IV medications and drips as needed.

C. Stop tPA infusion, but allow for permissive hypertension given improved exam.

D. Stop tPA infusion and treat with empiric antiepileptic medications given her presentation was likely a seizure.

6. An 86-year-old man develops acute hemiplegia and neglect with gaze preference, is found to have a large right MCA stroke with M-1 vessel occlusion, and is taken emergently for mechanical thrombectomy. During the procedure, groin access was complicated, but patient underwent successful TICI 3 recanalization. While in the ICU, patient develops acute hypotension overnight with decline in functional exam. What is the immediate next step in management?

A. Maintain MAP >65 with fluid resuscitation or IV pressors.

B. Perform groin check to evaluate for superficial groin hematoma at puncture site.

C. Perform CT abdomen/pelvis to evaluate for retroperitoneal bleed.

D. Start broad spectrum antibiotics and provide aggressive fluid resuscitation to treat for early septic shock.

7. A 55-year-old man presents with large right hemispheric stroke and is found to have a complete occlusion of the right carotid artery with a large perfusion deficit on CT perfusion imaging, and an ASPECTS of 8. He is deemed an appropriate mechanical thrombectomy candidate; however, despite numerous attempts, recanalization of the right carotid is not achieved. He is taken to the intensive care unit postprocedurally. What is the most important complication to monitor over the next several days?

A. Risk of acute groin hematoma post thrombectomy

B. Safety while swallowing given increased risk of aspiration and aspiration pneumonia

C. Malignant cerebral edema, with risk of cerebral herniation

D. Postcontrast anaphylaxis

8. A 75-year-old woman is transferred from an outside hospital after receiving IV alteplase for an NIHSS of 14. On arrival, her exam is reportedly mildly better, and she is noted to be moving her right arm more spontaneously though her NIHSS remains above 10. What is the next best step in her care?

A. Admission to an ICU or stroke step-down unit for close monitoring for alteplase

B. MRI of the brain for assessment of acute stroke

C. Urgent CTA and CT perfusion to evaluate for any LVO

D. Echocardiogram with continuous telemetry monitoring to evaluate for possible cardioembolic source

9. A 24-year-old male suffers a motor-vehicle accident after which he presents to an emergency room with a Glasgow Coma Scale score of 14. He has no focal neurologic deficits but does complain of some neck and leg pain. Tertiary survey reveals a femur fracture for which he is admitted to the trauma unit. The next day he is found to have confusion, shortness of

breath, and left-sided weakness. What is the most likely cause of his exam change?

A. Vertebral artery dissection

B. Fat embolism

C. Drug reaction

D. Small-vessel ischemic disease

10. A 67-year-old woman presents to the hospital with NIHSS 12 and a LVO. She satisfies alteplase administration criteria, completes the infusion, and undergoes mechanical thrombectomy under conscious sedation, during which multiple passes are required to aspirate the clot successfully. During the procedure, she develops frank angioedema and an urticarial rash with hypoxemia. What are the most likely cause and the next best step of management for this patient?

A. tPA; intubation, epinephrine, diphenhydramine, steroids

B. tPA; intubation

C. iodinated contrast; intubation

D. iodinated contrast; intubation, epinephrine, diphenhydramine, steroids

REVIEW QUESTION ANSWERS

1. C. In the setting of an acute neurologic symptoms during alteplase infusion should be stopped immediately in the setting of an acute neurologic symptom developing during infusion. An emergent CT scan of the head is indicated, and if a hemorrhage is discovered, blood pressure should be controlled tightly (generally less than 160 mmHg), and patients should have fibrinogen repleted either with cryoprecipitate or recombinant fibrinogen products. (39)

2. D. Postoperative strokes are a known complication of major cardiothoracic surgery. Close neurological examination post-procedurally is essential to identifying patients with LVO syndromes who may be eligible for mechanical thrombectomy. Major surgery is a contraindication to alteplase therapy regardless of timing.

3. C. This patient should undergo emergent mechanical thrombectomy if found to have a perfusion deficit and/or favorable ASPECTS. Patients may now be offered mechanical thrombectomy up to 24 hours from last seen well depending on perfusion deficits and mismatch of infarcted tissue based on recent clinical trial findings (32). She is not an appropriate systemic thrombolysis candidate given time from last known well.

4. D. The most appropriate anesthetic strategy for managing patients during mechanical thrombectomy should be decided by the team caring for the patient. Both conscious sedation or general anesthesia are accepted options; however, care must be maintained to prevent any episode of hypotension prior to recanalization as this may extend ischemic core and penumbra.

5. B. Blood pressure must be tightly controlled post alteplase with goals <180/105 mmHg during infusion. Sudden spikes in blood pressure can occur and should warrant

aggressive management with IV medications and necessary drips within minutes. Systolic blood pressures greater than 180 mmHg post alteplase have been associated with increased risk of symptomatic intracerebral hemorrhage and worse outcome.

6. A. Hypotension must be treated first in any critical care setting while subsequently assessing for etiology. Patient's postmechanical thrombectomy are at risk for development of groin hematoma and, in high-access sites, possible retroperitoneal hematoma. The decline in examination despite TICI 3 recanalization is not unexpected in setting of an acute systemic stressor, such as hypotension.

7. C. Although all of the listed choices are complications of AIS and mechanical thrombectomy, the unsuccessful recanalization and large perfusion deficit on initial CT perfusion raise the risk for a full-territory ischemic stroke. These patients are at increased risk for malignant cerebral edema and may warrant hyperosmolar therapies to manage edema or event evaluation for an urgent life-saving decompressive hemicraniectomy.

8. C. Although all of the choices are potentially correct, the best next step is to evaluate for an LVO. Despite improvement in the patient's examination, an NIHSS >6 still suggests and clinical exam with cortical signs still raises the suspicion for an LVO and, if confirmed on CTA, would potentially make this patient a candidate for mechanical thrombectomy.

9. B. Fat embolism syndrome is commonly associated with trauma to the femur, pelvis, and tibia. The core clinical features are skin petechiae, cerebral dysfunction, and respiratory failure although rarely do all three aspects of the triad present together. Fat embolism syndrome often occurs within 1 to 3 days of the event. The fat emboli likely lodge in vascular beds such as the brain and the lungs causing the symptomology observed. Arterial blood gas often show increases in the shunt fraction and an increased alveolar–arterial gradient. (40) Of note, although these patients are not eligible for tPA, the possibility for mechanical thrombectomy should be considered if an LVO is present.

10. D. This patient is suffering from anaphylaxis given the presence of angioedema and urticarial rash with impending airway distress. Although angioedema due to alteplase (often due to increased plasma kinins and activation of C1) is a known albeit rare occurrence, it occurs during infusion and not after. This patient already completed infusion and required more contrast than usual to achieve recanalization. As such, the most likely culprit is the iodinated contrast dye. Standard management of anaphylaxis, including administration of epinephrine, diphenhydramine, steroids, and airway protection, is appropriate as indicated. Epinephrine has been noted to be safe in the care of postalteplase patients (41).

12.

ELEVATED ICP WITH A SELLA TURCICA TUMOR WITH DIPLOPIA AND PANHYPOPITUITARISM

Payal Boss and Murtaza Diwan

STEM CASE AND KEY QUESTIONS

A 46-year-old female with past medical history significant for hypertension and atrial fibrillation on chronic warfarin therapy presents to the emergency department with sudden onset of severe retro-orbital headache, nausea, vomiting, and diplopia. When obtaining vital signs, it is noted that her blood pressure is 86/42 and her finger stick glucose is 45. She is given intravenous (IV) fluids and the blood pressure improves to 95/50.

The patient is then sent for a computed tomography (CT) for further evaluation of her symptoms.

WHAT IS THE DIAGNOSIS AND SUBSEQUENT WORKUP?

The patient had a CT scan which showed a heterogeneous, hyperdense, and intrasellar lesion, with the coexistence of solid and hemorrhagic areas, consistent with hemorrhage into a pituitary tumor.

Upon return to the emergency department, the patient was given IV fluids, and neurology was consulted. Neurology recommended intensive care unit admission, fluids, hydrocortisone, and obtaining laboratory work to help evaluate the mass. A complete blood count, comprehensive metabolic panel, and coagulation studies were sent. To evaluate endocrine hormone function—cortisol, prolactin, thyroid-stimulating hormone, and free T4 levels were all checked.

The serum cortisol level was 2.5 mcg/dL, which indicated the patient has cortisol deficiency. In addition, serum sodium level was noted to be 124 mEq/L. After the patient was stabilized, she was sent for diffusion weighted magnetic resonance imaging (MRI), which revealed a hyperdense 14 mm sellar mass, suggestive of hemorrhage within a pituitary adenoma—consistent with pituitary apoplexy.

WHAT IS THE INITIAL TREATMENT? WHAT ARE THE CONSEQUENCES OF HER ALTERED MENTAL STATUS? HOW DO YOU MANAGE ELEVATED INTERCRANIAL PRESSURE?

The patient was immediately given fluid resuscitation and hydrocortisone 100 mg IV bolus. Fluid resuscitation should

be done with normal saline as the hyponatremia should resolve with fluids and the hydrocortisone without aggressive therapy. Given her altered mental status and concern for elevated intracranial pressures (ICPs), the decision was made to intubate the patient. She was given fentanyl, etomidate and rocuronium and intubated via direct laryngoscopy.

Neurosurgery was consulted, and they recommended measures to reduce her ICP including elevation of head of her bed to 30 degrees, maintenance of normocapnia with a $PaCO_2$ goal of 35, and administration of mannitol for osmotic diuresis as well as continuation of the hydrocortisone. If these measures did not improve the patient's mental status, they recommended placement of external ventricular drain to decrease ICP and improve cerebral perfusion pressure.

Further history was obtained from the family, and they confirmed that the patient had been having vision problems for the past several weeks—specifically complaints of diplopia and ptosis.

WHAT DOES THE DIPLOPIA SIGNIFY?

The patient continued to have vision problems, and thus ophthalmology was consulted to evaluate the patient's vision. The ophthalmologist performed visual field assessment, checked visual acuity, and evaluated ocular motility. Diplopia was confirmed, which indicated upward compressive pressure on the oculomotor nerve (CN III) from the pituitary tumor.

SHOULD EMERGENT SURGERY BE PERFORMED? IS MEDICAL MANAGEMENT A SAFE ALTERNATIVE?

Given the patient's ongoing visual symptoms, after discussion with neurosurgery and ophthalmology, the patient was scheduled to undergo transphenoidal resection of her pituitary tumor. She was counseled on the benefits, which include immediate improvement of compressive symptoms and permanent removal of adenoma. The risks were thoroughly explained to the patient, which include postoperative cerebrospinal fluid (CSF) leak, CSF rhinorrhea, damage to posterior pituitary gland, and risk of permanent hypopituitarism from accidental resection of normal pituitary tissue.

The patient inquired about medical management and was told that while she could continue steroid treatment for the acute phase of her condition, she would likely need surgery for adenoma resection in the future. She was also told that her visual symptoms may not improve if she decides not to proceed with surgical intervention. She elected to proceed with surgery.

WHAT POSTOPERATIVE ISSUES ARE IMPORTANT TO MONITOR FOR IN THE INTENSIVE CARE UNIT AFTER TRANSPHENOIDAL RESECTION OF PITUITARY TUMOR?

Postoperative day 1, the patient was noted to have an abrupt increase in her urine output to greater than 2.5 mL/kg/hr as well as complaints of polydipsia. Serum lab work revealed a sodium of 151 mEq/L and urine lab work revealed low urine osmolality and low specific gravity of less than 1.001.

A diagnosis of central diabetes insipidus was made, and it was felt to be likely transient related to recent neurosurgery. The patient's urine output was replaced 1:1 with IV fluids and desmopressin was administered with resolution of her symptoms.

WHAT IS THE LONG-TERM PROGNOSIS AFTER PITUITARY APOPLEXY? WILL THE PATIENT REQUIRE HORMONE SUPPLEMENTATION?

Three months postoperatively, the patient was seen for follow-up. Her visual symptoms had resolved completely. However, she continued to have hypopituitarism and required hormone supplementation and has been prescribed levothyroxine and prednisone. She will undergo monitoring MRI on a yearly basis to evaluate for tumor regrowth.

DISCUSSION

Pituitary adenomas are the most common sellar masses in the adult population and account for 10% of intracranial mass lesions. They can arise from any cell population in the anterior pituitary and may result in increased secretion of the hormone produced by that cell or may result in decreased secretion secondary to mass compression of other cell types [1]. They are classified by size (>10 mm are considered macroadenomas, and <10 mm are microadenomas), as well as by the cell type they originate from [1].

Pituitary apoplexy is a clinical syndrome classified as abrupt onset of symptoms secondary to hemorrhage or infarction of a pituitary adenoma and complicates the course of 2% to 12% of patients who have pituitary adenomas [2]. This condition is associated with a number of precipitating factors, including recent surgery, recent angiography (cerebral angiography in particular), head trauma, use of anticoagulants, arterial hypertension, and size of pituitary adenoma, as well as an increase in ICP [3].

Nearly 80% of patients who present with pituitary apoplexy will display one or more deficiencies of anterior pituitary hormone secretion. Of these, 70% will display central hypoadrenalism, which can lead to hemodynamic shock [2]. The pathogenesis of hormone deficiencies is complex and may be related to chronic compromise from the pituitary adenoma, or it may be related to the sudden necrosis of pituitary tissue related to hemorrhage or infarction.

CLINICAL MANIFESTATION OF PITUITARY APOPLEXY

1. *Headache*: Most prominent symptom, usually due to dural traction from mass compression or extravasation of blood/necrotic material into the subarachnoid space, which causes meningeal irritation. Usually retro-orbital, but can be bifrontal or diffuse. Can mimic migraine or meningitis.

2. *Visual disturbances*: Related to sudden hemorrhage-related increase in mass size, which compresses nearby structures—optic chiasm or optic nerves, in particular. This results in visual-field impairment, with bitemporal hemianopsia being the classical finding. Oculomotor palsies are also common, due to functional compression of CN III, IV, and VI, which are very sensitive to changes in intracranial pressures. CN III palsies are the most common and present with ptosis, limited eye adduction, and mydriasis [2].

3. *Other neurological symptoms*: Photophobia from meningeal irritation, nausea/vomiting and altered mental status from increased intracranial pressure may also be presenting symptoms. Cerebral ischemia can also occur from mechanical compression or from cerebral vasospasm—this can lead to hemiparesis or dysphasia.

4. *Endocrine dysfunction*: Decreased libido, impotence, impaired fertility, menstrual disturbances, fatigue, or galactorrhea can occur due to mass compression on the normal pituitary [2]. Endocrine insufficiencies can also occur due to direct destruction of the anterior pituitary or to increased intrasellar pressure on the pituitary stalk, which impairs the release of hypothalamic and pituitary hormones.

- Corticotropic deficiency is the most common hormone dysfunction and is the most life-threatening. This presents as hypotension, hyponatremia, and hypoglycemia.

- Thyrotropic, gonadotropic, and growth hormone deficiencies can also be present, but do not have immediate clinical ramifications. Patients will require hormone supplementation long-term after the acute phase of pituitary apoplexy resolves.

DIAGNOSTIC MODALITIES

The clinical presentation of pituitary apoplexy may raise the concern for two other conditions, namely subarachnoid hemorrhage and bacterial meningitis [4]. Lumbar puncture with culture may be useful in ruling out bacterial meningitis, but both pituitary apoplexy and subarachnoid hemorrhage may present with xanthochromia. In this situation, the best modalities for diagnosing pituitary apoplexy include CT or MRI, which can reveal a pituitary tumor with evidence of infarction, hemorrhage, necrosis, or clot (see Figure 12.1).

CT scan will rule out subarachnoid hemorrhage expeditiously and will reveal intrasellar mass, which can be heterogeneously enhancing, indicating mixed hemorrhagic/necrotic features.

MRI is now considered the imaging modality of choice for pituitary apoplexy for a number of reasons. First, it can detect new bleeding; second, it will also show hemorrhage and necrosis very clearly. Third, MRI can identify structural relationships between optic chiasm, optic nerve, hypothalamus, and cavernous sinuses [5]. MRI can also be used for monitoring, as you may be able to see mass shrinkage over time with conservative management [1].

TREATMENTS

The course of pituitary apoplexy is variable, and is dependent on tumor hemorrhage versus tumor infarction. Infarction tends to produce milder symptoms with more rapid recovery. Recovery of altered consciousness can be expected after surgical decompression, and endocrine dysfunction can be alleviated with exogenous supplementation. However, optic nerve atrophy can lead to long-standing visual deficits. In the most severe cases, death can occur in the span of hours secondary to refractory hypotension from adrenal failure or from neurological complications.

The overall treatment goals are to improve patient symptoms and to relieve compression of neurologic structures, mainly the optic pathway. This can be accomplished via 2 pathways: conservatively with steroid and exogenous hormone administration or via neurosurgical decompression. The details of both approaches are summarized in the following discussion; however, it is important to note that pituitary apoplexy should be managed in a multidisciplinary setting with involvement of intensivist, endocrinologist, ophthalmologist, and neurosurgeon.

CONSERVATIVE TREATMENTS

Corticotropin deficiency is present in the vast majority of patients who present with pituitary apoplexy; thus, steroid administration is the mainstay of treatment. As soon as the diagnosis is confirmed via imaging or clinical suspicion, the patient should receive IV hydrocortisone 50 mg every 6 hours or IV hydrocortisone 2 to 4 mg/hour [6]. Mineralocorticoid supplementation is usually not necessary. In addition, patients in shock should receive fluid resuscitation and may require dextrose-containing fluid to treat hypoglycemia.

There have been reports of spontaneous recovery following pituitary apoplexy, and it may be appropriate to monitor some patients clinically. However, if patients develop neuro-ophthalmic signs of compression or altered mental status with reduced level of consciousness, then surgical decompression is recommended.

SURGICAL MANAGEMENT

When the presentation of pituitary apoplexy necessitates surgical decompression, a transsphenoidal approach is considered the gold standard. It is noninvasive and uses the nasal passages and sinuses to gain access to the sellar tumor. The goals are to reach the sella, visualize the tumor through a narrow window, and remove the tumor completely while avoiding damage to surrounding structures, specifically the normal nonadenomatous pituitary tissue.

The two main risks of surgery include hormonal deficiencies and damage to parasellar structures. Hormone deficiencies occur due to damage or resection of anterior pituitary or stalk of the pituitary and may necessitate long-term treatment with hormone replacement. Damage to the pituitary stalk or posterior pituitary can result in vasopressin deficiency, which leads to diabetes insipidus. Damage to parasellar structures can cause CSF rhinorrhea, which can lead to meningitis if not treated. Internal carotid artery injury during mobilization can cause life-threatening hemorrhage. Other complications include compression or direct damage to optic chiasm and optic nerves.

After surgical resection, adjunctive radiotherapy may be required in select patients. Postoperative MRIs done at 3 months and 1 year will evaluate for residual tumor or regrowth [1].

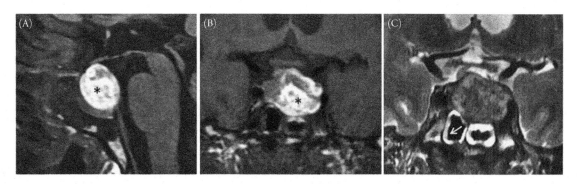

Figure 12.1 Typical MRI presentation of pituitary apoplexy, revealing hyperintense mass with hemorrhagic component (10).

PROGNOSIS AND OUTCOMES AFTER PITUITARY APOPLEXY

Patients with pituitary apoplexy will show quick improvement in acute symptoms if diagnosed appropriately. After surgical or medical management, most patients will experience ophthalmologic improvement with resolution of visual field defects. Long-term hormonal replacement will often be required, as patients will continue to have hypopituitarism. Approximately 50% of patients in one retrospective analysis required levothyroxine, while 67% required glucocorticoids. Men will require testosterone supplementation 50% of the time. More rarely, patients will have ongoing issues with vasopressin deficiencies after surgical resection, and 23% required desmopressin daily [7].

CONCLUSIONS

- Pituitary apoplexy complicates approximately 2% to 12% of pituitary adenomas and symptoms include headache, visual disturbances, and hemodynamic instability related to hormone deficiencies.

- Diagnosis involves high clinical suspicion, signs of central hypoadrenalism, and CT/MRI, which shows pituitary adenoma with evidence of hemorrhage, thrombus, or infarction.

- Treatment options include medical versus surgical management and are a matter of great debate. Broadly, the goals are to improve compressive ocular symptoms and establish hemodynamic stability. Surgical decompression provides the speediest way to these goals. However, some patients do recover normal endocrine as well as visual acuity after conservative management using steroids.

- If diagnosed appropriately, patients with pituitary apoplexy have a fair prognosis with improvement in visual symptoms, but most will require long-term hormone replacement.

REFERENCES

1. Molitch ME. Diagnosis and treatment of pituitary adenomas: a review. JAMA. 2017;317(5):516–524.
2. Albani A, Ferrau F, et al. Multidisciplinary management of pituitary apoplexy. Int J Endocrinol. 2016;2016:7951536.
3. Moller-Goede DL, Brandle M, et al. Pituitary apoplexy: re-evaluation of risk factors for bleeding into pituitary adenomas and impact on outcome. Eur J Endocrinol. 2011;164(1):37–43.
4. Ayuk J, McGregor EJ, et al. Acute management of pituitary apoplexy--surgery or conservative management? Clin Endocrinol (Oxf). 2004 Dec; 61(6):747–752.
5. Piotin M, Tampieri D, et al. The various MRI patterns of pituitary apoplexy. Eur Radiol. 1999; 9(5):918–923.
6. Rajasekaran S, Vanderpump M, et al. UK guidelines for the management of pituitary apoplexy. Clin Endocrinol (Oxf). 2011 Jan; 74(1):9–20.
7. Singh TD, Valizadeh N, et al. Management and outcomes of pituitary apoplexy. J Neurosurg. 2015 Jun;122(6):1450–1457.
8. Skljarevski V, Khoshyomn S, et al. Pituitary apoplexy in the setting of coronary angiography. J Neuroimaging. 2003. 13:276–279
9. Holness RO, Ogundimu FA, et al. Pituitary apoplexy following closed head trauma. Case report. J Neurosurg. 1983 Oct;59(4):677–679.
10. Briet C, Salenave S, et al. Pituitary apoplexy. Endocrine Rev. 1025;36,(6):622–645.

REVIEW QUESTIONS

1. Which of the following is not a risk factor for the development of pituitary apoplexy in a patient with a known pituitary adenoma?

    A. Recent cardiac surgery
    B. Use of dabigatran
    C. Recent cerebral angiography
    D. Adenoma size less than 10 mm
    E. Closed head trauma

D. Adenoma less than 10mm is not associated with greater risk of pituitary apoplexy. A larger tumor likely has a greater arterial supply and thus may have a higher propensity to bleed. However, even though the size of the adenoma appears to be a major factor, a microadenoma can still bleed. Cerebral angiography is associated with risk of precipitating apoplexy [8]. Other risk factors are well-established and include use of anticoagulation, surgery (especially which involves blood pressure variation), and recent head trauma, which could cause changes in intracranial pressure or intracerebral ischemia leading to apoplexy [9].

2. A patient presents with the following lab findings following transphenoidal resection of pituitary tumor. She complains of polyuria and confusion. What is the most likely diagnosis?

Plasma osmolality: 342
Urine osmolality: 102
Serum sodium: 152

    A. Syndrome of inappropriate antidiuretic hormone
    B. Central diabetes insipidus
    C. Nephrogenic diabetes insipidus
    D. Cerebral salt wasting syndrome
    E. Iatrogenic fluid overload

B. Central diabetes insipidus. A common postsurgical complication after transphenoidal resection of pituitary tumor, central diabetes insipidus is characterized by decreased secretion of ADH by the posterior pituitary. Characteristic findings include copious dilute urine output, hypovolemia, increased serum sodium, low urine sodium, and high plasma osmolality. Treatment includes administration of intravenous fluids and desmopressin.

3. A 32-year-old female with no known past medical history comes to the emergency room with progressive severe headaches, nausea, and fatigue during the 32nd week of her pregnancy. She is taken for a noncontrast MRI, which shows a diffusely enlarged pituitary that is 15 mm wide. Her labs are unremarkable except for a total T4 of 13.5 mcg/dL, thyroid-stimulating hormone of 1.5 mIU/L and a morning cortisol of 9 mcg/dL. Which of the following is indicated?

    A. Start hydrocortisone
    B. Emergency cesarean section

C. Transphenoidal decompression
D. Start bromocriptine
E. Start levothyroxine

A. Start hydrocortisone. This patient presents with pituitary apoplexy and steroids are a mandatory part of treatment. Steroid therapy replaces corticotropin deficiencies and may also cause pituitary adenoma shrinkage, which can alleviate compressive symptoms [2]. Transphenoidal decompression and plans for cesarean delivery should be considered after steroid administration and IV fluid resuscitation.

4. What imaging modality is considered superior in the subacute and chronic phases of pituitary apoplexy?

   A. Plain radiography
   B. CT scan
   C. MRI
   D. Angiography
   E. Transcranial doppler

C. MRI. In the subacute to chronic phases of pituitary apoplexy, MRI is the superior imaging tool as it can detect new bleeding, show hemorrhage and necrosis clearly, and can identify structural relationships between optic chiasm, optic nerve, hypothalamus, and cavernous sinuses [5]. Plain radiograph is quick and inexpensive and can show enlarging of the pituitary fossa and destruction of the sellar dorsum; however, it cannot exclude pituitary apoplexy. CT can be of great benefit acutely as it shows recent hemorrhage; however, it is less reliable in the subacute and chronic phases. Transcranial Doppler and angiography may be useful to diagnose cerebral vasospasm or cerebral aneurysm, but is not useful in diagnosis of the mass.

5. 42-year-old female presents with worsening headaches and vision loss. On examination she has a right temporal hemianopsia and decreased visual acuity. MRI shows a pituitary neoplasm that is displacing the optic chiasm superiorly and the pituitary stalk posteriorly. What are the indications for surgical intervention in this case?

   A. Severe headache
   B. Metastatic disease
   C. Elevated prolactin levels
   D. Compression of optic chiasm
   E. Decreased cortisol levels

D. Compression of the optic chiasm is an indication for surgical intervention. Other indications for surgical intervention include documented tumor growth and a symptomatic mass causing visual or endocrine symptoms [4]. Hormonal derangements should be medically managed, and patients will require hormone replacement even after surgical resection.

6. The patient in the previous question has agreed on surgery and transsphenoidal surgery was performed. Biopsy is performed during surgery, which is suspicious of meningioma, and approximately 90% of the tumor was resected. She had an uneventful postoperative hospital stay. Two weeks later, she returns with partial oculomotor palsy on the right side, an elevated white blood cell count and no fever. What is a potential cause of the patients delayed oculomotor palsy?

   A. Infection
   B. Inflammatory response
   C. Local trauma
   D. Intracranial hemorrhage
   E. All the above

E. Infection, inflammatory response, local trauma, and intracranial hemorrhage can all be potential causes of the oculomotor palsy. Inflammatory response is most likely secondary to inflammation from surgical entry into the cavernous sinus.

7. What is the expected outcome after appropriate management of pituitary apoplexy?

   A. Permanent ocular dysfunction
   B. Majority of patients will require endocrine replacement therapy
   C. Recurrent apoplexy after surgical treatment
   D. Minimal permanent sequela
   E. Majority of patients will require adjunctive radiotherapy

B. The majority of patients will require endocrine replacement therapy regardless of the management of the pituitary apoplexy. The overall outcome with appropriate management is good [7]. Visual symptoms are usually reversible and depend on the severity of the initial defect, appearance of the optic disk, and the timing of the decompression. Recurrent apoplexy has been documented in patients who have been treated conservatively; however, this outcome is rare after surgical treatment.

8. A 36-year-old female with a MRI that shows a pituitary neoplasm displacing the optic chiasm causing headaches and blurry vision elects to proceed with surgical intervention. What surgical approach would be the best choice.

   A. Transphenoidal approach
   B. Craniotomy pterional apprach
   C. Endoscopic nasal approach
   D. Craniotomy subfrontal approach
   E. Cerebral angiography approach

A. The transphenoidal approach is the preferred surgical choice as this allows the tumor to be directly accessible and also has the lowest morbidity and mortality as compared to more invasive options. It is done via transnasal septal displacement and can be performed using either a microscope or endoscope, depending on surgeon preference [10].

9. What is the most common initial symptom of pituitary apoplexy?

   A. Hypotension
   B. Severe Headache
   C. Nausea
   D. Hyponatremia
   E. Visual disturbances

B. Severe headache is present in over 95% of cases of pituitary apoplexy, and the causes include dural traction, mass compression, and meningeal irritation from blood or thrombus extravasation [10]. The headache is usually of sudden onset and is located retro-orbital, bifrontal, or bitemporal in region. The patients can also have hypotension, weakness, pain, and hyponatremia secondary to adrenal insufficiency.

10. A 44-year-old female with a past medical history of hypertension presents to the emergency department somnolent, cool, and hypotensive with a blood pressure of 75/43. Family reports that she had been complaining of severe headache and double vision the day prior. On physical exam, the patient has a Glasgow Coma Scale score of 5, as well as dilated, minimally reactive left pupil. with severe headache for 2 hours. Lab results reveal a sodium level of 126 and CT scan shows an intraseller mass with hemorrhagic component. Which of the following is the most appropriate first step in the management of this patient?

A. Secure the airway and administer IV fluids

B. Start IV hydrocortisone
C. Lumbar puncture
D. IV mannitol
E. Emergent craniotomy

A. Secure the airway and administer IV fluids. This patient presents in shock after development of pituitary apoplexy. Given her altered mental status and Glasgow Coma Scale of 5, immediate steps should be taken to secure her airway and stabilize her hemodynamics. Subsequently, STAT IV hydrocortisone should be administered, and emergent neurosurgery consultation should be obtained as this patient is exhibiting signs of elevated intracranial pressures due to pituitary apoplexy [6].

13.

POSTOPERATIVE MYOCARDIAL ISCHEMIA COMPLICATED BY CARDIOGENIC SHOCK

Ricardo Diaz Milian and Manuel R. Castresana

STEM CASE AND KEY QUESTIONS

A 65-year-old man with hypertension, chronic renal failure and peripheral vascular disease is admitted to the intensive care unit (ICU) for perfusion monitoring after a femoro-popliteal bypass. His home medications include metoprolol, furosemide, and aspirin. The surgery was complicated by significant blood loss and hypotension that resolved after surgical control of the bleeding and transfusion of packed red blood cells. Six hours postoperatively he became distressed and oliguric. His vital signs where blood pressure 90/50 mmHg, heart rate 80 bpm and pulse oximetry 90% on room air. He complained of mild incisional pain and shortness of breath. Physical exam was remarkable for cold, clammy skin, and jugular venous distention.

WHAT IS THE DEFINITION OF CARDIOGENIC SHOCK? WHICH CLINICAL AND LABORATORY FINDINGS SUPPORT THE DIAGNOSIS?

An electrocardiogram (ECG) was obtained (Figure 13.1). A chest X-ray was obtained but was unremarkable. An arterial blood gas results showed pH 7.30, PCO_2 40 mmHg, and PO_2 60 mmHg (fraction of inspired oxygen 0.4). Abnormal serum laboratory studies included creatinine 1.9 mg/dL, troponin I 0.09 ng/mL (the institution's 99th percentile reference is 0.01 ng/mL), lactate 3.0 mmol/L and a metabolic acidosis with an increased anion gap.

HOW DO YOU INTERPRET THE ECG IN FIGURE 13.1? WHAT CONSTITUTES A CRITICAL TROPONIN VALUE AND WHAT ARE COFOUNDING CONDITIONS THAT CAN CAUSE A MISLEADING ELEVATION?

A limited bedside echocardiogram was performed. The ejection fraction was 30% and isolated anterior wall motion akinesia was present. No gross valvular anomalies were identified with color Doppler. Cardiac output (CO) measured 3 L/min, which yielded a cardiac index (CI) of

1.67 L/min/m^2. These findings were new compared to a normal previous echocardiogram.

A subclavian central venous access was placed and a pulmonary artery catheter was then advanced. Pulmonary artery pressure measured 60/30 mmHg, with a pulmonary arterial occlusion pressure measured of 18 mmHg. The CO and index values were consistent with the echocardiogram. Epinephrine was started at 0.04 mcg/kg/min, which led to modest improvement of CO and pulmonary artery pressures. Follow-up troponin I was 0.8 ng/mL. The patient emergently underwent cardiac catheterization via percutaneous coronary intervention (PCI). He also received aspirin, a statin, a heparin infusion, and narcotics for pain control.

HOW ARE MYOCARDIAL INFARCTIONS CLASSIFIED? WHAT ARE THE INDICATIONS FOR EMERGENCY PERCUTANEOUS CORONARY INTERVENTION?

Nonocclusive stenosis of the left anterior descending coronary artery and right coronary artery were found during angiography. These lesions could not be entirely addressed via stenting alone. Therefore, adequate targets for a surgical grafting were identified and cardiothoracic surgery consultation was recommended. During the intervention the patient's respiratory status worsened, and he was intubated and placed on volume control ventilation mode. His cardiac index decreased despite increased inotropic support, and the metabolic acidosis worsened with an increased lactate.

IS THERE A ROLE FOR MECHANICAL DEVICES TO ASSIST VENTRICULAR FUNCTION IN REFRACTORY SHOCK? WHAT ARE THE OPTIONS? IS THERE A SURVIVAL BENEFIT WITH THE USE OF THESE DEVICES?

An intra-aortic balloon pump (IABP) was inserted via the axillary artery. The pump was programmed to provide 1:1 assistance. The cardiac index improved and inotropic support was weaned. Subsequent arterial blood gas showed improved oxygenation and resolution of the metabolic acidosis with a normal serum lactate.

WHAT ARE THE HEMODYNAMIC EFFECTS OF AN IABP? WHAT ARE THE ADVANTAGES/DISADVANTAGES IN COMPARISON WITH OTHER ASSIST DEVICES?

Cardiac surgery was consulted for urgent coronary artery bypass surgery (CABG). Pre-operative laboratory studies showed a decreased hemoglobin from 11 to 8 g/dL and a reduced platelet count of 50,000 per microliter. The CABG was scheduled for the next morning.

WHAT IS THE DIFFERENTIAL DIAGNOSIS OF ANEMIA AND THROMBOCYTOPENIA FOR THIS PATIENT? WHAT ARE THE COMPLICATIONS OF INTRA-AORTIC BALLOON COUNTERPULSATION?

The surgical incision was found to be clean, dry, and intact, lessening the suspicion for postsurgical hematoma. A haptoglobin value of 20 mg/dL was discovered, a heparin-induced thrombocytopenia antibody panel was negative. The anemia and thrombocytopenia were, therefore, attributed to hemolysis caused by the IABP. A platelet transfusion was administered prior to surgery. The patient underwent a successful CABG followed by gradual weaning of IABP over the next 24 hours. He was discharged from the ICU 48 hours after an uneventful recovery.

DISCUSSION

POSTOPERATIVE MYOCARDIAL INFARCTION

Myocardial infarction (MI) is defined as myocardial cell death that results from prolonged ischemia.[1] The current classification includes five types of MI; Type 1 results from coronary athero-thrombosis, Type 2 involves mismatch of oxygen supply and demand, Type 3 results in death with no documented ECG or cardiac biomarker, Type 4 relates to PCI or stent thrombosis, and Type 5 relates to CABG.[2]

It is estimated that 1% of surgeries in the United States are complicated by postoperative MIs (POMI), most of which happen during the first 48 hours after surgery.[3] This incidence is significantly higher (0.5%–20%) in patients undergoing vascular surgery, making it the leading cause of morbidity and mortality in this population.[4] Risk factors for POMI in patients undergoing major vascular surgery include advanced age, obesity, renal insufficiency, diabetes, anemia, and underlying cardiac disease.[4] Cardiogenic shock (CS) complicates up to 10% of acute MIs and is associated with a significant increase in mortality.[5]

CARDIOGENIC SHOCK

The components of CO are heart rate and stroke volume. Stroke volume is dependent on contractility, preload and afterload. Contractility is determined by the ability of cardiac muscle cells to generate a contraction, which is affected in patients suffering from POMI.

CO is the main factor that determines delivery of blood to peripheral tissue. This relationship is illustrated by the following formula: $DO_2 = CO \times CaO_2$ (DO_2 is oxygen delivery and CaO_2 is the oxygen content of blood.) CaO_2 is determined by oxygen saturation, hemoglobin, and the partial pressure of oxygen, although to a much lesser extent.

CS is a state of hypoperfusion caused by low CO^6 and therefore insufficient DO_2 required to meet the demand of oxygen consumption (VO_2) by peripheral tissues.[7] The most common cause of CS is acute MI.[8] Hemodynamic criteria used to define CS are systolic blood pressure ≤90 mmHg for more than 30 minutes (or need for catecholamine therapy) with end-organ hypoperfusion, CI ≤ 2.2 L/min^{-2}, and PAOP ≥15 mmHg. Laboratory anomalies consistent with CS include metabolic acidosis, elevated serum lactate, and creatinine.[5,9,10]

Clinical manifestations of CS are the consequence of DO_2/VO_2 mismatch and include altered mental status, hypotension, oliguria, and cold extremities.

PATHOPHYSIOLOGY

The hallmark pathophysiological mechanism of Type 1 POMI is an obstruction of a coronary artery by rupture or erosion of an atherosclerotic plaque, which leads to downstream ischemia and myocardial injury.[11] However, most patients with POMI after surgery suffer from a Type 2 MI rather than an obstructive infarction.[3,12] This occurs because an increase in myocardial oxygen demand (secondary to pain, stress of surgery, and anesthesia) is not met by an increase in coronary blood flow.

CS caused by POMI is characterized by a decrease in contractility of the ischemic left ventricle, which leads to a decreased CO and blood pressure. Peripheral vasoconstriction follows, in an effort to maintain coronary perfusion pressure, at the expense of increasing afterload on an already weakened myocardium. The entire vascular system is then affected by the release of vasodilatory inflammatory mediators (nitric oxide, tumor necrosis factor, and cytokines), further complicating the picture, as some cytokines have negative inotropic effects.[8] Peripheral tissues then convert to anaerobic metabolism due to hypoxia-induced mitochondrial dysfunction, which leads to an increased lactate and anion gap metabolic acidosis.

DIAGNOSIS

Typical signs and symptoms of MI are typically masked or absent in patients after surgery. Atypical presentations include hemodynamic instability, new arrhythmias, respiratory failure, and CS.

Identifying patients with Type 1 MI for revascularization is the most important goal after establishing the diagnosis. Electrocardiography, cardiac biomarkers, and echocardiography are used to make this distinction (Figure 3.2 provides a diagnostic and management algorithm for patients with a diagnosis of POMI).

ELECTROCARDIOGRAPHY

ECG is used to differentiate between ST-segment elevation MI (STEMI) and non-ST-segment elevation MI (NSTEMI). A STEMI typically corresponds to a Type 1 MI, and it is considered a medical emergency. New ST elevation in 2 contiguous leads defines ST-segment elevation. NSTEMI is characterized by ST depressions and/or T wave changes. Q-waves are late electrocardiographic changes of an acute MI.

CARDIAC BIOMARKERS

Serum troponins (cardiac troponin I and cardiac troponin T) have replaced other cardiac biomarkers that have lower specificity and sensitivity. A troponin increase above the laboratory's 99th percentile is considered significant.[2] Increased troponins without myocardial injury can occur in patients with pulmonary embolism, renal failure, heart failure, myocarditis, sepsis, cardiomyopathies, and arrhythmias. In the ICU, troponin levels are commonly elevated and associated with poor outcomes,[13] which in part may be explained by type 2 MI and myocardial injury via toxins and medications.

POINT-OF-CARE ECHOCARDIOGRAPHY

Limited bedside transthoracic echocardiography is an efficient method for intensivists to assess cardiac function and guide management of the critically ill.[14] Point-of-care echocardiographic evaluation in patients with shock includes assessment of pericardial effusion, measurement of right and left ventricular size and function, respiratory variations in vena cava dimensions (a predictor of volume responsiveness), and calculation of the aortic velocity-time integral, used to calculate stroke volume and CO.[15] Regional wall motion abnormality on imaging corresponds to a new loss of myocardial viability, which can be used to diagnose MI[2]; therefore, echocardiography is particularly useful in patients with equivocal ECG and troponin results.

PULMONARY ARTERY CATHETER

Pulmonary artery catheters, in use since 1970, provide direct continuous measurements of: pulmonary artery pressures, CO, and mixed venous saturation. An increase in pulmonary artery pressures can indicate an MI,[16] before ECG changes become evident. It is particularly sensitive for ischemia when combined with echocardiography.[16] Despite this, in recent years, their routine use has been disfavored due concern for complications and lack of evidence that shows improved outcomes.[17]

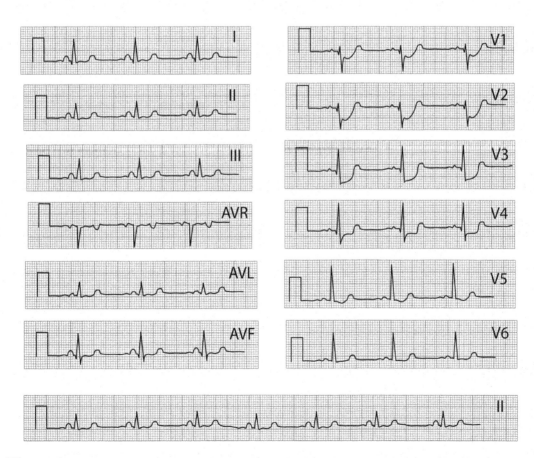

Figure 13.1 Initial Electrocardiogram.

12-lead electrocardiogram showing depressed ST-segment in leads V1-V4.

MANAGEMENT

Initial Medical Management of Postoperative Myocardial Infarction

Oxygen therapy has traditionally been administered to all patients presenting with acute coronary syndrome (ACS). However, no impact on outcomes has been demonstrated with this strategy in patients with normal oxygenation.[18] Therefore, oxygen should be given selectively to treat hypoxemia.

Nitroglycerin is indicated to relieve ischemic chest discomfort and can be sublingually administered and continued as an intravenous infusion if necessary. The use of beta blockers is favored to achieve heart rate control; nonetheless, it should be avoided during hypotension or shock. High-intensity statin therapy should be continued or initiated. Optimal pain control is particularly important in the postoperative period as pain increases myocardial oxygen demand through a sympathetic mediated response. Narcotics, multimodal analgesia and regional anesthesia should be optimized to achieve adequate pain control.

Antithrombotic therapy is essential in the management of patients with ACS. Aspirin should be given to all patients and continued daily indefinitely. Additionally, a second antiplatelet agent, usually clopidogrel, is recommended for patients that are considered high risk and for those treated with a stent, which is continued for up to a year.

Parenteral anticoagulation is recommended for patients with Type 1 MI, although a risk–benefit assessment to account the risk of bleeding is necessary in patients with POMI. Anticoagulation is usually stopped after a successful PCI. When a noninvasive strategy is chosen for the management of MI, anticoagulation is recommended for a few days during the hospital length of stay. Unfractioned heparin is usually the anticoagulant of choice as it is easily reversed if bleeding ensues.

Coronary Reperfusion

Coronary reperfusion therapy includes (i) PCI, which consists of angioplasty and stenting; (ii) CABG; and (iii) pharmacological thrombolysis; this last strategy is contraindicated in the perioperative period due to the risk of bleeding.

PCI is the recommended intervention for patients with STEMI when the onset of symptoms is within 12 hours, and in all patients with CS regardless of the onset of symptoms.[19]

Patients with NSTEMI that develop refractory angina, hemodynamic, or electrical instability should undergo immediate PCI.[20] Two treatment pathways exist for the management

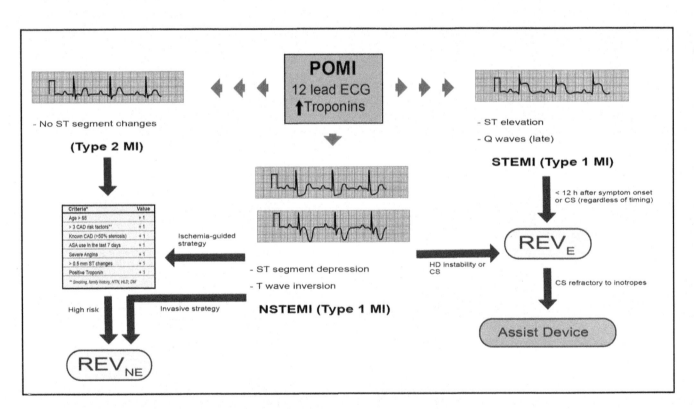

Figure 13.2 Management algorithm of Post-Operative Myocardial Infarction.

The figure illustrates the initial management algorithm of a patient with a diagnosis of postoperative myocardial infarction (POMI).
Electrocardiography is utilized to distinguish between STEMI and NSTEMI in patients with elevated troponins. The next step is determining which patients need revascularization therapy. Patients with refractory cardiogenic shock (CS) that is refractory to inotropes should be considered for an assist device.
* Thrombolysis in Myocardial Infarction (TIMI) score, a score of 5-7 is considered "high-risk".
REV_E: Emergency revascularization, includes percutaneous coronary intervention and coronary artery bypass grafting.
REV_NE: Non-Emergent revascularization, includes percutaneous coronary intervention and coronary artery bypass grafting. The timing is debatable but is usually performed 12-72 hours after the onset of symptoms.

of stable patients with NSTEMI: an *invasive strategy,* in which all patients undergo coronary angiography, and an *ischemia-guided* strategy, where invasive testing is reserved for patients that fail medical therapy, develop objective signs of ischemia, or have a high prognostic score.[20] The risk-stratification prognostic scores that have been validated for this purpose are the Thrombolysis in Myocardial Infarction and the Global Registry of Acute Coronary. The optimal timing of angiography in this clinical situation has not yet been elucidated; however, it is usually deferred to 12 to 72 hours while medical therapy is optimized. The rationale for this delay is that revascularization might be safer with a more stable plaque, which is achieved over time. Figure 13.2 provides a management algorithm for patients with POMI.

TYPE 2 MYOCARDIAL INFARCTION

The focus of the management of patients with a suspected Type 2 MI, is to reduce the precipitating factors that cause an increase in myocardial oxygen demand. This includes hypertension, hypotension, heart rate control, and postoperative pain.

There is no evidence to routinely recommend antithrombotic therapy, anticoagulation, or PCI in these patients.[12] Nonetheless, patients deemed high risk by prognostic scores should be considered for a nonemergent PCI.

SUPPORTIVE TREATMENT OF CARDIOGENIC SHOCK

Up to 10% of acute MI cases are complicated by CS, which dramatically increases mortality to 50% to 80%.[21,22] This has triggered the search for strategies to improve survival. Emergency revascularization is the priority in these patients, after which patients usually require supportive therapy with inotropes and vasopressors. Assist devices are used to support the failing contractility of the myocardium when shock remains refractory to medical therapy.

IABP is a widely used assist device, in which helium is pumped into a balloon that is inflated during diastole and deflated during systole (counterpulsation). Contraindications include aortic dissection, aneurysm, severe atherosclerotic disease, aortic graft, and aortic valve insufficiency. The procedure can be performed in the catheterization laboratory or at the bedside in the ICU. A balloon-tipped catheter is inserted in a peripheral artery via Seldinger technique and then advanced to the thoracic aorta. Placement is confirmed with fluoroscopy or transesophageal echocardiography. Proper position is 2 to 3 cm distal of the branching of the left subclavian artery. The balloon is triggered via an ECG (preferred) or by the arterial pressure waveform (Figure 13.3 shows a monitor of a patient with a 1:2 ECG triggered IABP). The hemodynamic effects of counterpulsation are (i) decreased left ventricular afterload, (ii) increased CO, (iii) decreased left ventricular systolic and end-diastolic pressures, (iv) reduction in ventricular wall tension, (v) increased coronary perfusion pressure, and (vi) decreased aortic systolic pressure and increased diastolic pressure.

The pump can be set to inflate at a cardiac cycle/counterpulsation ratio of 1:1, 1:2, or 1:3. Initially, the IABP should be programmed at 1:1 (maximum support) and then weaned as the patient improves. The pump should not be left in place while not counterpulsating as it increases the risk of cloth formation and embolism. Complications of IABP are related to malposition or aortic trauma and include limb ischemia, embolic events, compartment syndrome, aortic dissection, infection, balloon rupture causing gas embolism, hemolysis, thrombocytopenia, cerebral, mesenteric or renal ischemia, and cardiac tamponade.[23]

Despite early enthusiasm, the utilization of IABP to support shock after PCI has not been shown to improve prognostic ICU scores, 30-day, or 12-month mortality[10,21,24]; therefore, its routine use is not currently recommended. Other percutaneous assist devices (Impella-Abiomed, TandemHeart-Tandemlife, and extracorporeal membrane oxygenation) are gaining popularity as they have become more readily available.

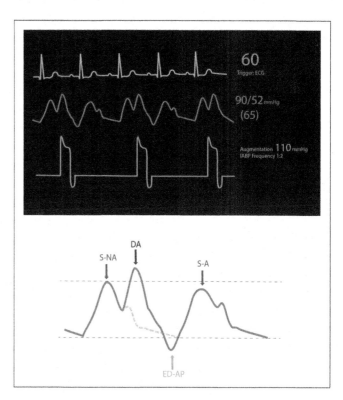

Figure 13.3 Intra-Aortic Balloon Counter-pulsation (IABP).

The upper figure shows an IABP monitor, of a pump programmed to provide 1:2 assistance, and triggered by the ECG. Note that the pump inflates (blue) during diastole in the middle of the ST segment (green), which corresponds to the dicrotic notch in the arterial pressure waveform (red).

The lower figure shows an arterial pulse waveform with an assisted pulse (DA), notice the increase in pressure caused by the IABP inflation (DA). When the pump deflates it causes a decrease in intra-aortic and end-diastolic pressures which constitutes a decrease in afterload. The following systolic pressure is also decreased (S-A).
S-NA: Systolic pressure (non-assisted)
DA: Diastolic Augmentation
ED-AP: End-diastolic pressure (assisted)
S-A: Systolic pressure (assisted)

Nonetheless, they have also failed to show a survival benefit,[22] and costs are significantly increased when compared to IABP. For this reason, IABP remains an initial reasonable choice for patients presenting with CS that is refractory to inotropic medications.[22]

CONCLUSIONS

- MI complicated by CS is a medical emergency and is associated with high mortality.

- Diagnosis is challenging in the postoperative period as atypical presentations are more common than chest pain.

- All patients with STEMI and unstable patients with NSTEMI are candidates for emergency PCI.

- The use of left ventricle assist devices is gaining widespread use, although a mortality benefit is yet to be demonstrated.

REFERENCES

1. Carroll I, Mount T, Atkinson D. Myocardial infarction in intensive care units: a systematic review of diagnosis and treatment. J Intensive Care Soc. 2016;17(4):314–325. doi:10.1177/1751143716656642.

2. Thygesen K, Alpert JS, Jaffe AS, et al. Third universal definition of myocardial infarction. Circulation. 2012;126(16):2020–2035. doi:10.1161/CIR.0b013e31826e1058.

3. Helwani M, Amin A, Lavigne P, et al. Etiology of acute coronary syndrome after noncardiac surgery. Anesthesiology. 2018;128(6):1084–1091. doi:10.1097/ALN.0000000000002107.

4. Juo YY, Mantha A, Ebrahimi R, Ziaeian B, Benharash P. Incidence of myocardial infarction after high-risk vascular operations in adults. JAMA Surg. 2017;152(11):1–8. doi:10.1001/jamasurg.2017.3360.

5. Hochman J, Sleeper L, Webb J, et al. Early revascularization in acute myocardial infarction complicated by cardiogenic shock. N Engl J Med. 1999;341(9):624–634. doi:10.1056/NEJMoa012295.

6. Patel H, Nazeer H, Yager N, Schulman-Marcus J. Cardiogenic shock: recent developments and significant knowledge gaps. Curr Treat Options Cardiovasc Med. 2018;20(2):15. doi:10.1007/s11936-018-0606-2.

7. Lim HS. Cardiogenic shock: failure of oxygen delivery and oxygen utilization. Clin Cardiol. 2016;39(8):477–483. doi:10.1002/clc.22564.

8. Van Diepen S, Katz JN, Albert NM, et al. Contemporary management of cardiogenic shock: a scientific statement from the American Heart Association. Circulation. 2017;136(16):e232–e268. doi:10.1161/CIR.0000000000000525.

9. Ponikowski P, Voors AA, Anker SD, et al. 2016 ESC Guidelines for the diagnosis and treatment of acute and chronic heart failure. Eur Heart J. 2016;37(27):2129–2200. doi:10.1093/eurheartj/ehw128.

10. Thiele H, Zeymer U, Neumann F-J, et al. Intraaortic balloon support for myocardial infarction with cardiogenic shock. N Engl J Med. 2012;367(14):1287–1296. doi:10.1056/NEJMoa1208410.

11. Anderson JL, Morrow DA. Acute myocardial infarction. N Engl J Med. 2017;376(21):2053–2064. doi:10.1056/NEJMra1606915.

12. Alpert JS, Thygesen KA, White HD, Jaffe AS. Diagnostic and therapeutic implications of type 2 myocardial infarction: review and commentary. Am J Med. 2014;127(2):105–108. doi:10.1016/j.amjmed.2013.09.031.

13. Guest TM, Ramanathan AV, Tuteur PG, Schechtman KB, Landenson JH, Jaffee AS. Myocardial injury in critically ill patients: a frequently unrecognized complication. JAMA. 1995;273(24):1945–1949. doi:10.1378/chest.128.4.2758.

14. Haji K, Haji D, Canty DJ, et al. The feasibility and impact of routine combined limited transthoracic echocardiography and lung ultrasound on diagnosis and management of patients admitted to ICU: a prospective observational study. J Cardiothorac Vasc Anesth. 2017;32:354–360. doi:10.1053/j.jvca.2017.08.026.

15. Vincent J-L, De Backer D. Circulatory shock. N Engl J Med. 2013;369(18):1726–1734. doi:10.1056/NEJMra1208943.

16. Boldt J. Clinical review: hemodynamic monitoring in the intensive care unit. Crit Care. 2002;6(1):52–59. doi:10.1186/cc1453.

17. Chatterjee K. The Swan-Ganz catheters: past, present, and future: a viewpoint. Circulation. 2009;119(1):147–152. doi:10.1161/CIRCULATIONAHA.108.811141.

18. Hofmann R, James SK, Jernberg T, et al. oxygen therapy in suspected acute myocardial infarction. N Engl J Med. 2017:NEJMoa1706222. doi:10.1056/NEJMoa1706222.

19. O'Gara PT, Kushner FG, Ascheim DD, et al. 2013 ACCF/AHA guideline for the management of st-elevation myocardial infarction: a report of the American College of Cardiology Foundation/American Heart Association Task Force on Practice Guidelines. Circulation. 2013;127(4):e362–e425. doi:10.1161/CIR.0b013e3182742cf6.

20. Amsterdam EA, Wenger NK, Brindis RG, et al. 2014 AHA/ACC guideline for the management of patients with non-st-elevation acute coronary syndromes: a report of the American College of cardiology/American Heart Association Task Force on Practice Guidelines. Circulation. 2014;130:2354–2394. doi:10.1161/CIR.0000000000000134.

21. Prondzinsky R, Lemm H, Swyter M, et al. Intra-aortic balloon counterpulsation in patients with acute myocardial infarction complicated by cardiogenic shock: the prospective, randomized IABP SHOCK trial for attenuation of multiorgan dysfunction syndrome. Crit Care Med. 2010;38(1):152–160. doi:10.1097/CCM.0b013e3181b78671.

22. Miller PE, Solomon MA, McAreavey D. Advanced percutaneous mechanical circulatory support devices for cardiogenic shock. Crit Care Med. 2017;45(11):1922–1929. doi:10.1097/CCM.0000000000002676.

23. Krishna M, Zacharowski K. Principles of intra-aortic balloon pump counterpulsation. Contin Educ Anaesthesia, Crit Care Pain. 2009;9(1):24–28. doi:10.1093/bjaceaccp/mkn051.

24. Thiele H, Zeymer U, Neumann F-J, et al. Intra-aortic balloon counterpulsation in acute myocardial infarction complicated by cardiogenic shock (IABP-SHOCK II): final 12 month results of a randomised, open-label trial. Lancet. 2013;382(9905):1638–1645. doi:10.1016/S0140-6736(13)61783-3.

25. Wutrich Y, Barraud D, Conrad M, et al. Early increase in arterial lactate concentration under epinephrine infusion is associated with a better prognosis during shock. Shock. 2010;34(1):4–9. doi:10.1097/SHK.0b013e3181ce2d23.

REVIEW QUESTIONS

1. A 53-year-old man is undergoing a percutaneous coronary intervention for a NSTEMI MI. An epinephrine infusion is started to support a CI of 1.8 L/min/m² at 0.04 mcg/kg/min. The CI improves, his blood pressure remains stable with a urine output of 1 cc/kg/hr. However, the lactate level (4 mmol/L) does not improve after 3 hours. What is the best next step?

    A. Continue current therapy
    B. Place an intra-aortic balloon pump
    C. Add a second inotrope
    D. Add a pressor

2. During a Bentall procedure to replace the aortic valve and ascending aorta of a woman with a bicuspid aortic valve, the

anesthesia team is having difficulties to separate from cardiopulmonary bypass as the myocardial function is severely depressed. The transesophageal echocardiogram shows global hypokinesis, an ejection fraction of 10% and a well-seated prosthetic valve with no significant stenosis or regurgitation. Mechanical assistance for the left ventricle is deemed necessary, which would be the most appropriate

A. IABP
B. Left ventricle assist device
C. Veno-venous extracorporeal membrane oxygenation
D. Veno-arterial extracorporeal membrane oxygenation

3. A patient with a history of diabetes mellitus, hypertension, and a transient ischemic attack presents for an elective femoro-popliteal bypass. He complains of chest pain just before the surgery. An ECG reveals ST elevation on the anterior leads. In addition to an emergency PCI, which is the most appropriate therapy?

A. Aspirin + heparin infusion
B. Aspirin + heparin infusion + prasugrel
C. Clopidogrel + heparin infusion
D. Aspirin + heparin infusion + clopidogrel

4. An ischemia-guided strategy is utilized to treat a NSTEMI, after the patient underwent a pancreatoduodenectomy. Cardiac index is 2.2 L/min/m², blood pressure 110/70 mmHg, heart rate 50 bpm, and oxygen saturation 96%. His laboratory results are significant for a hemoglobin of 7 g/dL the arterial blood gas shows pH 7.30, pCO_2 40 torr, pO_2 70 while breathing room air. Which of the following strategies will increase the oxygen delivery to the injured myocardium?

A. Oxygen supplementation
B. Norepinephrine administration to raise the systolic blood pressure above 120 mmHg
C. Transfusion of packed red blood cells
D. Administration of a chronotope

5. A 54-year-old-man with history of angina, smoking, diabetes, chronic renal failure, and hypertension is recovering from a thoracotomy and lobectomy, which were performed for lung cancer. He complains of chest pain immediately after surgery, which is attributed to surgery. Nonetheless, ECG and troponins are obtained. There are no ST segment changes, but the troponin I is marginally elevated at 0.04 ng/mL (institutional 99th percentile is 0.01 ng/mL). Which of the following would aid in the diagnosis of MI on this patient?

A. Repeating the troponin I measurement in 3 hours
B. Measurement of serum creatine kinase myocardial isoenzyme
C. Measurement of serum myoglobin
D. Measurement of troponin T

6. During a liver resection for cancer, a patient receives 10 units of packed red blood cells, 10 units of fresh frozen plasma, and 3 units of platelets. Shortly after arriving to the ICU, ST depression is detected on the monitor and confirmed in leads V1, V2, and V3 on a 12-lead ECG. Serum troponins are elevated. He complains of shortness of breath and is oriented to

person, but not to time or place. A chest X-ray reveals bilateral diffuse infiltrates, and his oxygen saturation is 90% on an inspired oxygen fraction of 30%. Urine output had been gradually declining during the surgery and stops for the last hour. What is the best next step?

A. Diuretic challenge
B. Endotracheal intubation and emergent PCI
C. Chest CT with intravenous contrast
D. Endotracheal intubation and ventilation with lung protective tidal volumes

7. Which of the following is not a hemodynamic effect of counter-pulsation by an intra-aortic balloon pump?

A. Increased left ventricle afterload
B. Increased CO
C. Increased aortic diastolic pressure
D. Increased coronary perfusion pressure

8. After a successful emergency PCI and stent placement for a STEMI complicated by CS, a 60-year-old man is recovering in the ICU. An intra-aortic balloon pump is in place with a counter-pulsation ratio of 1:2. A severe metabolic acidosis has resolved and the patient is producing adequate urine output. Suddenly, he becomes hypotensive and tachycardic. A transthoracic echocardiogram is performed and reveals a hyperdynamic left ventricle, no regional wall motion abnormalities and new onset of severe aortic regurgitation by color Doppler. What is the best next step?

A. Emergency surgery consultation
B. Set the IABP to a 1:1 ratio
C. Set the IABP to a 1:3 ratio
D. Amiodarone bolus

9. Which of the following triggers a well-functioning intra-aortic balloon pump?

A. T wave offset
B. S wave
C. T wave onset
D. Dicrotic notch

10. In patients with CS caused by an ST elevation MI, which assist device has been shown to improve mortality if instituted early?

A. Intra-aortic balloon pump
B. Left ventricle assist device (LVAD)
C. Extra-corporeal membrane oxygenation (ECMO)
D. None of the above

ANSWERS

1. A. Lactate is considered a surrogate marker of hypoperfusion during shock. Trending serum levels to monitor resolution or worsening of shock is common practice. However, epinephrine activates aerobic glycolysis of which lactate is a by-product. Therefore, increased lactate levels have been associated with high dose epinephrine infusions used for treating shock. In fact, this trend has been shown to indicate

an improved prognosis.[25] Escalating therapy is not necessary as long as other indicators of hypoperfusion are not present (decreased urine output, altered mental status).

2. D. Failure of separating from cardiopulmonary bypass occurs when the contractility of the left ventricle is impaired, and it cannot support organ perfusion. Assist devices provide temporary support until the myocardium recovers. They may also serve as a bridge to transplant, or they may become destination therapy (LVAD). IABP would be contraindicated in this patient with a recent aortic graft due to the risk of anastomotic rupture with counter-pulsation (A). An LVAD is not the best option in this patient as myocardial stunning is usually reversible in the short term (B). Veno-venous extracorporeal membrane oxygenation assists with oxygenation but does not assist contractility (C). Venous-arterial extracorporeal membrane oxygenation can provide full support to the heart and lung and would be the most appropriate choice in these patient (D).

3. D. Primary PCI is recommended for patients presenting with a STEMI: with less than 12 hours of symptoms; with more than 12 hours of onset of symptoms but with contraindication to thrombolysis; or in patients with heart failure/shock secondary to the STEMI regardless of the time of presentation (level 1 recommendation).[19] Aspirin should be given to all patients presenting with ACS. Anticoagulation and antiplatelet agents (clopidogrel, prasugrel, or ticagrelor) should be given as well unless there is a strong contraindication (level 1 recommendation).[19] Prasugrel is a more potent antiplatelet agent than clopidogrel (B); however, it is contraindicated in patients with a history of stroke or transient ischemic attack.

4. C. Oxygen delivery is determined by the CO and the oxygen content in blood ($DO_2 = CO \times CaO_2$); oxygen is carried in blood mostly bound to hemoglobin; therefore, the oxygen content of blood (CaO_2) is dependent on hemoglobin and oxygen saturation. Oxygen supplementation (A), will not increase the CaO_2 in this patient because his oxygen saturation is already 97%. Clinical trials have also shown no advantage of oxygen supplementation in patients without hypoxemia.[18] Increasing the blood pressure will not increase DO_2 and could be detrimental because the increase in afterload would increase the oxygen demands of the myocardium (B). Chronotropic drugs will increase the heart rate, which would modestly increase the CO and DO_2; however, it would also increase the oxygen demands of the myocardium. Packed red blood cell transfusion (C) will increase the oxygen carrying capacity of the blood and, therefore, DO_2.

5. A. With the advent of contemporary troponin assays, other cardiac biomarkers are not recommended for the diagnosis of MI (B and C). Chronic renal failure can cause an elevation in troponins in patients that are not experiencing myocardial ischemia. Troponin I is less affected than troponin T (D), therefore, measuring a troponin I improves sensitivity in patients with renal failure. The sensitivity of elevated troponins increases with a rising "trend," and it is recommended to repeat troponin levels at 3 and 6 hours (class 1 recommendation).[20]

6. B. Impeding respiratory failure in patients with CS necessitates endotracheal intubation and ventilation, since the ability to maintain a patent airway becomes compromised. An NSTEMI complicated by CS should undergo emergency PCI (B). Volume overload can cause hypoxemia and usually responds to diuretic therapy (A); however, the cause in this case is cardiogenic pulmonary edema. Immobilization, recent surgery, and history of cancers are risk factors for pulmonary embolism (PE) and are present in this case. Of note, PE can also cause elevated troponins; however, the most likely cause of hypoxemia in this case is CS caused by an NSTEMI, and therefore a PCI should not be delayed to rule out the less likely diagnosis of PE. The standard of care treatment for acute respiratory distress syndrome involves protective lung ventilation with low tidal volumes (D); however, explanation of the X-ray abnormalities in this case is cardiogenic pulmonary edema.

7. A. In summary, the physiological effects of IABP therapy are (i) decreased aortic systolic pressure; (ii) increased aortic diastolic pressure; (iii) decreased left ventricle systolic pressure, end diastolic pressure and wall tension; (iv) decreased afterload and preload; (v) increased CO; and (6) increased coronary blood flow by an increase in coronary perfusion pressure.[23]

8. A. Complications of intra-aortic balloon pump counterpulsation are related to malposition or aortic trauma. If an aortic dissection travels proximal to the ascending aorta (Type A), aortic valve regurgitation ensues; the treatment is emergency surgery (Bentall procedure). Changing the counterpulsation ratio will increase the assistance of the left ventricle (B) but is not be the best option in this case. Decreasing the counterpulsation ratio to 1:3 is chosen to wean off the IABP and is not appropriate in this case (C). Amiodarone is a class III antiarrhythmic, useful in the management of some tachyarrhythmias and is not the treatment in this case (D).

9. D. An IABP can be triggered by the ECG or the arterial pressure waveform. ECG is the preferred trigger. The pump is programmed to inflate during the middle of the T wave (early diastole). If the arterial pressure waveform is chosen, the pump is inflated at the dicrotic notch, the small increment in pressure that results from closure of the aortic valve (Figure 13.3 shows a correlation between ECG, balloon pressure waveform, and arterial pressure waveform).[23]

10. D. Despite advances in medical device technology, including ventricular assist devices, a mortality advantage is yet to be demonstrated for any of these devices. Intra-aortic balloon counterpulsation had a class 1 recommendation downgraded as clinical trials failed to show reduced early[10] and late mortality.[24] There is also no survival advantage when comparing LVADs and IABP[6]; there are no clinical trials on ECMO for this pathology.

14.

IN-HOSPITAL ACUTE CORONARY SYNDROME

Dennis Wells and Suzanne Bennett

STEM CASE AND KEY QUESTIONS

A 78-year-old woman presented to the hospital for video assisted thoracoscopic left lower lobectomy for resection of a stage 1A nonsmall cell lung cancer. Her past medical history included a 50-pack year smoking history and quit smoking 1 month prior to her operation, hypertension, hyperlipidemia, diet-controlled diabetes mellitus, and coronary artery disease (CAD) with a prior drug-eluting stent (DES) to the right coronary artery (RCA) 5 years ago. She was taking daily aspirin but had stopped taking clopidogrel a few years prior to the surgery. She was also taking metoprolol and atorvastatin, which were continued perioperatively. Pulmonary function testing demonstrated adequate pulmonary reserve and stress echocardiography demonstrated normal left ventricular function and no evidence of ischemia.

The patient underwent a left lower lobectomy via video-assisted thoracoscopic surgery under general anesthesia with a thoracic epidural placed for postoperative pain management. There were no complications, and she was transferred to the intensive care unit (ICU) for postoperative care. On postoperative day 1, the patient developed hypotension, mild tachycardia, and oliguria with a metabolic acidosis. She transiently improved with fluid boluses and a reduction of her epidural dose. Soon, however, with ongoing hypotension, tachycardia, and oliguria, a phenylephrine infusion was initiated. Despite improvement in blood pressure and urine output, she began to complain of left-sided chest pain. A change in the ST segments on her bedside telemetry was noted. A 12-lead electrocardiogram (ECG) demonstrated significant ST elevations in leads II and III, and arteriovenous fistula. Initial troponin was 4.3 ng/L. A focused bedside echocardiogram demonstrated inferior hypokinesis and an estimated left ventricular ejection fraction (LVEF) of 40%. The most likely diagnosis was a postoperative acute inferior wall myocardial infarction, concerning for in-stent thrombosis.

WHAT SHOULD WE CONSIDER IN THE DIFFERENTIAL DIAGNOSIS OF CHEST PAIN?

A change in the ST segments on her bedside telemetry was noted. A 12-lead ECG demonstrated significant ST elevations in leads II and III and arteriovenous fistula. Initial troponin was 4.3 ng/L.

WHAT IS ACUTE CORONARY SYNDROME? WHAT OTHER CLINICAL PROBLEMS OR DISEASES MAY CAUSE ST SEGMENT CHANGES OR ELEVATIONS IN CARDIAC ENZYMES?

ECG changes without symptoms or without elevation of cardiac biomarkers may be related to improper lead placement or other inflammatory changes such as pericarditis. While it should not be overlooked, bedside or remote telemetry changes in ST segments are not reliable, and any suspicious changes should be evaluated with a 12-lead ECG. Elevated cardiac biomarkers without ischemic ECG patterns or typical symptoms of angina may be related to other causes of myocardial injury or muscle injury such as after significant trauma, blunt cardiac injury, myocarditis, or even some major surgery. It is common for cardiac biomarkers to be elevated after cardiac surgery. The combination of typical angina, ischemic ECG changes, and elevated cardiac biomarkers should prompt an immediate further workup with a focus on the etiology of the ischemia rather than looking for an alternative diagnosis. Given this history, a focused bedside echocardiogram demonstrated inferior hypokinesis and an estimated LVEF of 40%. The diagnosis of postoperative acute inferior wall myocardial infarction was made with suspected in-stent thrombosis.

WHAT FACTORS ARE ASSOCIATED WITH THE PATIENT'S PROGNOSIS IF SHE IS HAVING ACS?

The factors that increase her morbidity and mortality are in-hospital ACS, ST segment elevation myocardial infarction (STEMI) presentation, and likely in stent thrombosis (1–3).

WHAT DIAGNOSTIC TESTS ARE NECESSARY TO DIAGNOSE ACS AND WILL SHE BENEFIT FROM ANGIOGRAPHY?

After multidisciplinary discussions, the anesthesiology pain team removed the epidural catheter to reduce the risk of epidural hematoma given the patient's possible need for anticoagulation and dual antiplatelet therapy. Given the risk of epidural hematoma and surgical bleeding, dual antiplatelet therapy, and intravenous unfractionated heparin were delayed until angiography.

WHAT ARE INITIAL TREATMENT MEASURES TO TREAT ACS AND HOW DO THEY DIFFER WHEN IT OCCURS IN THE HOSPITAL SETTING?

The patient was placed on bedrest with telemetry and continuous pulse oximetry and supplemental oxygen was administered. Nitroglycerin was prescribed with caution given the setting of hypotension, bradycardia, and suspected right ventricular (RV) infarct, and her chest pain was alleviated with the administration of morphine. She subsequently underwent a left heart catheterization, which revealed an in-stent thrombosis of the RCA. A percutaneous coronary intervention (PCI) with DES to RCA was performed with resolution of chest pain. The remainder of the left heart catheterization showed nonobstructive coronary disease. Following catheterization, she was given aspirin and Plavix. In addition, beta blocker therapy titrated to a heart rate of 50 to 60 and an angiotensin converting enzyme inhibitor due to her reduced LVEF were prescribed as well as a high-intensity statin (80 mg atorvastatin).

DISCUSSION

A patient with chest pain presents a complicated diagnostic challenge. The differential diagnosis of chest pain is vast and includes cardiovascular and non-cardiovascular etiologies that can be imminently life-threatening (Table 14.1).

Table 14.1 DIFFERENTIAL DIAGNOSIS OF CHEST PAIN

CARDIOVASCULAR ETIOLOGIES	NONCARDIOVASCULAR ETIOLOGIES
Acute coronary syndrome	Trauma
Inflammatory: • Pericarditis • Myocarditis	Musculoskeletal pain: • Costochondritis • Postoperative pain
Aortic Catastrophe: • Dissection • Intramural hematoma • Rupture	Pleuritic chest pain related to • Pneumonia • Pneumothorax • Pulmonary embolism
	Esophageal pathology • Gastroesophageal reflux • Esophageal spasm • Motility disorder • Perforation
	Abdominal pathology (referred pain) • Cholecystitis • Peptic ulcer disease • Pancreatitis
	Panic attacks

DEFINITION AND CLINICAL MANIFESTATIONS OF ACS

ACS refers to one of the following presentations of myocardial ischemia (4):

STEMI, defined as clinical symptoms of myocardial infarction associated with ECG findings of new ST elevation in at least 2 contiguous leads of at least 2 mm in men or 1.5 mm in women in leads V2–V3 and/or 1 mm in other contiguous chest leads or the limb leads, or a new left bundle branch block. Cardiac biomarkers will be positive.

Non-ST segment elevation myocardial infarction (NSTEMI) defined as elevation in cardiac biomarkers without associated ECG findings that meet STEMI criteria although may still be associated with some degree of ST segment elevation, ST segment depression, or T-wave inversion.

Unstable angina, which typically refers to angina at rest, new onset severe angina, or crescendo angina (angina which increases in intensity, frequency, or duration) and is not associated with ECG findings that meet STEMI criteria. This may still be associated with some degree of ST segment elevation, ST segment depression, or T-wave inversion but not associated with laboratory findings of elevated cardiac biomarkers (4–6).

"Typical" or "stable" angina is described as chest pain or pressure that is exacerbated by exertion and relieved by rest or antianginal medications such as nitroglycerin. The chest pain may radiate to the left shoulder, arm, or jaw. It may also be associated with other symptoms including diaphoresis or dyspnea.

Atypical angina or chest pain usually refers to any other type of chest pain or discomfort that does not meet the previous criteria; often practitioners may cite dyspnea as atypical angina as well.

In addition to chest pain, the patient having ACS may present with other associated signs and symptoms (Box 14.1). Echocardiography is the best diagnostic tool to confirm presence of one of the listed mechanical complications as it is often readily available, and a competent practitioner can identify one of the structural changes quickly as these patients may be in shock and too unstable to be transported for other studies.

Box 14.1 SIGNS AND SYMPTOMS ASSOCIATED WITH ACS

Cardiogenic shock
Arrhythmia
RV infarct
Mechanical complications of AMI:
• Papillary muscle rupture
• Ventricular free wall rupture
• Postinfarction ventricular septal defect

DIAGNOSTIC MODALITIES FOR ACS

Electrocardiogram and cardiac biomarkers are the fundamental tests for making the diagnosis. Echocardiography demonstrates changes in cardiac function, regional wall motion abnormalities, pericardial effusion, or new mechanical complications and can be quite helpful although not always necessary prior to angiography. A comprehensive echocardiogram will always be warranted prior to surgical intervention. Stress testing should be reserved for patients who present without any evidence of hemodynamic instability. Patients that have evidence of unstable angina that resolves and does not recur over a period of several hours with only a mild troponin elevation may be considered to have a NSTEMI from "demand ischemia" from a transient imbalance of myocardial oxygen demand and supply. The clinical findings typically resolve quickly without recurrence. Angiography is indicated for most cases of ACS with STEMI requiring immediate intervention and NSTEMI/unstable angina timing dependent upon a risk assessment of the patient.

Currently, angiography with PCI of the culprit lesion is recommended within 90 minutes of STEMI presentation.

Current recommendations for NSTEMI and unstable angina include angiography as soon as possible for high-risk patients (Box 14.2). Low risk patients may undergo a conservative evaluation with angiography reserved for those low-risk patients with persistent or recurrent symptoms or rising troponins (7).

EPIDEMIOLOGY AND MORTALITY

Several factors are of prognostic value in patients with ACS from STEMI with the highest 30-day mortality. Troponin level correlates with severity of myocardial injury and correlates with poor prognosis. Elevated brain natriuretic peptide, white blood cell count, and C-reactive protein also correlate with poor prognosis. Increasing age and diabetes mellitus are associated with worse outcomes. In the setting of unstable angina or NSTEMI, ECG changes, particularly ST segment elevations, less than those that meet STEMI criteria, are associated with worse outcomes

Box 14.2 HIGH RISK FACTORS FOR PATIENTS PRESENTING WITH NSTEMI OR UNSTABLE ANGINA

- Recurrent angina
- Elevated biomarkers
- New ST-segment depression
- New or worsening congestive heart failure or mitral regurgitation
- Prior PCI within 6 months
- Prior CABG
- Reduced LVEF <40%
- High-risk stress test
- Sustained VT or hemodynamic instability

Recently, more attention has been directed at in-hospital occurrence of ACS and STEMI. In-hospital STEMI more commonly occurs in older patients with more comorbid conditions. The presentation is more frequently atypical and patients often have contraindications to anticoagulation or fibrinolytics. As such, delays in diagnosis and treatment are common. One review reported only 34% to 71% of patients with in-hospital STEMI undergo angiography, only 22% to 56% have PCI performed, and in-hospital mortality in these patients ranges from 31% to 42% (1).

While the patient, in the aforementioned case, had delayed in-stent stenosis, early in-stent stenosis also occurs and carries significant risk. Studies have indicated that in-stent stenosis is more common after an episode of ACS than in patients treated with PCI for stable CAD. Early in-stent stenosis rates after ACS have been reported as high as 1.4% with both DES and bare metal stents (BMS) and is associated with significant morbidity and mortality: 80% recurrent myocardial infarction, 66% need for repeat revascularization, and 25% mortality. In addition, higher mortality rates are associated with in-hospital versus out-of-hospital in-stent thrombotic events (27.8% vs. 10.8%, respectively) at 1 year (2, 8). Predictors of early in-stent stenosis include small coronary arteries with diffuse disease, inadequate pharmacotherapy, or noncompliance, as well as associated insulin dependent diabetes or renal insufficiency (3). This supports the concept of "optimization" of medical therapy prior to surgery as mentioned in this case.

GUIDELINE RECOMMENDATIONS FOR INTERVENTION

For all patients with STEMI including those patients presenting in shock, culprit lesion PCI is the primary treatment modality recommended. Culprit lesion PCI is also the treatment for high-risk patients presenting with unstable angina and NSTEMI.

Coronary Artery Bypass Surgery Versus PCI

- Urgent coronary artery bypass surgery (CABG) is recommended for patients with STEMI and coronary anatomy not amenable to PCI *and if* there is

  - Ongoing ischemia.
  - Severe heart failure.
  - Cardiogenic shock.
  - Other high-risk features or mechanical defects that require surgery.

- Emergency CABG within 6 hours can be considered for a stable patient who is not a candidate for PCI or fibrinolytics.

There are no prospective randomized controlled trials comparing outcomes of PCI versus CABG for revascularizations strategy in patients presenting with ACS.

- Multiple studies have shown long-term benefits of CABG including many randomized controlled trials comparing patients undergoing elective revascularization (9).

- A recent retrospective study demonstrated improved short- and long-term outcomes in diabetic patients presenting with ACS (but not STEMI) who underwent CABG versus PCI (10).

Despite long-term benefits of CABG compared to PCI, the primary treatment goal for a patient presenting with acute coronary syndrome, particularly STEMI, is to treat the culprit lesion, limit myocardial injury, and prevent other organ injury. In most settings, initial PCI accomplishes this most efficiently with limited morbidity.

In patients with multivessel disease, multivessel PCI has been reported to be safe and effective for patients presenting with ACS. It may be considered for patients with high surgical risk and low SYNTAX score, but it is not currently recommended (11).

Specific Recommendations for Treatment of In-Stent Stenosis Presenting With ACS

PCI remains the current recommendation for in-stent stenosis related ACS events. Several studies have evaluated various catheter-based treatments. Two large meta-analysis evaluating randomized controlled trials treating in-stent restenosis concluded that a DES or drug-coated balloon yields superior results both clinically and angiographically to other modalities (12, 13). The lack of an additional stent layer provided by treatment with a drug-coated balloon may be desirable in certain instances such as small target vessels.

Timing of Intervention

Culprit lesion PCI should be performed as soon as possible in patients with STEMI and high-risk patients with unstable angina and NSTEMI.

CABG may be warranted for patients with coronary anatomy not suitable to PCI or after culprit lesion PCI in patients with significant additional coronary disease.

The best timing of CABG after acute coronary syndrome is difficult to determine across patients and will vary based on the specific presentation and risk profile. Many studies have produced conflicting data. Several studies have demonstrated poor outcomes with early CABG after ACS. Studies that evaluate this question with risk stratification of patients demonstrated no significant increased mortality risk in low-risk patients, such as stable patients after NSTEMI without active ischemia at time of surgery (14). Mortality is likely more related to the patient's overall acuity and not timing of CABG.

While some factors such as inability to perform PCI and ongoing ischemia may predispose practitioners to recommend early surgical revascularization, patients without an emergent indication definitely benefit from stabilization and medical optimization.

CONCLUSION

In-hospital acute coronary syndrome represents a complex problem generally occurring in a high-risk patient population.

Outcomes are worse when patients present with ACS as an in-hospital complication compared to presentation to the emergency department. This is likely due to diagnostic and treatment delays related to atypical presentations and comorbid conditions that present contraindications to standard therapies.

Practitioners need a high index of suspicion for myocardial ischemia in patients with significant risk factors or known CAD. Outcomes may be improved if ICUs and hospitals develop protocols for early assessment and rapid intervention for suspected in-hospital ACS. Collaboration between a critical care based rapid response team and the cardiology service in conjunction with the cardiac catheterization lab to establish protocols that mimic the guidelines for ACS patients presenting to the emergency department could improve results.

In all cases, proper management of in-hospital ACS will require effective communication and cooperation between multidisciplinary teams.

REFERENCES

1. Levine GN, Dai X, Henry TD, et al. In-hospital ST-segment elevation myocardial infarction improving diagnosis, triage, and treatment. JAMA Cardiology. Published online February 21, 2018. doi:10.1001/jamacardio.2017.5356
2. Dangas GD Claessen BE, Mehran R, et al. Clinical outcomes following stent thrombosis occurring in-hospital versus out-of-hospital: results from the HORIZONS-AMI (Harmonizing Outcomes with Revascularization and Stents in Acute Myocardial Infarction) trial. Journal of the American College of Cardiology. 2012;59(20):1752–1759.
3. Aoki J, Lansky AJ, Mehran R, et al. Early stent thrombosis in patients with acute coronary syndromes treated with drug-eluting and bare metal stents. Circulation 2009;119(5):687–698.
4. Kumar A, Cannon CP. Acute coronary syndromes: diagnosis and management, Part I. Mayo Clinic Proceedings. 2009;84(10):917–938.
5. Thygesen K, Alpert JS, Jaffe AS, et al. Third universal definition of myocardial infarction. Circulation. 2012;126:2020–2035.
6. O'Gara PT, Kushner FG, Ascheim DD, et al. 2013 ACCF/AHA guideline for the management of ST-elevation myocardial infarction: a report of the American College of Cardiology Foundation/American Heart Association Task Force on Practice Guidelines. Circulation. 2013;127:1–88.
7. Anderson JL, Adams CD, Antman EM, et al.; American College of Cardiology, American Heart Association Task Force on Practice Guidelines (Writing Committee to Revise the 2002 Guidelines for the Management of Patients With Unstable Angina/Non-ST-Elevation Myocardial Infarction), American College of Emergency Physicians, Society for Cardiovascular Angiography and Interventions, Society of Thoracic Surgeons., American Association of Cardiovascular and Pulmonary Rehabilitation, Society for Academic Emergency Medicine. J Am Coll Cardiol. 2007 Aug 14; 50(7):e1–e157.
8. Dangas GD, Schoos MM, Steg PG, et al. early stent thrombosis and mortality after primary percutaneous coronary intervention in ST-segment–elevation myocardial infarction. Circulation: Cardiovascular Interventions. 2016;9:e003272.
9. Head SJ, Milojevic M, Daemen J, et al. Mortality after coronary artery bypass grafting versus percutaneous coronary intervention

with stenting for coronary artery disease: a pooled analysis of individual patient data. *The Lancet.* 2018;*391*(10124):939–948.

10. Ramanathan K, Abel JG, Park JE, et al. Surgical versus percutaneous coronary revascularization in patients with diabetes and acute coronary syndromes, *Journal of the American College of Cardiology.* 2017;*70*(24):2995–3006.

11. Brener SJ, Milford-Beland S, Roe MT, Bhatt DL, Weintraub WS, Brindis RG. Culprit-only or multivessel revascularization in patients with acute coronary syndromes: an American College of Cardiology National Cardiovascular Database Registry report. *American Heart Journal.* 2008;*155*(1):140–146.

12. Giacoppo D, Gargiulo G, Aruta P, Capranzano P, Tamburino C, Capodanno D. Treatment strategies for coronary in-stent restenosis: systematic review and hierarchical Bayesian network meta-analysis of 24 randomised trials and 4880 patients. BMJ. 2015;351:h5392. doi:10.1136/bmj.h5392.

13. Siontis GC, Stefanini GG, Mavridis D, et al. Percutaneous coronary interventional strategies for treatment of in-stent restenosis: a network meta-analysis. *The Lancet.* 2015;*386*(9994):655–664.

14. Manuel Caceres MD, Weiman DS. Optimal timing of coronary artery bypass grafting in acute myocardial infarction. Annals of Thoracic Surgery. 2013;*95*:365–372.

REVIEW QUESTIONS

1. A patient complains of substernal chest pain at rest, initial workup demonstrates an ECG with ST segment elevations of 1 mm in leads V1 and V2, and troponin level is normal. What is this presentation classified as?

   A. STEMI
   B. NSTEMI
   C. Unstable angina
   D. Stable angina

2. A patient presents with severe chest pain; he is hemodynamically stable with normal blood pressure, heart rate, and oxygen saturations. ECG demonstrates significant ST segment elevations in lateral leads and troponin level is 5.7 ng/L. The most important next step in management of the options given is

   A. contacting the cardiac catheterization lab.
   B. morphine administration.
   C. adding supplemental oxygen via face mask.
   D. angiotensin converting enzyme inhibitor administration.

3. A patient with a history of CAD who presents with unstable angina should be given what medication immediately, even prior to ECG completion and troponin results?

   A. Heparin infusion
   B. Atorvastatin
   C. Esmolol infusion
   D. Aspirin

4. A patient with known CAD who presents with unstable angina and has increasing symptoms despite initial medical therapy. What intervention should be performed next?

   A. Continued medical therapy
   B. Angiography as soon as possible

   C. Angiography within the next 24 hours
   D. Noninvasive stress test

5. A patient with normal neurologic status suffers a STEMI complicated by ventricular fibrillation cardiac arrest. Return of spontaneous circulation is achieved after 10 minutes of resuscitation. PCI to the proximal left anterior descending artery is performed but the patient remains comatose. Additional interventions for this patient should include

   A. cardiac magnetic resonance imaging to evaluate function and viability.
   B. therapeutic hypothermia for 24 and 48 hours.
   C. continuous video EEG for 48 hours.
   D. magnetic resonance imaging and magnetic resonance angiography of the head and neck.

6. A patient who complains of substernal chest pain, dyspnea, and malaise is found to have an elevated troponin level and ECG demonstrated ischemic changes in inferior leads. He is hypotensive and bradycardic. In addition, he seems to feel worse after administration of aspirin and sublingual nitroglycerin. The next best steps include

   A. Nitroglycerin and Lasix infusion.
   B. Esmolol infusion.
   C. Digoxin administration.
   D. Fluid bolus and transcutaneous pacing.

7. A patient presents with STEMI and cardiogenic shock. This patient should have which of the following interventions?

   A. Emergency CABG
   B. Urgent PCI
   C. Medical stabilization in the ICU prior to PCI
   D. Immediate administration of fibrinolytics

8. A 55-year-old male patient who presented with chest pain occurring 1 hour ago at 6:30 AM and was found to have a STEMI is now in the cardiac catheterization lab where angiography demonstrates 3-vessel disease with a culprit lesion at the left main coronary artery bifurcation. The SYNTAX score is high, and the patient is a low surgical risk. He continues to have angina despite heparin and nitroglycerin infusions. The best treatment option for this patient is

   A. PCI.
   B. emergent CABG.
   C. fibrinolytics.
   D. continued medical therapy with CABG in 72 hours.

9. In-stent stenosis presenting as an ACS event is best treated with

   A. CABG because PCI for in-stent stenosis events yields poor results.
   B. Fibrinolytics because PCI yields poor results and CABG is too invasive.
   C. PCI with a drug-coated balloon or DES if amenable.
   D. Medical management with heparin and low dose fibrinolytic infusion.

10. A patient who presented with ACS was found to have a STEMI resulting from 3-vessel disease with a culprit lesion in the RCA. Given that her surgical risk is low, and her SYNTAX score is moderate, she should have which of the following therapies?

A. Emergent PCI to the RCA lesion followed by CABG later this admission
B. Emergent PCI to the RCA lesion followed by PCI to the LAD and circumflex lesion within 24 hours
C. Emergent PCI to the RCA lesion and simultaneous PCI to the LAD and circumflex lesions
D. Emergent PCI to the RCA lesion and medical therapy for her remaining disease

ANSWERS

1. C. Unstable angina. Unstable angina can present without ECG changes meeting STEMI criteria and without positive cardiac biomarkers.

2. A. Contacting the cardiac catheterization lab. Prompt intervention to restore myocardial blood flow is the most important next step.

3. D. Aspirin. In the absence of a contraindication, aspirin should be administered as soon as the diagnosis of ACS is suspected.

4. B. Angiography as soon as possible. Progressive unstable angina is an indication for angiography and should be completed as soon as possible.

5. B. Therapeutic hypothermia. Guideline recommendations for patients who are comatose after a ventricular fibrillation/ventricular tachycardia arrest include therapeutic hypothermia for 24 hours.

6. D. Fluid bolus and transcutaneous pacing. Inferior lead ischemia, hypotension, and bradycardia are consistent with an RV infarct. The patient worsening after nitroglycerin administration is another clue that RV preload may be insufficient. A fluid bolus and pacing is needed in this setting.

7. B. Urgent PCI. Even in the setting of cardiogenic shock, current guidelines recommend urgent PCI as soon as possible. Medical therapy and mechanical therapy for shock can be implemented in the cardiac catheterization lab. Emergency CABG is reserved for patients not suitable for PCI or fibrinolytics.

8. B. Emergent CABG. In a capable center this is one of the rare instances in which emergent CABG is likely the best option. The patient is young and otherwise low risk, with poor PCI options. In addition, it is less than 6 hours since the onset of chest pain and he is having progressive ischemia.

9. C. PCI with drug coated balloon or drug eluting stent if amenable. Recommendations for treatment of in-stent stenosis are the same as for native vessel disease. DES and drug-coated balloons have been shown to yield superior results to other catheter-based interventions.

10. A. Emergent PCI to the RCI lesion followed by CABG during this admission. STEMI treatment should be emergent PCI of the culprit lesion, but a patient with additional coronary disease including LAD occlusion should undergo CABG surgery for the best long-term results. Timing of the surgery is dependent on patient risk factors and condition.

15.

HYPERTROPHIC OBSTRUCTIVE CARDIOMYOPATHY WITH SYSTOLIC ANTERIOR MOTION OF THE MITRAL VALVE

Justin Daniels

STEM CASE AND KEY QUESTIONS

A 43-year-old male patient is transferred to the emergency department following an outside the hospital cardiac arrest. CPR was performed until emergency medical services arrived. Upon arrival, paramedics found the patient in ventricular fibrillation and were able to obtain return of spontaneous circulation following direct current cardioversion. The patient received endotracheal intubation in the field due to cardiac arrest with a low initial Glasgow Coma Scale score. Initial workup includes serum chemistries, complete blood count, troponin, electrocardiogram (EKG), and echocardiography. The cardiology team is consulted for concern of hypertrophic cardiomyopathy (HCM).

WHAT FINDINGS WOULD YOU EXPECT ON EKG FOR A PATIENT WITH HCM? WHAT ARE THE TYPICAL PHYSICAL EXAM FINDINGS FOR PATIENTS WITH HCM? WHAT ARE THE ECHOCARDIOGRAPHIC REQUIREMENTS FOR DIAGNOSING HCM?

The echocardiography for the patient demonstrates a thick basal septal region of the LV with a maximum thickness of 19 mm. The initial EKG illustrates a left axis deviation with evidence of left ventricular hypertrophy and non-specific ST-T changes in various leads.

The patient remains intubated and is admitted to the intensive care unit (ICU). On arrival to the unit, the patient is noted to be agitated, tachycardic, and hypertensive. He is assessed for extubation and fails to meet criteria. The critical care team administers propofol for sedation. After the propofol drip is started, the patient becomes profoundly hypotensive. On physical exam, a new heart murmur is noted by the team.

WHAT ARE THE CLASSIC CHARACTERISTICS OF THE MURMUR ASSOCIATED WITH HCM OBSTRUCTION? WHAT FACTORS CONTRIBUTE TO THE DEVELOPMENT OF LEFT VENTRICULAR OUTFLOW TRACT OBSTRUCTION? WHAT ARE THE MANAGEMENT PRIORITIES WITH ACUTE LEFT VENTRICULAR OUTFLOW TRACT OBSTRUCTION AND HYPOTENSION? WHAT IS THE VASOPRESSOR OF CHOICE IN THIS CASE?

The patient is given a bolus of lactated Ringer's and started on a phenylephrine drip. The propofol infusion is switched to Precedex to prevent the vasodilation associated with propofol. The patient's blood pressure improves, and the phenylephrine is slowly weaned off. The next day the patient undergoes his daily spontaneous awakening trial and spontaneous breathing trial, resulting in successful extubation. After extubation a medical history is obtained, which includes progressive dyspnea on exertion and easy fatigability over the last year.

WHAT CLASS OF MEDICATIONS ARE FIRST-LINE TREATMENT FOR SUBACUTE OR CHRONIC SYMPTOMS ASSOCIATED WITH HCM? WHAT ARE SECOND-LINE AND ADJUNCT MEDICATIONS THAT CAN BE USED IN HCM?

The patient is started on oral metoprolol, which improves his symptoms. The cardiology team places an automatic internal cardiac defibrillator for secondary prevention of sudden cardiac arrest from ventricular arrythmias.

WHAT ARE RISK FACTORS FOR DEVELOPING SUDDEN CARDIAC DEATH IN HCM? WHAT ARE THE INDICATIONS FOR ICD IN PLACEMENT IN PATIENTS WITH HCM?

Prior to discharge, there is a family meeting to discuss the diagnosis of HCM and the implications for the patient's first-degree relatives concerning the genetic basis of the disease.

WHAT MODE OF INHERITANCE DOES HCM HAVE? WHAT ARE THE MOST COMMON GENES INVOLVED AND THE MOST COMMON TYPE OF MUTATION ASSOCIATED WITH HCM? WHAT TESTING IS APPROPRIATE FOR FIRST-DEGREE RELATIVES OF PATIENTS WITH HCM?

At a follow-up appointment, the patient is told that he has a mutation to the *MYH7* gene encoding the beta myosin heavy chain of the sarcomere. It is recommended that his first-degree family members should all undergo genetic testing. Additional testing may be necessary based on their results.

After approximately 3 years the patient returns to the hospital due to increased fatigue, dyspnea, and new-onset orthopnea. The patient denies any anginal chest pain or irregular heartbeat. As an outpatient over the past several years, the man's symptoms were controlled with disopyramide and metoprolol. Now, with the progressive symptoms, a new echocardiogram is ordered.

WHAT ADDITIONAL THERAPIES ARE AVAILABLE FOR HCM PATIENTS WITH SYMPTOMS REFRACTORY TO MEDICAL THERAPY? WHAT ARE THE COMPLICATIONS ASSOCIATED WITH HCM?

On the new echocardiogram the patient has evidence of left ventricular outflow tract obstruction with systolic anterior motion of the mitral valve present at rest. His maximal left ventricular wall thickness of the basal septum has increased to 32 mm and his outflow tract gradient is >50 mmHg at rest. Other findings on the echocardiography include an elongated anterior leaflet of the mitral valve and moderate to severe mitral regurgitation. The cardiothoracic surgery team is consulted for evaluation. The patient asks about nonsurgical interventions available.

WHAT WOULD BE THE PREFERRED INVASIVE PROCEDURE TO HELP REDUCE HIS OBSTRUCTION AND RELATED SYMPTOMS? WHY IS SURGICAL MYECTOMY PREFERRED TO ALCOHOL SEPTAL ABLATION? FOR WHICH PATIENTS WOULD ALCOHOL SEPTAL ABLATION BE RECOMMENDED OVER A SURGICAL MYECTOMY?

The patient undergoes a surgical myectomy and has a mitral valve repair done at the same time. He tolerates the surgery well and has significant improvement in his symptoms. On postoperative day 4, the patient is discharged home with cardiac rehab.

DISCUSSION

INTRODUCTION

HCM is defined as the presence of left ventricular hypertrophy with wall a thickness of >15 mm in at least 1 left ventricular (LV) myocardial segment in the absence of another cardiac or systemic disease capable of producing the magnitude of hypertrophy present, or a wall thickness of >13 mm in at least 1 segment with a first-degree relative with confirmed HCM.[1-3] It is a disease process associated with diastolic dysfunction, sudden cardiac death (SCD) due to ventricular tachyarrhythmias, outflow tract obstruction, development of atrial fibrillation, progressive heart failure, and myocardial ischemia.[1,4-6]

EPIDEMIOLOGY

HCM is the most common genetic cardiovascular disease and affects people across the globe.[1,3] This disease process affects at least 1 in 500 people with up to 1 in 200 having the genotype to develop the clinical disease with variable penetrance.[1,3,7,8] The natural history of HCM is extremely variable. Frequently individuals diagnosed with HCM have a normal life expectancy, and many have no functional disability or disease-related complications.[3,9,10] The overall mortality rate for patients with HCM is estimated at 0.5% to 1% per year, which is similar to the mortality rate of the general population.[3,4,8,9]

The most devastating sequelae of HCM is the prevalence of SCD among young individuals, including athletes. One in 3 athletic field deaths of US high school and college athletes is results from HCM.[10] SCD is the most common cause of mortality among patients with HCM but is found mostly in younger patients under the age of 30.[1,6,10,11] SCD is uncommon in HCM patients above the age of 60 where the mortality from stroke increases.[10,11] SCD may be the presentation of HCM in an otherwise asymptomatic young patient.

GENETICS

HCM is a genetic disease that is predominantly inherited in a Mendelian autosomal dominant pattern with incomplete penetrance and variable phenotypic expression.[3,4,7,10,13] Although rare, autosomal recessive and x-linked modes of inheritance have been described.[8,13] Around 1500 different mutations have been identified affecting at least 9 causative genes that encode components of the cardiac sarcomere, the functional unit that causes contraction of cardiac muscle; see Figure 15.1.[9,14] The most common type of mutation is a missense mutation which is found in 90% of known cases.[3,9,10]

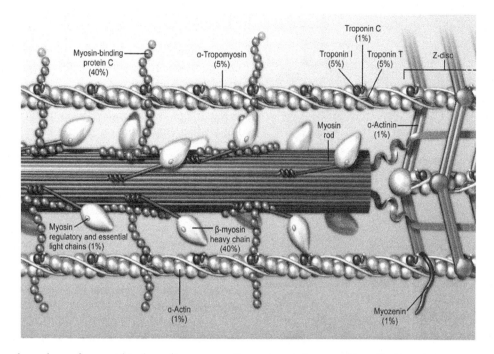

Figure 15.1 Location and prevalence of genes within the cardiac sarcomere known to cause hypertrophic cardiomyopathy.
Used with permission from Maron BJ, Maron MS. Hypertrophic cardiomyopathy. The Lancet. 2013;381(9862):242–255. doi:10.1016/S0140-6736(12)60397-3

A mutation to the *MYH7* gene, which encodes the sequence for the β-myosin heavy chain, was the first identified mutation causing HCM.[1,14] A mutation in *MYBCC3*, which encodes for the cardiac myosin binding protein C, also results in HCM. Together, these two mutations account for over half of familial HCM cases.[1,3,9,14] Along with the 9 genes identified as causative, an additional 11 genes have been implicated as causative or reported in HCM but currently have no clear causal role.[1,9,15]

Genetic testing plays a role in the evaluation of a patient with HCM; however, the test only discovers a mutation in about half of all cases. There is no clear correlation between mutation type and clinical outcome.[4,6,14,16] The discovery of a gene mutation allows screening of a patient's first-degree family members to aid in identifying and monitoring affected relatives.[1] If a causative mutation is unable to be identified, there is no indication for genetictesting first degree relatives.[1,2,4] The family members of patients with HCM should undergo routine screening assessments including a clinical exam, EKG, and echocardiography on a periodic basis starting at the age of 12 or earlier if the child has signs of early puberty, has accelerated growth, develops symptoms, or is involved in high-intensity sports.[1,2,4,9] With the increasing use of genetic testing, a new subgroup of HCM patients has emerged who are asymptomatic gene carriers without any left ventricular hypertrophy, known as genotype-positive phenotype-negative patients.[2,3,7] These patients should still undergo serial EKGs, transthoracic echocardiogram, and clinical assessments at periodic intervals as the penetrance of HCM can be age related and the patient may develop hypertrophy after a normal initial evaluation.[2,3]

PATHOPHYSIOLOGY

HYPERTROPHY/OBSTRUCTION

Hypertrophy associated with HCM can vary from diffuse wall thickening to focal, asymmetric thickening. The hypertrophy predominatly involves the basal interventricular septum below the aortic valve. The hypertrophy can also involve only the LV free wall, predominantly the apex of the LV, and rarely the posterior or lateral wall; see Figure 15.2.[3,7,9,13] The increased wall thickness present is due to hypertrophic myocytes with bizarre shapes, in disarray with loss of normal alignment. Over time these regions can develop fibrosis likely due to ischemia from microvascular disease.[3,9,13,16,17]

Patients with HCM can also have elongation of the leaflets of the mitral valve, anterior displacement of the mitral apparatus, and abnormal insertion of the papillary muscles.[1,5,9] The mitral valve morphology and the location of the hypertrophy in the basal septal region increases the likelihood of developing a left ventricular outflow tract obstruction (LVOTO) and systolic anterior motion of the mitral valve (SAM).[1,5,9] SAM describes the dynamic movement of the mitral valve during systole anteriorly toward the LVOT due to drag forces and to a lesser extent the Venturi effect.[5,18] Factors that may precipitate obstruction include hypovolemia with reduced left ventricular end diastolic volume and tachycardia with reduced ventricular filling as seen during prolonged intense exercise. Other aggravating factors include a hyperdynamic LV from inotrope excess, tachyarrhythmias with reduced ventricular filling or loss of atrial kick, and reduction in systemic vascular resistance resulting in increased systolic function.[1,4]

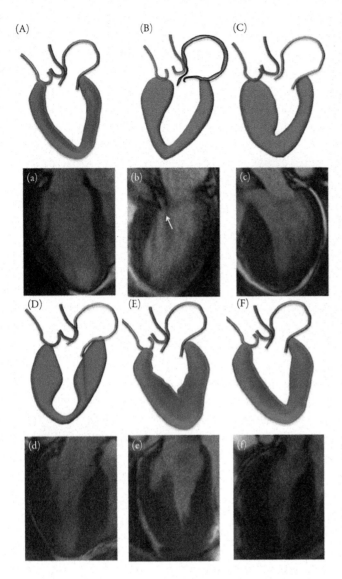

Figure 15.2 Left ventricular patterns in HCM. Each drawing is accompanied by its corresponding image, (A,a) normal LV; (B,b) sigmoid septum showing SAM of mitral valve (white arrow); (C,c) reversed septal contour (note that there is no signs of LVOT); (D,d) mid-ventricular hypertrophy; (E,e) Apical HCM; and (F,f) symmetric HCM.
Used from open access article, Noureldin RA, Liu S, Nacif MS, et al. The diagnosis of hypertrophic cardiomyopathy by cardiovascular magnetic resonance. Journal of Cardiovascular Magnetic Resonance. 2012;14(17). doi:10.1186/1532-429X-14-17.

on auscultation, harsh midsystolic murmur, and bifid carotid pulse.[4,9] The classic murmur heard is a mid-systolic, crescendo-decrescendo murmur at the left lower sternal border.[4] This murmur is due to turbulent flow through the aortic outflow tract and will be louder with a Valsalva maneuver that reduces preload and softer with maneuvers that increase preload, such as squatting.[4] The dynamic changes to the murmur with varying loading conditions can help differentiate a murmur of HCM from that of aortic stenosis.

HCM can cause nonspecific changes to EKGs including voltage changes consistent with left ventricular hypertrophy, ST-T wave changes, and deep Q waves in the lateral and inferior leads.[4,9,12] If apical hypertrophy is present, diffuse symmetric T-wave inversions across the precordium may be seen.[12] Although the findings are nonspecific, these EKG abnormalities are sensitive for HCM and are present in 95% of patients with the disease.[4] The few HCM patients with a normal EKG will typically have less severe disease and an improved survival rate.[12]

IMAGING

Two-dimensional echocardiography is the gold standard imaging modality for diagnosing HCM. It can be used to assess the myocardial walls for hypertrophy, measure the outflow tract gradients for evidence of obstruction, and diagnose valvular abnormalities.[2,4] If no resting outflow gradient is present, provocative maneuvers such as exercise may be used to look for latent left ventricular outflow tract obstruction that may occur with dynamic changes in contractility and loading conditions.[2,4]

Cardiac magnetic resonance imaging (CMR) has been used extensively in the HCM population to assist with risk stratification and as an adjunct to echocardiography.[2] CMR provides precise LV wall measurements to aid in identifying focal hypertrophy and atypical hypertrophic distribution.[1,4,5,7,10] CMR also allows for the identification of fibrosis with late gadolinium enhancement.[1,10] The identification of fibrosis helps with risk stratification as significant fibrosis has been associated with higher rates SCD, progressive heart failure, and increased cardiac and all-cause mortality.[1,2,13]

MANAGEMENT

Noninvasive

Acute hypotension in patients with HCM with obstruction is best treated with volume resuscitation, pure vasoconstrictors such as phenylephrine or vasopressin, and a reduction in heart rate.[2] The beta adrenergic effect of drugs such as norepinephrine, epinephrine, and dopamine may exacerbate the outflow obstruction by increasing contractility. Inotropes are relatively contraindicated in HCM patients with obstruction. If tachycardia is present, adding a beta blocker can alleviate LVOTO by reducing the heart rate to increase the diastolic filling time and providing negative inotropy.[5]

In patients who have persistent symptoms, dyspnea on exertion, orthopnea, fatigue, and chest pain, a course of

Presence of LVOTO is defined as having a peak LVOT gradient >30 mmHg on echocardiogram, which occurs in 25% to 33% of patients at rest and another 25% to 33% with exercise or hemodynamic stressors.[1,3,5,19] The outflow obstruction may be well tolerated. There is some evidence of patients surviving with large gradients for many years with little or no negative effects.[3]

PHYSICAL EXAM/EKG

Like the natural history of the disease, the presenting physical exam findings can vary from no significant findings to severe abnormalities. Physical exam findings that may indicate HCM include a forceful precordial impulse, prominent S4

medical therapy is generally recommended for long-term management.[3,4,10,16] The symptoms can be caused by LVOTO at rest or attributed to progressive diastolic dysfunction. Non-vasodilating beta blockers are the cornerstone of pharmacologic therapy as they reduce outflow obstruction, increase diastolic filling time, decrease inotropy, and may reduce ventricular stiffness, which are the goals of medical therapy.[1,2,4,9,10]

If beta blockers are not well tolerated, second-line therapy includes non-dihydropyridine calcium channel blockers (CCB). CCBs are used to help reduce myocardial inotropy and chronotropy. These agents must, however, be used cautiously in patients with a severe outflow tract obstruction. CCBs have vasodilatory effects that could acutely increase the obstruction and decrease the patient's cardiac output.[1,2,4,9,10]

Disopyramide, an antiarrhythmic drug that blocks sodium channels, may be used as adjunct therapy added to either beta blockers or calcium channel blockers. Used to prevent ventricular tachyarrhythmias, it provides additional negative inotropic effects. Of the pharmacologic treatments available, disopyramide most consistently reduces LVOT gradients and improves symptoms in patients with obstruction.[1,4,9,10] However, there are concerns with long-term use of the drug including prolonged QTc and anticholinergic side effects.[4,10]

Besides pharmacological management, lifestyle adjustments can reduce the morbidity and mortality of patients with HCM. Avoidance of any moderate to high-intensity sports is highly recommended.[2,4] Patients should be encouraged to continue low-intensity exercise programs and competitive sports such as golfing and bowling.[2]

Invasive

HCM patients with LVOT gradients of >50 mmHg with symptoms refractory to optimized medical management are candidates for either surgical myectomy or alcohol septal ablation therapy (ASA).[1–3,10,20] Septal reduction therapies help by reducing outflow obstruction and restoring normal left ventricular pressures.[10]

Surgical septal myectomy is considered the gold standard of invasive therapy. It has been shown to reliably reverse heart failure symptoms related to significant LVOTO as well as reduce mitral valve insufficiency, if present.[1,2,4,10,20] The procedure involves resection of the hypertrophied tissue from the ventricular septum causing the outflow obstruction.[1] If the mitral valve anatomy is abnormal, the surgeon can also perform a mitral valve repair or replacement to reduce SAM and concurrent mitral regurgitation.[4,5] If the surgical risk is high and septal myectomy is contraindicated, ASA is an alternative procedure that may be performed and is effective therapy for reducing symptoms from LVOTO.[2–4] ASA is a catheter-based procedure where absolute alcohol is injected into a septal perforating artery to induce myocardial necrosis. This reduces contractility of the septum and the amount of septal tissue present.[1,4,10] ASA has been shown to be effective in reducing outflow gradients, but comparative analyses have shown surgical myectomy to be superior in reducing

resting and exercise-induced LVOT gradients.[4,21] The primary complication associated with ASA is the development of a high-grade AV block requiring the placement of a permanent pacemaker.[1,3,20,21] Long-term survival for both procedures have been shown to be nearly equivocal.[1,21]

SCD AND PREVENTION

SCD is the most prevalent cause of mortality in patients with HCM.[3] SCD is typically related to ventricular tachyarrhythmias and often occurs without any warning signs or symptoms. It may be associated with vigorous physical activity as seen in athletes with extreme training regimes.[9,10] Fibrosis present within the LV as evidenced on CMR has been associated with a 2-fold increased risk for ventricular arrhythmias resulting in SCD.[10] The placement of an implantable cardioverter-defibrillator (ICD) is the only nonsurgical therapy proven to reduce mortality in HCM patients.[1,4,10] ICD placement is absolutely recommended for SCD patients who have experienced sustained ventricular tachycardia or suffered cardiac arrest. The placement of an ICD may also be recommended based on the patient's life expectancy and the presence of risk modifiers as outlined in Box 15.1.[2] Patients who meet the criteria for ICD placement should have at least a 1-year life expectancy.

Box 15.1. ICD RECOMMENDATIONS

Class I

• Prior cardiac arrest

or

• Sustained VT

Class IIa

• First-degree family member with sudden death

or

• LV wall thickness of >30 mm

or

• Recent unexplained syncope

Class IIb

• Nonsustained VT

or

• Abnormal BP response to exercise

with

• Other risk modifiers (LVOTO, high LGE on MRI, apical aneurysm)

From Gersh BJ, Maron BJ, Bonow RO, et al. 2011 ACCF/AHA Guideline for the diagnosis and treatment of hypertrophic cardiomyopathy: a report of the American College of Cardiology Foundation/American Heart Association task force on practice guidelines. *Circulation.* 2011;*124*(24):2761–2796. doi:10.1161/CIR.0b013e318223e2bd.

COMPLICATIONS

Atrial Fibrillation

Atrial fibrillation is the most common complication associated with HCM with an incidence of 2% to 3% per year affecting 20% to 25% of all HCM patients.[3,4,9,10] Initial management of atrial fibrillation focuses on rate control with beta blockers and verapamil. Often, atrial fibrillation is poorly tolerated due to comorbid diastolic dysfunction and impaired left ventricular filling. In this case, rhythm control is preferred and the use of amiodarone is recommended.[3,10] If patients continue to have atrial fibrillation with symptoms despite medical management, AV nodal ablation with placement of a permanent pace maker has been shown to be effective treatment.[1–3,22] Paroxysmal, persistent, and chronic atrial fibrillation should also be treated with anticoagulation using a vitamin K antagonist to prevent stroke.[1,2,4]

Myocardial Ischemia

Anginal chest pain is a common symptom suffered by patients with HCM. These patients have intramural coronary arteries that have thickened walls and narrow lumens and are imbedded in interstitial fibrous tissue leading to microvascular dysfunction.[1,3,4] The presence of diastolic dysfunction from thickened and fibrotic walls leads to increased end diastolic pressure, resulting in increased compression of the narrowed vessels.[1] Due to this microvascular disease and increased diastolic pressure, there is limited reserve and an inability to increase blood flow under stress as evidenced by a poor response to dipyridamole infusion on stress tests. The severity of the microvascular disease and poor response to dipyridamole infusion has been associated with increased risk of death and clinical deterioration.[1,23]

Heart Failure

Diastolic dysfunction leading to heart failure symptoms is the most common form of heart failure observed in patients with HCM. Up to 50% of HCM patients will have some degree of heart failure with exertional dyspnea, fatigue, orthopnea, or paroxysmal nocturnal dyspnea.[3,10] Between 3.5% and 5% of patients will then progress to a "burnt-out" end-stage heart failure associated with reduced ejection fraction, dilation of the LV, and remodeling with myocardial scarring.[3,4,24,9,10] This subgroup of patients is at increased risk of death with mortality rates over 10% per year. This cohort can benefit from ICD placement to prevent life threatening ventricular arrhythmias.[4,24]

FUTURE INTERVENTIONS

The drug Ranolazine is a selective late sodium current inhibitor that reduces myocardial energy expenditure. It has shown efficacy in reducing angina and increasing functional capacity and may improve myocyte diastolic function through modulation of calcium sensitivity.[1,4,25] MYK-461 is a molecular inhibitor of sarcomeric contraction. It inhibits myosin ATPase, which can reduce fractional shortening increasing end systolic diameter, reducing the severity of obstruction and the presence of SAM.[1,4,19] In addition to new medical therapies, endocardial radiofrequency ablation of the hypertrophied septum is being utilized with increased frequency. Similar to ASA, it induces cellular necrosis of the hypertrophied tissue to reduce contractile force and systolic excursion. This may be an alternative to ASA for patients who are not candidates for surgical myectomy.[1,26]

CONCLUSIONS

- HCM is the most common genetic cardiomyopathy associated with an autosomal dominant inheritance of a defect resulting in hypertrophied myocytes in disarray histologically.

- The ventricular hypertrophy can affect various regions of the ventricle including basal septal, which is the most common, mid-ventricular with obstruction, apical, or either the posterior or lateral free walls. The disease can rarely affect the right ventricle.

- These patients often have abnormal morphology of the mitral valve or papillary insertion leading to systolic anterior motion of the mitral valve. These anatomical changes to the mitral valve coupled with the basal septal hypertrophy leads to LVOTO.

- The disease is associated with SCD from ventricular tachyarrhythmias in young patients.

- Acute treatment of SAM and LVOTO include volume resuscitation, vasoconstrictors, and treatment of tachycardia/arrythmias.

- Long-term treatment of HCM includes ICD placement in patients at risk for SCD, beta blockers, calcium channel blockers, disopyramide, and septal reduction therapies in patients with symptoms refractory to medical management.

- HCM is also associated with diastolic heart failure, development of atrial fibrillation, cardiac ischemia from microvascular disease, and a burnt-out LV with systolic heart failure.

REFERENCES

1. Liew AC, Vassiliou VS, Cooper R, Raphael CE. Hypertrophic cardiomyopathy: past, present and future. *Journal of Clinical Medicine.* 2017;6(12):118. doi:10.3390/jcm6120118.

2. Gersh BJ, Maron BJ, Bonow RO, et al. 2011 ACCF/AHA guideline for the diagnosis and treatment of hypertrophic cardiomyopathy: a report of the American College of Cardiology Foundation/American Heart Association task force on practice guidelines. *Circulation.* 2011;*124*(24):2761–2796. doi:10.1161/CIR.0b013e318223e2bd.

3. Maron BJ. Hypertrophic cardiomyopathy a systematic review. *JAMA.* 2002;*287*(10):1308–1320.

4. Houston BA, Stevens GR. Hypertrophic cardiomyopathy: a review. *Clinical Medicine Insights Cardiology*. 2014;8(Suppl 1):53–65. doi:10.4137/CMC.S15717.

5. Ibrahim M, Rao C, Ashrafian H, Chaudhry U, Darzi A, Athanasiou T. Modern management of systolic anterior motion of the mitral valve. *European Journal of Cardio-Thoracic Surgery*. 2012;6(41):1260–1270. doi:10.193/ejcts/ezr232.

6. Trivedi A, Knight BP. ICD therapy for primary prevention in hypertrophic cardiomyopathy. *Arrhythmia & Electrophysiology Review*. 2016;5(3):188–196. doi:10.15420/aer.2016:30:2.

7. Semsarian C, Ingles J, Maron MS, Maron BJ. New perspectives on the prevalence of hypertrophic cardiomyopathy. *Journal of the American College of Cardiology*. 2015;65(12):1249–1254. doi:10.1016/j.jacc.2015.01.019.

8. Maron BJ, Gardin JM, Flack JM, Gidding SS, Kurosaki TT, Bild DE. Prevalence of hypertrophic cardiomyopathy in a general population of young adults. *Circulation*. 1995;92(4):785–789. doi:10.1161/01.CIR.92.4.785.

9. Marian AJ, Braunwald E. Hypertrophic cardiomyopathy: genetics, pathogenesis, clinical manifestations, diagnosis, and therapy. *Circulation Research*. 2017;121(7):749–770. doi:10.1161/CIRCRESAHA.117.311059.

10. Maron BJ, Ommen SR, Semsarian C, Spirito P, Olivotto I, Maron MS. Hypertrophic cardiomyopathy: present and future, with translation into contemporary cardiovascular medicine. *Journal of the American College of Cardiology*. 2014;64(1):83–99. doi:10.1016/j.jacc.2014.05.003.

11. Maron BJ, Olivotto I, Spirito P, et al. Epidemiology of hypertrophic cardiomyopathy-related death: Revisited in a large non-referral-based patient population. *Circulation*. 2000;102(8):858–864.

12. McLeod CJ, Ackerman MJ, Nishimura RA, Tajik AJ, Gersh BJ, Ommen SR. Outcome of patients with hypertrophic cardiomyopathy and a normal electrocardiogram. *Journal of the American College of Cardiology*. 2009;54(3):229–233. doi:10.1016/j.jacc.2009.02.071.

13. Noureldin RA, Liu S, Nacif MS, et al. The diagnosis of hypertrophic cardiomyopathy by cardiovascular magnetic resonance. *Journal of Cardiovascular Magnetic Resonance*. 2012;14(17): doi:10.1186/1532-429X-14-17.

14. Landstrom AP, Ho CY, Ackerman MJ. Mutation type is not clinically useful in predicting prognosis in hypertrophic cardiomyopathy. *Circulation*. 2010;122(23):2441–2450. doi:10.1161/CIRCULATIONAHA.110.954446.

15. Olivotto I, Ashley EA. INHERIT (INHibition of the renin angiotensin system in hypertrophic cardiomyopathy and the Effect on hypertrophy: a Randomised Intervention Trial with losartan). *Global Cardiology Science and Practice*. 2015;2015;7. doi:10.5339/gcsp.2015.7

16. Marian AJ. Hypertrophic cardiomyopathy: from genetics to treatment. *European Journal of Clinical Investigation*. 2010;40(4):360–369.

17. Varnava AM, Elliot PM, Sharma S, McKenna WJ, Davies MJ. Hypertrophic cardiomyopathy: the interrelation of disarray, fibrosis, and small vessel disease. *Heart*. 2000;84(5):476–482.

18. Sherrid MV, Chu CK, Delia E, Mogtader A, Dwyer EM. An echocardiographic study of the fluid mechanics of obstruction in hypertrophic cardiomyopathy. *Journal of the American College of Cardiology*. 1993;22(3):816–825.

19. Stern JA, Markova S, Ueda Y, et al. A small molecule inhibitor of sarcomere contractility acutely relieves left ventricular outflow tract obstruction in feline hypertrophic cardiomyopathy. PLoS ONE. 2016;11(12). doi:10.1371/journal.pone.0168407.

20. Veselka J, Jensen MK, Liebregts M, et al. Long-term clinical outcome after alcohol septal ablation for obstructive hypertrophic cardiomyopathy: results from the Euro-ASA registry. *European Heart Journal*. 2016;37(19):1517–1523. doi:10.1093/eurheartj/ehv693.

21. Agarwal S, Tuzcu EM, Desai MY, et al. Updated meta-analysis of septal alcohol ablation versus myectomy for hypertrophic cardiomyopathy. *Journal of the American College of Cardiology*. 2010;55(8):823–834. doi:10.1016/j.jacc.2009.09.047.

22. Providencia R, Elliott P, Patel K, et al. Catheter ablation for atrial fibrillation in hypertrophic cardiomyopathy: a systematic review and meta-analysis. *Heart*. 2016;102(19):1533–1543. doi:10.1136/heartjnl-2016-309406.

23. Cecchi F, Olivotto I, Gistri R, Lorenzoni R, Chiriatti G, Camici PG. Coronary microvascular dysfunction and prognosis in hypertrophic cardiomyopathy. *New England Journal of Medicine*. 2003;349(11):1027–1035.

24. Harris KM, Spirito P, Maron MS, et al. Prevalence, clinical profile, and significance of left ventricular remodeling in the end-stage phase of hypertrophic cardiomyopathy. *Circulation*. 2006;114(3):216–225. doi:10.1161/CIRCULATIONAHA.105.583500.

25. Gentry JL, Mentz RJ, Hurdle M, Wang A. Ranolazine for treatment of angina or dyspnea in hypertrophic cardiomyopathy patients (RHYME). *Journal of the American College of Cardiology*. 2016;68(16):1815–1817. doi:10.1016/j.jacc.2016.07.758.

26. Lawrenz T, Borchert B, Leuner C, et al. Endocardial radiofrequency ablation for hypertrophic obstructive cardiomyopathy. *Journal of the American College of Cardiology*. 2011;57(5):572–576. doi:10.1016/j.jacc.2010.07.055.

27. Maron BJ, Maron MS. Hypertrophic cardiomyopathy. *The Lancet*. 2013;381(9862):242–255. doi:10.1016/S0140-6736(12)60397-3.

REVIEW QUESTIONS

1. A 16-year-old previously healthy male admitted to the hospital after syncope was diagnosed with HCM via echocardiography. What EKG finding is most likely to be found?

   A. Q1S3T3
   B. Normal EKG
   C. Left axis deviation
   D. ST elevation in inferior leads

2. A family member of a patient just diagnosed with HCM without an identified gene asks if she needs to have any testing done. What testing/follow-up would you recommend?

   A. All first-degree family members should follow routinely with their primary care physician for surveillance of development of symptoms prior to any lab testing or imaging.
   B. No testing is required as the disease is most likely sporadic and not familial.
   C. All first-degree relatives should undergo genetic testing to evaluate for the presence of the mutation.
   D. All first-degree relatives should undergo clinical assessment including an echocardiograph for evidence of HCM.

3. All of the following are factors that increase the risk of LVOTO *except*

   A. elongated mitral valve leaflets.
   B. abnormal insertion of the papillary muscle.
   C. severe apical hypertrophy.
   D. increased systolic function.

4. A 46-year-old man presents with worsening fatigue and orthostasis over the last 3 months associated with his HCM. He was previously asymptomatic and not on any medications. Which pharmaceutical agent would be

your first-line treatment of his progressive heart failure symptoms?

    A. Metoprolol
    B. Verapamil
    C. Carvedilol
    D. Propranolol

5. A 55-year-old woman with HCM has had worsening of fatigue, dyspnea on exertion, and paroxysmal nocturnal dyspnea while on metoprolol and disopyramide. She has no additional significant medical problems. On echocardiography her LVOT gradient is 65 mmHg but her mitral valve shows no gross abnormalities and she has preserved ejection fraction. She asks about additional therapies to help reduce symptoms. What is your first recommendation?

    A. Endocardial radiofrequency ablation of the septum
    B. Alcohol septal ablation
    C. Heart transplantation
    D. Surgical myectomy

6. A 48-year-old woman with known HCM is in the ICU after a motor vehicle collision that resulted in polytrauma. She begins to develop tachycardia with fever and progressive hypotension. While she is undergoing fluid resuscitation, what would be the vasopressor of choice to treat her hypotension?

    A. Dopamine
    B. Norepinephrine
    C. Phenylephrine
    D. Epinephrine

7. A 16-year-old male with HCM, discovered after a cardiac arrest during a basketball game, had an ICD placed for secondary prevention. Now that he has an ICD in place, he asks if he is able to resume playing basketball. What is your response?

    A. Even though he has an ICD in place, he should limit activity to low-intensity activities.
    B. He should limit his activity to moderate-intensity activities since he has an ICD in place.
    C. With an ICD in place he can play basketball recreationally.
    D. He should develop a sedentary lifestyle to help prevent further episodes of SCD or progression of his disease.

8. A 63-year-old man with HCM develops paroxysmal atrial fibrillation. He has failed an attempt at rate control management. What is the best antiarrhythmic medication for this patient?

    A. Digoxin
    B. Amiodarone
    C. Flecainide
    D. Propafenone

9. A 29-year-old man was diagnosed with HCM after a recent syncopal episode while at home. He has been researching HCM and asks if he needs an ICD now. What do you tell him?

    A. Yes, he should have an ICD since he had a recent unexplained syncopal episode and a positive diagnosis of HCM.

    B. No, he needs additional testing to wear a holter monitor to assess for presence of life-threatening ventricular arrhythmias.
    C. Yes, all patients with HCM who are less than 30 years old are at risk of SCD and should have an ICD.
    D. No, ICDs are only required in patients who have sustained ventricular tachycardia or prior cardiac arrest.

10. Benefits of CMR when compared to echocardiography include all of the following *except*

    A. can be used to better define the presence of fibrosis.
    B. reduces exposure to radiation.
    C. improved visualization of endocardial borders.
    D. more precise measurement of ventricular wall thickness.

ANSWERS

1. D. In the presence of HCM, 95% of patients will have abnormal EKG findings. Typical EKG findings include criteria for LVH, left axis deviation, and non-specific ST-T wave changes.[4,9,12] Patients may have Q waves in precordial leads, which is more typical if hypertrophy is predominantly in the apex.[12]

2. D. Without a known mutation, there is no role for first-degree relatives undergoing genetic testing.[2] Screening for first-degree relatives should include periodic testing based on age with echocardiography, clinical assessment, and EKG as the phenotypic penetrance can increase with age.[2,3]

3. C. Anatomical risk factors that increase the likelihood of LVOTO include hypertrophy of the basal septal region; elongated mitral leaflets, especially anterior leaflet with an anterior to posterior leaflet ratio >1.3; abnormal insertion of the papillary muscles; and anterior displacement of the mitral apparatus.[1,5,9] Other factors that can increase the risk of developing LVOTO include hypovolemia, tachycardia, increased inotropy, and decreased afterload.[1,4]

4. A. For symptomatic LVOTO and diastolic heart failure symptoms, the first-line treatment of choice is nonvasodilating beta blockers, like metoprolol.[1,2,4,9,10] Labetalol and carvedilol have vasodilating properties with their alpha antagonism and should be avoided due to the risk of worsening the LVOTO. Verapamil is second-line treatment and can be used in patients who do not tolerate beta blocker therapy. Disopyramide can be added to either beta blocker or verapamil for reduction in obstructive symptoms.[2,4,9,10]

5. D. For patients who have refractory heart failure symptoms on appropriate medical therapy secondary to obstruction with LVOT gradients >50 mmHg, the gold standard treatment is surgical myectomy as it has shown benefit to reduce LVOTO and improve symptoms.[1–3,10,20] In patients who are high surgical risk or otherwise contraindicated in surgery, then alcohol septal ablation would be the next choice. Endocardial radiofrequency ablation is a therapy that may have benefit but is not a current recommended therapy.[2–4,21]

6. C. This patient has tachycardia with known HCM. The tachycardia is likely worsening a left ventricular outflow obstruction with SAM. Fluid resuscitation to increase the left ventricular end diastolic diameter and a pure vasoconstrictor like phenylephrine or vasopressin would be effective treatments.[2] Norepinephrine, epinephrine, and dopamine all have beta agonist effects that can increase inotropy and worsen the outflow obstruction. If the patient had tachycardia not in the presence of hypotension, beta blocker therapy could be used to reduce the heart rate, decease inotropy, and help prevent a significant LVOTO.[5]

7. A. Patients with HCM should not participate in intense competitive sports even if they have an ICD in place but can participate in low-intensity competitive sports and recreational activities, such as golf, bowling, snorkeling, and nonfree weight use.[2]

8. B. The antiarrhythmic drug of choice in patients with atrial fibrillation is amiodarone with disopyramide as a reasonable alternative.[1-3,22] Digoxin should be avoided as it could have positive inotropic effects that could worsen outflow tract obstruction. Flecainide and propafenone should be avoided in patients with ventricular hypertrophy as they can be proarrythmic.[1,3]

9. A. The class I recommendation for ICD placement includes patients with prior cardiac arrest or sustained VT. Class IIa evidence indicates that it is reasonable to place an ICD in patients with a family history of HCM in a first-degree relative, LV wall thickness >30 mm or recent unexplained syncope. Patients with NSVT or abnormal blood pressure response to exercise, if they have other risk modifiers, are class IIb evidence for ICD placement.[2]

10. B. Echocardiography is still considered the initial imaging test of choice for evaluation of HCM.[1-3] CMR has several benefits over echocardiography and is a reasonable option, especially in patients with suboptimal echocardiography images. Benefits of CMR include better visualization of endocardial walls, allowing for more precise measurement of the wall thickness, identification of hypertrophy in atypical locations and distribution, and ability to define fibrosis with the use of LGE.[1,4,5,7,10] Downsides of using CMR include increased cost, possible need for anesthesia in patients who cannot tolerate undergoing the procedure, and availability of scanners.

16.

REFRACTORY VT/VF TO ECLS/ECMO

WITH DISCUSSION OF VV VERSUS VA AND CANNULATION STRATEGIES

Brent Barta and Jared Staab

STEM AND KEY QUESTIONS

A 57-year-old male presents to the emergency department (ED) with complaints of recent-onset shortness of breath, palpitations, nausea, and lightheadedness. He has a past medical history significant for an ST-elevation infarct 8 months prior that required placement of 2 drug-eluting stents to the proximal right coronary artery and mid-circumflex. Physical exam reveals pallor, cannon A waves, tachycardia, and hypotension. Labs are drawn in the ED and are remarkable for mild metabolic acidosis and elevated creatinine. A chest X-ray is taken and is unremarkable. An electrocardiogram (EKG) reveals a regular, monomorphic wide complex rhythm with a rate of 175 beats per minute.

WHAT IS THE MOST LIKELY IMMEDIATE CAUSE OF THIS PATIENT'S SYMPTOMS? WHAT IS THE MOST APPROPRIATE INITIAL INTERVENTION FOR THIS CONDITION?

The patient is given conscious sedation with etomidate, undergoes cardioversion, and is loaded with amiodarone. After 5 unsuccessful cardioversions in the ED, the patient is continued on an amiodarone infusion and norepinephrine is initiated. The blood pressure improves modestly, but there is no immediate change in the heart rate or rhythm, and the patient's symptoms persist. Cardiology is consulted and the patient is transferred to the cardiac intensive care unit (CICU) for continuing management of his refractory ventricular tachycardia (VT) and cardiogenic shock.

WHAT ARE SOME OF THE UNDERLYING CONDITIONS THAT MIGHT CONTRIBUTE TO REFRACTORY VT IN THIS PATIENT? WHAT ARE THE NEXT MOST REASONABLE STEPS IN MANAGEMENT OF THIS PATIENT?

Prior to transfer to the CICU the patient is transported to the cardiac cath lab for left heart catheterization. Both of the patient's stents are found to be patent, and there are no new areas of stenosis or occlusion when compared to his catheterization 8 months earlier. In the CICU the patient requires escalating doses of norepinephrine and additional vasopressors to support his blood pressure. As his hypotension becomes refractory to medication, the patient's mental status begins to deteriorate. Subsequently, endotracheal intubation is performed for airway protection. An emergent echocardiogram is obtained and shows severely reduced left ventricular function, with an ejection fraction of 20%. Additionally, there is evidence of concentric hypertrophy with an area of thinning in the inferolateral wall. In the absence of acute ischemic findings and the patient's progressive cardiogenic shock, the electrophysiology (EP) service is consulted for assistance in controlling the sustained unstable VT.

ARE THERE ADDITIONAL PHARMACOLOGIC TREATMENT OPTIONS FOR THIS CONDITION? WHAT ARE SOME DISADVANTAGES TO DRUG THERAPY AT THIS POINT? WHAT OTHER OPTIONS EXIST FOR TREATING THE PATIENT'S CARDIOGENIC SHOCK?

The patient has been anuric since hospital admission, and on repeat serum chemistries the creatinine has markedly increased. In addition, the patient's liver enzymes are rising, the lactate is now 4, and the mixed venous oxygen saturation is 48. The EP service assesses the patient in the CICU and concludes that, with evidence of multiorgan dysfunction, the patient is too unstable at this time to perform an electrophysiology study. Cardioversion is attempted again but is unsuccessful after 2 attempts. The cardiothoracic surgery service is subsequently consulted to evaluate the patient for mechanical support to restore organ perfusion and "bridge" the patient to a VT mapping/ablation procedure.

WHAT ARE THE AVAILABLE OPTIONS FOR MECHANICAL SUPPORT IN THIS PATIENT? WHAT ARE THE CONTRAINDICATIONS FOR EACH MECHANICAL SUPPORT DEVICE? WHAT ARE THE COMPLICATIONS OF THESE DEVICES? WHAT ARE THE DIFFERENCES BETWEEN VENOUS-ARTERIAL EXTRACORPOREAL MEMBRANE OXYGENATION AND VENO-VENOUS ECMO? WHICH WOULD BE MORE APPROPRIATE?

The patient is taken to the hybrid-operating room where venous-arterial extracorporeal membrane oxygenation (VA

ECMO) via percutaneous access of the left femoral artery and right femoral vein is instituted without complication. There is immediate improvement of the patient's hemodynamics and acidosis. Vasopressor requirements decline drastically. The EP service proceeds to map the right and left ventricle and finds a large area of scarring with a reentrant circuit. This is successfully ablated, and the patient regains a normal sinus rhythm.

WHAT IS VT ABLATION, AND WHAT IS THE SUCCESS RATE OF THE PROCEDURE? WILL THE ABNORMAL RHYTHM REOCCUR? WHAT OPTIONS EXIST FOR THE PREVENTION A RECURRENCE OF VT IN THIS PATIENT? FOR HOW LONG SHOULD MECHANICAL SUPPORT BE CONTINUED? IF CONTINUED, WHAT ANTICOAGULATION STRATEGY SHOULD BE USED?

After completion of the procedure, ECMO support is continued. The patient is taken back to the unit where he continues to improve. He begins to produce urine shortly after return to the unit, and within a few hours his metabolic acidosis has completely resolved. After some hemodynamic stability and recovery of end-organ function as evidenced by declining lactate, increased urine output and falling creatinine the process of ECMO weaning is started. Baseline left ventricular internal dimension-diastole and overall function is recorded by echocardiography. ECMO flow and FiO_2 are gradually decreased. Mixed venous oxygenation, arterial blood gasses, and right ventricle/left ventricle systolic function are monitored during this time to ensure the patient will tolerate liberation from VA ECMO. He tolerates the wean from ECMO, and, upon trial discontinuation, he is decannulated. The following day the patient is extubated and has no vasopressor requirement. He remains in sinus rhythm, and a follow-up echocardiogram evidences a normal right ventricle and a left ventricular ejection fraction of 50%. His liver enzymes and creatinine return to normal ranges. An implantable cardiac defibrillator is placed, and, after a relatively short hospital stay, he is discharged home neurologically and functionally intact.

WHAT ARE THE OUTCOME DATA FOR MECHANICAL SUPPORT IN REFRACTORY VT/VF?

DISCUSSION

VT that is refractory to initial treatment or that recurs frequently (VT storm) can be difficult to treat and has a high morbidity and mortality. If not successfully treated, the rhythm can degenerate to ventricular fibrillation and death. In the United States, VT and ventricular fibrillation (VF) are the most common causes of sudden death at a rate of 300,000 out-of-hospital deaths[1] and 200,000 in-hospital deaths per year.[2]

VT can be divided into several types and is defined as 3 or more consecutive QRS complexes arising from the ventricle

with a frequency of greater than 100 bpm. Sustained VT is 30 seconds or more of VT or any VT with hemodynamic instability requiring intervention. VT/VF storm (arrhythmogenic storm or electrical storm) is defined as 3 or more sustained VT/VF events, each requiring intervention and all within 24 hours of the initial event. The term *refractory* is used when the arrhythmia is not abated by appropriate therapy. It is often used interchangeably with VT/VF storm or when VF persists after 5 attempts at defibrillation in conjunction with appropriate pharmacotherapy and advanced cardiac life support (ACLS) treatment.[3]

VT can also be classified as stable or unstable depending on the patient's symptoms (angina) and hemodynamics. Stable VT is defined as sustained VT without hemodynamic compromise or angina. Unstable VT occurs with any signs of hemodynamic instability or symptoms of angina.[2] VF by definition is unstable. The disorganized electrical activity in VF is unable to produce a mechanical contraction that results in a meaningful stroke volume. VT is further subdivided by its morphology into monomorphic, polymorphic, and bidirectional rhythms. Monomorphic VT consists of a QRS repeatedly originating from a single focus in the ventricle. In polymorphic VT there is a "moving" focus or multiple foci that drive the arrhythmia which creates a QRS morphology that changes over time and includes torsades de pointes.[4] Bidirectional VT has QRS complexes that have 2 distinct and separate axes that alternate after each QRS. This subtype is associated digitalis toxicity and catecholaminergic VT.[3,5]

ETIOLOGY/PATHOGENESIS OF VT

The incidence of refractory VT/VF has increased, with 10% to 20% of patients who receive an implantable cardiac defibrillator possessing the diagnosis.[6] The overall incidence, however, is lower and varies depending on the group being studied.[4]

Ventricular arrhythmias develop when the automaticity of a normal electrical system increases, abnormal automaticity develops, or a re-entry circuit exists. An aberrant re-entry pathway is the most common cause of monomorphic VT in the presence of structural heart disease.[3,4,7] For a re-entry arrhythmia to occur there must be a triggering event, often a premature ventricular contraction that activates the pathway allowing an electrical wave front to create a complete circuit. This commonly occurs within scar tissue from a previous myocardial infarction.[4,7]

Causes of ventricular tachycardia may be divided into 2 broad categories: those with presence of structural heart disease and those without. Structural heart disease includes scar formation from prior myocardial infarction (MI), dilated or hypertrophic cardiomyopathy, and congenital heart disease. A re-entry pathway, as discussed earlier, is commonly present in this category. VT without structural disease has many causes and can be further subdivided into ischemic, exercise-induced, and inheritable and idiopathic causes. Ischemic-related VT is more often polymorphic in nature than not. Of those patients who present to the hospital with acute coronary syndrome, 5% to 10% will have witnessed sustained VT or VF prior to arrival and 5% to 8% during a hospital admission.[3] Heritable causes of VT include long QT syndrome, short QT syndrome, channelopathies (Brugada syndrome, etc.), and arrhythmogenic right ventricular cardiomyopathy. Other causes of VT include electrolyte disturbances and drug-induced long QT.

The prognosis for refractory VT/VF is poor. Several studies have demonstrated an increase in mortality as high as 700% in patients with a history of refractory VT. The risk of death appears to be highest within the first 3 months after the initial presentation of the arrhythmia. Patients who survive the initial VT/VF event have a significant ongoing risk of morbidity including progressive systolic heart failure.[4]

DIAGNOSTIC MODALITIES

As with any diagnostic evaluation, a thorough history is important and can identify risk factors and narrow the differential diagnosis. The history should focus on previous cardiac, pulmonary, thyroid, and renal disease. A family history of cardiac disease or sudden death should increase clinical suspicion. In addition, a history of seizures or unexplained motor vehicle accidents may also be due to undiagnosed cardiogenic syncope.

Electrocardiogram (ECG) is the primary diagnostic tool for assessment of VT/VF. A rudimentary 3 or 5 lead ECG will evidence a wide complex tachycardia or fibrillation. To confirm the diagnosis and evaluate for underlying cardiac morbidity a follow-up 12-lead ECG should be performed. The 12-lead ECG can identify risk factors for VT including myocardial ischemia, prior cardiac infarct, left atrial enlargement, or inherited disorders.[3] The ECG accompanied by a rhythm strip will also differentiate VT from a supraventricular with aberrancy. If the 12-lead ECG is inconclusive, patients with a prior MI will have VT in 95% of the cases.[8]

After the initial identification of the malignant rhythm, it is important to determine the underlying cause so that the appropriate treatment can be delivered. Refractory VT/VF is a relatively common complication of ischemic heart disease. Patients should be evaluated for ongoing myocardial ischemia using echocardiography, cardiac enzymes, and coronary angiography where appropriate. Renal failure and its associated metabolic disorders are another common cause of malignant arrhythmias, and serum electrolyte abnormalities should be corrected and renal function assessed.[2] If the aforementioned workup is negative, further investigation may be warranted including ambulatory monitoring, implantable recorders, exercise testing for exercise induced arrhythmias, or electrophysiology studies to identify a re-entry pathway.

TREATMENT SUPPORTED BY THE MEDICAL LITERATURE

Medical Treatment

The treatment of refractory VT/VF begins with the appropriate application of the ACLS algorithm. For the hemodynamically stable patient with VT, rate control and rhythm conversion using pharmacotherapy is the primary treatment strategy. Calcium channel blockers such as verapamil and beta blockers may be used in the absence of structural heart disease. In monomorphic VT, if there is structural heart disease present, then amiodarone or procainamide have greater efficacy.[2] Patients with polymorphic VT should be evaluated for QT prolongation, which is frequently associated with medication toxicity or drug-drug interactions. If the VT converts to a benign rhythm, then long-term pharmacologic therapy may be prescribed while the evaluation to identify the cause proceeds. If the VT does not convert, then direct current cardioversion (DCCV) should be performed.[2]

Patients with hypotension or evidence of organ ischemia have unstable VT/VF and are treated with defibrillation followed by antiarrhythmic and vasoactive medications. Defibrillation should be repeated if the malignant rhythm fails to convert. After the 5th failed attempt at DCCV, the rhythm is referred to as refractory VT/VF. This can be divided into 2 subtypes. The first category of patients has an unstable rhythm accompanied by cardiovascular collapse that is refractory to 5 defibrillation attempts, whereas the second group of patients have an episode of VT storm where there is an urgent need for intervention but there is no immediate threat of death. The patient in the case study in this chapter has unstable monomorphic VT but is "stable" enough to move through some of the diagnostic and treatment phases of the second category of refractory VT.

Mechanical Circulatory Support

Several mechanical devices exist for the purpose of circulatory support in the failing heart. The most common of these include intra-aortic balloon pumps (IABP), Impella™ devices, and ECMO devices. IABPs are inserted into the aorta, most commonly from the femoral artery, and counter pulsate with the heart to provide forward aortic blood flood during diastole. This counter pulsation is achieved by rapid inflation of a long slim balloon to force blood out of the aorta when the aortic valve closes. Once diastole has ended, the balloon deflates and the aorta is left empty, which allows the left ventricle to eject blood under lower than normal pressure and volume condition, which both decreases left ventricle wall tension and increases stroke volume. IABPs are contraindicated with aortic insufficiency, aortic aneurysm or dissection, severe sepsis, and severe peripheral vascular disease. The Impella device by Abiomed is a percutaneous self-contained impeller that can either be placed across the aortic valve or across the pulmonic valve. The device (in the aortic position) is inserted, most commonly from the femoral artery, continuously pumps blood from the left ventricle cavity to the aorta at a rate of 2.5 to 5 liters per minute depending on the actual device type. This device is contraindicated in aortic stenosis or insufficiency, intra-cardiac mural thrombus, mechanical aortic valve replacement, and severe peripheral vascular disease. Both the IABP and the Impella are unable to provide supplemental-oxygenation by the device itself.

For patients who present in complete cardiovascular collapse with refractory VT/VF, extracorporeal life support (ECLS) is being used with increasing frequency as an emergency intervention for both in-hospital and out-of-hospital arrest.

There are several studies that have compared CPR with ECLS/ECMO rescue in the setting of refractory VT/VF to conventional cardiopulmonary resuscitation.[9] Unfortunately, there are no large prospective randomized controlled trials evaluating ECLS. The majority of available studies have been observational.[10] With the current available evidence, the use of mechanical support in cardiopulmonary collapse receives a class IIa American College of Cardiology/American Heart Association indication when used as a bridge-to-decision or bridge-to-recovery.[10] (It is recommended and reasonable to use ECMO in this setting as the benefits outweigh the risk.)

Most observational studies have shown some benefit with ECLS. In a recent meta-analysis there was a 13% increase in the absolute survival rate at 30 days post-arrest and 15% increase at long-term follow-up, were long-term was defined as the longest available data collection point from the included studies.[9] Favorable neurologic outcomes increased by 14% and 11% over traditional CPR at 30-day and long-term follow-up, respectively. At this observed rate, the number needed to treat is 9 for a favorable long-term neurologic outcome.[9] Other benefits have been observed with ECLS rescue including a reduced rate of renal failure from 7% in patients surviving cardiac arrest to 1.9% in patients that survived and received ECLS.[12]

When applied to specific population, such as short arrest to ECLS time or young patients even with extended CPR times, there does appear to be a dramatic survival benefit with the use of ECLS.[13] If the initial cardiac rhythm after cardiac arrest was refractory VT/VF following 3 attempts at defibrillation, amiodarone, and effective CPR, ECLS placement resulted in a 50% survival rate and favorable neurologic outcomes beyond discharge.[14] In a subsequent larger study of the same population, there was a 42% rate of favorable neurologic outcomes at hospital discharge.[15] It is important to note that both patient cohorts received immediate percutaneous coronary intervention, if indicated, following the initiation of ECLS.

Several scoring tools have been developed to predict survival rates in patients that receive ECLS rescue following cardiopulmonary arrest. The PREDICT VA-ECMO uses arterial pH, bicarbonate, and lactate levels making is simple to calculate; however, it useful only to predict 12-hour mortality after ECMO initiation.[16] A more useful predictor may be the SAVE (Survival After Va ECMO) score, which includes more variables but will predict percentage survival at discharge. The validating studies for the SAVE score, however, did not include ECLS use post-arrest.[17] Yet another tool that may be helpful but that was also not developed specifically for rescue following arrest is the ENCOURAGE score, which estimates survival at 6 months post-ECLS.[18]

Making the emergent decision to place a patient on ECLS is difficult and depends on many factors including the availability of resources within a hospital system. While rescue of patients with refractory VT/VF due to acute coronary syndrome appears to convey a survival benefit, placement of ECLS in the setting of septic shock, advanced age, or after

inadequate/prolonged CPR (greater than 60 minutes) results in poor outcomes with little or no demonstrated benefit.[9,19] Patients with advance end-stage organ disease, significant vascular disease, polytrauma, or hostile anatomy not conducive to cannula placement should not be considered candidates for ECLS.[9] It is also important to remember that VA ECMO is contraindicated in aortic valve insufficiency and aortic dissection.

For the patient in the case study here, VA ECMO is the appropriate ECLS modality. VA ECMO takes blood from the systemic venous circulation and pumps it to the systemic arterial circulation after it has been oxygenated and carbon dioxide removed. In the case of refractory VT, the patient requires mechanical support to augment his cardiac output in addition to oxygenation and ventilatory support. Veno-venous (VV) ECMO would not provide effective augmentation of the cardiac output.[20] Cannulation strategy varies widely with percutaneous access of the femoral vessels, most common in patients without comorbid vascular disease or aberrant anatomy. Flow rates of up to 4 L/min are often achieved. Serious vascular complications of VA ECMO placement include limb ischemia (1%–7%), cannulation site infection (8%), and compartment syndrome (3%). However, with emergent cannula placement the rates are likely higher.[9] Bleeding is a common complication that occurs in up to 40% of patients, and cannula infection rates are significant in up to 30% of cases.[21]

North-south syndrome/harlequin syndrome is a complication that deserves special consideration. This phenomenon is seen when oxygenated blood is returned to the arterial circulation distal to the aortic arch such as from a femoral artery cannula. At some point in the aorta, the poorly oxygenated blood from coming anterograde from the heart mixes with the well oxygenated blood flowing retrograde up the aorta from the arterial limb of the ECMO. If this point is distal to the carotid arteries, deoxygenated blood is delivered to the brain, increasing the risk for anoxic brain injury. This can be prevented by increasing the arterial flow of the ECMO or moving the arterial cannula proximally to the axillary artery. The oxygen content at the right radial artery should be monitored, as this artery receives blood from the proximal aortic arch and reflects the oxygen content in the right common carotid. Of note, some level of native anterograde flow through the patient's heart should be maintained to prevent intracardiac thrombus formation.

The goal of VA ECMO is to maintain adequate end-organ perfusion, maintain acid base balance, and unload the patient's damaged ventricles to "rest" the myocardium. Flow rates are generally set between 2 to 3 liters per minute. A minimum critical flow of approximately 2 liters per minute is maintained to prevent thrombotic events. To prevent thrombotic events, most patients are anticoagulated with heparin while on ECMO support. The specific protocols will vary from institution to institution, but generally for adults an activated clotting time of 160 to 200 sec, an activated partial thromboplastin time of 40 to 80 sec, or an anti-Xa of 0.3 to 0.7 IE/ml will be maintained for the duration of the ECMO run.[22] If renal replacement therapy is required, it may often be placed in-line with the ECMO circuit.[9]

Weaning of ECMO support should be performed as soon as possible to prevent the complications mentioned here. ECMO is no longer necessary once the patient can maintain adequate circulation, oxygenation, and ventilation. This often requires correction of the underlying condition. In the case of the previously discussed patient, a VT ablation procedure was performed in the catheterization lab. This can be demonstrated though a prolonged period of relative hemodynamic stability with minimal inotropic or vasoconstrictive support coupled with adequate metabolic function on mechanical ventilatory support. Staged reduction in ECMO flow while monitoring arterial blood gases, mixed venous oxygen saturation, and native cardiac output help in the weaning process. Once ECMO support is discontinued, the ability to reinitiate support should close at hand should the patient's condition deteriorate.

VT Ablation Therapy

VT ablation procedures are performed by an electrophysiologist with a catheter-based radio frequency ablation device that can either be introduced into the heart via peripheral vascular sites (femoral vein with or without interatrial septal puncture if left ventricular access is needed) or by pericardial access through a sub-xiphoid puncture. The myocardium is first mapped by attempting to induce the abnormal rhythm and then ablating the offending tissue in that area with radio frequency energy. These ablation procedures are a useful treatment strategy when medical and pharmacologic therapy fail or are not well tolerated.[2] Those patients with structural heart disease as the ideology for their VT have higher success rates with ablation procedures than those without.[23] In patients with electrical storm, like the patient in the case study, this strategy is the therapy of choice as it has a low failure rate of between 0% and 10%.[24] However, at 1 year the recurrence rate has been reported to be as low as 6%[24] or high as 32%.[22] The mortality risk remains elevated even after ablation, likely due to the fact that recurrent VT is a symptom of an advanced-disease state of the heart. For those with VT from structural heart disease without electrical storm, the 1-year recurrence has also been reported to be as high as 23%.[22] The overall success rate for VT ablation with other etiologies of heart disease vary.[23,24] VT ablation procedures do carry risk, including vascular injury, ventricular perforation, pericardial tamponade, conduction blocks, and stroke with the risk of major complications (death, stroke, tamponade) at less than 1% to 4%.[22–25]

CONCLUSIONS

- In the United States, VT and VF are the most common cause of sudden death at a rate of 300,000 out-of-hospital deaths with another 200,000 in-hospital deaths per year.

- VT/VF can easily be diagnosed from an EKG.

- VT is defined as 3 or more consecutive QRS complexes arising from the ventricle that are 100 bpm or greater.

- Sustained VT is 30 seconds or more of VT or any VT that requires intervention due to patient instability.

- VT/VF storm (arrhythmogenic storm or electrical storm) is defined as 3 or more sustained VT/VF events, each requiring intervention and all within 24 hours of the initial event.

- The term *refractory* is used when the arrhythmia is not abated by appropriate therapy and is often used interchangeably with *VT/VF storm* or when VF persists after 5 defibrillations in conjunction with the appropriate ACLS treatment.

- VT/VF is a medical emergency commonly associated with ischemic heart disease. Initial treatment should focus on the advanced cardiac life support algorithm including early defibrillation and pharmacologic support of the circulation

- In appropriately selected patients with refractory VT/VF, early ECLS has survival benefits and contributes to better neurologic outcomes.

- In the setting of hemodynamic collapse, VA ECMO is the appropriate strategy, commonly through femoral artery and vein.

- Harlequin (north-south) syndrome occurs when there is competing blood flow from the left ventricle and the ECMO circuit in the femoral artery. Deoxygenated blood from the left ventricle flows to carotid arteries, putting the brain at risk for ischemic injury. This can be detected with a sampling of blood from the right radial arterial.

- VT ablation is a useful therapy for recurrent VT.

- Long-term survival is significantly decreased even after successful VT ablation in patients who develop VT storm.

REFERENCES

1. Myerburg RJ, Junttila MJ. Sudden cardiac death caused by coronary artery disease. *Circulation.* 2012;*125*:1043–1052.
2. Al-khatib SM, Stevenson WG, Ackerman MJ, et al. 2017. AHA/ACC/HRS guidelines for management of patients with ventricular arrhythmias and the prevention of sudden cardiac death. *Circulation.* 2017;*138*(13):e210–e271. doi:CIR.0000000000000549.
3. Slovis CM, Wrenn KD. The technique of reversing ventricular fibrillation: improve the odds of success with this five-phase approach. *J Crit Illn.* 1994;*9*:873–889.
4. Eifling M., Razavi M. The evaluation and management of electrical storm. *Tex Heart Inst J.* 2011;*38*(2):111–121.
5. Buxton AE, Calkins H, Callans DJ, et al. ACC/AHA/HRS 2006 key data elements and definitions for electrophysiological studies and procedures: a report of the American College of Cardiology/American Heart Association Task Force on Clinical Data Standards. *J Am Coll Cardiol.* 2006;*48*:2360–2396.
6. Emkanjoo Z, Alihasani N, Alizadeh A, et al. Electrical storm in patients with implantable cardioverter-defibrillators: can it be forecast? *Tex Heart Inst J.* 2009;*36*(6):563–567.

7. El-Sherif N, Smith RA, Evans K. Canine ventricular arrhythmias in the late myocardial infarction period. 8. Epicardial mapping of reentrant circuits. *Circ Res.* 1981;*49*:255–265.

8. Baerman JM, Morady F, DiCarlo LA Jr, de Buitleir M. Differentiation of ventricular tachycardia from supraventricular tachycardia with aberration: value of the clinical history. *Ann Emerg Med.* 1987;*16*(1):40–43.

9. Ouweneel DM, Schotborgh JV, Limpens J, et al. Extracorporeal life support during cardiac arrest and cardiogenic shock: a systematic review and meta-analysis. *Intens Care Med.* 2016;*42*(12):1922–1934. doi:10.1007/s00134-016-4536-8.

10. Meuwese CL, Ramjankhan FZ, Braithwaite SA, et al. Extracorporeal life support in cardiogenic shock: indications and management in current practice. *Netherlands Heart J.* 2018;*26*(2):58–66. doi:10.1007/s12471-018-1073-9.

11. Yancy C, Jessup M, Bozkurt B, et al. 2013 ACCF/AHA guideline for the management of heart failure: a report of the American College of Cardiology Foundation/American Heart Association Task Force on Practice Guidelines. *J Am College Card.* 2013;*62*(16):e147–e239.

12. Blumenstein J, Leick J, Liebetrau C, et al. Extracorporeal life support in cardiovascular patients with observed refractory in-hospital cardiac arrest is associated with favourable short and long-term outcomes: a propensity-matched analysis. *Eur Heart J Acute Cardiovasc Care.* 2016;*5*(7):13–22. doi:10.1177/2048872615612454.

13. Aubin H, Petrov G, Dalyanoglu H, et al. A suprainstitutional network for remote extracorporeal life support: a retrospective cohort study. *JACC: Heart Failure.* 2016;*4*(9):698–708.

14. Yannopoulos DA, Bartos JA, Raveendran G, et al. Coronary artery disease in patients with out-of-hospital refractory ventricular fibrillation cardiac arrest. *JACC.* 2017;*70*(9):1109–1117.

15. Wengenmayer T, Duerschmied D, Graf E, et al. Development and validation of a prognostic model for survival in patients treated with venoarterial extracorporeal membrane oxygenation: the PREDICT VA-ECMO score. *Eur Heart J Acute Cardiovasc Care.* 2019;*8*(4):350–359. doi:10.1177/2048872618789052.

16. Schmidt M, Burrell A, Roberts L, et al. Predicting survival after ECMO for refractory cardiogenic shock: the survival after veno-arterial-ECMO (SAVE)-score. *Eur Heart J.* 2015;*36*(33):2246–2256. doi:10.1093/eurheartj/ehv194.

17. Muller G, Flecher E, Lebreton G, et al. The ENCOURAGE mortality risk score and analysis of long-term outcomes after VA-ECMO for acute myocardial infarction with cardiogenic shock. *Intense Care Med.* 2016;*42*(3):370–378. doi:10.1007/s00134-016-4223-9.

18. Kim DH, Kim JB, Jung SH, Choo SJ, Chung CH, Lee W. Extracorporeal cardiopulmonary resuscitation: predictors of survival. *Kor J Thoracic Cardiovasc Surg.* 2016;*49*(4):273–279. doi:10.5090/kjtcs.2016.49.4.273.

19. Conrad SA, Rycus P.T. Extracorporeal membrane oxygenation for refractory cardiac arrest. *Ann Cardiac Anaesth.* 2017;*20*(Suppl 1):S4–S10. doi:10.4103/0971-9784.197790.

20. Cheng R, Hachamovitch R, Kittleson M, et al. Complications of extracorporeal membrane oxygenation for treatment of cardiogenic shock and cardiac arrest: a meta-analysis of 1,866 adult patients. *Ann Thorac Surg.* 2014;*97*(2):610–616.

21. Koster A, Ljajikj E, Faraoni D. Traditional and non-traditional anticoagulation management during extracorporeal membrane oxygenation. *Ann Cardiothorac Surg.* 2019;*8*(1):129–136. doi:10.21037/acs.2018.07.03

22. Vergara P, Tung R, Vaseghi M, et al. Successful ventricular tachycardia ablation in patients with electrical storm reduces recurrences and improves survival. *Heart Rhythm.* 2018;*15*(1):48–55.

23. Markman T, McBride D, Liang J. Catheter ablation for ventricular tachycardias in patients with structural heart disease. *US Cardiology Review.* 2018;*12*(1):51–56.

24. Leal RT, Monteiro GC, da Silva Menezes Júnior A. Catheter ablation in the treatment of electrical storm: integrative review. *Indian Pacing Electrophysiol J.* 2017;*17*(5):140–145.

REVIEW QUESTIONS

1. A 68-year-old male arrives in the intensive care unit (ICU) in normal sinus rhythm with a history of 4 episodes of unstable VT within the last 12 hours. The first 2 episodes resolved with an amiodarone bolus and infusion. The third episode was abated with lidocaine. The fourth episode required cardioversion. Which of the following would best describe the patient's condition?

   A. VT storm
   B. Refractory VT
   C. Sustained VT
   D. None of the above

2. A 52-year-old female with a history of coronary artery disease, current smoker, obstructive sleep apnea, and insulin-dependent diabetes mellitus presents to the ICU directly from the emergency department for non-ST segment elevation myocardial infarction. When moving the patient to the ICU bed, you witness a wide complex tachycardia on the transport monitor. Which of the following is the best first initial diagnostic tool?

   A. 5-lead KEG
   B. Troponin
   C. 12-lead ECG
   D. Basic metabolic panel

3. A 64-year-old male presents to the emergency department in monomorphic VT. His blood pressure is 142/86 and he remains asymptomatic. Which of the following drugs are acceptable initial therapies?

   A. Metoprolol
   B. Verapamil
   C. Amiodarone
   D. All of the above

4. Which of the following locations would be *most* helpful to draw an arterial blood gas to assess adequate oxygenation in a patient currently being managed with femoral VA ECMO?

   A. Femoral artery
   B. Left radial artery
   C. Right radial artery
   D. All of the above

5. You are called to assess a patient in the emergency department with refractory VT. The patient is unstable. You decide to initiate ECLS. Which of the following represents the most appropriate cannulation strategy?

   A. Right femoral artery and right femoral vein
   B. Avalon catheter
   C. Bi-femoral venous cannulation
   D. None of the above.

6. A 65-year-old female was placed on ECLS in the emergency department for refractory VT. She is cannulated in the right femoral artery and left femoral vein. She regains normal sinus rhythm 6 hours after initiation of VA ECMO. You notice that

her upper extremities seem pale in comparison to her lower extremities. Which of the following is the most likely cause?

    A. Decrease in venous congestion
    B. Distal movement of previous mixing zone.
    C. Failing oxygenator
    D. None of the above

7. An 81-year-old male placed on VA ECMO for refractory V-tach is admitted to your ICU from the emergency department. The patient's wife inquiries about the likelihood of survival. Which of the following may assist in outcomes prediction with VA ECMO?

    A. SAVE score
    B. Encourage score
    C. Both A and B
    D. None of the above

8. You are seeing a 38-year-old male placed on VA ECMO. The patient was percutaneously cannulated via the right and left femoral artery and vein, respectively. The left lower extremity is cool to the touch, and pulses are no longer palpable. Which of the following complications should be included in your differential?

    A. Limb ischemia related to catheter placement
    B. Compartment syndrome
    C. Thrombosis
    D. All of the above

9. A 59-year-old patient with ischemic cardiomyopathy was placed on VA ECMO for refractory VT. After successful VT ablation, the patient continues to improve clinically. In addition to tolerating a weaning trial, which of the following indicate successful weaning from VA ECMO?

    A. Ejection fraction greater than 30%
    B. Hemodynamic stability in the presence of low inotropic/vasopressor infusions
    C. Left ventricular outflow tract VTI greater than 10 cm/s
    D. All of the above

10. Of the following which is a contraindication to femoral VA ECMO?

    A. Severe mitral stenosis
    B. Severe mitral regurgitation
    C. Severe aortic regurgitation
    D. Severe aortic stenosis

ANSWERS

1. A. VT storm is defined at 3 or more episodes of VT within a 24-hour period. Refractory VT describes VT that does not respond to standard treatment, whereas sustained VT describes unstable VT and/or duration greater than 30 seconds.

2. B. The 12-lead EKG is the gold standard for the diagnosis of cardiac arrhythmias.

3. D. A patient presenting with stable VT should be evaluated by formal EKG, electrolytes, and cardiology consult to determine the history of structural disease and determine correct treatment. Control of both rate and rhythm are a part of the management strategy.

4. C. The right radial artery represents the area most distal to femoral arterial retrograde flow provided by femoral VA ECMO and therefore acts as a surrogate for cerebral flow.

5. A. The patient is in cardiogenic shock and requires VA ECMO for resuscitation. Choices B and C represent cannulation strategies for VV ECMO and would not provide mechanical circulatory support or allow for organ perfusion.

6. B. Femoral VA ECMO forces blood up the arterial tree in retrograde fashion. As the intrinsic cardiac function returns, the area where the antegrade blood flow from intrinsic cardiac function and retrograde blood flow provided by the ECMO circuit moves distally along the arterial tree. This can result in inadequate delivery of oxygenated blood upstream from the mixing zone.

7. C. The SAVE and Encourage scoring systems are useful in predicting survival for patients on ECLS. These scores were not designed, however, for prediction of survival in patients for whom ECLS was initiated after cardiac arrest.

8. D. Limb ischemia, hyperperfusion, compartment syndrome, and thrombosis are all known complications of ECMO and should be monitored for in all patients receiving this therapy.

9. D. All of these can indicate that adequate perfusion will likely take place after cessation of mechanical circulatory support.

10. C. Femoral VA ECMO in patients with severe aortic regurgitation can decrease coronary perfusion and myocardial oxygen demand by increasing left ventricular end diastolic pressures.

17.

ANAPHYLAXIS PRESENTING FROM HOME

Jared Staab and Brent Barta

STEM CASE AND KEY QUESTIONS

A 34-year-old female presents to the emergency department with severe abdominal pain and hypotension. Paramedics report that upon arrival to the patient's home she was in acute distress, warm, and diaphoretic. Oxygen was delivered to the patient via a non-rebreather mask. Intravenous (IV) access was initially difficult to obtain; however, fluids were administered as soon as access was established. Further history from the patient revealed that she became ill after eating food at a neighborhood BBQ. She endorsed a history of mild asthma with infrequent inhaler use. Upon arrival to the emergency department the patient's blood pressure is 80/40, her heart rate is 120, and her respiratory rate is 35. Her SpO$_2$ is 95% on 100% O$_2$ via facemask. She is administered nebulized albuterol with minimal improvement.

WHAT IS ANAPHYLAXIS? WHAT SHOULD BE INCLUDED IN YOUR DIFFERENTIAL DIAGNOSIS?

She is admitted to the intensive care unit (ICU) for treatment of hypoxemia and vasodilatory/distributive shock. Her chest X-ray is normal, the computer tomography scan of the chest is negative for pulmonary embolism, and troponins and electrocardiogram are normal. The patient is resuscitated with an additional 2 liters of intravenous normal saline and an arterial blood pressure line is placed. She continues to have dyspnea and new onset of diarrhea. An hour later there is no clinical improvement with the nebulizer treatments and fluids. There is wheezing on exam and her skin is noted to have numerous urticaria. Her oropharynx is now markedly edematous consistent with angioedema.

HOW IS ANAPHYLAXIS DIAGNOSED? ARE THERE ANY LAB TESTS THAT MAY AID IN THE DIAGNOSIS?

Given the acute onset of hypotension, gastrointestinal symptoms, including diarrhea, urticaria, and angioedema, the patient meets criteria for a diagnosis of anaphylaxis based on the World Allergy Organization's (WAO) 2011 guidelines. A serum tryptase level is ordered to confirm the clinical diagnosis. The patient's condition continues to deteriorate. She is increasingly tachycardic and complains of worsening dyspnea and diarrhea.

HOW DO YOU MANAGE THE AIRWAY OF A PATIENT WITH ANGIOEDEMA?

With this degree of respiratory failure, the critical care team performs an awake fiberoptic endotracheal intubation and the patient is placed on a ventilator.

WHAT IS THE PRIMARY TREATMENT FOR THE PATIENT'S ANAPHYLACTIC REACTION?

The patient is given a bolus of 100 micrograms IV epinephrine, and an epinephrine infusion is started at 2 mcg/kg/min. IV fluids are also administered via infusion and intermittent bolus to maintain hemodynamic stability. Mechanical ventilatory support is continued with albuterol nebulizer treatments as needed for wheezing.

WHAT ARE THE BASIC PATTERNS OF ANAPHYLACTIC REACTIONS? ARE THERE ANY ANCILLARY TREATMENTS FOR ANAPHYLAXIS?

Thirty minutes after administration of epinephrine, the patient's blood pressure has improved and wheezing is notably less on the physical exam. Her urticarial rash appears also to have improved. Over the next several hours, however, increasing amounts of epinephrine and IV fluid are required to maintain her blood pressure. With sedation holiday she endorses pruritus. Steroids are started to help ameliorate the biphasic reaction. In addition, diphenhydramine and famotidine are started to assist with pruritus. Methylene blue is considered for refractory shock; however, she ultimately responds to epinephrine and fluids.

WHAT ARE COMMON TRIGGERS FOR ANAPHYLAXIS?

A more thorough history is obtained, which reveals a patient history of eczema and an allergy to eggs as a child. Family history is notable for a mother with an allergy to penicillin and a father with a history of anaphylaxis to bee venom.

HOW DO YOU COUNSEL YOUR PATIENT ABOUT PREVENTION OF ANAPHYLAXIS?

The patient continues to improve with epinephrine, IV fluids, steroids, and H1 and H2 antagonists and is extubated. In preparation for discharge she is counseled to avoid triggers until confirmatory testing can take place.

WHAT MEDICATIONS AND/OR SUPPLIES SHOULD THE PATIENT BE DISCHARGED WITH? WHEN SHOULD FOLLOW-UP OCCUR?

On discharge, the patient's asthma medications are optimized to include an inhaled steroid, leukotriene inhibitor, prednisone taper, and albuterol measured dose inhaler as needed. In addition, she is discharged with an epinephrine auto injector, an anaphylaxis action plan, and a medical alert bracelet. The patient and her family also receive training in administration of the epinephrine auto injector. A follow-up appointment is made with an allergist within 3 to 4 weeks of discharge.

HOW ARE ANAPHYLACTIC TRIGGERS DIAGNOSED? WHAT CAN BE DONE TO PREVENT FUTURE ANAPHYLACTIC REACTIONS?

Four weeks after the anaphylactic episode, the patient is seen by an allergist. A baseline tryptase is drawn at this time to be compared with her peak tryptase while hospitalized. The patient undergoes allergen skin testing at this visit that evidences a positive reaction to nuts. The patient is counseled on avoidance of tree nuts and decides to pursue oral immunomodulation therapy. She eventually develops immunotolerance to tree nuts and continues to follow up with her allergist yearly.

DISCUSSION

The diagnosis of anaphylaxis has evolved over the past 100 years. Portier and Richet first noted increasingly severe reactions with repeated exposure to injected purified sea anemone toxins. Instead of conferring immunity on survivors of initial exposure, subsequent exposure resulted in fatal reactions.(1) Today, although definitions vary slightly, anaphylaxis is a life-threatening allergic reaction that can result in death if not identified and treated immediately (2). The incidence of anaphylaxis is estimated to be between 0.05% and 2%, although is likely underestimated due to underreporting, poor recognition, and differing definitions of what constitutes a reaction. (3, 4). The incidence has, however, increased over the past 10 years, including more than doubling among patients under 18 from 2000-2009 (3). Greater distance from the equator is associated with an increased prevalence based on epinephrine auto injector prescriptions (2, 4).

ETIOLOGY AND PATHOGENESIS

Anaphylaxis develops from repeat exposure to an allergen that has previously sensitized the immune system. Upon initial contact with an allergen, antigen presenting cells present processed allergen to T cells, which then mature into TH2 cells that activate B cells to produce immunoglobulin E (IgE) specific to the allergen. These IgE antibodies are then bound to high-affinity receptors on basophils and mast cells. Upon reexposure to the allergen, cross-linking of IgE receptors then results in mast cell degranulation. Mast cells and basophils release many mediators of inflammation, including early-acting mediators such as histamine and tryptase and later-acting mediators such as leukotrienes. This secretion of mediators may continue for several hours (1).

SIGNS AND SYMPTOMS

Signs and symptoms of anaphylaxis are broad and involve many organ systems including skin, mucosa, respiratory, cardiac, and central nervous system. Skin manifestations include diffuse itching, urticaria, flushing, edema, angioedema, and erythema. Involvement of the respiratory system may cause congestion, wheezing, rhinorrhea, stridor, cough, and respiratory failure. Involvement of the cardiac system may lead to arrhythmias (most commonly tachycardia), hypotension, shock, and cardiac arrest. Food allergies commonly present with involvement of the gastrointestinal system including nausea, vomiting, diarrhea, cramping, and abdominal pain. Anaphylaxis may also present as dizziness, syncope, sense of impending doom, headache, and irritability when involving the nervous system. Other symptoms may include low back pain, uterine pain, and vaginal bleeding in women (1, 2).

TRIGGERS AND RISK FACTORS

Risk factors for anaphylaxis are many and varied. The incidence and severity of anaphylaxis is higher in certain demographics. For instance, pediatric, geriatric, and obstetric patients are at increased risk for severe anaphylactic episodes. In addition, certain conditions such as atopy and asthma are associated with severe food allergies in infants and children. These patients have a higher incidence of anaphylaxis. Other systemic diseases such as mastocytosis may predispose those afflicted to severe anaphylactic reactions from insect stings/venom (2, 3, 5). Most cases of anaphylaxis are triggered by foods, drugs, insect venom, or exercise. Causes vary by geographic region; however, food allergies are the most common. Anaphylaxis to foods is more common in children, with an overall incidence of 7 per 100 in ages 0 to 4, in contrast to 0.12 in patients of all ages (3). In North America and Europe, milk, eggs, peanuts, tree nuts, shellfish, and fin fish represent the majority of food-related cases of anaphylaxis. Sesame is a more predominant trigger in the Middle East, and buckwheat, chickpeas, and rice disproportionately trigger anaphylaxis in Asia (2–5). Interestingly, wheat allergy is a known risk factor for severity of exercise-induced anaphylaxis.

Anaphylaxis triggered by drugs also displays regional variation based on exposure. Anaphylaxis to antibiotics for management of tuberculosis (TB) is more common in areas where TB is endemic. History of anaphylaxis to antibiotics is a vexing problem. Patients with a history of penicillin allergy have been shown to have longer hospital stays and a higher incidence of antibiotic-resistant infections (3). Drugs associated with perioperative anaphylaxis include neuromuscular blockers, antibiotics, and sedative hypnotics. Ethanol and nonsteroidal anti-inflammatory drugs may also synergistically lead to leaky gut and systemic exposure to gut allergens. Beta blockers and ACE inhibitors have been shown to increase severity of anaphylactic reactions by priming mast cells to release histamine. Insect venom remains another common cause of anaphylaxis related to the local insect population. Similar to other triggers, patients become sensitized during the initial exposure and manifest anaphylaxis upon the second exposure (2–5).

DIAGNOSIS

A careful history and physical are the mainstays of diagnosis when evaluating a patient for anaphylaxis. Details surrounding stress, changes in diet, habits, and possible exposures should be elicited. The diagnosis of anaphylaxis is primarily clinical. A consensus statement from the National Institute of Allergy and Infectious Diseases/Food Allergy and Anaphylaxis Network outlines the diagnosis of anaphylaxis and divides the diagnosis into 1 of 3 categories with some caveats: (1) Patients with unknown exposure who exhibit sudden onset of mucocutaneous symptoms and either respiratory impairment or cardiac collapse; (2) known exposure to a likely allergen and any 2 of the following: cardiovascular collapse, respiratory compromise, mucocutaneous involvement, or gastrointestinal distress; (3) verified exposure to a known allergen with a sudden decline in the systolic blood pressure by at least 30%. Clinicians must be vigilant, however, and proceed with standard treatment in patients with known allergy exposures who may only manifest involvement of 1 organ system (2, 4). Concomitant cardiopulmonary disease, sedative use, altered mental status, and extremes of age may obscure signs or symptoms and delay the diagnosis of anaphylaxis. Laboratory testing of serum tryptase and histamine levels are commonly used to confirm anaphylaxis but should not delay treatment once the clinical diagnosis is suspected. Tryptase is a serine protease abundant in mast cells and basophils. Tryptase levels continue to rise after the onset of anaphylaxis and therefore should be measured between 15 to 30 minutes and 2 to 3 hours after the suspected triggering event to determine the peak concentration. Serum tryptase remains elevated for 24 to 48 hours. A tryptase level 2 weeks after recovery is needed to establish baseline tryptase levels for comparison. Importantly, tryptase may not be released in anaphylaxis to foods or in normotensive patients. Histamine has a faster rise and earlier peak level. It is ideally measured within 15 to 60 minutes of the triggering event (6).

TREATMENT

Anaphylaxis is a medical emergency and requires prompt treatment. Epinephrine remains the first-line treatment for anaphylaxis. It counteracts vasogenic and cardiogenic shock by increasing systemic vascular resistance and increasing cardiac output through its effect on alpha 1 and beta 1 receptors, respectively. Bronchodilation is mediated by agonism at the beta 2 receptor. Importantly, epinephrine also decreases mast cell degranulation through activation of beta 2 receptors on these cells. Epinephrine has a rapid onset and achieves systemic concentration within 10 minutes. Failure to rescue with epinephrine during anaphylaxis is associated with increased mortality. Recommendations are to administer epinephrine at 0.01 mg/kg up to 0.5 mg in adults and 0.3 mg in children intramuscularly. Repeated dosing may be necessary, and close monitoring is advised. Side effects from epinephrine administration include arrhythmia, hypertension, and coronary ischemia (2, 4). Although not recommended as first-line treatment by the WAO and the National Institute of Allergy and Infectious Diseases, various antihistamines and steroids are commonly given in addition to epinephrine.

H1 antihistamines are the most common drug given for anaphylaxis in emergency departments; however, there is scant evidence to support their efficacy. Diphenhydramine takes up to 80 minutes to antagonize 50% of histamine release during an anaphylactic episode. Importantly, many mediators other than histamine are released in an anaphylactic reaction. There are also concerns that these drugs cause excessive sedation and may be harmful in patients with respiratory compromise (2, 4).

Glucocorticoids are the second most common drug given for anaphylaxis. The onset of glucocorticoid action takes hours. This decreases their utility in acute anaphylaxis management. Glucocorticoids decrease many inflammatory mediators and may be beneficial for decreasing the occurrence and severity of biphasic anaphylactic reactions; however, further study is needed. Administration of steroids as a priority may delay epinephrine administration and therefore is not recommended as a first-line therapy at this time (2, 4).

H2 antihistamines are sometimes used in anaphylaxis and may decrease flushing and itching; however, there is currently a lack of quality evidence to recommend their use in anaphylaxis (2, 4).

Beta 2 agonists are often used to decrease bronchoconstriction in anaphylaxis. Though potentially helpful, these agents should not be used instead of, or prior to, epinephrine. Beta 2 agonists are unable to treat shock and oropharyngeal edema due to their lack of alpha 1 antagonism (2).

Refractory anaphylactic shock presents a challenging scenario. The importance of rapid epinephrine administration cannot be understated. Isotonic fluids and supplemental oxygen should also be administered, and invasive hemodynamic monitoring may be necessary. Patients with refractory anaphylactic shock often require large amounts of IV fluid, which may result in fluid overload during organ perfusion and after organ perfusion has been restored. Methylene blue is a nitric oxide scavenger and may be useful when given in anaphylactic shock not responding to epinephrine and isotonic fluids. Ultimately, refractory anaphylactic shock may require multiple vasoactive infusions as well as airway and ventilatory management by experts in anesthesiology and critical care. Select patients who do not respond to these therapies may be rescued by veno-arterial extracorporeal membrane oxygenation support (3).

FOLLOW-UP AND LONG-TERM MANAGEMENT

Patients with anaphylaxis are at risk of a biphasic reaction, as mentioned earlier. Monitoring for patients with moderate to severe reactions should be continued for at least 4 hours following resolution of hypotension and potentially longer. Prior to discharge, suspected allergens may be confirmed by IgE titers. Close follow-up with an allergist is recommended within 1 month. At this time supervised skin testing may help identify the allergen and assist in prevention of anaphylaxis through avoidance of the specific allergens. All patients should be discharged with an epinephrine auto-injection device and instructions on its usage as part of an anaphylaxis action plan. Barriers to use of epinephrine auto-injectors include cost, availability, and improper use/education (3). Immunomodulatory therapy may be available for prevention and management of anaphylaxis. Patients with venom and food-triggered anaphylaxis benefited from immunotherapy as evidenced by lower IgE levels and smaller wheels after skin prick tests. Patients with anaphylaxis to drugs benefit from testing to prevent recurrent administration of the offending agents. Follow-up with an allergist at yearly intervals is recommended in addition to management of coexisting medical conditions that can complicate anaphylaxis such as cardiac disease, COPD, and asthma (3).

CONCLUSIONS

Anaphylaxis is a common and dangerous condition manifested by rapidly progressive involvement of the cardiac, respiratory, integumentary, and digestive systems. Delayed recognition and improper treatment may result in distributive shock, leading to multiorgan failure. The diagnosis of anaphylaxis is primarily a clinical one, which may be confirmed by laboratory tests. Epinephrine is the first-line treatment and should be given without delay. Second-line treatments may include H1 and H2 blockers, glucocorticoids, and beta 2 agonists. All patients should be discharged with an epinephrine-containing autoinjector, education, and follow-up with an allergist within a month of discharge. Avoidance of triggers, immunomodulatory therapy, and management of coexisting disease are effective in the long-term prevention and management of anaphylaxis.

REFERENCES

1. Boden, S. and Wesley Burks, A. Anaphylaxis: a history with emphasis on food allergy. *Immunological Reviews*, 2011;*242*(1), 247–257.
2. Simons, F., Ardusso, L., Bilò, M., et al. World Allergy Organization Guidelines for the assessment and management of anaphylaxis. *World Allergy Organization Journal*, 2011;*4*(2), 13–36.
3. Simons, F., Ebisawa, M., Sanchez-Borges, M., et al. 2015 update of the evidence base: World Allergy Organization anaphylaxis guidelines. *World Allergy Organization Journal*, 2015;*8*(1), 1–16.
4. Lieberman, P. Recognition and First-Line Treatment of Anaphylaxis. *The American Journal of Medicine*, 2014;*127*(1), S6–S11.
5. Simons, F., Ardusso, L., Dimov, V et al. World Allergy Organization anaphylaxis guidelines: 2013 update of the evidence base. *International Archives of Allergy and Immunology*, 2013;*162*(3., 193–204.
6. Jimenez-Rodriguez, T., Garcia-Neuer, M., Alenazy, L. and Castells, M. Anaphylaxis in the 21st century: phenotypes, endotypes, and biomarkers. *Journal of Asthma and Allergy*, 2018;11, 121–142.

REVIEW QUESTIONS

1. A 74-year-old female with a history of coronary artery disease, type 2 diabetes, hypertension, and COPD is being treated in the emergency department for a severe anaphylactic reaction. Which of the following medications can increase the severity of anaphylactic reactions?

   A. Albuterol
   B. Amlodipine
   C. Insulin
   D. Lisinopril

2. A 4-year-old male presents to the emergency department with a sudden onset of tachycardia, hypotension, and angioedema. He is successfully treated with epinephrine. By which of the following mechanisms does epinephrine exert its effects in anaphylaxis?

   A. Beta 2 mediated mast cell and basophil stabilization
   B. Alpha 1 mediated increase in vascular tone
   C. Beta 1 mediated increase in chronotropy and inotropy
   D. All the above

3. A 30-year-old female is undergoing laparoscopic cholecystectomy and suddenly develops increased peak inspiratory pressures, hypotension, and urticaria. A presumptive diagnosis of anaphylaxis is made. Which of the following drugs is most commonly associated with anaphylaxis in the perioperative period?

   A. Propofol
   B. Rocuronium
   C. Cefazolin
   D. Fentanyl

4. A 20-year-old male presents to the emergency department intubated and sedated. He was found by emergency medical

services in respiratory distress with concomitant angioedema. Which of the following biomarkers could be helpful in confirming an anaphylactic reaction?

    A. C1 esterase
    B. Tryptase
    C. Urine metanephrines
    D. ADAMSTS13

5. You are discharging a 43-year-old female from the emergency department after successful treatment of anaphylaxis. Which of the following medications must you send home with her to prevent or treat recurrent anaphylaxis?

    A. Diphenhydramine
    B. Albuterol
    C. Epinephrine auto-injector
    D. Cimetidine

6. You are discharging a 50-year-old male home after an extended ICU stay for the treatment of a severe anaphylactic reaction. How soon should the patient see an allergist?

    A. 48 hours
    B. 1 week
    C. 1 month
    D. 1 year

7. A 5-year-old boy is diagnosed with a peanut allergy after skin prick testing. Which of the following treatments could help prevent anaphylaxis from a repeat exposure to peanuts?

    A. Sublingual immunomodulating therapy
    B. Daily Pepcid
    C. Daily Benadryl
    D. Daily prednisone

8. A 65-year-old female is being treated in the ICU for a severe anaphylactic reaction requiring mechanical ventilation, steroids, and infusions of epinephrine, vasopressin, norepinephrine, and IV fluids. She remains hypotensive. Which of the following may be helpful in restoration of her blood pressure?

    A. Diphenhydramine
    B. Famotidine
    C. Aminophylline
    D. Methylene blue

9. A 90-year-old male is evaluated in the emergency department for anaphylaxis associated with multiple bee stings. You decide to administer epinephrine. Which of the following adverse reactions is most likely?

    A. Hypotension
    B. Seizure
    C. Ventricular tachycardia
    D. Dyspnea

10. Which of the following conditions is most associated with elevated tryptase levels?

    A. Hereditary angioedema
    B. Coronary ischemia
    C. COPD
    D. Mastocytosis

ANSWERS

1. D. ACE inhibitors such as Lisinopril have the potential to increase severity of anaphylactic reactions by priming mast cells to release histamine.

2. D. Epinephrine, a cathecholamine with effects on apha 1, beta 1, and beta 2 receptors, is the treatment of choice for anaphylaxis. Acting on the beta 2 receptor, epinephrine stabilizes mast cells, preventing degranulation and release of histamine. Bronchial dilation also is induced by beta 2 agonism. Beta 1 agonism and alpha 1 agonism increase cardiac output and vasomotor tone, respectively.

3. B. Non-depolarizing neuromuscular blockers of the amino-steroid class such as Rocuronium are the most common medication-associated cause of intraoperative anaphylaxis. Other triggers of anaphylaxis in the perioperative period include latex exposure and antibiotics.

4. B. Tryptase, which is released by mast cells during degranulation, is associated with anaphylaxis. C1 Esterase deficiency is associated with hereditary angioedema. Urine metanephrines can assist in the diagnosis of pheochromocytoma. ADAMTS13 deficiency is associated with thrombotic thrombocytopenic purpura.

5. C. A epinephrine auto-injector is recommended for all patients with a history of anaphylaxis. Cimetidine, diphenhydramine, and albuterol may assist in the management of anaphylaxis but are not recommended for first-line therapy.

6. C. Patients with presumed anaphylaxis should see an allergist around 1 month after the anaphylactic reaction, which allows time for tryptase levels to return to baseline and repletion of mast cell granules, both of which help confirm anaphylaxis and allow for further testing.

7. A. Sublingual immunomodulating therapy is an important therapy in prevention of anaphylactic reactions to peanuts. Pepcid, Benadryl, and prednisone can be ancillary treatments for anaphylaxis but do not reliably prevent anaphylaxis.

8. D. Methylene blue can be used in refractory vasoplegia and shock to increase systemic vascular resistance.

9. C. Ventricular tachycardia and other arrhythmias can be caused by administration of beta antagonists such as epinephrine.

10. D. Mastocytosis is associated with elevations in baseline tryptase levels. Episodes of anaphylaxis require follow up with an allergist to reassess for the presence of continued elevation of tryptase levels to diagnose mastocytosis.

18.

SEVERE THERMAL BURN INJURY, GREATER THAN 80% TOTAL BODY SURFACE AREA

Joshua Trester

STEM CASE AND KEY QUESTIONS

A 36-year-old man with no past medical history was performing yard work and raking leaves at his home. Upon finishing the job, he chooses to dispose of the leaves and grass clippings by burning them in a nearby open field. After starting the fire with some gasoline from a handheld can he uses to fill his lawn mower, he attempts to add more gasoline to the fire by tossing it from the can onto the fire. While doing this, the gasoline fumes create a flash fire, which causes him to fall to the ground and spill a large amount of gasoline on himself that immediately ignites. He screams for help, and his wife, who was nearby, runs to his aid. She takes him by the arm and pulls him away from the fire and tells him to roll to extinguish the blaze. Unfortunately, the man loses consciousness and continues to burn. As quickly as she can, his wife grabs a nearby garden hose to extinguish her burning husband. She calls 911 and emergency medical services arrive approximately 10 minutes later. On arrival, the patient is moaning and following simple commands with rapid respirations with burns over his head, face, chest, back, and legs. Vitals signs on arrival are heart rate 125, noninvasive blood pressure 105/40, respiratory rate 27, oxygen saturation (SpO_2) 85%. Two 16-gauge intervenous (IV) needles are placed in bilateral antecubital fossae and he is placed on a non-rebreather mask with 100% oxygen with improvement of his SpO_2 to 100%. A bag of lactated Ringer's solution connected to the patient's IV and is hung to gravity; he is covered with mylar blankets and transferred to the local level 1 trauma center, which is also an American Burn Association (ABA) Verified Burn Center, located 25 minutes away by ambulance.

WHAT INITIAL CONSIDERATIONS SHOULD BE PAID TO PATIENTS WITH LARGE TBSA BURNS ON ARRIVAL TO A MEDICAL CENTER, AND SHOULD THIS PATIENT BE INTUBATED?

The patient arrives to the medical center now with a SpO_2 of 100% on 100% FiO_2 via a non-rebreather mask with a respiratory rate of 29. He has burns to his face as well as singed nasal hairs and blisters on his tongue. He has some hoarseness with groaning. His blood pressure is 104/65 with a heart rate of 105. He is not oriented but is following simple commands in 4 extremities. He has no obvious distracting injuries on primary assessment after all of his clothing is removed. The patient is intubated and subsequently vented with a FiO_2 of 1.0 on assist control mandatory ventilation with a tidal volume of 450 mL and a respiratory rate of 18. His oxygen saturation remains stable post-intubation and arterial blood gas reveals a $PaCO_2$ of 42.

HOW DOES ONE APPROACH THE INITIAL RESUSCITATION OF SEVERELY BURNED PATIENTS?

The patient's blood pressure starts to decrease to 80s/40s in the subsequent hour and a chest X-ray reveals a mid-tracheal endotracheal tube (ETT) without acute complication. A Foley catheter and central and arterial lines are placed. He is not clinically bleeding and has no other distracting injuries. His exam is otherwise unchanged. The patient's burns are surveyed, revealing 81% total body surface area (TBSA) partial and full thickness burns. The burns on his lower extremities are noted to be circumferential. He weighs 85 kg. His 24-hour crystalloid requirements are estimated using the Parkland Formula (4 mL/kg/TBSA burn) to be 27.5 L, with 13.8 L to be administered in the first 8 hours. He has already received 2 L of crystalloid in the first hour since arrival and is now subsequently normotensive. You estimate per Parkland he will require approximately 1.5 L each hour over the next 7 hours. You order those fluids to begin as he arrives to his room in the intensive care unit (ICU).

DOES FLUID RESUSCITATION HAVE COMPLICATIONS?

Over the ensuing hours his left lower extremity becomes increasingly tense with pallor. The nurse notes decreased posterior tibial and dorsalis pedal pulses (now only "1" from "4"), and the patient withdraws rapidly to pain when the leg is palpated. He subsequently undergoes measurement of compartment pressures by the in-house burn surgeon, which are elevated. The surgeon elects to perform bilateral lower extremity escharotomies to relieve pressure in the left leg and to prevent development of compartment syndrome in the right leg.

ARE TOXINS SUCH AS CARBON MONOXIDE AND CYANIDE A CONCERN IN THIS PATIENT?

The initial blood gas with co-oximetry reveals a carboxyhemoglobin (COHb) level of 14%. The patient is still following simple commands, and his serum lactic acid is 1.4 mmol/L. Electrocardiogram (EKG) reveals sinus tachycardia and a serum troponin is <0.04 ng/mL. He is continued on 100% oxygen via the ventilator circuit and a repeat COHb level normalizes 2 hours later. No therapy for cyanide toxicity is administered, and a cyanide level is sent but is not expected to return from the lab for 2 to 3 days.

SHOULD SUPPLEMENTAL NUTRITION BE CONSIDERED FOR THIS PATIENT?

The patient remains hemodynamically stable over the next 18 hours. His urine output remains adequate on Parkland Formula–guided fluid estimates. In consultation with the ICU dietician, a nasogastric tube is placed, and the patient is started on enteral nutrition.

DISCUSSION

INITIAL EVALUATION OF SEVERELY BURNED PATIENTS

All burn patients should undergo a primary trauma survey, often approached using the acronym ABCDE: Airway, Breathing, Circulation, Disability (neurologic examination), and Exposure. IV access should be established, and the airway should be examined and supported (see following discussion). Patients should be completely undressed and examined head to toe for a secondary survey of any accompanying injuries as well as a complete examination of the burn injury. A focused medical history should be obtained followed by routine trauma labs and imaging including complete blood count, basic metabolic panel, coagulation studies, blood gas with COHb level, serum lactate, creatine kinase, alcohol and toxicology screen, blood type and antibody screen, chest X-ray, and EKG. Patients with the considerations in Box 18.1 should immediately be stabilized, intubated if necessary, and transferred to a verified burn center for subspecialty care.

DECISION TO INTUBATE/ESTABLISH AN ARTIFICIAL AIRWAY

As with all injured patients, the inability to adequately oxygenate or ventilate without the ability to protect the airway are obvious indications for intubation emergently. Burn patients require a more conservative assessment of their injuries as inhalation injury can predispose to rapid and unpredictable upper airway edema that can lead to airway loss. Large-volume fluid resuscitation can also lead to worsening upper airway edema. Additionally, inhalation injury can lead to rapid development of acute respiratory distress syndrome. Early,

Box 18.1. BURN/INJURIES THAT SHOULD BE REFERRED TO A BURN CENTER

1. Partial thickness burns greater than 10% total body surface area (TBSA).

2. Burns that involve the face, hands, feet, genitalia, perineum, or major joints.

3. Third degree burns in any age group.

4. Electrical burns, including lightning injury.

5. Chemical burns.

6. Inhalation injury.

7. Burn injury in patients with pre-existing medical disorders that could complicate management, prolong recovery, or affect mortality.

8. Any patient with burns and concomitant trauma (such as fractures) in which the burn injury poses the greatest risk of morbidity or mortality. In such cases, if the trauma poses the greater immediate risk, the patient may be initially stabilized in a trauma center before being transferred to a burn unit. Physician judgment will be necessary in such situations and should be in concert with the regional medical control plan and triage protocols.

9. Burned children in hospitals without qualified personnel or equipment for the care of children.

10. Burn injury in patients who will require special social, emotional, or rehabilitative intervention.

Adapted from American College of Surgeons. Guidelines for the operation of burn centers. In *Resources for Optimal Care of the Injured Patient*, 79-86. Chicago, IL: American College of Surgeons, Committee on Trauma 2006.

preemptive intubation prior to development of upper airway edema is necessary in patients in whom there is concern for inhalation injury. Approximately two-thirds of patients with >70% TBSA burns have inhalation injury (1). Potential indications that patients need intubation (in addition to altered mental status, respiratory distress, hypoxemia, and hypercapnia) include hoarseness, stridor, singed nasal hairs, circumferential neck burns, wheezing, swollen lips, carbonaceous material in the oropharynx or nose, and visible blisters in the mouth or oropharynx. Of note, succinylcholine as part of a rapid sequence intubation—while considered to be contraindicated in burn patients due to concern for development of hyperkalemia—can be used within the first 24 to 48 hours after injury. After that, there is some discrepancy as to the exact time post-burn when succinylcholine can induce exaggerated hyperkalemia and should no longer be used. This is thought to be due to delayed development of upregulated of extra junctional nicotinic acetylcholine receptors in burn patients (2).

BURN SHOCK RESUSCITATION

Burn shock is a complicated pathophysiologic process that is comprised of a distributive shock caused by the inflammation induced from the burn injury as well as hypovolemia from the profound insensible losses that accompany large TBSA burns. Fluid administration is a tenant of initial resuscitation and requires an assessment of the percentage of TBSA of partial and full-thickness burns as well as an estimate of the patient's IV fluid requirements. Estimating burn TBSA can be accomplished by using a Lund and Browder chart for adults and children (Figure 18.1).

A Lund-Browder chart is thought to be the most accurate method to assess TBSA of burns (3). The palmar method can also be used to quickly evaluate surface burns, where the patient's palm of the hand plus palmar surface of the fingers represents slightly less than approximately 1% of their TBSA. For resuscitation formulas, calculations of TBSA are based on areas with second- and third-degree burns. Different formulas have been used to estimate initial fluid resuscitation volumes for burn patients over the first 24 hours of their resuscitation. The most widely utilized formula in the United States is the Parkland Formula (4). The Parkland Formula estimates the total 24-hour crystalloid volume requirements for these patients, half of which is administered over the first 8 hours and the remaining half administered over the next 16 hours from the time of the burn injury.

The Parkland Formula:

24-hour crystalloid requirement = TBSA % burned × Weight (in kg) × 4 mL

It is our institution's protocol to utilize the Parkland Formula for all burn patients with >20% TBSA burns. Burns with TBSA <20% can frequently be resuscitated with oral rehydration or standard maintenance rates of IV crystalloids. It is important to stress that the Parkland Formula, as well as other documented resuscitation formulas, are simply starting points to guide and estimate IV fluid requirements. One principle that is critical in guiding resuscitation of these patients is following markers of end-organ perfusion with continuous reassessment of progress. The gold standard for monitoring resuscitation is to accurately measure hourly urine output with a target of 0.5 to 1 ml/kg/hr (4). A Foley catheter is indicated for all severely burned patients who necessitate acute volume resuscitation. Constant monitoring and serial readjustments of fluid administration rate are critical in the first hours following acute burns. Subsequent changes in fluid rate in response to patients' urine output and markers of end-organ perfusion are critical to a successful resuscitation as well as to prevent over-resuscitation. Our institution favors

Estimating Percentage Total Body Surface Area in Children Affected by Burns

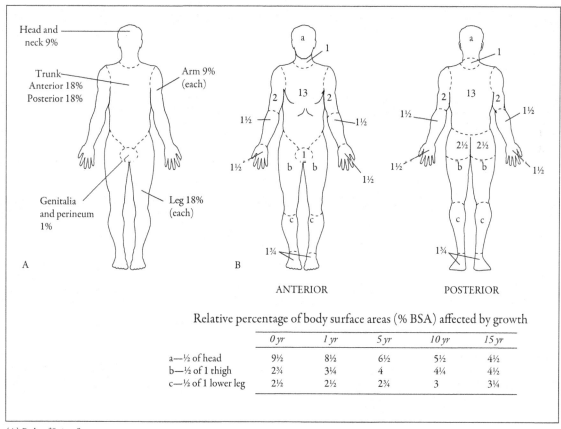

Relative percentage of body surface areas (% BSA) affected by growth

	0 yr	1 yr	5 yr	10 yr	15 yr
a—½ of head	9½	8½	6½	5½	4½
b—½ of 1 thigh	2¾	3¼	4	4¼	4½
c—½ of 1 lower leg	2½	2½	2¾	3	3¼

(A) Rule of "nines"

(B) Lund-Browder diagram for estimating extent of burns

Figure 18.1 Lund–Browder chart.

Source: U.S. Department of Health and Human Services. http://www.remm.nlm.gov/burns.htm. Accessed May 30, 2018. This image is in the public domain in the United States.

administration of a "balanced salt" solution as the crystalloid of choice instead of normal saline. Balanced salt solutions such as Plasma-lyte® or lactated Ringer's solution provide an electrolyte composition closer to that of plasma than normal saline. Additionally, large-volume administration of normal saline has been shown to promote development of a hyperchloremic metabolic acidosis (5) and can exacerbate the metabolic acidosis from hypovolemia that is present in many burn patients. Use of colloids in burns remains a controversial topic. A recent meta-analysis demonstrated no effect on mortality for patients resuscitated acutely with albumin solutions but did demonstrate total volumes of fluid administered were overall lower than those resuscitated with crystalloid (6, 10). Albumin-containing solutions are significantly more expensive than crystalloid solutions. It is our institutional practice to consider the addition of albumin-containing solutions as a rescue technique when patients being resuscitated with crystalloid solutions fail to reach hourly urine output targets with significantly higher than expected crystalloid volumes after the first 12 hours following injury.

COMPLICATIONS OF VOLUME RESUSCITATION

Excessive parenteral fluid resuscitation is accompanied by significant morbidity. Of concern in the management of severely burned patients is the sequalae of large-volume fluid resuscitation. Nearly all severely burned patients develop pulmonary edema of some variety from extravasation of administered crystalloid volume. "Third spacing" of administered IV fluids results in eventual development of whole body interstitial edema with severely burned patients nearly always having grossly net positive volume status during their ICU stays. Large-volume resuscitation can result in gross volume overload that can predispose patients to develop compartment syndrome, which is defined as an intra-abdominal pressure (for which intravesicular/bladder pressures are often are used as a surrogate) >20 mmHg and new organ dysfunction (7). Falling urine output/worsening acute kidney injury, rising serum lactic acid, and high peak airway pressures on the ventilator, among other acute changes, all should prompt the clinician to consider this life-threatening pathology, check bladder pressures, and consult a surgeon. Circumferential burns of the extremities should also prompt the clinician to monitor for compartment syndrome of the extremities, particularly as ongoing fluid resuscitation continues. Pain out of proportion (in awake patients) with the injury or severe pain with passive motion, palpable tenseness in skin overlying the extremity, pallor, and decreased pulses should all prompt the clinician, in consultation with a surgeon, to evaluate compartment pressures. For deep partial thickness and full-thickness circumferential burns, the treatment is often escharotomy of the affected circumferential burned limb to release the compartment pressure that results from the dermis becoming stiff and less elastic, forming an "eschar." Emergent escharotomy of the neck or chest may be warranted in patients with circumferential burns of

those areas, as restriction from the eschar can cause airway and respiratory compromise.

CARBON MONOXIDE

All patients with moderate to severe burns should have carboxyhemoglobin (COHb) levels measured as standard pulse oximetry is not reliable to detect elevated COHb levels. Carbon monoxide rapidly binds to hemoglobin with significantly greater affinity than oxygen. This binding significantly diminishes oxygen unloading from hemoglobin to the peripheral tissues and can result in tissue hypoxia. Patients with elevated levels of carbon monoxide should be maintained on 100% oxygen either via artificial airway (if indicated) or non-rebreather mask if not intubated until COHb until levels normalize. Oxygen at 100% significantly decreases the half-life of COHb when compared to room air, with studies showing a half-life of COHb of approximately 75 minutes at atmospheric pressure while patients were being treated with 100% oxygen (8). Very high levels of carbon monoxide (>25%) should prompt consideration (in consultation with a medical toxicologist and burn team) for hyperbaric oxygen treatment, which further rapidly decreases the half-life of COHb and decreases the overall time patients experience tissue hypoxia from carbon monoxide. Similarly, patients with signs of end-organ ischemia, encephalopathy, or signs of EKG changes/elevated troponin in the setting of elevated COHb levels should also prompt evaluation for hyperbaric oxygen therapy if available.

CYANIDE

Cyanide toxicity should be considered in any burn patient with an elevated lactic acid level, altered mental status, and/or altered hemodynamics. Low levels of end-tidal CO_2 measured via capnography post-intubation can also be indicative of cyanide toxicity. Cyanide compounds are used in the production of plastics, acrylics, and rubber compounds, as well as in metal processing and fumigation. Cyanide binds cytochrome oxidase C in mitochondria blocking aerobic cellular respiration, ultimately causing tissue hypoxia. It has a half-life of approximately 1 to 3 hours. Treatment of choice is hydroxocobalamin 5 g IV, which classically discolors the urine of patients to whom it was administered. Hydroxocobalamin binds cyanide forming cyanocobalamin, which is renally excreted. Empiric therapy should be administered to all patients in whom cyanide toxicity is suspected, particularly as laboratory measurement of cyanide levels are not widely available, the side effect profile of hydroxocobalamin is relatively mild, and, when left untreated, cyanide toxicity has significant accompanying morbidity and is potentially fatal (9).

NUTRITION

Severe burns cause a hypermetabolic and catabolic state. Obviously, intubated/vented patients are unable to swallow, necessitating enteral access and nutrition. For severely burned patients who are not intubated, often the daily caloric requirements from their hypermetabolic state exceed what they are able to eat, thus necessitating placement of enteral access and supplemental nutrition. Given their large, complex wounds, optimizing nutritional support in burned patients is important to optimizing conditions for wound healing. Guidelines from the Society of Critical Care Medicine and the American Society for Parenteral and Enteral Nutrition advocate for enteral nutrition initiation within 48 hours of hospital admission for all critically ill patients (10). A meta-analysis of early (less than 24 hours after presentation) versus late (greater than 24 hours after presentation) enteral nutrition in burn patients demonstrated no difference in length of stay or mortality (11). It is our institution's practice to establish enteral access and begin supplemental nutrition in hemodynamically stable burn patients within 24 to 48 hours after admission. Patients should be carefully evaluated for feeding intolerance, with concern for intra-abdominal complications associated with burns such as a necrotizing enterocolitis, development of abdominal compartment syndrome, and stress ulcer formation. Major burns are a known risk factor for the development of gastric stress ("Curling's") ulcers (12), and severely burned patients in the ICU should receive stress ulcer prophylaxis (13). Enteral nutrition is the preferred route for patients who do not have contraindications to enteral feeds and who can tolerate enteral feeds—burn patients receiving parenteral nutrition have been shown in studies to have overall increased rates of complications compared to those receiving only enteral feeds (14).

MORBIDITY AND MORTALITY

Severe burn injuries have significant accompanying morbidity and mortality. Mortality from burns has steadily improved over the past 50 years due to advances in critical care. Multiple prediction models have been developed to estimate mortality after burn injury; however, the widespread use of these models has been limited due to concerns regarding their accuracy in prediction of mortality as well as regional discrepancies in care. A meta-analysis from *Burns* in 2013 evaluated 45 studies that developed or assessed mortality models after burn injury (15). That meta-analysis showed only 8 of the published studies adhered to methodological standards for the construction of prediction models. Among those 8 studies, the Modified Baux score was noted to be the best predictor of survival in elderly (>60 years of age) burn patients. In a 1998 retrospective review of 1665 patients admitted to a tertiary care hospital, 3 independent risk factors for death were identified: age >60 years, partial and full-thickness burns>40% TBSA, and the presence of inhalation injury (16). The decision to continue critical and heroic medical care for severely burned patients should be a mutual discussion with the patient (if able), the patient's surrogate decision-makers, and the multidisciplinary burn care team to ascertain the patient's wishes. Particularly, concern should be paid to the prolonged hospital course that severely burned patients experience, the potential need for multiple operative interventions, accompanying disability, and quality of life after injury. In a 2001 review of 363 burn patients in the United States who were employed

prior to their injury, 66% and 90% of survivors had returned to work at 6 and 24 months post-burn; however, only 37% had returned to the same employer as prior to their burn at 24 months post-injury (17). Interestingly, a study from China in 2011 evaluated long-term health-related quality of life in 20 patients surviving more than 2 years with burns >70% TBSA. These patients were noted to have insignificant differences from chronic hemodialysis patients in the domains of mental health, physical function, bodily pain, and role limitations due to physical functions as assessed per a self-administered Short Form-36 Medical Outcomes Survey (18). That aside, the mental health consequences and changes to quality to life that occur for patients because of severe burns cannot be understated.

CONCLUSIONS

- Severely burned patients are among the most acutely ill patients among the general critical care population.

- Careful immediate concern should be paid to the airway of each severely burned patient, assessing for signs of inhalation injury, with a low threshold to intubate early prior to the development of life-threatening upper airway edema.

- Patients should be immediately stabilized and transferred to a burn center if they have severe or complicated burns, as noted in Box 18.1.

- Burn shock resuscitation in the first 24 hours following burn injury requires continuous critical care involvement and constant assessment of fluid status and volume administration.

- The Parkland Formula is the most widely used formula for fluid resuscitation of burned patients in the first 24 hours after injury.

- Large-volume fluid resuscitation is accompanied by multiple potential complications, and over-resuscitation has accompanying morbidity.

- Patients should be evaluated and treated for concomitant carbon monoxide and cyanide toxicity if present.

- As for all critically ill patients, critical care of the burn patient focuses on preservation of vital organ function. However, burn patients are unique in that they have complex wounds that must be managed by a surgeon and wound care team with burn expertise. The critical care of these patients should focus on optimizing the healing conditions of these life-threatening wounds.

REFERENCES

1. Monafo WW. Initial management of burns. N Engl J Med. 1996; 335(21):1581–1586.
2. Gronert GA. Succinylcholine hyperkalemia after burns. *Anesthesiology*. 1999;91(1):320–322.

3. Hettiaratchy S, Papini R. Initial management of a major burn: II—assessment and resuscitation. *BMJ*. 2004;*329*(7457):101–103.
4. Lundy JB, Chung KK, Pamplin JC, Ainsworth CR, Jeng JC, Friedman BC. Update on severe burn management for the intensivist. J Intensive Care Med. 2016;*31*(8):499–510.
5. Lira A, Pinsky MR. Choices in fluid type and volume during resuscitation: impact on patient outcomes. Ann Intensive Care. 2014;*4*:38.
6. Eljaiek R, Heylbroeck C, Dubois MJ. Albumin administration for fluid resuscitation in burn patients: A systematic review and meta-analysis. *Burns*. 2017;*43*(1):17–24.
7. Kirkpatrick AW, Ball CG, Nickerson D, D'amours SK. Intraabdominal hypertension and the abdominal compartment syndrome in burn patients. World J Surg. 2009;*33*(6):1142–1149.
8. Weaver LK, Howe S, Hopkins R, Chan KJ. Carboxyhemoglobin half-life in carbon monoxide-poisoned patients treated with 100% oxygen at atmospheric pressure. *Chest*. 2000;*117*(3):801–808.
9. Maclennan L, Moiemen N. Management of cyanide toxicity in patients with burns. *Burns*. 2015;*41*(1):18–24. https://www.ncbi.nlm.nih.gov/pubmed?term=19373044.
10. Wasiak J, Cleland H, Jeffery R. Early versus delayed enteral nutrition support for burn injuries. *Cochrane Database Syst Rev*. 2006;(3):CD005489.
11. Choi YH, Lee JH, Shin JJ, Cho YS. A revised risk analysis of stress ulcers in burn patients receiving ulcer prophylaxis. Clin Exp Emerg Med. 2015;*2*(4):250–255.
12. EAST Practice Management Guidelines Committee. *Practice Management Guidelines for Stress Ulcer Prophylaxis*. Eastern Association for the Surgery of Trauma. 2008. https://www.east.org/education/practice-management-guidelines/stress-ulcer-prophylaxis
13. O. Basaran, M.H.F., S. Uysal, E. Kesik, A. Kut. Comparison of frequency of complications in burn patients receiving enteral versus parenteral nutrition. *Burns*. 2007;*33*(1):S44.
14. Hussain A, Choukairi F, Dunn K. Predicting survival in thermal injury: a systematic review of methodology of composite prediction models. *Burns*. 2013;*39*(5):835–50.
15. Ryan CM, Schoenfeld DA, Thorpe WP, Sheridan RL, Cassem EH, Tompkins RG. Objective estimates of the probability of death from burn injuries. N Engl J Med. 1998;*338*(6):362–366.
16. Brych SB, Engrav LH, Rivara FP, et al. Time off work and return to work rates after burns: systematic review of the literature and a large two-center series. J Burn Care Rehabil. 2001;*22*(6):401–405.
17. Xie B, Xiao SC, Zhu SH, Xia ZF. Evaluation of long term health-related quality of life in extensive burns: a 12-year experience in a burn center. *Burns*. 2012;*38*(3):348–355.

REVIEW QUESTIONS

1. Which of the following burn patients should be immediately stabilized and transported to an ABA Verified Burn Center?

   A. A 24-year-old man with 4% TBSA second-degree burns to his left chest
   B. A 50-year-old man with 25% TBSA second- and third-degree burns to the face, neck, and chest
   C. A 45-year-old woman who has extensive electrical burns to her right hand
   D. B and C

Answer: D. Both answers B and C meet recommended criteria for transfer to an ABA Verified Burn Center.

2. Which is considered to be the most accurate method for estimating TBSA of burns in burned patients?

   A. Rule of 9s
   B. Palmar Method
   C. Lund and Browder Chart
   D. Capnography

Answer: C—The Lund and Browder Chart is thought to be the most accurate method for estimating TBSA of burns. The Rule of 9s and the Palmar Method can also be used but are not thought to be as accurate.

3. For the initial fluid resuscitation for patients with burn shock, which formula to estimate fluid requirements in the first 24 hours after injury is the most widely used in the United States?

   A. Monafo Formula
   B. Parkland Formula
   C. Brooke Formula
   D. Evans Formula

Answer: B. The Parkland Formula is the most widely used formula in the United States to estimate 24-hour fluid requirements in acute burns.

4. The Parkland Formula recommends _____ mL of crystalloid/kg/%TBSA burn to be administered in the first 24 hours after injury.

   A. 1
   B. 2
   C. 4
   D. 8

Answer: C. The Parkland Formula recommends 4 mL of crystalloid × weight (in kg) × %TBSA burned. Only second- and third-degree burns are included in the calculation.

5. Per the Parkland Formula, an 80 kg man with 50% TBSA second- and third-degree burns from a house fire can be estimated to require how much crystalloid resuscitation in the first 24 hours after injury?

   A. 5 liters
   B. 10 liters
   C. 13 liters
   D. 16 liters

Answer: D. 80 × 50 × 4 mL = 16,000 mL or 16 L of crystalloid volume in the first 24 hours after injury.

6. A 60-year-old 75-kg man is 18 hours into resuscitation from a 75% TBSA second-degree burn from a house fire. He has no circumferential burns. He is intubated and sedated. The respiratory therapist notes elevated peak and plateau airway pressures on the ventilator. A previous bronchoscopy revealed no inhalation injury, and a repeat chest X-ray is unchanged from his previous film a few hours ago showing generally clear lungs and a mid-tracheal ETT. On exam, the patient's abdomen is tense and distended. His serum lactate initially decreased with resuscitation but over the last 4 hours has risen to 2.5 and his urine output was most recently decreased from adequate to 0.1 mL/kg for the last 2 hours despite IV lactated Ringer's solution running at 1 L per hour. The most recent mean arterial pressure per arterial line is 65 mmHg. What should be your next steps?

A. Perform another bronchoscopy to reassess for inhalation injury.
B. Measure bladder pressures, and, if elevated, consult a surgeon to evaluate for abdominal compartment syndrome.
C. Start broad-spectrum antibiotics for community acquired pneumonia.
D. Consult pulmonology.

Answer: B. This patient has clinical signs that could be indicative of abdominal compartment syndrome. The clinician should check bladder pressures, and, if elevated, consult a surgeon.

7. A 24-year-old female is rescued from a house fire where she is severely burned with 55% TBSA partial and full-thickness burns and suspicion for inhalation injury. She is intubated on arrival to the emergency department for respiratory distress. Her measured COHb level on arrival is 18%. She follows simple commands and her EKG reveals sinus tachycardia. Her serum lactate on presentation is normal. She is sedated with a propofol infusion. What should be your next steps?

A. Wean to ventilator to pressure support, FiO_2 of 0.4 and positive-end expiratory pressure of 5.
B. Maintain an FiO_2 of 0.1 until carboxyhemoglobin levels normalize.
C. Administer sodium thiosulfate IV.
D. Administer hydroxocobalamin IV.

Answer: B. This patient has carbon monoxide toxicity that does not require consideration for hyperbaric therapy. She should be maintained on 100% oxygen until COHb levels normalize.

8. A 64-year-old man has sustained 25% TBSA partial and full-thickness burns from a brush fire. He has circumferential third-degree burns to his left lower extremity. He is on 2 L nasal cannula and had ongoing fluid resuscitation for the last 18 hours. Over the last 2 hours, he notes increasing pain in his left leg with severe pain with passive range of motion that was not present earlier that shift. The leg is tense. DP and PT pulses are palpable but are slightly diminished from prior per the nursing staff. What should be your next step?

A. Administer a dose of fentanyl and tell the patient his pain is from his burns.
B. Administer broad-spectrum antibiotics.
C. Consult with the in-house burn surgeon to measure compartment pressures of the leg and consider escharotomy for compartment syndrome.
D. ACE wrap the leg.

Answer: C. This patient may be developing compartment syndrome of the leg as a result of circumferential burns. Compartment pressures should be measured, and the patient may need escharotomy if they are elevated.

9. Which of the following are indications for early intubation in a patient with burns on arrival to the emergency department?

A. Facial burns with singed nasal hairs, hoarse voice, and pharyngeal erythema
B. Agitation
C. A home oxygen requirement of 4 L by nasal cannula currently at baseline
D. A new oxygen requirement of 2 L in a patient with 10% TBSA lower extremity burns

Answer: A. This patient has the potential to have inhalation injury and could subsequently develop life-threatening airway edema. This patient should be electively intubated.

10. Large-volume normal saline administration is associated with

A. hyperkalemia.
B. hypercalcemia.
C. hyperchloremia.
D. hyperphosphatemia.

Answer: C. Large-volume normal saline administration can cause hyperchloremia, which can contribute to a hyperchloremic metabolic acidosis.

19.

ABDOMINAL PAIN FOLLOWING A MOTOR VEHICLE CRASH

Eric Leiendecker, Jonathan Ketzler, and Douglas Coursin

STEM CASE AND KEY QUESTIONS

A 46-year-old man with an unknown medical history presents to the emergency department following a motor vehicle collision at highway speeds. No loss of consciousness was noted, but the patient arrives with a hard cervical collar in place with spinal precautions being followed on transfer. He has bilateral 16 g intravenous lines in the antecubital fossae, has received 2 liters of lactated ringers, and is complaining of dyspnea and severe abdominal pain. Vital signs are: 88/46 mmHg, 112 bpm, 24 respirations/min, 96% SpO$_2$ on 10 lpm via non-rebreather mask. He is alert and oriented but diaphoretic with cool skin.

IS THIS PATIENT IN SHOCK? WHAT DEFINES SHOCK, AND WHAT LABORATORY TESTS MIGHT BE USEFUL IN BOTH GUIDING THIS PATIENT'S THERAPY AND PREDICTING OUTCOMES?

Along with baseline laboratory values including a type and screen for blood products, complete blood count, complete metabolic profile, and coagulation studies (aPTT, PT/INR), the team performs a point of care arterial blood gas analysis and confirms a pH of 7.29 and a lactate of 4.2 mmol/L. The patient's hemoglobin results as 6.2 g/dL, and an order for multiple packed red blood cells (pRBCs), fresh frozen plasma (FFP), and platelets is placed as well.

WHAT DOES THE EVALUATION OF THE TRAUMA PATIENT ENTAIL?

The team starts going through the primary survey. The patient is awake and alert, his Glasgow Coma Score is 15, and he remains in his hard collar but is able to move all his extremities without any significant pain on palpation of his head, neck, or limbs. While he is breathing relatively rapidly, his breath sounds are clear bilaterally and his oxygen saturation is 100% albeit on a simple facemask. There appears to be no tenderness along his chest wall, but he both winces and calls out when both the upper quadrants of his abdomen are examined. A large contusion, almost like a stripe, is seen along his lower abdomen as well, although there is no pain elicited on rocking his pelvis but there is blood noted at his urethral meatus.

An abdominal computed tomography (CT) is ordered, but the team performs a focused assessment with sonography in trauma (FAST) exam at bedside.

WHAT MIGHT A FAST EXAM REVEAL IN THIS PATIENT?

Thoracic ultrasound (U/S) reveals lung sliding appropriately on both sides, and posteriorly there does not appear to be any significant pleural fluid collections. However, abdominal U/S demonstrates fluid in the haptorenal and splenorenal spaces. Based on the U/S findings in the setting of his severe anemia and shock picture, the decision is made to rush him to the operating room for exploratory laparotomy.

WHAT ARE THE MAJOR INJURY PATTERNS OF TRAUMA?

An arterial monitoring line is placed prior to beginning, and both induction of anesthesia and intubation are successful with some mild hemodynamic perturbations that are treated with low-dose vasopressors and transfusion of 2 pRBCs and 2 FFP. On first assessment, his liver has a small subcapsular hematoma and 1 cm laceration, both overall not very impressive, and 4 quadrants of the liver are packed to apply compression to the area. Further examination of the spleen reveals a very large subcapsular hematoma and a near complete transection. The decision is made to perform a splenectomy. Once controlled, a further surgical examination reveals no other significant sites of bleeding, and the grade 1 liver laceration is repaired directly and without incident. Now stabilized and with a decreasing arterial lactate on point of care assessment, the patient is closed, extubated, and transported to the intensive care unit (ICU) for postoperative care and monitoring.

DISCUSSION

THE DEFINITION OF SHOCK

Unfortunately, there is no discrete vital sign parameter that delineates or defines shock. Rather, it is a pathophysiologic state that develops when oxygen delivery to the tissues is outstripped by the oxygen demand. Unlike medical patients, where the shock state may be undifferentiated, the trauma patient should be assumed to be in hypovolemic shock until proven otherwise. Be aware however, some patient populations may not present with the stereotypical vital sign changes one would expect for a certain degree of hypovolemia. For example, young patients may maintain a relative normotensive state due to high vascular tone, or, conversely, patients on higher doses of beta blockers may not manifest the tachycardia one would expect.

An alteration in mental state in the absence of a head injury, a rising lactate or worsening base deficit, significant and sustained drop in urine output, as well as paradoxical bradycardia are all good predictors of shock in the trauma patient. While a decrease from baseline blood pressure of more than 30% is associated with worse outcomes in the emergency department, more predictive of worsening shock is a narrowing of the pulse pressure as a predictor of hypoperfusion.[17] It is important to always consider hemorrhagic shock as the cause for a trauma patient's hypoperfusion as it is the most common etiology; other states must be ruled out during the primary survey to ensure the appropriate treatment is initiated.

ABCS/PRIMARY SURVEY

The emphasis of the initial cursory examination is to rule out immediate threats to life. The patient should be confirmed to have an intact and unobstructed airway; if this is found to not be true then immediate action should be taken to secure the airway. This may require clearance of debris from the airway to ensure immediate patency. The necessity of maintaining cervical spine precautions while assessing and managing a compromised airway can complicate what would otherwise not be a challenging airway scenario.

Once the airway is confirmed to be patent/secured, ventilation may remain impaired due to the presence of air or blood in the thoracic cavity. An absence of breath sounds, or chest radiograph or ultrasound findings suggestive of pneumothorax or hemothorax, should prompt tube thoracostomy placement to evacuate the pleural space and restore adequate ventilation. Blunt trauma to the chest may result in pulmonary contusions that impair gas exchange. Supportive care with lung protective ventilatory strategies should be employed in these situations to limit the development of ventilator-induced acute lung injury.

Hemodynamic instability is generally thought to be due to hemorrhage until proven otherwise. As such, external evidence of hemorrhage should be detected and addressed expeditiously. There are generally thought to be 5 major areas of blood loss: external, chest, abdomen and pelvis,

retroperitoneum, and due to long bone fractures. The FAST exam detailed in the following discussion can aid in identifying sources of hemorrhage.

Neurologic exam should be performed with special attention to identify signs of brain or neuraxial spine injury. This exam may consist of discerning the Glasgow Coma Scale (GCS), a brief cranial nerve exam, and a brief motor/sensory exam of the periphery, which may show evidence of spinal cord injury.

Physical Exam

Blunt abdominal trauma can have a wide range of presentations from mild abdominal pain in the hemodynamically stable patient to those patients dying and obtunded from hypovolemic shock. Importantly, one should be cognizant of the fact that the absence of abdominal pain or tenderness does not exclude the presence of intra-abdominal injury. While the negative predictive value of the absence of pain or tenderness is low, the presence of peritoneal signs, pain, or tenderness are the most reliable physical indicators of intra-abdominal injury. There will occur instances where non-abdominal injuries cause distracting pain, masking the presence of abdominal injuries.[1] Thus, patients with distracting injuries should be viewed as having intra-abdominal injuries until proven otherwise. The 3 findings most predictive of an abdominal injury following blunt trauma are the seat belt sign, which carries a likelihood ratio approaching 10; rebound tenderness with a likelihood ratio of 6.5; and hypotension, carrying a likelihood ratio of over 5.[2] Given the high predictive value of these signs, they (especially in combination with one another) should prompt expeditious investigation.

SECONDARY SURVEY

The secondary survey is focused on the detailed exam aimed to find injuries that may not be an immediate threat to life. This is also the point in the exam where ancillary testing (CT scan, radiographs) may be performed. Here, it is also important to acquire the rest of the patient's relevant medical and surgical history.

Ancillary Testing

There is no substitute for clinical assessment, though laboratory testing can add supplemental information. For instance, a hemoglobin or hematocrit drawn following trauma may be falsely elevated as the patient is losing whole blood, and a normal value should offer no consolation. However, a hematocrit under 30 increases the likelihood of abdominal injury. Liver enzymes may be elevated due to pre-existing disease or as the result of direct trauma or from hypotension and are thus relatively nonspecific. Likewise, pancreatic enzymes may be elevated for a variety of reasons and can be nonspecific; conversely, normal values offer little solace as they do not rule out pancreatic injury. The expectation would be to find a leukocytosis due to demargination as result of stress response, so this lab test is of little use. Essentially, though labs are drawn routinely on presentation, they generally offer little insight into the presence or character of intra-abdominal injuries.

FAST Exam

The FAST exam is a focused U/S exam done to answer the dichotomous question: "Does this patient have an intra-abdominal or thoracic injury causing the apparent hemodynamic instability?" This easy and noninvasive procedure involves image acquisition at the perihepatic and hepatorenal space, splenic space, pelvis, and subxiphoid view of the heart and pericardium. This noninvasive and rapidly performed exam is a reliable tool for identifying the presence of an abdominal injury.

THE PATTERNS OF TRAUMA

Splenic

Incidence. Splenic injury remains the most frequent solid organ injury sustained following blunt abdominal trauma. Estimates of the incidence vary widely though it is thought to be 30% to 50%.[3] The intensivist should have a high index of suspicion based on history and mechanism of injury as splenic injuries carry a mortality rate as high as 18% depending on grade.[3]

Findings. FAST exam can show a dark hypoechoic rim around the spleen representing free fluid (blood) in the hepatorenal space or intraperitoneal perisplenic fluid. Additionally, this may represent subcapsular fluid from hematoma. Figure 19.1 shows the normal FAST exam findings as well as a positive exam with hypoechoic fluid in the splenorenal space. As mentioned previously, these findings in the hemodynamically unstable patient should prompt emergent intervention.

Management. Management of splenic injuries largely is dependent on the grade (Table 19.1) and hemodynamic status of the patient. Hemodynamic instability in this instance is defined as systolic blood pressure less than 90 mmHg, heart rate over 120 bpm with altered mental status, dyspnea, and/or evidence of vasoconstriction (cool, clammy skin).[4] Hemodynamically stable patients should be managed nonoperatively regardless of grade of injury, with angiography/embolization being

considered for management. This is especially beneficial in those "rapid responders" or those who though initially hypotensive respond well and are rapidly stabilized following resuscitation. Operative management is reserved for 2 specific populations. First, the hemodynamically unstable patient who is not a rapid responder and those with evidence of peritonitis or other bowel injury should be managed operatively.[5] Second, operative management is indicated in those managed initially nonoperatively who continue to bleed and become unstable (i.e., failing nonoperative management).

The asplenic patient is at especially high risk of sepsis from encapsulated organisms, specifically, *S. pneumoniae,* which is by the far the most common causative organism, followed by *H. influenzae* and *N. meningitidis*. While the incidence of post-splenectomy sepsis is relatively low at <0.5%, sepsis from these organisms carries a substantial risk of mortality (30% to 70%).[4] As such, asplenic patients should be vaccinated against these organisms prior to hospital discharge.

Hepatic

Incidence. The liver is a vascular abdominal organ that is frequently injured following blunt trauma, most commonly motor vehicle crashes. Mortality is rare with low-grade (I and II) injuries though, in the event of needing surgical management (or failing nonoperative management), mortality can be as high as 60%.[6]

Findings. Both U/S and CT are useful in diagnosing hepatic injury. U/S is sensitive for showing blood in the hepatorenal space consistent with liver injury, while CT is optimal for better characterizing the extent and character of the injury.[7] Figure 19.2 shows the FAST exam images for both a negative and normal exam of the hepatorenal space.

Grading. The American Association for the Surgery of Trauma has devised a grading system, similar to that for splenic injuries, based on anatomical findings of the injury. Roughly two-thirds of hepatic injuries are found to be lower grade (I to III) injuries with low mortality; however, one-third remain high grade with significant mortality. Table 19.2 displays injury grades with their associated findings.

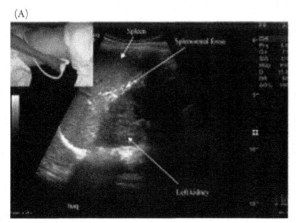
(A)

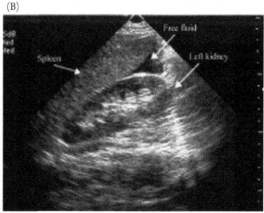
(B)

Figure 19.1 FAST exam findings of the splenorenal space.
Grading: The American Association for the Surgery of Trauma has published a scoring system that uses anatomic appearances of the injured spleen to grade and prognosticate. These can be seen in Table 20.1

Table 19.1. GRADING OF SPLENIC INJURIES

GRADE	INJURY TYPE	DESCRIPTION
I	Hematoma	Subcapsular <10%
	Laceration	Tear <1 cm deep
II	Hematoma	Subcapsular 10%–50% of surface area, or parenchymal <5cm
	Laceration	Tear 1–3 cm deep not involving trabecular vessels
III	Hematoma	Subcapsular >50% surface area, or expanding, or rupture of hematoma
	Laceration	>3 cm deep, or involvement of trabecular vessels
IV	Laceration	Involvement of segmental or hilar vessels resulting devascularization (>25%)
V	Laceration	Shattered spleen
	Vascular	Hilar injury resulting in complete devascularization

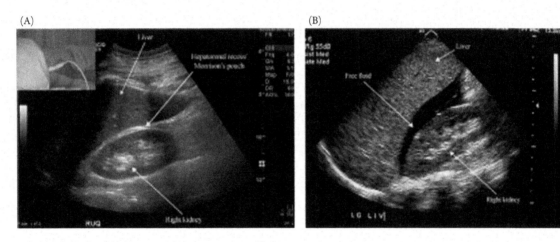

(A)   (B)

Figure 19.2 FAST exam findings of the hepatorenal space.

Table 19.2 GRADING OF HEPATIC INJURIES

GRADE	INJURY	DESCRIPTION
I	Hematoma	Subcapsular: <10% of surface area
	Laceration	Capsular Tear: <1 cm deep
II	Hematoma	Subcapsular: 10%–50% of surface area or intra-parenchymal <10 cm diameter
	Laceration	Capsular tear 1–3 cm deep and <10 cm long
III	Hematoma	Subcapsular >50% of surface area, or intra-parenchymal lesion >10 cm and expanding. Or, any hematoma that ruptures through the liver capsule.
	Laceration	Laceration >3 cm deep
IV	Laceration	Parenchymal disruption affecting 25%–75% of hepatic lobe, or 1–3 segments
V	Laceration	Parenchymal disruption of >75% of hepatic lobe or involvement of >3 segments
	Vascular	Juxtahepatic vascular injury
VI	Avulsion	Hepatic avulsion

Management. Management of traumatic liver injuries mimics that of splenic injuries in the emphasis on nonoperative management for those patients who remain hemodynamically stable.[8] The vast majority of hepatic injuries may be cared for noninvasively with resuscitation and monitoring. Hepatic embolization may be used to increase the odds of successful nonoperative management in those patients who are stable though show contrast extravasation on CT imaging.[9] In specialized trauma centers capable of salvage surgery, this modality may be expanded to those patients with borderline hemodynamic status and contrast extravasation. While embolization is an effective therapy, there is the possibility for treatment failure leading to operative management; generally, higher grade injuries are thought to be at higher risk.

Reserved largely for hemodynamically unstable patients with higher grade hepatic injury, operative management should focus on damage control through obtaining surgical hemostasis. The abdomen may be left open or temporarily closed with planned reexploration performed within 48 hours.[6]

Bladder

Incidence. Bladder injury occurs at a low rate compared to that of splenic or hepatic; however, it must be ruled out following blunt abdominal trauma. While the bladder is well protected by the bony pelvis, the dome of the bladder is simply covered by the peritoneum and may rise into the peritoneal cavity when filled with urine. It should come as no surprise that bladder injuries are often associated with pubic ramus and obturator ring fractures.

Findings. Mechanism of injury and associated pelvic fracture should prompt evaluation for bladder injury. Blood at the urethral meatus should raise the concern for bladder/urethral injury prompting further investigation. Pelvic fracture and hematuria are each highly associated with bladder injury and when found together are viewed as an absolute indication for imaging. Note, however, that this statement holds true only in reference to gross hematuria. Often, trauma patients will have a CT scan of the abdomen, which may show bladder injury or rupture. However, a dedicated CT cystogram should be performed to confirm the presence of an injury.[10,11] One component of the FAST exam is investigating for free fluid in the pelvis, which may or may not be related to bladder injury. These findings are displayed in Figure 19.3.

Grading. As with solid organ injury, the American Association for the Surgery of Trauma has published a grading scale for bladder injuries. Also similar to hepatic or splenic injury, bladder injuries are graded based on anatomic findings. Table 19.3 displays this grading system.

Management. The management of bladder injuries is dependent on the anatomic classification. Extraperitoneal injuries are further divided into simple and complex injuries. Largely, simple extraperitoneal injuries self-heal with simple bladder drainage. Complex extraperitoneal injuries are characterized by associated injury to the rectum or vagina, the presence of an open pelvic fracture, persistent hematuria, or an injury to the bladder neck. Patients with such complex bladder

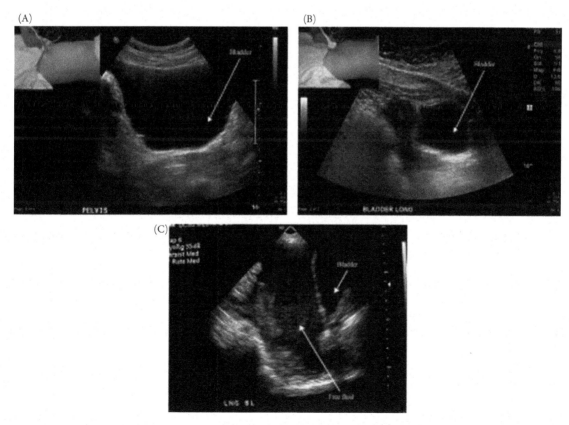

Figure 19.3 FAST exam of the bladder and pelvis.

Table 19.3. GRADING OF BLADDER INJURIES

GRADE	INJURY TYPE	DESCRIPTION
I	Hematoma Laceration	Contusion, intramural hematoma Partial thickness
II	Laceration	Extraperitoneal bladder wall laceration <2 cm
III	Laceration	Extraperitoneal >2cm or intraperitoneal <2 cm
IV	Laceration	Intraperitoneal >2 cm
V	Laceration	Any laceration extending into the bladder neck or ureteral orifice

Table 19.4. GRADING OF DIAPHRAGMATIC INJURIES

GRADE	FINDINGS
I	Contusion
II	Laceration <2 cm
III	Laceration 2–10 cm
IV	Laceration >10 cm, tissue loss <25 cm^2
V	Tissue loss >25 cm^2

injuries require urgent surgical management and should not be expected to heal with simple drainage. Additionally, those with additional rectal or vaginal injuries are at elevated risk for fistula formation.[12]

Surgically, bladder injuries (both extra- and intraperitoneal) are repaired in a 2-layer fashion. This is followed by catheter drainage for multiple weeks. Often, the bladder is full at the time of blunt injury, which can lead to a large intraperitoneal defect. In addition to necessitating surgical correction, the spillage of urine into the peritoneal cavity can predispose the patient to intra-abdominal sepsis/peritonitis.[12]

Diaphragm

Incidence. The diaphragm is a musculotendinous barrier between the negative pressure thorax and positive pressure abdominal cavity and is a major driver of ventilation. While the diaphragm is less often injured compared to the liver or spleen, diaphragmatic injuries are found in up to 7% of cases following blunt trauma and between 10% to 15% of cases following penetrating trauma Physicians must be aware of and rule out these injuries on presentation. Classically, the left diaphragm is injured more often, with the right being injured roughly half as often as the left.[13]

Findings. Because of the wide excursion of the diaphragm with ventilation, virtually any penetrating injury from the mid-thorax to the upper abdomen should raise concern for diaphragmatic injury. While these penetrating injuries make up the bulk of diaphragmatic injuries, blunt trauma can lead to a massive increase in pressure gradient across the diaphragm, resulting in rupture. Because of the force required to result in rupture, it is rare to find an isolated diaphragmatic injury.

Of note, diaphragmatic injuries may be relatively occult and in extreme cases are missed on initial laparotomy. In these patients, the positive intraperitoneal pressure will cause herniation of the abdominal organs into the thoracic cavity over time. Thus patients with recent thoracic trauma with new-onset abdominal pain or nausea/vomiting should be examined for diaphragmatic injury.[14]

Commonly, diaphragmatic injuries can be diagnosed with plain films, which may show herniation of the stomach or bowel into the thoracic cavity. CT imaging, generally performed as part of a trauma evaluation, can show a plethora of findings suggestive or confirmatory of a diaphragmatic injury. Most striking of course will be the presence of abdominal organs in the thorax. This modality can also elucidate the precise character and location of the injured diaphragm.[15]

Grading. The American Association for the Surgery of Trauma has released a grading scale analogous to that of solid organs. As with those, morbidity and mortality increases with the increasing grade of injury. Table 19.4 shows this grading scheme.

Management. Unlike solid organ injury, diaphragmatic injuries have no viable endovascular treatment options. These injuries must be addressed through a surgical approach. Generally, this will entail a laparotomy, though in select cases laparoscopy or thoracoscopy may be sufficient.[13]

Kidney

Incidence. The kidney is a relatively well-protected organ that lies in the retroperitoneum, guarded by the rib cage and musculature of the back with additional protection afforded by fat surrounding the organ itself. This protection requires a large force to cause renal damage. Renal injuries may be caused by fractured lower ribs, which can cause direct trauma to the kidney. Additionally, deceleration injury may lead to avulsion of the renal pedicle or dissection of the renal vasculature.

Findings. Signs and symptoms of renal injury are largely nonspecific and may consist of such findings as flank pain or tenderness, bruising, rib fractures, or gross hematuria. CT imaging is the modality providing the most robust information and allows for grading of the injury.[16]

Grading. Once again, the American Association for Surgery of Trauma has published guidelines for the grading of traumatic kidney injuries. This is displayed in Table 19.5.

Management. The management of renal trauma falls in line with the management of other abdominal solid organ trauma in that there is dichotomy between stable and unstable patients. As expected, hemodynamically stable patients can and should be managed nonsurgically. Depending on the injury, this may mean expectant management or embolization. Controversy surrounds the management of higher-grade (IV or V) injuries but is beyond the scope of this discussion. Those patients that are hemodynamically unstable will require emergent surgical intervention.[12,16]

Table 19.5. GRADING OF TRAUMATIC RENAL INJURY

GRADE	TYPE	DESCRIPTION
I	Contusion	Hematuria (gross or microscopic), normal urologic studies
	Hematoma	Subcapsular, nonexpanding hematoma
II	Hematoma	Nonexpanding hematoma confined to the retroperitoneum
	Laceration	<1 cm deep in the renal cortex with no urinary extravasation
III	Laceration	>1 cm deep in the renal cortex without urinary extravasation or rupture of the collecting system
IV	Laceration	Laceration of the parenchyma extending through the cortex, medulla, and collecting system
	Vascular	Main renal vein or artery injury with contained hemorrhage
V	Laceration	Shattered kidney
	Vascular	Devascularization or avulsion

CONCLUSIONS

The patient with abdominal pain following a motor vehicle crash poses both diagnostic and treatment challenges. The immediate focus, as with any trauma patient, will be addressing threats to life through ensuring adequate ventilation and circulation. The subsequent physical exam should be paired with a FAST exam in order to identify those patients in need of emergent surgical intervention. Generally, hemodynamically stable patients with lower grade injuries can be managed nonoperatively, either expectantly or with embolization. However, those patients who are unstable will require emergent operative procedures to manage their injury.

REFERENCES

1. Ferrera P, Verdile V, Bartfield J, Snyder H, Salluzzo R. Injuries distracting from intraabdominal injuries after blunt trauma. *Am J Emerg Med*. 1998;*16*:145–150.
2. Nishijima D, Simel D, Wisner D, Holmes J. Does this adult patient have a blunt intra-abdominal injury? *JAMA*. 2012; *307*(14):1517–1527.
3. El-Matbouly M, Jabbour G, El-Menyar A, et al. Blunt splenic trauma: assessment, management and outcomes. *The Surgeon*. 2016;*14*: 52–58.
4. Coccolini F, Montori G, Catena F, et al. Splenic trauma: WSES classification and guidelines for adult and pediatric patients. World J Emerg Surg. 2017;*12*:40.
5. Olthof DC, van der Viles CH, Goslings JC. Evidence-based management and controversies in blunt splenic trauma. Cur Trauma Rep. 2017;*3*:32–37.
6. Doklestic K, Stefanovic B, Gregoric P, et al. Surgical management of AAST grades III-V hepatic trauma by damage control surgery with perihepatic packing and definitive hepatic repair-single centre experience. World J Emerg Surg. 2015;*10*:34.
7. Parks RW, Chrysos E, Diamond T. Management of liver trauma. Brit J Surg. 1999;*86*:1121–1135.
8. Stassen N, Bhullar I, Cheng JD, et al. Nonoperative management of blunt hepatic injury: an Eastern Association for the Surgery of Trauma practice management guideline. J Trauma Acute Care Surg. 2012; *73*: S288–S293
9. Letoublon C, Morra I, Chen Y, Monnin V, Voirin D, Arvieux C. Hepatic arterial embolization in the management of blunt hepatic trauma: indications and complications. J Trauma. 2011;*70*:1032–1037.
10. Morey A, Iverson A, Swan A, et al. Bladder rupture after blunt trauma: guidelines for diagnostic imaging. J Trauma. 2001;*51*;683–686.
11. Morgan D, Nallamala L, Kenney P, Mayo M, Rue L. CT cystography: radiographic and clinical predictors of bladder rupture. AJR. 2000;*174*:89–95.
12. Morey A, Brandes S, Dugi D, et al. Urotrauma: AUA guideline. *J Uro*. 2014;*192*:327–335.
13. Scharff J, Naunheim K. Traumatic diaphragmatic injuries. Thorac Surg Clin. 2007;*17*:81–85
14. Feliciano D, Cruse P, Mattox K, et al. Delayed diagnosis of injuries to the diaphragm after penetrating wounds. J Trauma. 1988;*28*(8):1135–1144.
15. Panda A, Kumar A, Gamangatti S, Patil A, Kumar S, Gupta A. Traumatic diaphragmatic injury: a review of CT signs and the difference between blunt and penetrating injury. Diagn Interv Radiol. 2014;*20*:121–128.
16. Chouhan J, Winer A, Johnson C, Weiss J, Hyacinthe L. Contemporary evaluation and management of renal trauma. *Can J Urol*. 2016;*32*(2):8191–8197.
17. Lilitsis E, Xenaki S, Athanasakis E, et al. Guiding management in severe trauma: reviewing factors predicting outcome in vastly injured patients. J Emerg Traum Shock. 2018;*11*(2):80–87.

REVIEW QUESTIONS

1. What finding is most predictive of an intra-abdominal injury?

    A. Hypotension
    B. Associated long bone fracture
    C. Seatbelt sign
    D. Rebound tenderness

2. Which of the following patients should be considered for operative management of a splenic injury?

    A. An initially stable patient who underwent embolization, now with hemoglobin of 5 g/Dl, which is down from 9g/dL
    B. A patient with hemodynamic stability though with GCS of 6 and evidence of intracranial injury
    C. A patient with hemodynamic stability though with hypoxic respiratory failure necessitating endotracheal intubation

D. A patient who is hemodynamically stable with evidence of contrast extravasation

3. What is the goal of damage control surgery for hepatic injuries?

A. To provide definitive and permanent correction of injury
B. To achieve immediate surgical hemostasis with the plan to return within 48 hours
C. To increase the likelihood of successful embolization
D. To remove a damaged liver in preparation for transplant evaluation

4. Who should undergo CT cystogram?

A. Any patient with intra-abdominal injury
B. A patient with blood at the urethral meatus and known pelvic fracture
C. A hypotensive patient with a positive FAST exam
D. Any patient requiring a Foley catheter

5. Which patient should be considered for delayed presentation of diaphragmatic injury?

A. A patient with post damage control surgery for hepatic injury, now hypotensive
B. A patient with post splenic embolization, now with fever, leukocytosis, and hypotension
C. A patient with known pulmonary contusions, now with hypoxemia
D. A patient with known thoracic injury, now with abdominal pain, nausea, and vomiting

6. Which patients should undergo surgical intervention for their traumatic renal injury?

A. Hemodynamically unstable patients with positive FAST exams
B. Patients with associated pulmonary injury
C. Stable patients with blood in the retroperitoneum
D. Patients with blood at the urethral meatus

7. Which patients require prophylactic vaccination against encapsulated organisms?

A. Patients now asplenic following embolization or surgery
B. Multisystem trauma patients now leaving the ICU
C. Patients with traumatic injuries now with intra-abdominal sepsis
D. Patients with intracranial injuries

ANSWERS

1. C. As mentioned in the text, the 3 findings most predictive of an abdominal injury following blunt trauma are the seat belt sign, rebound tenderness, and hypotension.

2. A. All hemodynamically stable patients can be managed nonoperatively but hemodynamically unstable patients that are not responding to appropriate therapy or those managed non-operatively who continue to bleed or become unstable, such as this patient with a decreasing hemoglobin after embolization, should be taken to the operating room emergently.

3. B. In the setting of hemodynamic instability, damage control surgery's goal is to obtain hemostasis and allow the team to "catch up" on resuscitation. Once stabilized, the patient can be re-explored later for definitive surgery and closure.

4. B. Pelvic fractures, hematuria, and blood at the urethral meatus should raise the concern for bladder/urethral injury prompting further investigation by CT cystography.

5. D. Diaphragmatic injuries can often be small, subtle, and masked by much larger and emergent surgical needs. The patient with recent thoracic trauma that has new-onset abdominal pain or nausea/vomiting should be examined for diaphragmatic injury that has resulted in an internal hernia.

6. A. A positive FAST exam in the hemodynically unstable patient should always prompt surgical intervention.

7. A. Asplenic patients are high risk of sepsis from encapsulated organisms and therefore should be vaccinated against these organisms prior to hospital discharge.

20.

PREECLAMPSIA AND HELLP SYNDROME IN THE PARTURIENT

Erik Romanelli and Laurence Ring

STEM CASE AND KEY QUESTIONS

A 22-year-old G1P0 woman at 38 weeks gestation presents to labor and delivery triage with premature rupture of membranes. Her pregnancy has been otherwise uncomplicated, and she has received good prenatal care. On triage evaluation, her vital signs are noted to be: blood pressure 155/105, heart rate 102, and SpO$_2$ 98% on room air.

ARE THESE VITAL SIGNS NORMAL FOR A TERM PREGNANT WOMAN? WHAT FURTHER WORKUP IS INDICATED?

While the patient's heart rate and oxygen saturation are normal for a term pregnant woman, the blood pressure is hypertensive. She is admitted for further workup preeclampsia (PEC), which includes regular blood pressure checks as well as a urine dipstick for protein. On obtaining a further history, the patient indicates that she has a headache that has been unresponsive to pharmacological treatment. She denies visual changes, dyspnea, or abdominal pain. Her lab tests are within normal range with the exception of a hematocrit of 42%.

HOW IS PEC DEFINED? DOES THE PATIENT MERIT A DIAGNOSIS OF PEC? WHAT OTHER ORGAN SYSTEMS MAY BE INVOLVED?

The patient meets the criteria for PEC with severe features (new hypertension after 20 weeks and headache). As prophylaxis against progression to eclampsia, the patient is loaded and started on a magnesium infusion. The patient's hypertension is treated with labetalol to bring the systolic blood pressure to 130 to 140 mmHg. Her labs are checked with some frequency every 6 hours to monitor for impaired hepatic function, coagulation, renal function, and thrombocytopenia. Lastly, delivery is indicated in this patient and induction of labor is started. Several hours into the patient's induction, she requests neuraxial analgesia.

IS PEC, EVEN WITH SEVERE FEATURES, A CONTRAINDICATION TO NEURAXIAL ANALGESIA? ARE FURTHER LABORATORY STUDIES WARRANTED?

The patient's labs from 2 hours prior are reviewed. There are no new abnormalities. While the anesthesiologist is preparing to initiate epidural analgesia, a prolonged late deceleration is noted on the fetal heart rate monitor. After 3 minutes, with oxygen and repositioning, the fetal heart rate returns to its baseline in the 140s. Approximately 30 minutes later, again prior to placing an epidural, the fetal heart rate tracing loses its baseline variability demonstrates recurrent late decelerations.

WHAT IS THE SIGNIFICANCE OF THE FETAL HEART RATE RACING? IS THERE TIME TO PLACE AN ELECTIVE EPIDURAL IN THIS SITUATION?

This is an unresolving category III fetal heart rate tracing that indicates recurrent bradycardia. Fearing imminent fetal injury, the obstetrician decides the patient requires an urgent cesarean delivery.

IT IS SAFE TO PERFORM AN EMERGENT SPINAL ANESTHETIC ON A PATIENT WITH PEC?

The patient's coagulation studies have remained normal, and her platelet level is 150,000/mcl. She is taken emergently to the operating room (OR) where a spinal anesthetic is performed without complication. Just as the incision is made, the patient is noted to have jerking movements of the upper extremities. Her mouth is shut tight, and she seems unresponsive.

WHAT IS THE MANAGEMENT OF ECLAMPSIA?

The patient is diagnosed as having an eclamptic seizure. She is treated with high flow oxygen and 5 mg of midazolam. The anesthetic team prepares to support the patient's airway and induce general anesthesia with propofol. Her seizure breaks 5 minutes after benzodiazepine; however, she remains unresponsive, with SpO_2 at 86%, and general endotracheal anesthesia is administered without issue. The neonate is delivered, after which the patient develops uterine atony and bleeds at least 3.5 L.

WHAT IS UTERINE ATONY? WHAT ARE THE RISK FACTORS, AND HOW IS IT TREATED?

The patient is stabilized in the OR using an arterial blood pressure line, low-dose vasopressors, and blood product transfusion. The decision is made to keep the patient intubated postoperatively and transfer her to the intensive care unit for 24 hours of magnesium therapy and close monitoring until it is determined that her eclampsia has resolved.

DISCUSSION

PEC DEFINITION AND ETIOLOGY

As defined by the American College of Obstetricians and Gynecologists (ACOG), there are 4 classifications of hypertension noted during pregnancy:

1. Chronic hypertension, a pre-existing diagnosis of hypertension predating pregnancy (or prior to 20 weeks of gestation)

2. Gestational hypertension, defined as an elevation of blood pressure after 20 weeks of gestation in the absence of proteinuria

3. Preeclampsia/eclampsia

4. Superimposed PEC (chronic hypertension in association with PEC)

The most recent ACOG executive summary recommends classifying PEC as either being "preeclampsia without severe features" or "preeclampsia with severe features" (akin to "severe preeclampsia"). Under the most recent definition provided by ACOG [1], a diagnosis of "preeclampsia without severe features" requires the following:

Systolic blood pressures ≥140 mmHg *or* diastolic blood pressures ≥90 mmHg on 2 occasions, 4 hours apart, noted after 20-weeks gestational age in a previously normotensive patient

AND

Proteinuria ≥300 mg/24 hours *or* protein:creatinine ratio ≥0.3
The diagnosis of "preeclampsia with severe features" is made if the new-onset hypertension is accompanied by any

one of the following features indicative of progression towards significant end-organ dysfunction:

- Severely elevated blood pressures of systolic blood pressure (SBP) ≥160 mmHg and/or diastolic (DBP) ≥110 mmHg on 2 occasions, 4 hours apart

- Thrombocytopenia of <100,000/mcl

- Renal insufficiency—defined as serum creatinine concentrations >1.1 mg/dL *or* doubling of serum creatinine concentrations in the absence of other renal disease

- Liver function tests with transaminases twice normal and/or severe persistent right upper quadrant or epigastric pain

- Pulmonary edema

- Cerebral or visual changes

Preeclampsia is a hypertensive condition that is unique to human pregnancy wherein global vascular hyperreactivity can lead to a state of intravascular volume depletion, high systemic vascular resistance, uterine vasoconstriction within the myometrium, and decreased uterine and placental blood flow. Although of unclear etiology, the disease has been related to poor placentation and subsequent abnormal vascular remodeling at the level of the maternal myometrial spiral arteries leading to angiogenic imbalances (i.e., increased endothelin, increased thromboxane, decreased prostacyclin, decreased nitric oxide) [2]. This leads to subsequent generalized endothelial dysfunction and systemic maternal disease.

Preeclampsia affects 3% to 4% of all pregnancies [3, 4]. Risk factors include, but are not limited to, primiparity, multiple gestation, history of PEC, history of chronic hypertension, obesity, systemic lupus erythematosus, and type I diabetes mellitus. Screening for PEC risk factors (particularly development of early-onset PEC in the patient with PEC in a previous pregnancy) should be performed early in gestation to identify patients who may benefit from taking low-dose aspirin, which has been shown to reduce the risk of developing the disease [5]. PEC and eclampsia rank among the top causes of maternal morbidity and mortality, accounting for 12% of maternal deaths in the United States and 15% of preterm births [6, 7]. Low-dose aspirin administration after the first trimester of pregnancy has been estimated to reduce the risk of developing PEC by approximately 10%, with reductions in births complicated by prematurity reduced by 14% and intrauterine growth restriction reduced by 20% [6].

CLINICAL MANIFESTATIONS OF PEC

Potential systemic manifestations of PEC may include:

Airway: increased risk of difficult intubation secondary to edematous airway

Cardiovascular: decreased circulating blood volume (intravascular hypovolemia), increased sensitivity to vasopressors, increased systemic vascular resistance, susceptibility to pulmonary edema (secondary to increased pulmonary capillary permeability, low capillary oncotic pressure, and increased inflammatory response)

Neurologic: potential for seizures (progression to eclampsia), cerebral hemorrhage, cerebral edema, posterior reversible encephalopathy syndrome

Renal: oliguria (decreased glomerular filtration rate and renal blood flow), acute kidney injury

Hepatic: increased liver enzymes (liver inflammation), synthetic failure of the liver (coagulopathy), subcapsular hematoma, hepatic rupture

Hematologic: thrombocytopenia

With regards to the fetus of a preeclamptic patient, there is the concern for decreased uteroplacental perfusion with the risk of fetal hypoxia and intrauterine growth restriction. Recent meta-analyses have demonstrated that patients who develop PEC prior to 37 weeks gestation have an 8-fold higher risk for the development of cardiovascular disease later in life [8].

EVALUATION

It has been suggested that approximately 40% of parturients who initially present (at any gestational age) with either new-onset hypertension or new-onset proteinuria will go on to develop classic PEC [9]. Thus, any new onset of hypertension, proteinuria, or vague symptoms (i.e., headache, abdominal pain, dyspnea, generalized swelling, complaint of "I just don't feel right") [10] should warrant immediate evaluation for PEC. Laboratory evaluation for PEC is aimed at detecting abnormalities indicative of end-organ dysfunction. This includes complete blood count with platelet count, liver function tests (alanine transaminase, aspartate aminotransferase, Lactate dehydrogenase), creatinine, glucose, uric acid, and bilirubin. For patients complaining of abdominal pain, serum amylase, lipase, and ammonia levels should be obtained. Because PEC onset may be insidious and the diagnosis easily missed, the California Maternal Quality Care Collaborative Preeclampsia Task Force has also developed a diagnostic algorithm in an effort to aid providers in recognizing early signs of PEC, allowing for early intervention [11] (Figure 20.1). The fullPIERS (Preeclampsia Integrated Estimate of Risk) model has recently been developed as a means for predicting adverse maternal outcomes within 48 hours for parturients admitted with PEC at any gestational age [12]. Predictors of adverse maternal outcome include gestational age, presence of chest pain or dyspnea, decreased oxygen saturation, decreased platelet count, increased serum creatinine, and aspartate transaminase concentrations.

MANAGEMENT

The ACOG consensus opinion holds that any acute onset severe systolic (>160 mmHg) or diastolic (>110 mmHg) blood pressures lasting more than 15 minutes in pregnant and postpartum women constitutes a *hypertensive emergency.* Treatment should be initiated immediately (as opposed to waiting 4 hours to confirm a diagnosis of PEC with urine and blood testing). It is suggested that, in these cases, antihypertensive treatment should be initiated *within 30 to 60 minutes* [13]. It has been shown that the degree of *systolic* hypertension is the most important predictor of cerebral injury and infarction. The goal of treatment is not to normalize the patient's blood pressure (which could be poorly tolerated by the fetus) but to merely lower the blood pressure below the severe range to prevent the greater potential for morbidity.

First-line therapy recommendations for acute treatment of critically elevated blood pressures in pregnant women [13] include

- Intravenous (IV) labetalol (initial 10–20 mg IV, then 20–80 mg every 20–30 minutes to a maximum dose of 300 mg)

  - Contraindicated in active reactive airway disease, heart block, and severe bradycardia

- Hydralazine (initial 5 mg IV, then 5–10 mg IV every 20–40 minutes)

- Oral nifedipine (10–20 mg orally, repeated in 30 minutes if necessary, and then 10–20 mg every 2–6 hours) can be used when there is no IV access available

Magnesium sulfate infusion is recommended in all cases of PEC with severe features (initiated with a 4–6 gm bolus, followed by an infusion of 1–2 g/hr). There is no universal consensus on the use of magnesium sulfate therapy in PEC without severe features. The ACOG has published a low-quality evidence yet qualified recommendation that magnesium sulfate should not be administered universally to women with PEC who are asymptomatic and have SBP<160 and DBP<110 [1]. The use of magnesium sulfate therapy in patients with PEC has demonstrated a 58% reduction in the incidence of seizures, a 45% reduction in maternal mortality, and a 33% reduction in the incidence of placental abruption [14]. Its primary mechanism of action consists of central nervous system (CNS) depression and improvement of blood flow to the CNS by vasodilating small vessels [15]. Notwithstanding its vasodilatory properties, magnesium sulfate should not be considered, or used in lieu of, an antihypertensive medication in the treatment of PEC. Should a cesarean delivery become necessary, it is recommended that the magnesium infusion is maintained throughout surgery, as subtherapeutic levels could result from premature discontinuation (magnesium has a half-life of approximately 5 hours). Important considerations for patients maintained on magnesium infusions include an increased sensitivity to nondepolarizing muscle relaxants; decreased platelet aggregation, thereby increasing the risk of bleeding; increased uterine blood flow; decreased uterine tone, thereby increasing the risk of uterine atony;

Preeclampsia Early Recognition Tool (PERT)

ASSESS	NORMAL (GREEN)	WORRISOME (YELLOW)	SEVERE (RED)
Awareness	Alert/Oriented	• Agitated/Confused • Drowsy • Difficulty speaking	• Unresponsive
Headache	None	• Mild headache • Nausea, Vomiting	• Unrelieved Headache
Vision	None	• Blurred or impaired	• Temporary blindness
Systolic BP (mmHG)	100–139	140–159	≥160
Diastolic BP (mmHG)	50–89	90–105	≥105
HR	61–110	111–129	≥130
Respiration	11–24	25–30	<10 or >30
SOB	Absent	Present	Present
O2 Sat (%)	≥95	91–94	≤90
Pain: Abdomen or Chest	None	• Nausea, Vomiting • Chest Pain • Abdominal Pain	• Nausea, Vomiting • Chest Pain • Abdominal Pain
Fetal Signs	• Category I • Reactive NST	• Category II • IUGR • Non-Reactive NST	• Category III
Urine Output (ml/hr)	≥50	30–49	≤30 (in 2 hrs)
Proteinuria	Trace	• +1/+2 • ≥300mg/24 hours	• >+3 • ≥5g/24hrs*
Platelets	>100	50–100	<50
AST/ALT	<70	>70	>70
Creatinine	<0.8	0.9–1.2	>1.2
Magnesium Mag Sulfate Toxicity	• DTR +1 • Respiration 16–20	• Depression of patellar reflexes	• Respiration <12

*Level of Proteinuria is not an accurate predictor of pregnancy outcome

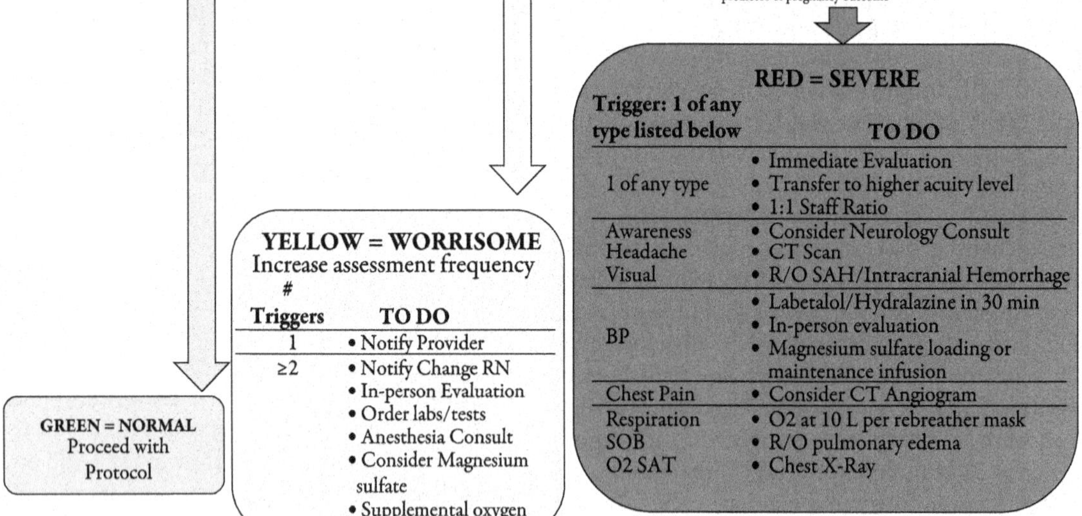

GREEN = NORMAL
Proceed with Protocol

YELLOW = WORRISOME
Increase assessment frequency

# Triggers	TO DO
1	• Notify Provider
≥2	• Notify Change RN • In-person Evaluation • Order labs/tests • Anesthesia Consult • Consider Magnesium sulfate • Supplemental oxygen

RED = SEVERE

Trigger: 1 of any type listed below	TO DO
1 of any type	• Immediate Evaluation • Transfer to higher acuity level • 1:1 Staff Ratio
Awareness Headache Visual	• Consider Neurology Consult • CT Scan • R/O SAH/Intracranial Hemorrhage
BP	• Labetalol/Hydralazine in 30 min • In-person evaluation • Magnesium sulfate loading or maintenance infusion
Chest Pain	• Consider CT Angiogram
Respiration SOB O2 SAT	• O2 at 10 L per rebreather mask • R/O pulmonary edema • Chest X-Ray

Figure 20.1 Schema for the early identification, stratification and treatment of PEC.
Used with permission from the California Maternal Quality Care Collaborative (CMQCC) Preeclampsia Task Force.

and increased risk for neonatal respiratory depression and hypotonia.

When treating PEC with a magnesium sulfate infusion, it is not necessary to aggressively check serum magnesium levels as there is no clear therapeutic range for seizure prophylaxis. However, a typical loading dose of 6 grams of magnesium sulfate, followed by an infusion of 2 g/hr (unless renal dosing is required) is commonly recommended to achieve therapeutic magnesium level of 4 to 6 mEq/L or 5 to 9 mg/dL. During magnesium therapy, it is necessary to periodically assess the patient for signs and symptoms of magnesium toxicity every 1 to 2 hours. Maintenance dosing should be discontinued if there is loss of patellar reflexes, respiratory depression, muscle weakness, or alterations in cardiac conductance (which may progress to cardiac arrest) [1].

While the definitive treatment for PEC is delivery of the fetus and placenta, strategies differ depending upon the timing of presentation.

- *If the patient presents at a gestational age where there is no fetal viability,* delivery is always recommended in any case of PEC with severe features.

- *If the patient is stable and presents prior to 34 weeks,* it is recommended that antenatal corticosteroids are administered for fetal lung maturity. If there are no severe features, patients can be ideally delivered at 37 weeks.

- *If severe features are present prior to 34 weeks,* patients should be delivered by the 34-week mark (delivery should not be delayed if maternal or fetal status becomes unstable).

Onset of PEC prior to 34 weeks gestation typically portends a severe diagnosis, with highly unpredictable progression. These patients should be managed in a facility capable of providing the appropriate resources to treat both maternal *and* fetal complications. Table 20.1 lists potential "trigger criteria" for which obstetricians and/or anesthesiologists may find it necessary to engage additional consulting services.

There has been considerable debate about neuraxial anesthesia techniques for the PEC patient. Although no longer a diagnostic feature, the capillary leak physiology that is present in cases of PEC can often lead to local or generalized edema as well as intravascular hypovolemia. Historically, placing a spinal anesthetic, with its expected rapid-onset lower extremity sympathectomy and peripheral vasodilation, was considered contraindicated in patients with PEC. However, modern practice has shown that, in the absence of coagulopathy or severe thrombocytopenia, epidural and spinal anesthesia, is quite safe and appropriate in patients with PEC. Additional

coagulation studies such as prothrombin time, partial thromboplastin time, and fibrinogen should be considered in patients with platelet counts less than 100,000/mcl, and neuraxial anesthesia should be generally considered contraindicated in patients with a platelet count less than 50,000/mcl [16–19]. Ultimately, the risk of developing a spinal or epidural hematoma must be weighed against the risks associated with the administration of general anesthesia, including a difficult edematous airway in the parturient and the possibility of exacerbated hypertension on induction. For cesarean deliveries, a spinal anesthetic may be an appropriate choice as it has been shown to cause only modest decreases in afterload and less hypotension in the preeclamptic patient compared to normotensive parturients [18].

General anesthesia may become necessary in the PEC patient most commonly for acute fetal distress. Late decelerations are a reduction in fetal heart rate that begin after the start of a uterine contraction and are thought to be a sign of uteroplacental insufficiency. When late decelerations are said to be recurrent, they occur with every or almost every contraction. When this occurs with a loss of baseline variability, the tracing is considered to be a category III, the most concerning category of tracing, considered to be a sign of imminent fetal injury. The category III tracing should be resolved before any elective procedure (labor analgesia) is considered. In addition to fetal distress, coagulopathy or patient refusal of regional anesthesia may also necessitate administration of general anesthesia for delivery of the PEC patient. In this case it is prudent to utilize a smaller endotracheal tube to reduce the potential for laryngeal edema in these patients. Antihypertensive agents such as labetalol, esmolol, or remifentanil may also be used in addition to an induction agent to blunt sympathetic stimulation upon laryngoscopy [13, 20]. Because the PEC placenta has shifted blood flow autoregulation to conform with a higher maternal blood pressure, it is recommended to maintain intraoperative

Table 20.1 PREECLAMPSIA TRIGGER CRITERIA TO ENGAGE SUBSPECIALTY CONSULTATION. FROM [11].

PULMONARY/FLUIDS	CARDIAC	NEUROLOGIC	HEMATOLOGIC
- Pulmonary edema - Fluid overload, leaky membrane, low Colloid Oncotic Pressure - Not responding to one dose of diuretic - Shortness of breath—DDx includes r/o pulmonary embolism (spiral CT scan preferred)	- Cardiac pump failure—(DDx) includes peripartum cardiomyopathy, preeclarmpsia induced—need echo. - Arrhythmia (e.g., SVT, atrial fibrillation) - Difficulty breathing, (might need intubation: DDx: pulmonary edema, stridor from swelling fluids/allergic, asthmatic not responsive to initial medications, magnesium toxicity, occult Mitral Stenosis for new onset asthma in labor - Hypoxia, any cause (decreased O2Sat)—(e.g., oxygen saturation < 95% on oxygen). Trauma history (possible pneumothorax—chest tube required) - Intrinsic—cardiac pump failure, leaky membrane, COP low, bronchospasm, Extrinsic—PTX, ETT kink, FB in airway, Swelling/stridor—fluid/preeclampsia progression labor, allergic reaction	- Repeated seizures, unresponsive to initial therapy (DDx includes SAH/intracranial hemorrhage—CT required) - Altered mental status (DDx—metabolic, toxic, etc.) - Acute stroke/neurologic changes (r/o intracranial bleed) - Cortical vein thrombosis	- DIC - HELLP syndrome (e.g., platelets <50,000) - Coagulopathy, any cause - Massive transfusion/OB hemorrhage - On anticoagulants (e.g., LMWH)—timing dosing, when to hold, when to restart

DDx, Differential Diagnosis; r/o, Rule Out; CT, computed tomography; SVT, Supraventricular Tachycardia; COP, colloid osmotic pressure; PTX, Pneumothorax; ETT, Endotrachial tube kink; FB, foreign body; SAH, subarachnoid haemorrhage; DIC, Disseminated Intravascular Coagulopathy; HELLP, Hemolysis, Elevated Liver Enzymes Low Platelet; LMWH, low molecular weight heparin.

maternal systemic blood pressure within 20% of preoperative blood pressures. Magnesium sulfate infusions should be continued throughout the cesarean delivery and following parturition for 24 hours. While delivery is often considered the definitive treatment for PEC, resolution of the PEC does not necessarily happen with delivery; PEC may persist and may even worsen, thus close postpartum monitoring is necessary. It is also worth noting that providers should exercise considerable caution in fluid resuscitating the PEC patient. While the patient is intravascularly depleted, this results from a capillary leak phenomenon that may result in anasarca and increased susceptibility for pulmonary and/or cerebral edema. Medications that can precipitate elevations in blood pressure such as ketamine and methylergonovine should be avoided in the preeclamptic patient. Whereas the ACOG has previously cautioned against the use of ketorolac and other nonsteroidal anti-inflammatory drugs in the setting of PEC with severe features due to concerns that their use may cause postpartum hypertension [1], Blue et al. found that use of ibuprofen (as compared to acetaminophen) did not lengthen the duration of severe-range hypertension in parturients with PEC with severe features [21].

ECLAMPSIA

Eclampsia is defined as new-onset grand mal seizures or unexplained coma in a preeclamptic patient having no pre-existing neurologic disorder. Seizures are typically self-limiting, and there may not be immediate cause to perform endotracheal intubation and/or emergency delivery by cesarean section. The treatment algorithm in Figure 20.2 details additional considerations in the management of the eclamptic patient, emphasizing that prior to making decisions regarding delivery, consideration must be given to controlling blood pressure, seizure treatment, and seizure prophylaxis.

In the peripartum period, benzodiazepines (i.e., midazolam, lorazepam) are most commonly used for seizure control (although propofol is another option is airway support is available). In addition, a magnesium sulfate infusion should be initiated for prevention of further seizures. Progression to eclampsia should prompt a more expeditious delivery; however, labor and vaginal delivery may still be viable options. While fetal bradycardia may accompany maternal seizures, it is typically transient and does not mandate cesarean delivery in all cases.

A retrospective review of 254 consecutive cases of eclampsia over 12 years [22] noted that, at the time of seizure onset, 19% of parturients did not have proteinuria, 23% did not have hypertension, and 29% occurred in the postpartum period (over half of which occurred beyond 48 hours postpartum). Studies finding an increased incidence of eclampsia in the postpartum period (even occurring up to 4 weeks postpartum) has recently prompted the ACOG to refine its recommendations for women in whom gestational hypertension, PEC, or superimposed PEC is diagnosed. In these patients, blood pressure monitoring should continue for at least 72 hours postpartum and checked again 7 to 10 days after delivery.

HELLP SYNDROME

HELLP syndrome is a variant of PEC defined by the presence of hemolysis (increased LDH or total bilirubin levels, decreased haptoglobin level), elevated liver enzymes (increased AST and/or ALT), and a low platelet count (<100,000/mcl). HELLP syndrome has a 0.9% incidence in all pregnancies, occurring in approximately 25% of preeclamptic patients [23], and has similar increased risk of adverse outcomes (i.e., placental abruption, disseminated intravascular coagulation, renal failure, preterm delivery, subcapsular hepatic hematoma, recurrent eclampsia, maternal/fetal death). It is possible to have HELLP syndrome without having markedly elevated blood pressure readings, and, like PEC, it can occur in the antepartum or postpartum period. If occurring antenatally, delivery represents the only definitive treatment of HELLP syndrome and should be performed promptly in gestational ages less than 23 weeks or greater than 34 weeks, following maternal stabilization [1]. Antihypertensive treatment and seizure prophylaxis with magnesium sulfate are additional mainstay therapies.

Compared to PEC and eclampsia, a diagnosis of HELLP syndrome has been associated with an increased risks for maternal death and other maternal morbidities (i.e., acute renal failure, pulmonary edema, disseminated intravascular coagulation, Acute respiratory distress syndrome, stroke) [24]. Fetal perinatal death rates have ranged from 7.4% to 20.4% in various case series, and the rate of preterm delivery is estimated at approximately 70% with 15% occurring before 28 weeks gestation [24, 25]. Because of these higher maternal and perinatal morbidity and mortality rates, there is less consideration toward expectantly managing patients presenting between >23 and <34 weeks gestation, and delivery will often not be delayed any longer than 48 hours to allow for antenatal corticosteroids (so long as maternal or fetal status does not deteriorate) [1, 24]. Some experts posit that, should a cesarean delivery be necessary, a platelet count of 40,000 to 50,000/mcl is required. A platelet transfusion is indicated in the setting of active bleeding and/or platelet counts <20,000/mcl; however, it is controversial whether transfusion should be administered for platelet counts between 20,000 and 50,000/mcl [24].

CONCLUSION

- Vigilance with a high index of suspicion is required to recognize and diagnose PEC. Early treatment in order to prevent disease progression and risk for life-threatening complications such as cerebral hemorrhage, pulmonary edema, hepatic failure or rupture, placental abruption, and fetal compromise is tantamount.

- PEC is defined as new-onset hypertension after 20 weeks gestation, in addition to either proteinuria or significant end-organ dysfunction.

- With diagnosis confirmed, management includes maternal stabilization, fetal status assessment to decide if delivery is

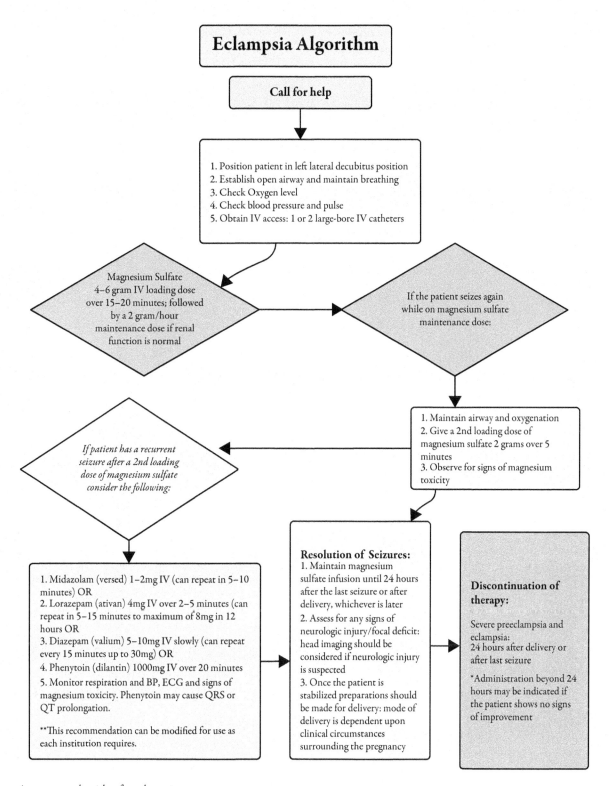

Figure 20.2 A treatment algorithm for eclampsia.
Used with permission from the California Maternal Quality Care Collaborative (CMQCC) Preeclampsia Task Force.

necessary, and treatment of severe hypertension (SBP ≥160 mmHg and/or DBP ≥110 mmHg) to prevent cerebral insult. Magnesium sulfate infusion should be administered for seizure prophylaxis.

• The minimum platelet count for neuraxial anesthesia placement is controversial, and ultimately an assessment of risks

and benefits should be taken into consideration for platelet counts between 50,000 and 70,000 /mcl. A platelet count of less than 50,000 /mcl should preclude placement of a spinal or epidural anesthetic.

• Progression to eclampsia entails the occurrence of new-onset generalized tonic-clonic seizures. Management is similar to that of PEC, including treatment of severe hypertension (if present), seizure treatment, preventing seizure recurrence with magnesium sulfate infusions, and evaluation for prompt delivery.

- HELLP syndrome is a PEC variant in which there is multiorgan dysfunction and greater risk of morbidity and mortality. Delivery is indicated regardless of gestational age.

REFERENCES

1. American College of Obstetricians and Gynecologists; Task Force on Hypertension in Pregnancy. Hypertension in pregnancy: report of the American College of Obstetricians and Gynecologists' Task Force on Hypertension in Pregnancy. *Obstet Gynecol,* 2013. *122*(5): p. 1122–1131.
2. Maynard, S.E. and S.A. Karumanchi, Angiogenic factors and preeclampsia. *Semin Nephrol,* 2011. *31*(1): p. 33–46.
3. Hutcheon, J.A., S. Lisonkova, and K.S. Joseph, Epidemiology of preeclampsia and the other hypertensive disorders of pregnancy. Best Pract Res Clin Obstet Gynaecol, 2011. *25*(4): p. 391–403.
4. Ananth, C.V., K.M. Keyes, and R.J. Wapner, Pre-eclampsia rates in the United States, 1980-2010: age-period-cohort analysis. *BMJ,* 2013. *347*: p. f6564.
5. Askie, L.M., et al., Antiplatelet agents for prevention of pre-eclampsia: a meta-analysis of individual patient data. *Lancet,* 2007. *369*(9575): p. 1791–1798.
6. Henderson, J.T., et al. *Low-Dose Aspirin for the Prevention of Morbidity and Mortality From Preeclampsia: A Systematic Evidence Review for the U.S. Preventive Services Task Force.* Rockville, MD: Agency for Healthcare Research and Quality, 2014.
7. MacKay, A.P., C.J. Berg, and H.K. Atrash, Pregnancy-related mortality from preeclampsia and eclampsia. *Obstet Gynecol,* 2001. *97*(4): p. 533–538.
8. Bellamy, L., et al., Pre-eclampsia and risk of cardiovascular disease and cancer in later life: systematic review and meta-analysis. *BMJ,* 2007. *335*(7627): p. 974.
9. Barton, J.R. and B.M. Sibai, Prediction and prevention of recurrent preeclampsia. *Obstet Gynecol,* 2008. *112*(2 Pt 1): p. 359–372.
10. Sibai, B.M. and C.L. Stella, Diagnosis and management of atypical pre-eclampsia-eclampsia. *Am J Obstet Gynecol,* 2009. *200*(5): p. 481 e1–7.
11. Druzin, M., N.L. Peterson, and V. Cape, *Preeclampsia Toolkit: Improving Health Care Response to Preeclampsia (California Maternal Quality Care Collaborative Toolkit to Transform Maternity Care).* Developed under contract #11-10006 with the California Department of Public Health; Maternal, Child and Adolescent Health Division; Published by the California Maternal Quality Care Collaborative, November 2013. https://www.cmqcc.org/resources-tool-kits/toolkits/preeclampsia-toolkit.
12. von Dadelszen, P., et al., Prediction of adverse maternal outcomes in pre-eclampsia: development and validation of the fullPIERS model. *Lancet,* 2011. *377*(9761): p. 219–227.
13. American College of Obstetricians and Gynecologists. Emergent therapy for acute-onset, severe hypertension during pregnancy and the postpartum period (Committee Opinion Summary, Number 692). *Obstet Gynecol* 2017. *129*: p. 769–770.
14. Altman, D., et al., Do women with pre-eclampsia, and their babies, benefit from magnesium sulphate? The Magpie Trial: a randomised placebo-controlled trial. *Lancet, 2002.* 359(9321): p. 1877–1890.
15. Belfort, M., J. Allred, and G. Dildy, Magnesium sulfate decreases cerebral perfusion pressure in preeclampsia. *Hypertens Pregnancy,* 2008. *27*(4): p. 315–327.
16. Ankichetty, S.P., et al., Regional anesthesia in patients with pregnancy induced hypertension. *J Anaesthesiol Clin Pharmacol,* 2013. *29*(4): p. 435–444.
17. Dennis, A.T., Management of pre-eclampsia: issues for anaesthetists. *Anaesthesia,* 2012. *67*(9): p. 1009–1020.
18. Henke, V.G., B.T. Bateman, and L.R. Leffert, Focused review: spinal anesthesia in severe preeclampsia. *Anesth Analg,* 2013. *117*(3): p. 686–693.
19. Lee, L.O., et al., Risk of epidural hematoma after neuraxial techniques in thrombocytopenic parturients: a report from the multicenter perioperative outcomes group. *Anesthesiology,* 2017. 126(6): p. 1053–1063.
20. Pant, M., R. Fong, and B. Scavone, Prevention of peri-induction hypertension in preeclamptic patients: a focused review. *Anesth Analg,* 2014. *119*(6): p. 1350–1356.
21. Blue, N.R., et al., Effect of ibuprofen vs acetaminophen on postpartum hypertension in preeclampsia with severe features: a double-masked, randomized controlled trial. *Am J Obstet Gynecol,* 2018. *218*(6): p. 616 e1–616 e8.
22. Sibai, B.M., Eclampsia. VI. Maternal-perinatal outcome in 254 consecutive cases. *Am J Obstet Gynecol,* 1990. *163*(3): p. 1049–1054; discussion: 1054–1055.
23. Aloizos, S., et al., HELLP syndrome: understanding and management of a pregnancy-specific disease. *J Obstet Gynaecol,* 2013. *33*(4): p. 331–337.
24. Sibai, B.M., Diagnosis, controversies, and management of the syndrome of hemolysis, elevated liver enzymes, and low platelet count. *Obstet Gynecol,* 2004. *103*(5 Pt 1): p. 981–991.
25. Sibai, B.M., et al., Maternal morbidity and mortality in 442 pregnancies with hemolysis, elevated liver enzymes, and low platelets (HELLP syndrome). *Am J Obstet Gynecol,* 1993. *169*(4): p. 1000–1006.

REVIEW QUESTIONS

1. Which of the following is consistent with a diagnosis of PEC with severe features?

   A. Platelet count of 140,000/mcl
   B. Systolic blood pressure of 155 mmHg
   C. Proteinuria of 7 g/day
   D. New-onset visual disturbances

Answer: D. Severe features of PEC include systolic blood pressures of 160 mmHg or higher, or diastolic blood pressure of 110 mmHg or higher on 2 occasions at least 4 hours apart (unless antihypertensives are initiated prior to this time), thrombocytopenia (platelet count less than 100,000/mm³), impaired liver function tests, progressive renal insufficiency, pulmonary edema, and new cerebral or visual disturbances. Massive proteinuria (previously requiring 5 g/day for a diagnosis of "severe preeclampsia") is not recognized as a severe feature of PEC.

2. A 28-year-old G1P0 woman is at 30 weeks' gestation with superimposed PEC. Her blood pressure is 150/100. The platelet count is 95,000 and liver function tests demonstrate transaminase levels twice the normal value. The patient's biophysical profile is 10/10. What is the best immediate management plan?

   A. Antihypertensive agent
   B. Magnesium sulfate and delivery
   C. Continued observation
   D. Corticosteroids

Answer: D. Corticosteroid therapy is the single most important intervention to impact on the neonatal outcome in a pregnancy <34 weeks when delivery is expected imminently (within 7 days). Magnesium sulfate is often given during this time of carefully monitoring the platelet count and liver function tests, but not necessarily delivery. This change in carefully observing patients with stable mild thrombocytopenia and stable elevated LFTs is based on the knowledge of antenatal corticosteroid impact on neonatal outcome.

3. A 30-year-old G2P1 woman is at 31 weeks with chronic hypertension, using oral labetalol. Her blood pressure in the office is 160/95. The urine protein is negative. What is the best immediate management plan?

   A. Additional antihypertensive agent
   B. Magnesium sulfate and delivery
   C. Continued observation
   D. Corticosteroids

Answer: A. This patient has severely elevated blood pressure and must receive an antihypertensive agent as soon as possible to reduce the risk of stroke. This may be IV labetolol, IV hydralazine, or oral nifedipine. Although corticosteroids and BPP are viable answer choices, the highest priority is to lower the blood pressure.

4. A 25-year old woman is undergoing a cesarean section for arrest of dilation following an induction for significant hypertension and proteinuria. She had received 18 hours of oxytocin infusion prior to cesarean delivery. After delivery of the placenta, the obstetrician reports poor uterine tone and uncontrolled bleeding. Which of the following is *not* appropriate in the treatment of uterine atony?

   A. Carboprost 250 mcg intramuscularly
   B. Methylergonovine 0.2mg intramuscularly
   C. Misoprostol 800 mcg rectally
   D. Oxytocin 30 units/hr infusion

Answer: B. Administration of methylergonovine should be used with extreme caution in any patient with PEC or a history of hypertension. If oxytocin proves ineffective in this situation, carboprost should first be considered. If this fails to improve hemorrhage, other considerations could include administration of misoprostol (either rectally, orally, or sublingually), ligation, or embolization of the uterine arteries, and finally hysterectomy.

5. A woman presents to labor and delivery triage at 29 weeks' gestation with complaint of new-onset headache. Her blood pressure is elevated to 175/110 and heart rate is 70. Urinalysis reveals 4+ proteins. Which of the following is the *best* medication for treating her hypertension?

   A. Esmolol
   B. Lisinopril
   C. Labetalol
   D. Magnesium sulfate

Answer: C. Labetalol and hydralazine are considered first-line therapies in the treatment of acute hypertension in pregnancy. Esmolol is a pure beta-1 blocker, and, when given to pregnant patients, has been associated with fetal bradycardia

and subsequent hypoxia and acidosis, making labetalol (with a safer drug profile) a more appropriate choice. While magnesium sulfate can cause transient vasodilation, its indication is solely for seizure prophylaxis and is not intended for use as an antihypertensive. Lisinopril, and all other angiotensin-converting-enzyme inhibitors, are contraindicated in pregnancy because of risk of fetal renal damage.

6. A parturient diagnosed with PEC with severe features requires cesarean section because of breech presentation. Platelet count is 105,000/mm^3 and had been 110,000/mm^3 24 hours earlier. Her most recent blood pressure was 151/91. Which of the following is true with regard to her anesthetic management for cesarean delivery?

   A. Epidural anesthesia is contraindicated.
   B. General anesthesia is the technique of choice for delivery.
   C. Compared to a normotensive patient, less hypotension would be expected with a spinal anesthetic.
   D. Additional coagulation studies must be obtained before neuraxial placement is attempted.

Answer: C. General anesthesia may be more appropriate in some situations (i.e., fetal distress, precipitous drop in platelet count); however, one must also weigh the risks of the airway concerns of PEC, concerns for hypertension on induction/laryngoscopy, and intraoperative hypotension causing compromised uteroplacental perfusion). In the scenario described, the patient has a sufficient platelet count and the indication for delivery is for breech presentation. A spinal, epidural, or combined spinal-epidural are all appropriate choices. Whereas, historically, it was worrisome that spinals in preeclamptic patients would cause profound hypotension (secondary to sympathectomy), studies have not found any increased incidence of hypotension when comparing spinals versus epidurals, and hypotension is overall more profound in a normotensive patient as compared to a preeclamptic patient.

7. Following a rapid-sequence induction in a known pre-eclamptic patient, blood pressure is noted to be 230/110 and remains elevated for 5 minutes before adequate control is obtained. During the operation, the patient loses 2 L of blood, receives 4 L crystalloid, and requires transfusion with 2 units of packed red blood cells. A total of 8 mg morphine is given throughout the case. At the end of the case, muscle relaxation is reversed and vitals are noted to be blood pressure 175/85, heart rate 48, oxygen saturation of 95% on 100% O$_2$. What is the *most* likely cause of the failure to emerge?

   A. Cerebral edema
   B. Hyponatremia
   C. Seizure
   D. Cerebral hemorrhage

Answer: D. The most common cause of mortality in a preeclamptic patient is from cerebral hemorrhage and should be high on the list of differential diagnoses for patients who fail to emerge, particularly in this patient in whom there was inadequate sympathetic blunting of hypertension on induction. The patient's hypertension and bradycardia at the end of the case may represent criteria for Cushing's triad. Despite the patient's likely intravascular depletion, low oncotic state, and potential renal dysfunction from PEC, somewhat aggressive fluid resuscitation with crystalloid and packed red blood cells are unlikely to precipitate either hyponatremia or cerebral edema to the extent to cause this presentation. The possibility of progression to development of an eclamptic seizure is certainly a possibility, though unlikely to have emerged during general anesthesia.

8. A 29-year old woman at 32 weeks' gestation is diagnosed with PEC. Her blood pressure on admission to labor and delivery is 175/95 mmHg. She is experiencing uterine contractions every 4 minutes and has a cervical dilation of 5 cm. A magnesium sulfate infusion is begun. Which of the following statements about magnesium therapy is *most* likely true?

   A. It will cause a decrease in uterine blood flow.
   B. It will reliably increase the time to optimal intubating conditions when using succinylcholine.
   C. It will have no effect on uterine vascular resistance.
   D. Complete heart block may be seen with higher plasma levels of magnesium

Answer: D. Loss of deep tendon reflexes and generalized weakness are usually seen first when reaching toxic levels of serum magnesium. At higher levels of plasma magnesium levels, sinoatrial nodal block, atrioventricular nodal block, and complete heart block can be seen, which can be followed by cardiac or respiratory arrest or comatose state. Magnesium sulfate infusions have been shown to increase uterine blood flow and decrease uterine vascular resistance. While magnesium can potentiate the effect of nondepolarizing muscle relaxants, it does not have a definitive effect on depolarizing muscle relaxants and hence there should be no adjustment made to intubating doses of succinylcholine (1.0–1.5 mg/kg).

9. A 25-year-old G1P0 female at 35 weeks' gestation with known ideopathic thrombocytopenic purpura (ITP) presents to triage complaining of right upper quadrant pain, nausea, and vomiting. Her blood pressure is newly elevated at 143/75. Her platelet counts throughout pregnancy have consistently ranged from 85,000 to 100,000 /mm³. Labs are obtained in triage and are notable for a platelet count of 52,000 /mm³, AST of 155 IU/L, 3+ urine protein on dipstick, and schistocytes are seen on a peripheral blood smear. Physical exam is notable for bilateral ankle edema. What is the most appropriate next step in management?

   A. Right upper quadrant ultrasound
   B. Immediate delivery
   C. Monitoring on antepartum service
   D. IV labetalol

Answer: B. While the patient has a known history of ITP, her now significantly decreased platelet count, elevated liver enzymes, and schistocytes (indicative of a microangiopathic hemolytic anemia) are more consistent with HELLP syndrome rather than a worsening of ITP. The most appropriate management is thus immediate delivery of the fetus. Consideration might be given to trying to raise the platelet count (especially for a cesarean delivery) with either intravenous immune globulin or a platelet transfusion. While a right upper quadrant ultrasound could indicate a subcapsular hematoma or hepatic infarction, it does not have a role in the acute management of this patient. Antihypertensives could certainly be utilized but should not be considered the "treatment" in this scenario (had the patient presented with SBP >160 mmHg and/or DBP >110 mmHg, however, blood pressure stabilization to prevent cerebral insult would be first-line therapy). Consideration might be given to a delaying delivery for a parturient with a gestational age <34 weeks to give antenatal corticosteroids for fetal lung maturity; however, in this patient there is no reason to delay delivery.

10. Immediately following the treatment of an eclamptic seizure in a patient with known PEC, the fetal heart rate is found to be 100 bpm. What is the most appropriate action?

   A. Intubate the patient
   B. Emergent cesarean section
   C. Clinical exam to assess for magnesium level
   D. Maternal supportive care and fetal heart rate observation

Answer: D. Following an eclamptic seizure, the best strategy is to ensure maternal stability and monitor the fetal heart rate. Intubation is not necessary if a patient is maintaining her airway and vital signs. Reductions in fetal heart rate seen after eclamptic seizure are often transient. If, after several minutes, the fetal heart rate has not returned to its baseline, consideration should be given to urgent delivery.

21.

POSTPARTUM HEMORRHAGE

Haley Goucher Miranda

STEM CASE AND KEY QUESTIONS

A 32-year-old (gravida 1, para 0 woman) at 37.0 weeks estimated gestational age presents for induction of labor for severe preeclampsia. For induction of labor, she initially receives dinoprostone and then an oxytocin infusion with artificial rupture of membranes. Oxytocin dose requirements continue to escalate to maintain an acceptable contraction pattern on tocometer. After 24 hours, her obstetrician calls for a semi-urgent caesarean section for nonreassuring fetal heart tones. Following delivery of the fetus, the obstetrician states the uterus is "boggy" and requests uterotonics from the anesthesia team.

WHAT IS POSTPARTUM HEMORRHAGE? HOW DOES IT CONTRIBUTE TO MATERNAL MORBIDITY AND MORTALITY IN THE UNITED STATES VERSUS THE REST OF THE WORLD?

A 40 U oxytocin/500 ml N saline infusion is commenced. Uterine tone continues to be poor, and the obstetrician asks for additional uterotonic medication. Prostaglandin F2α 0.25mg intramuscular (IM) is administered, given the patient's severe preeclampsia. Current estimated blood loss is 1500 ml—the patient is being resuscitated with crystalloid, a total of 3000 ml at this point, and a phenylephrine infusion is commenced to maintain mean arterial pressure >65 mmHg.

WHAT ARE THE RISK FACTORS FOR POSTPARTUM HEMORRHAGE? HOW DOES THE COAGULATION PROFILE OF A TERM PARTURIENT DIFFER FROM THAT OF A NONPREGNANT PATIENT? WHAT HEMATOLOGIC AND COAGULATION LAB TESTING IS MOST HELPFUL IN THE PERIPARTUM PERIOD?

Large-bore peripheral venous access is placed, and resuscitation with packed red blood cells (pRBCs) is commenced. Massive transfusion protocol is activated, and as blood products arrive in the operating room, resuscitation continues with

PRBCs/fresh frozen plasma (FFP)/platelets in a 1:1:1 ratio. Cryoprecipitate is administered approximately every 8 units of pRBCS. A further dose of prostaglandin F2α is administered, 15 minutes after the first. A radial arterial line is also placed.

WHAT MEDICATIONS SHOULD BE CONSIDERED IN THE IMMEDIATE POSTPARTUM SETTING TO HELP CONTROL ONGOING HEMORRHAGE? HOW SHOULD MASSIVE TRANSFUSION BE DIRECTED IN THE OBSTETRIC PATIENT? ARE RECOMBINANT FACTOR VII OR ANTIFIBRINOLYTIC THERAPY INDICATED FOR POSTPARTUM HEMORRHAGE? WHAT IS THE PATHOPHYSIOLOGY OF DISSEMINATED INTRAVASCULAR COAGULATION, AND HOW IS IT DIAGNOSED? HOW SHOULD IT BE MANAGED?

Uterine tone appears somewhat better; however, bleeding is ongoing, and the obstetric team feels that, clinically, the patient does not seem to be forming clot. Tranexamic acid 1g intravenous (IV) is given. A thromboelastogram is performed, and, based upon the result, additional cryoprecipitate is administered. At this time, the patient exhibits oxygen desaturation, with altered mentation, and is intubated for these reasons. A central venous line is placed to help with resuscitation and central administration of pressors.

WHAT INTERVENTIONS SHOULD BE CONSIDERED IF HEMORRHAGE IS UNRESPONSIVE TO PHARMACOTHERAPY?

A Bakri balloon is inserted into the uterus to provide tamponade. Uterine tone seems to have improved significantly. Clinical coagulopathy has improved, although the patient remains "oozy." She is on a stable dose of norepinephrine 5 mcg/min via her central line. The team transfers the patient intubated to the intensive care unit (ICU), where she requires further transfusion to correct coagulopathy. She is successfully extubated the following morning, and the Bakri balloon is removed 24 hours after placement with no evidence of further bleeding.

DISCUSSION

PPH is defined as greater than 500 cc of estimated blood loss (EBL) for a vaginal delivery or greater than 1000 cc for a caesarean delivery.[1] However, many organizations have advocated that the presence of hemodynamic instability automatically qualifies as PPH regardless of estimated blood loss, as visual EBL is notoriously variable and is typically underestimated by as much as 33% to 50%.[1,2] PPH complicates 2% to 10% of births and is the world's leading cause of maternal death, claiming more than 140,000 lives every year.[3] Most of these fatalities occur in low- or middle-income countries, but PPH remains the leading preventable cause of maternal death in the United States.[4] Despite best efforts, analysis of nationwide inpatient data trends from 2001 to 2012 suggested the rate of severe PPH in the United States requiring transfusion, hysterectomy, or uterine tamponade use may be increasing.[5] This may be due to improved recognition and definitions of PPH but may be partially attributable to increasing patient comorbidities and an increase in the rate of caesarean deliveries in the United States. PPH continues to remain a leading cause of morbidity and mortality in the United States.[1] Given the more than 200 million pregnancies worldwide each year, primary prevention of PPH has been an important aim of the World Health Organization (WHO). The WHO has recognized the active management of the third stage of labor as the single best management tool in the primary prevention of PPH. The WHO PPH update in 2012 defined this as the administration of uterotonics, late cord clamping (1 to 3 minutes seconds after delivery), and controlled traction on the umbilical cord by an experienced provider while awaiting placental delivery.[6] The use of oxytocin alone, considered the first-line uterotonic medication, reduces the rate of PPH by more than 40%, and by more than 68% when it is used in conjunction with the other components of the active management of the third stage of labor.[4]

RISK FACTORS

The risk factors for PPH recognized by the American College of Obstetricians and Gynecologists (ACOG) and other professional obstetric societies worldwide are listed in Box 21.1.[3] Risk factors are broken down into pre-existing factors, placental factors, and intrapartum factors. Of these, only pre-existing factors may be modifiable, though placenta previa or suspected abnormal placentation (i.e., placenta accreta, increta, or percreta) should also indicate the patient is high risk before presentation to the labor and delivery unit. In these cases, antepartum multidisciplinary consultation with anesthesiology, transfusion medicine, gynecologic oncology, or urology may be indicated to help best determine a care plan to minimize patient risk. When present, appropriate and management of iron-deficiency anemia should be corrected during pregnancy by the obstetrician. Type and screen should determine the patient's blood type and rule out the presence of antibodies. If antibodies are found, consultation with the blood bank should occur to ensure sufficient compatible units are available during the anticipated window of delivery.

Box 21.1 RISK FACTORS FOR POST-PARTUM HEMORRHAGE

Risk Factors
Preexisting Conditions

- History of post-partum hamorrhage
- Preeclampsia
- Overdistended uterus (i.e multiple gestation, macrosomia, polyhydramnios)
- Asian or Hispanic ethnicity
- Uterine anomalies
- Hereditary coagulopathies
- High parity

Placental Factors

- Placenta previa
- Abnormal placentation (placenta accreta, increta, or percreta)
- Retained placenta

Intrapartum

- Prolonged labor
- Induction or augmentation of labor (with oxytocin)
- Precipitous labor
- Episiotomy
- Operative delivery
- Infection

RESUSCITATION AND COAGULATION

The ACOG recommends that centers that deliver obstetric care should have a well-defined massive transfusion protocol (MTP) in place. Low-volume hospitals without sufficient resources should have protocols in place to transfer patients to tertiary care centers.[7] Such MTPs have been previously well described.[8,9] Four units of type-O negative uncross-matched pRBCs should ideally always be available for emergency transfusion. Activation of the MTP in a bleeding patient should result in the expedient release of compatible or type-specific blood products, including 6 units of pRBCs and 4 units of FFP. One apheresis pack of platelets should also be available upon request. Previously, the initial recommended transfusion ratio of pRBCs to FFP to platelets was 1.5:1:1, up to a total dose of 6 units of pRBCs, 4 units of FFP, and 1 "six-pack" unit of platelets.[9] However, a 1:1:1 transfusion ratio is now recommended by the ACOG to better approximate transfusion of whole blood and avoid dilutional coagulopathy.[7] STAT labs (including complete blood count, prothrombin time/partial thromboplastin time, and fibrinogen) should be drawn immediately when the MTP is activated and for every 30 minutes thereafter until the hemorrhage has been controlled and the patient is stabilized.[10] pRBCs are indicated to maintain a hematocrit 21% to 24%, though additional empiric transfusions may be needed if hemorrhage is ongoing. Cryoprecipitate should be administered if hemorrhage is ongoing and fibrinogen levels are <150 to 200 mg/dL despite adequate FFP replacement.[11]

Across the coagulation cascade, serum factor concentrations increase throughout gestation. Abbassi-Ghanavati et al. helpfully compiled a comprehensive reference table of standard laboratory values in pregnancy.[12] Like the physiologic anemia of pregnancy, platelet counts similarly decrease, as the increase in both cell lines does not match the increase in circulating plasma volume. This physiologic decline however rarely results in increased bleeding. Thromboelastographic (TEG) laboratory analysis allows for real-time functional assessment of primary and secondary hemostasis. This can be beneficial when coagulation labs such as platelet count, prothrombin time (PT or INR), partial thromboplastin time (PTT), or fibrinogen levels may take longer than 30 minutes to result, and TEG may provide a more complete assessment of the patient's physiological coagulation profile.[13] The presence of hyperfibrinolysis, as in the case of disseminated intravascular coagulation (DIC), can also be determined based on the TEG appearance. In addition, standard transfusion goals, such as maintaining a fibrinogen level >100 mg/dL, may not be sufficient resuscitation targets for the parturient. Conversely, the patient may have a low fibrinogen level but a normal TEG appearance, suggesting that ongoing hemorrhage may not necessarily improve with the administration of cryoprecipitate. A typical TEG is seen in Figure 21.1. Notably, when compared to nonpregnant values, R-time and K-time decreased, and alpha angle and maximum amplitude both increased by 6% to 20%; LY30 also decreased by approximately 70%.[13,14] The increased clot formation and strength with reduced fibrinolysis reflect the hypercoagulability of pregnancy that develops in preparation for childbirth.

The use of recombinant factor VIIa in the obstetric population is controversial. There are case reports of its successful use in PPH with doses of 90 mcg/kg, but due to the high risk of potentially life-threatening thrombosis, it is not routinely recommended unless multiple rounds of massive transfusion agents have been unsuccessful.[7,11] The WHO now recommends that tranexamic acid be incorporated into the treatment of PPH.[15] The WOMAN trial, a prospective randomized controlled trial published in 2017, demonstrated that tranexamic acid reduced death due to PPH when compared to placebo. Additionally, no increase in adverse effects such as renal failure

or thromboembolic events were seen.[16] Initial tranexamic acid doses consist of a bolus of 10 mg/kg or a 1 g dose given as an intravenous infusion.[11,16]

DIC is a syndrome in which uncontrolled systemic activation of coagulation occurs due to an underlying disorder. The subsequent formation of diffuse microvascular fibrin clots results in consumptive coagulopathy, organ dysfunction, and the perpetuation of severe bleeding due to impaired synthesis of coagulation factors. Acute severe hemorrhage is the most likely etiology of DIC in this obstetric patient, though placental abruption, preeclampsia, retained stillbirth, intrauterine infection, and amniotic fluid embolism are also potential causes.[17] DIC from these conditions may arise from a common mechanism in which systemic endothelial activation results from disruption or separation of the placenta, releasing tissue factor into the maternal circulation.[17] Consumptive coagulopathy can quickly result from this subsequent systemic activation, leading to later stages of DIC characterized by exhaustion of clotting factors and worsening hemorrhage.[11,17] This condition may quickly lead to exsanguination if not aggressively corrected by the anesthesia or critical care teams.

Diagnosis of DIC in the parturient is often based on clinical assessment, as no single test is sensitive nor specific enough to confirm the diagnosis.[17] Thrombocytopenia is generally cited as the most common abnormal laboratory parameter in DIC, though platelet counts may be normal in its early stages. A decreasing trend is thus used as a marker in these cases. PTT and activated partial thromboplastin time are typically prolonged. This prolongation may, however, not be appreciated if using nonpregnant reference ranges, as PT and PTT times both shorten during gestation. Similarly, serum fibrinogen levels should be significantly elevated in pregnancy,[12] and even low-normal values may reflect severe coagulopathy in the parturient. A fibrinogen level <150 mg/dL has been suggested as a transfusion threshold in the obstetric patient, though one study demonstrated that even fibrinogen levels <200 mg/dL conferred a positive predictive value for risk of postpartum hemorrhage of 100%.[11,17,18]

Multiple scoring systems have been developed to help identify high-risk patients, most notably by the International Society for Thrombosis and Hemostasis;[19] modifications have been suggested for the pregnant population.[17,20] In acute hemorrhage, however, waiting on a score-based diagnosis of DIC is not appropriate, and massive resuscitation should be initiated according to institutional protocols.[17,19] As previously discussed, point-of-care testing for serum hemoglobin and hematocrit or TEG should be used if available, as they may most expeditiously guide appropriate resuscitation.

Management of DIC should always be directed at the underlying cause.[11,17,20] In cases of massive obstetric hemorrhage, controlling any surgical bleeding, appropriately treating uterine atony, and ensuring adequate blood product resuscitation are the mainstays of treatment.

UTEROTONICS

WHO guidelines for postpartum hemorrhage mandate oxytocin as a first-line treatment. Dosing regimens vary significantly

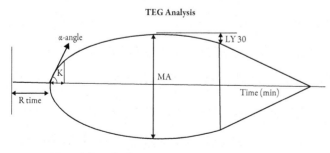

TEG Analysis

Figure 21.1 Normal thromboelastogram

by institution, and oxytocin may be given as an IV bolus, an IM injection or as an infusion in ranges of 5 to 40 units/hr.[3] Large IV boluses can, however, result in significant hypotension; other side effects include nausea and vomiting.

Second-line therapy consists of the ergot methyl-ergonovine (Methergine), which is administered in 0.2 mg IM injections every 2 to 4 hours as needed. Ergot alkaloids are vasoconstrictors that are relatively contraindicated in patients with a history of hypertension, as severe elevations in blood pressure can be induced.[21] Nausea and vomiting are other common side effects.

The prostaglandins F_{2a}-carboprost (Hemabate), E_2-dinoprostone (Cervidil), or E_1-misoprostol are additional uterotonic agents that may be considered for refractory hemorrhage. Hemabate may be given intramuscularly as a 0.25 mg dose every 15 to 90 minutes with a maximum cumulative dose of 2 mg. Cervidil may be given in doses of 20 mg per vagina or rectum, and misoprostol is given in 800 to 1000 mcg doses per rectum. Side effects of the prostaglandins include bronchospasm, diarrhea, abdominal pain, nausea, vomiting, shivering, and fever.[22]

SURGICAL INTERVENTIONS

Failing response to medical therapy, several procedural or surgical interventions are available and are discussed here. In general, in the interest of preserving fertility, uterine-sparing techniques should be attempted before considering definitive therapy with caesarean hysterectomy.

1. Uterine balloon tamponade

   One of the first-line procedures considered by the obstetric team is the use of uterine balloon tamponade. The Bakri balloon is perhaps the most common device used for this purpose. It is a silicone balloon that is inserted up into the uterus and inflated up to a maximum 500 cc capacity by the obstetrician. Notably, it was designed with a tip like a Foley catheter to allow drainage of any surrounding fluid collections, as a historical concern with use of uterine packing was that it may conceal hemorrhage rather than treat it. The balloon is typically left in place for 12 to 24 hours. Deflation and removal should be performed after appropriate notification of the anesthesia or critical care teams, as resuscitation and further management may be required if bleeding recurs.

2. Arterial ligation

   Direct ligation of the hypogastric or internal iliac vessels is an option, though ureteral injury and injury of the external iliac arteries is a risk. If PPH is suspected preoperatively, consultation with urology and placement of ureteral stents may improve surgical exposure and reduce the risk of subsequent ureteral injury. Blood pressure after arterial ligation may be reduced by as much as 85%, theoretically allowing for improved hemostasis and clot formation. Few randomized controlled trials using this technique are available, though one of the largest retrospective studies reported post-procedural uterine

viability of less than 15% and an efficacy of only 25% to 40%.[23] Ligation of the uterine artery is also an option for experienced providers, with reported efficacy rates in 1 case series of greater than 90%, with case reports of successful subsequent pregnancies.[24,25]

3. Arterial embolization or balloon occlusion

   If the patient is a high preoperative risk for hemorrhage, as in cases of suspected abnormal placentation, placement of balloon catheters into the internal iliac arteries may be a consideration. If PPH is observed, the catheters may be inflated to reduce blood flow and associated blood loss. Most cases of PPH are, however, unanticipated. In these cases, uterine artery or internal iliac artery embolization are options if the patient is hemodynamically stable to tolerate transport to the interventional radiology suite. Potential complications include pain; lower extremity ischemia; pseudoaneurysm formation; and uterine, bladder, or rectal wall necrosis. If uncomplicated, fertility is typically preserved, with reported success rates of 77%.[26]

4. Compression sutures

   The B-lynch suture technique was initially reported in 1997 and was designed to function as extrinsic compression of the uterus to combat uncontrolled hemorrhage due to uterine atony.[26] Other compression suture techniques have since been described. They offer the ease of placement during a caesarean section, when the uterus is obviously exposed. A Pfannenstiel incision would be required if considered in a patient who underwent vaginal delivery, making it a less attractive option than other less invasive methods. The suture material is, however, absorbable, theoretically preserving future fertility.

5. Caesarean hysterectomy

   In the United States, abnormal placentation has replaced uterine atony as the most common indication for peripartum hysterectomy, likely due to the increase in the number of caesarean deliveries.[26] The estimated rate of caesarean hysterectomy required for postpartum hemorrhage is likely lower than 1 in 1000 deliveries, but patient risk increases significantly with the number of prior caesarean sections (0.65% risk for first vs. 8.99% risk for a history of 6 or more caesarean deliveries).[26] Surgical dissection similarly becomes more challenging with an increasing number of deliveries. If the potential need for hysterectomy is anticipated preoperatively, placement of ureteral stents may help reduce the risk of injury.

   Although thought of as the last therapeutic resort, retrospective studies demonstrated a trend toward decreased morbidity and reoperation in women who underwent hysterectomy as the initial therapeutic intervention.[27] Associated maternal mortality can be as high as 6%, with median operative transfusion requirements of 10 units of red blood cells and 4 units of FFP.[26,27] These patients are typically admitted to the ICU postoperatively, and many will require mechanical ventilation. Given the massive resuscitation required, pulmonary edema may be significant and may be due to transfusion-associated circulatory overload, with transfusion-related lung injury (TRALI) as another possible etiology of postoperative hypoxemia.

SUMMARY

Even with impressive reductions in the incidence of PPH, however, it continues to be a significant public health problem. Multiple quality improvement initiatives have been implemented over the last decade, including the comprehensive maternal safety bundle developed by the Partnership for Maternal Safety in 2015.[10] Studies from institutions that have applied these bundles have shown promising reductions in transfusion requirements and death,[28,29] though the results have not yet been consistent.[30] Management of severe PPH requires a multidisciplinary approach built upon early recognition and activation of institutional PPH protocols. Uterine atony remains the most common cause of PPH. Awareness of the full range of uterotonics as described in this chapter is imperative, as is familiarity with the common procedures and surgical interventions that may be necessary if pharmacotherapy fails.

The critical care provider plays an important role in the postoperative care of patients with severe PPH. Understanding the physiologic changes of pregnancy is an important first step. Clinical markers of shock may not be sensitive in the parturient, as blood volume and cardiac output in pregnancy increase by almost 50% by term, both to provide sufficient oxygen delivery to the fetus and in anticipation of parturition.[1] Patients may thus be able to compensate well up to 1500 cc of blood loss, making hypotension and tachycardia relatively late signs of hypovolemia in severe postpartum hemorrhage.[31] Delayed recognition in such cases can result in a worsening spiral of consumptive coagulopathy. Intensivists should also be aware of the physiologic alterations in the coagulation profile of the parturient, as many will require ongoing resuscitation in the ICU. Fibrinogen levels should be closely monitored, and cryoprecipitate should be considered for transfusion thresholds <200 mg/dL if PPH is ongoing.[11] Hemorrhage is one of the most common causes of DIC in the obstetric patient, and treatment requires aggressive correction of consumptive coagulopathy to prevent further deterioration and death.

Consequences of massive transfusion, such as volume overload or tissue edema, may result in the need for endotracheal intubation and mechanical ventilation in the ICU.[27] Transfusion-associated circulatory overload and transfusion-related lung injury are other important considerations if the patient remains hypoxemic postoperatively.[32] Additionally, if emergency release platelets were required prior to patient type and crossmatch availability, the critical care team should check with the blood bank to ensure that no Rh-D maternal alloimmunization occurred. Rh immunoglobulin should be administered if Rh-negative patients received Rh-positive platelets due to the risk of hemolytic disease of the fetus during subsequent pregnancies.

Obstetricians are generally in favor of dedicated obstetric ICUs due to the special considerations involved with managing the parturient patient.[33] However, most hospitals lack the volume or resources to support this. Intensivists from all disciplines should thus familiarize themselves with the physiologic and laboratory changes unique to pregnancy and should be prepared to manage the complications of severe PPH and massive transfusion.

CONCLUSIONS

- PPH continues to be the leading cause of preventable maternal death in the United States.

- Active management of the third stage of labor may help reduce the risk of PPH.

- Oxytocin is the uterotonic agent of choice for management of PPH. Methylergonovine, carboprost, and misoprostol are additional second-line agents that may be considered.

- Intensivists should be aware of the complications of invasive procedures that may be indicated for PPH.

- Critical care providers should be aware of the national recommendations included in the obstetric hemorrhage safety bundle and should be included as part of their institution's maternal response team.

- Disseminated intravascular coagulopathy from obstetric causes is often a clinical diagnosis and typically requires aggressive blood product resuscitation to avoid life-threatening hemorrhage.

REFERENCES

1. Borovac-Pinheiro A, Pacagnella RC, Cecatti JG, et al. Postpartum hemorrhage: new insights for definition and diagnosis. American Journal of Obstetrics and Gynecology. Aug 2018;219(2):162–168.
2. Al Kadri HM, Al Anazi BK, Tamim HM. Visual estimation versus gravimetric measurement of postpartum blood loss: a prospective cohort study. Archives of Gynecology and Obstetrics. Jun 2011;283(6):1207–1213.
3. Dahlke JD, Mendez-Figueroa H, Maggio L, et al. Prevention and management of postpartum hemorrhage: a comparison of 4 national guidelines. American Journal of Obstetrics and Gynecology. Jul 2015;213(1):76 e71–10.
4. Devine PC. Obstetric hemorrhage. Seminars in Perinatology. Apr 2009;33(2):76–81.
5. Ahmadzia HK, Thomas SM, Murtha AP, Heine RP, Brancazio LR. Obstetric hemorrhage survey: Attitudes and practices of maternal-fetal medicine fellows. Journal of Neonatal-Perinatal Medicine. May 17 2016;9(2):133–137.
6. World Health Organization. WHO recommendations for the prevention and treatment of postpartum hemorrhage. 2012; http://www.who.int/reproductivehealth/publications/maternal_perinatal_health/9789241548502/en/.
7. Committee on Practice Bulletins-Obstetrics. Practice Bulletin No. 183: postpartum hemorrhage. Obstetrics and Gynecology. Oct 2017;130(4):e168–e186.
8. Barr J, Fraser GL, Puntillo K, et al. Clinical practice guidelines for the management of pain, agitation, and delirium in adult patients in the intensive care unit. Critical Care Medicine. Jan 2013;41(1):263–306.

9. Burtelow M, Riley E, Druzin M, Fontaine M, Viele M, Goodnough LT. How we treat: management of life-threatening primary postpartum hemorrhage with a standardized massive transfusion protocol. Transfusion. Sep 2007;47(9):1564–1572.

10. Main EK, Goffman D, Scavone BM, et al. National Partnership for Maternal Safety Consensus Bundle on Obstetric Hemorrhage. Journal of Midwifery & Women's Health. Jul–Aug 2015;60(4):458–464.

11. James AH, Grotegut C, Ahmadzia H, Peterson-Layne C, Lockhart E. Management of Coagulopathy in Postpartum Hemorrhage. Seminars in Thrombosis and hemostasis. Oct 2016;42(7):724–731.

12. Abbassi-Ghanavati M, Greer LG, Cunningham FG. Pregnancy and laboratory studies: a reference table for clinicians. Obstetrics and Gynecology. Dec 2009;114(6):1326–1331.

13. Macafee B, Campbell JP, Ashpole K, et al. Reference ranges for thromboelastography (TEG®) and traditional coagulation tests in term parturients undergoing caesarean section under spinal anaesthesia. Anaesthesia. Jul 2012;67(7):741–747.

14. Karlsson O, Sporrong T, Hillarp A, Jeppsson A, Hellgren M. Prospective longitudinal study of thromboelastography and standard hemostatic laboratory tests in healthy women during normal pregnancy. Anesthesia and Analgesia. Oct 2012;115(4):890–898.

15. Vogel JP, Oladapo OT, Dowswell T, Gulmezoglu AM. Updated WHO recommendation on intravenous tranexamic acid for the treatment of post-partum haemorrhage. Lancet: Global Health. Jan 2018;6(1):e18–e19.

16. Collaborators WT. Effect of early tranexamic acid administration on mortality, hysterectomy, and other morbidities in women with post-partum haemorrhage (WOMAN): an international, randomised, double-blind, placebo-controlled trial. Lancet. May 2017;389(10084):2105–2116.

17. Erez O, Mastrolia SA, Thachil J. Disseminated intravascular coagulation in pregnancy: insights in pathophysiology, diagnosis and management. American Journal of Obstetrics and Gynecology. Oct 2015;213(4):452–463.

18. Collins P, Abdul-Kadir R, Thachil J; Subcommittees on Women's Health Issues in Thrombosis and Haemostasis and on Disseminated Intravascular Coagulation. Management of coagulopathy associated with postpartum hemorrhage: guidance from the SSC of the ISTH. Journal of Thrombosis and Haemostasis. Journal of Thrombosis and Haemostasis. Jan 2016;14(1):205–210.

19. Levi M, Toh CH, Thachil J, Watson HG; British Committee for Standards in Haematology. Guidelines for the diagnosis and management of disseminated intravascular coagulation. British Journal of Haematology. Apr 2009;145(1):24–33.

20. Erez O, Novack L, Beer-Weisel R, et al. DIC score in pregnant women—a population based modification of the International Society on Thrombosis and Hemostasis score. PloS ONE. 2014;9(4):e93240.

21. Liabsuetrakul T, Choobun T, Peeyananjarassri K, Islam QM. Prophylactic Use of ergot alkaloids in the third stage of labour. Cochrane Database of Systematic Reviews. Apr 2007(2):CD005456.

22. Tuncalp O, Hofmeyr GJ, Gulmezoglu AM. Prostaglandins for preventing postpartum haemorrhage. Cochrane Database of Systematic Reviews. Aug 2012(8):CD000494.

23. Papp Z, Toth-Pal E, Papp C, et al. Hypogastric artery ligation for intractable pelvic hemorrhage. International Journal of Gynaecology and Obstetrics. Jan 2006;92(1):27–31.

24. O'Leary JL, O'Leary JA. Uterine artery ligation for control of postcesarean section hemorrhage. Obstetrics and Gynecology. Jun 1974;43(6):849–853.

25. Doumouchtsis SK, Papageorghiou AT, Arulkumaran S. Systematic review of conservative management of postpartum hemorrhage: what to do when medical treatment fails. Obstetrical & Gynecological Survey. Aug 2007;62(8):540–547.

26. Shah M, Wright JD. Surgical intervention in the management of postpartum hemorrhage. Seminars in Perinatology. Apr 2009;33(2):109–115.

27. Knight M, Ukoss. Peripartum hysterectomy in the UK: management and outcomes of the associated haemorrhage. BJOG. Nov 2007;114(11):1380–1387.

28. Main EK, Cape V, Abreo A, et al. Reduction of severe maternal morbidity from hemorrhage using a state perinatal quality collaborative. American Journal of Obstetrics and Gynecology. Mar 2017;216(3):298 e291–298 e211.

29. Shields LE, Wiesner S, Fulton J, Pelletreau B. Comprehensive maternal hemorrhage protocols reduce the use of blood products and improve patient safety. American Journal of Obstetrics and Gynecology. Mar 2015;212(3):272–280.

30. Hamm RF, Wang E, O'Rourke K, Romanos A, Srinivas SK. Institution of a Comprehensive Postpartum Hemorrhage Bundle at a Large Academic Center does not Immediately Reduce Maternal Morbidity. American journal of perinatology. Feb 19 2018.

31. Lockhart E. Postpartum hemorrhage: a continuing challenge. Hematology. American Society of Hematology. Education Program. 2015;2015:132–137.

32. Roubinian NH, Hendrickson JE, Triulzi DJ, et al. Contemporary risk factors and outcomes of transfusion-associated circulatory overload. Critical Care Medicine. Apr 2018;46(4):577–585.

33. Kaur MD, Sharma J, Gupta P, Singh TD, Mustafi SM. Obstetric critical care requirements felt by the obstetricians: An experience-based study. Journal of Anaesthesiology Clinical Pharmacology. Jul–Sep 2017;33(3):381–386.

34. Stanworth SJ. The evidence-based use of FFP and cryoprecipitate for abnormalities of coagulation tests and clinical coagulopathy. Hematology: American Society of Hematology Education Program. 2007;2007:179–186.

35. Middelburg RA, Van Stein D, Zupanska B, et al. Female donors and transfusion-related acute lung injury: a case-referent study from the International TRALI Unisex Research Group. Transfusion. Nov 2010;50(11):2447–2454.

36. Celi LA, Scott DJ, Lee J, et al. Association of hypermagnesemia and blood pressure in the critically ill. Journal of Hypertension. Nov 2013;31(11):2136–2141; discussion 2141.

37. Kovacs K. Sheehan syndrome. Lancet. Feb 8 2003;361(9356):520–522.

38. Fitzsimons KJ, Modder J, Greer IA. Obesity in pregnancy: risks and management. Obstetric Medicine. Jun 2009;2(2):52–62.

39. Kim J, Na S. Transfusion-related acute lung injury; clinical perspectives. Korean Journal of Anesthesiology. Apr 2015;68(2):101–105.

REVIEW QUESTIONS

1. Which of the following coagulation factors is not present in significant amounts in cryoprecipitate?

    A. Factor V
    B. Factor I
    C. Factor XIII
    D. Factor VIII

2. A 39-year-old G2P2 with preeclampsia requires ICU admission for management of severe hypertension post-delivery. She is on nicardipine and magnesium infusions. Which of the following uterotonics would be relatively contraindicated in a parturient with a history of hypertension?

    A. Hemabate (carbaprost tromethamine)
    B. Methergine (methylergovine maleate)
    C. Pitocin (oxytocin)
    D. Cytotec (misoprostol)

3. A prolonged R time on TEG in a hypotensive parturient who required 4 units pRBCs for resuscitation during PPH would be best treated with the administration of which of the following?

    A. Platelets
    B. FFP

C. Cryoprecipitate

D. Desmopressin

4. A 35-year-old G5P5 woman is admitted to the ICU after undergoing emergent caesarean hysterectomy for placenta percreta. She received 14 units of pRBC and 6 units of FFP. She was left-intubated due to significant hypoxemia noted by the anesthesia team. PaO_2 on arterial blood gas is 69 mmHg on ventilator settings of AC 14/450/7/70%. The treatment team suspects transfusion-related acute lung injury. Which of the following is most likely to be associated with this diagnosis?

A. pRBCs from a male donor

B. pRBCs from a female donor

C. FFP from a male donor

D. FFP from a female donor

5. A 32-year-old woman with a history of severe asthma is undergoing caesarean delivery for non-reassuring fetal heart tones. After delivery of the fetus and removal of the placenta, uterine atony is noted by the obstetrician and uterotonics are administered with improvement in bleeding. The patient, however, starts to complain of shortness of breath, and diffuse wheezing is heard on auscultation. Vitals are otherwise stable. Her symptoms are most likely due to which of the following?

A. Amniotic fluid embolism

B. Anaphylaxis

C. Carboprost administration

D. Oxytocin

6. A 33-year-old G3P3 patient is admitted to the ICU with severe preeclampsia on a magnesium infusion for prophylaxis. She required 6 units of pRBC and 2 units of FFP for resuscitation after suffering from PPH with an EBL of 2.5 liters. The ICU nurse calls you for progressive hypotension over the past 10 minutes. No bleeding is seen, and uterine tone is adequate on fundal exam. Which action is most likely to improve the patient's hemodynamics?

A. Stop the magnesium infusion

B. Administer calcium chloride 1 g IV

C. Administer 2 units of pRBC

D. Administer stress-dose steroids

7. Which of the following blood products would be inappropriate to emergently transfuse to a hemorrhaging obstetric patient without an available type and crossmatch?

A. Type O-negative pRBCs

B. Type O-positive platelets

C. Group AB plasma

D. Type A-negative platelets

E. Type A-positive cryoprecipitate

8. Which of the following is *not* associated with an increased risk of postpartum hemorrhage?

A. Morbid obesity

B. Elective induction of labor

C. Twin gestation

D. Chorioamnionitis

E. Placenta previa

9. A patient is brought to the ICU intubated and sedated after receiving 6 units of pRBCs and 2 units of FFP required during D&C for postpartum hemorrhage. The nurse notes significant bleeding after fundal exam. Reduced maximum amplitude (MA) on TEG is noted; other parameters are within normal limits. In addition to escalation of uterotonic therapy, what other intervention is most indicated?

A. Caesarean hysterectomy

B. Transfusion of 1 to 2 units of platelets

C. Administration of 1 g calcium chloride IV

D. Transfusion of 1 unit of FFP

10. A 38-year-old patient with preeclampsia is brought to the ICU intubated after undergoing an emergent caesarean section for non-reassuring fetal heart tones. Past medical history consists of hypertension and chronic kidney disease. She required 2 units of pRBCs for an EBL of 2000 cc. Bilateral infiltrates are seen on chest X-ray postoperatively. Transfusion-associated circulatory overload (TACO) is suspected. Which of the following is most likely to be consistent with a diagnosis of TACO instead of TRALI?

A. Hypoxemia

B. Normal ejection fraction on echocardiogram

C. Serum brain natriuretic peptide level of 245

D. Hypertension

ANSWERS

1. Answer: A. Cryoprecipitate is a concentrated product consisting of fibrinogen (factor I), factor VIII, von Willebrand factor, factor XIII, and fibronectin. An adult dose consists of 10 units, which contains more than 150 mg of fibrinogen and can be expected to raise the serum fibrinogen level by 60 to 100 mg/dL.[11,34]

2. Answer: B. Methergine would be relatively contraindicated in a patient with a history of hypertension and should be avoided in patients with severe preeclampsia or elevated blood pressures in the peripartum setting. It is an ergot alkaloid that results in vasoconstriction.[21]

3. Answer: B. A prolonged R time suggests reduced initial clotting factor activation. For a hypotensive, hemorrhaging patient, the most appropriate initial therapy would be administration of 15 to 30 cc/kg of FFP. In a volume-overloaded patient, 1 to 2 bags of cryoprecipitate may be considered instead.

4. Answer: D. Transfusion of FFP from female donors has been associated with an increased incidence of TRALI.[35] The same association was not demonstrated for transfusions of pRBCs. The development of acute respiratory distress syndrome within 6 hours after transfusion in the absence of circulatory overload is consistent with a diagnosis of TRALI. This reaction is thought to be mediated by white blood cell antibodies that result from prior donor exposure to alloantigens, which most commonly result from past pregnancies or blood transfusions. TRALI occurs with an estimated incidence of approximately 1 in every 5000 transfusions. Treatment is supportive.

5. Answer: C. Hemabate, a prostaglandin, has been associated with inducing significant bronchospasm in asthmatic patients. It should be avoided as a uterotonic agent in patients with uncontrolled or severe asthma.[22] Both amniotic fluid embolism and anaphylaxis can be associated with wheezing, but these are less common causes of bronchospasm and the patient's vitals are otherwise stable, making these diagnoses unlikely. Oxytocin is not associated with bronchospasm.

6. Answer: B. Hypocalcemia is commonly seen with massive transfusion and may require correction. This hypocalcemia may be potentiated by magnesium therapy.[36] The associated hypotension will typically be improved by appropriate correction of serum ionized calcium. While pausing the magnesium infusion may be appropriate if other signs of hypermagnesemia are seen after discussion with the obstetric team or after checking serum magnesium levels, it may risk provoking seizure activity in an eclamptic patient. No information is given on the patient's Hb/Hct, so transfusion of 2 units of pRBCs is not appropriate. Stress-dose steroids may be helpful if Sheehan's syndrome is suspected, but no peripartum history of severe hypotension is reported, making postpartum hypopituitarism unlikely.[37] Steroids thus likely have little utility in this scenario and would only increase the risk of hyperglycemia, infection, and impaired wound-healing.

7. Answer: B. Only Type O-negative pRBCs are appropriate to transfuse in an emergency without an available crossmatch. Group AB plasma is also safe to use in emergency release protocols. Cryoprecipitate does not strictly require compatibility testing, but ABO compatible units are generally preferred for transfusion. Platelets do not need to be type-specific unless large volumes of platelets are required, but they should be RhD-antigen negative given the risk of Rh alloimmunization that may impact subsequent pregnancies.[11]

8. Answer: A. Although obesity is associated with an increased risk of a host of peripartum complications including preeclampsia, venous thromboembolism, and gestational diabetes, it has not been associated with an increased risk of PPH.[38] Significant risk factors for PPH are listed in Box 21.1 and notably include a history of PPH, preeclampsia, an overdistended uterus (i.e., twin gestation, polyhydramnios), placenta previa, abnormal placentation, infection such as chorioamnionitis, and induction of labor.[3]

9. Answer: B. A reduced MA in the setting of ongoing hemorrhage suggests that platelet transfusion may be warranted. Calcium chloride may be separately indicated if hypocalcemia is noted due to massive transfusion, but it is unlikely to address the principal cause of the ongoing hemorrhage. FFP or cryoprecipitate transfusion should be considered with a prolonged R or K time or a reduced alpha-angle.

10. Answer: D. Hypertension is most likely to be associated with transfusion-associated circulatory overload than with TRALI.[39] Patients with TACO may also have a depressed ejection fraction and an elevated brain natriuretic peptide in addition to other systemic signs of volume overload, such as jugular venous distention or lower extremity edema. Pre-existing hypertension, congestive heart failure, and acute or chronic kidney injury were found to be independent risk factors for the development of TACO.[32]

22.

AMNIOTIC FLUID EMBOLISM

Xiwen Zheng and Laurence Ring

STEM CASE AND KEY QUESTIONS

A 42 year-old G1P0 woman at 38 weeks gestation presents to the labor and delivery triage area with elevated blood pressure. The patient's pregnancy has been uncomplicated to date. Her medical history is notable for hypothyroidism successfully treated with replacement therapy. In triage, the patient has a blood pressure of 150/95 and 2+ protein in her urine. She is diagnosed with preeclampsia and admitted for induction of labor. Laboratory studies including serum chemistries, complete blood count coagulation studies, and liver function tests are normal. As Induction of labor proceeds, the patient requests and receives epidural analgesia at 2 cm dilation. At 5 cm dilation, the patient undergoes artificial rupture of membranes. Several minutes later, the patient reports feeling lightheaded. Her blood pressure decreases from 135/89 to 100/70.

WHAT IS THE DIFFERENTIAL DIAGNOSIS FOR MATERNAL HYPOTENSION DURING INDUCTION OF LABOR? WHAT STEPS SHOULD BE TAKEN AT THIS POINT?

The patient is given a liter of intravenous of lactated ringers solution, and a phenylephrine infusion is started to raise her systolic blood pressure to the high normal range (120s–130s mmHg). Continuous fetal monitoring shows a normal tracing. After this treatment, the patient's blood pressure fails to respond and decreases to 80/50 with a heart rate of 120 despite significant doses of phenylephrine and ephedrine. Her oxygen saturation is 90% on 4 liters per minute of oxygen delivered by nasal cannula. She becomes increasingly anxious and agitated. The obstetricians note the patient is bleeding per vagina. He exam is now 8 cm dilated. The fetal heart tracing, which previously was found to be category 1 in the 140s, is now in the 70s and difficult to trace.

HOW ARE FETAL HEART TRACINGS CATEGORIZED? WHAT IS THE DIFFERENTIAL DIAGNOSIS, AND HOW SHOULD TREATMENT PROCEED?

After 2 minutes, the maternal condition has not improved. Given the nonreassuring category 3 fetal heart tracing, a fetal scalp electrode is placed and the fetal heart rate is found to be around 65 bpm. The obstetrician wishes to do an emergent cesarean section. A differential diagnosis is formulated including pulmonary thromboembolism, anaphylactic reaction, amniotic fluid embolism, placental abruption, and uterine rupture. The patient's blood pressure is supported with additional fluid boluses and intermittent doses of 10 micrograms of epinephrine and she is placed on 10 liters per minute of oxygen by non-rebreather mask (NRB). Her epidural is quickly loaded with 3-chloroprocaine and she is rushed to the operating room. The fetus is successfully delivered, but the maternal condition continues to deteriorate. Her blood pressure is 70/30 mmHg, her heart rate is 140 bpm, and her oxygen saturation is 88% on 100% FiO_2 by NRB. The patient is somnolent. The surgeons are reporting uterine atony and some oozing in the operative field.

HAS THE DIFFERENTIAL DIAGNOSIS NARROWED? WHAT IS UTERINE ATONY? SHOULD THIS PATIENT RECEIVE ENDOTRACHEAL INTUBATION, AND WHAT ARE THE RISKS?

At this point, amniotic fluid embolism (AFE) is strongly suspected, although other diagnoses, including disseminated intravascular coagulation (DIC) not related to AFE, uterine atony related to the induction of labor, and pulmonary embolism cannot be ruled out. The patient is hemodynamically unstable, and several actions are now taken concurrently. The patient undergoes successful endotracheal intubation for hypoxic respiratory failure. An arterial line and central line are placed, and the patient is started on norepinephrine and vasopressin infusions to treat distributive shock. A dose of 1 g tranexamic acid is administered, and blood samples are sent to the lab for coagulation studies and a complete blood count. After 15 minutes, the obstetricians report improved uterine tone but continued blood oozing in the operative field. Blood pressure is maintained at 80/40, and oxygen saturation remains 90% on FiO_2 of 100%.

WHAT IS TRANEXAMIC ACID, AND HOW DOES IT HELP IN THIS SITUATION? WHAT WOULD YOU EXPECT TO SEE ON THE RESULTS OF SERUM COAGULATION STUDIES AND COMPLETE BLOOD COUNT IN A PATIENT WITH AFE?

Lab results show a Hb of 9.5 mg/dL and platelets of 129,000. The activated partial thromboplastin time (aPTT) and prothrombin time (PT) are above readable limits, and the fibrinogen is below the readable limit. With this constellation of signs including refractory hypotension, hypoxia, and severe coagulopathy, a provisional diagnosis of AFE is made. Multiple units of red blood cells (RBCs), fresh frozen plasma (FFP), platelets, and cryoprecipitate are transfused. A transesophageal echocardiogram (TEE) is performed, and the right ventricle is found to be dilated with severely reduced function and end-systolic septal flattening. The patient's urine output is also noted to be only 10 ml over the prior hour. The obstetricians report that some mild oozing remains. Due to generalized edema, the wound is packed, and the fascia remains open.

WHAT IS DIC, AND HOW IS IT TREATED? WHAT IS THE SIGNIFICANCE OF THE TEE FINDINGS?

The patient is started on infusions of epinephrine and milrinone to treat her distributive and cardiogenic shock. A pulmonary artery catheter is placed to monitor her pulmonary hypertension, and inhaled nitric oxide therapy is initiated at 20 ppm. The patient is transferred to the intensive care unit. Where further transfusion of blood products is guided by thromboelastography (ROTEM) to correct her coagulopathy.

DISCUSSION

AFE, or anaphylactoid syndrome of pregnancy, is a rare and often devastating obstetric complication. With a reported incidence of 1.9 to 7.7 per 100,000 pregnancies (1, 2) it has a high mortality rate of 11% to 43% (1). AFE classically presents with the triad of hypoxia, right heart failure, and coagulopathy. However, since the syndrome is uncommon, consistent data about the disorder are often inconsistent. Many of the signs and symptoms of AFE are shared with other common comorbid diseases of pregnancy; it is therefore critical to exclude other disease entities (Box 22.1) before ultimately making the diagnosis of AFE. Recently, clinical criteria have been proposed for diagnosis (Box 22.2) but have not been universally adopted as some studies found that a significant number of patients ultimately diagnosed with AFE do not fulfill all

Box 22.1 DIFFERENTIAL DIAGNOSES FOR AFE

Eclampsia
High spinal anesthesia
Peripartum cardiomyopathy
Hemorrhage
Anaphylaxis
Air embolism
Pulmonary thromboembolism
Uterine rupture
Abruptio placentae
Septic shock

Box 22.2 PROPOSED CRITERIA FOR RESEARCH REPORTING OF AFE (ADAPTED FROM (3))

- Sudden onset of cardiorespiratory arrest or both hypotension (systolic blood pressure < 90 mm Hg) and respiratory compromise (dyspnea, cyanosis, or peripheral capillary oxygen saturation [SpO2] < 90%)

- Documentation of overt DIC following appearance of these initial signs or symptoms, using scoring system of Scientific and Standardization Committee on DIC of the ISTH modified for pregnancy.* Coagulopathy must be detected prior to loss of sufficient blood to itself account for dilutional or shock-related consumptive coagulopathy

- Clinical onset during labor or within 30 min of delivery of placenta

- No fever (greater than 38.0∘C) during labor

*ISTH: International Society on Thrombosis and Hemostasis. Scoring system includes assigning points as follows: platelet count >100,000/mL3 = 0; <100,000/mL3= 1; <50,000/mL3 = 2. PT or INR <25% increase from baseline = 0; 25-50% increase = 1; >50% increase = 2. Fibrinogen level >2 g/L = 0; <2 g/L = 1. Total score of 3 or more points is compatible with overt DIC in pregnancy.

the proposed criteria (3, 4). Notably, AFE has been reported in patients who presented hours after delivery, and, in some cases, hemorrhage accompanied by DIC were the only clinical manifestations (4). In addition, diagnosis of DIC before sufficient blood loss and transfusion is often not clinically practical or possible, while sources of fever such as chorioamnionitis or other infection may be present alongside AFE.

ETIOLOGY AND PATHOGENESIS

Historically, the pathophysiology of AFE was thought to be related to a physical embolus of fetal or amniotic material (hence its name) that, once in the pulmonary circulation, causes obstruction of blood flow and circulatory collapse. This idea was supported by autopsy results in the 1940s that showed fetal squamous cells in maternal pulmonary tissue in patients whose death was otherwise unexplained. However, the increased use of pulmonary artery catheters in the 1980s allowed identification of squamous cells in maternal pulmonary vasculature among patients with disorders unrelated to AFE (5). Thus, it has been concluded, that the presence alone of fetal material in the maternal circulation is not enough to explain the disorder. AFE is now better understood to be an abnormal maternal inflammatory response to fetal material that has crossed the maternal-fetal barrier. Proposed sites of a compromised barrier include the endocervix, lower uterine segment, sites of uterine trauma, and placental attachments (6). Once in the maternal circulation, fetal tissue triggers the release of proinflammatory mediators, an increase in circulating catecholamines, and activation of the coagulation cascade. This leads to the classic triad of respiratory distress with hypoxia, hypotension leading to cardiovascular collapse, and coagulopathy from DIC (Figure 22.1). It is important to note that while it is relatively common for amniotic or fetal matter to enter the maternal circulation, AFE is a rare disorder. Animal studies have shown that injection of amniotic or fetal

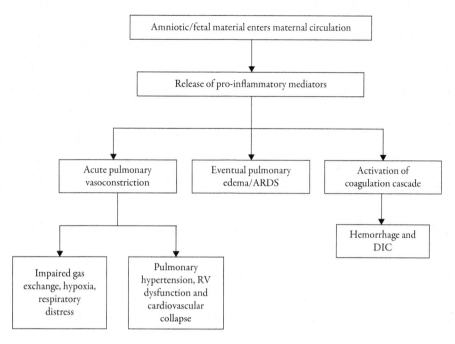

Figure 22.1 Pathophysiology and presentation of AFE

material into maternal circulation alone does not necessarily cause adverse physiologic effects (7). It is believed that AFE is the result of an *abnormal* maternal proinflammatory and coagulopathic response to fetal material. Why there should be an abnormal response in any specific patient is unknown.

Several biomarkers have been proposed to aid in diagnosis of AFE. Zinc coproporphyrin is a component of meconium, and serum sialyl-Tn is a fetal antigen found in both meconium and amniotic fluid. Raised levels of both substances are often found in pulmonary blood samples of patients with AFE. Insulin like growth factor can also be elevated whereas complement levels are often decreased. Unfortunately, none of these labs are definitive for the diagnosis of AFE, thus basing diagnosis on any specific laboratory test is not recommended (6, 8, 9).

RISK FACTORS

Due to the rare nature of the disorder, data on risk factors for AFE vary across the literature. Interventions that facilitate passage of fetal tissue into the maternal circulation, such as cesarean section, instrumental delivery, and artificial rupture of membranes, are thought to be associated with the disease. Disorders including placenta previa, placenta accreta, and abruptio placentae have also been suggested as risk factors. Other commonly proposed risk factors include advanced maternal age, preeclampsia and other maternal hypertensive disorders, induction and augmentation of labor, polyhydramnios, male gender fetus, and multiparity (5, 6, 8, 10).

CLINICAL PRESENTATION

Cardiovascular and respiratory manifestations are seen in the first stage of AFE, although maternal mental status changes or nonreassuring fetal heart tracings may precede overt signs of systemic decompensation (6). Specific presenting signs and symptoms may include tachypnea, dyspnea, hypoxia, tachycardia, or hypotension (anywhere from mild to profound). The patient may exhibit mental status changes ranging from anxiety and confusion to abrupt somnolence with obtundation. The maternal inflammatory response to fetal material leads to release of catecholamines and inflammatory mediators that result in significant pulmonary vasoconstriction. This results in hypoxia, pulmonary hypertension, increased right ventricular afterload, and subsequent right ventricular (RV) failure. Echocardiography typically reveals end-systolic septal flattening with a dilated hypokinetic RV from pressure overload. Invasive monitoring should include central venous access for with strong consideration of pulmonary artery catheter placement to measure pulmonary artery pressure and cardiac output. Arterial access should be obtained for systemic blood pressure monitoring and frequent laboratory bloodwork including arterial blood gases. Large-bore venous access for rapid transfusion of blood products should also be obtained. The airway should be secured and mechanical ventilation initiated to reduce hypoxia and hypercapnia.

Often RV failure will lead to left ventricular failure with subsequent cardiogenic pulmonary edema. Fluids and blood products at this stage should be administered with care to avoid volume overload on the heart. Pulmonary hypertension is often attenuated with milrinone, inhaled nitric oxide, prostacyclin, and/or sildenafil. Cardiac contractility and systemic blood pressure are supported with dobutamine, norepinephrine, epinephrine, and vasopressin. Notably, milrinone has the dual effect of both inotropy and pulmonary vasodilation, but its reduction of systemic vascular resistance must also be considered in the setting of hypotension.

Activation of the coagulation cascade in AFE results in DIC in up to 83% of cases and may occur without cardiovascular and respiratory signs (8). DIC is an accelerating consumptive coagulopathy that results in embolic/thrombotic complications of the microvasculature as well as hemorrhage. Thus it may present as both thrombosis and bleeding, particularly oozing in both the surgical field and around vascular access sites. Workup usually reveals thrombocytopenia, elevated PTT and PT/international normalized ratio, and low fibrinogen. D-dimer levels may be less useful as they are often already elevated during pregnancy. ROTEM may be helpful to elucidate specific coagulation cascade deficiencies and hyperfibrinolysis (11). Treatment of DIC often involves large volume transfusion of FFP and RBCs. The antithrombolytic drug tranexamic acid may be administered to help decrease clot breakdown. It is important to differentiate surgical blood loss, postpartum hemorrhage, and uterine atony from DIC, although they may occur simultaneously. Communication with the obstetrician can identify potential sources of surgical bleeding including occult lacerations, abnormal placentation, and poor uterine tone. Uterine atony should be treated with uterotonics such as oxytocin, methylergonovine, and carboprost tromethamine.

While replacement of RBCs during hemorrhage is clearly indicated, massive RBC transfusion can cause dilutional coagulopathy. Modern transfusion protocols often recommend 1:1:1 replacement of RBCs, plasma, and platelets, but adjustments to this ratio may be needed on a case-by-case basis. Some centers recommend a greater FFP to RBC replacement ratio (12–14). Cryoprecipitate should be used to treat hypofibrinogenemia while hyperfibrinolysis may benefit from tranexamic acid or aminocaproic acid. As mentioned earlier, ROTEM may be especially helpful for guiding transfusion and antifibrinolytics (12). Use of factor VII for AFE is controversial due to concerns about thrombosis, but it may be considered as a last resort in cases of refractory bleeding (8, 15).

Electrolyte derangements are common with transfusion, and close monitoring of arterial blood gases and blood chemistry is warranted during resuscitation. Profound acidemia can occur in the setting of poor perfusion, tissue hypoxia, rising lactate, and drug administration (e.g., boluses or infusions of epinephrine). Bicarbonate administration to normalize pH is controversial as bicarbonate is eventually converted to carbon dioxide, which can further exacerbate acidemia. Increased minute ventilation may need to be increased in this setting to help clear CO_2 and, if needed, induce respiratory alkalosis to offset metabolic acidosis. Large volumes of RBC transfusion can cause severe hyperkalemia, which can prevent successful resuscitation and recovery of cardiac function (16, 17). Kidney function may be compromised due to microvascular damage from thrombosis and ischemic damage from hypoperfusion. Calcium, bicarbonate, insulin, and glucose administration may help treat hyperkalemia, but renal replacement therapy in the form of continuous veno-veno hemodialysis may be necessary to treat acidemia and refractory hyperkalemia. Both RBC and plasma transfusion can significantly decrease levels of ionized calcium, further compromising cardiac activity and vascular tone, and calcium must be repleted aggressively during massive transfusion (17).

CARDIAC ARREST IN AFE

Cardiac arrest may quickly follow initial presentation of AFE due to acute systemic pulmonary hypertension, resulting in heart failure. In these cases, for parturients who have not yet delivered, standard Advanced Cardiac Life Support (ACLS) protocol should be modified to include left lateral tilt of the supine patient or manual lateral displacement of the gravid uterus to decrease aortocaval compression. When left lateral tilt is used, it is important to remember that chest compressions may be less effective since the heart is shifted laterally (18). Current recommendations are for delivery of the fetus at 4 minutes of cardiopulmonary resuscitation if return of spontaneous circulation has not been achieved. Box 22.3 includes current recommendations for ACLS for the parturient. Extracorporeal membrane oxygenation (ECMO) as a component of resuscitation is controversial as anticoagulation required for ECMO may exacerbate bleeding and profound coagulopathy, the third stage of the classic AFE triad (8).

NOVEL TREATMENTS

While management of AFE is largely supportive, there are case reports of novel therapies and approaches. There has been recent focus on treatment with ondansetron, ketorolac, and atropine (19). It is hypothesized that serotonin and thromboxane are components of the initial proinflammatory response in AFE and contribute to the development of acute pulmonary hypertension and the platelet aggregation that is an early step in the coagulation cascade (20). By blocking these interactions with a serotonin receptor antagonist such as ondansetron and a thromboxane inhibitor like ketorolac, further inflammation, cardiovascular collapse, and coagulopathy may be attenuated. The addition of

---

Box 22.3 MANAGEMENT OF CARDIAC ARREST IN THE PARTURIENT (ADAPTED FROM (9))

- Patient should be placed supine with continuous manual left lateral displacement of the uterus. When manual uterine lateral displacement is not available, left lateral tilt of the patient may be used but chest compressions may be less effective

- Early bag-mask ventilation at FiO2 100%. Due to airway changes during pregnancy including edema, equipment such as oral airways may be especially helpful for mask ventilation until advanced airway is secured

- Standard chest compression rate of at least 100 compressions per minute with a depth of at least 2 in (5 cm) with compression:ventilation ratio of 30:2

- Standard placement of hand position at lower half of the sternum for chest compressions

- Standard initial defibrillation energy setting of 120-200 J with subsequent escalation

- Anterolateral defibrillator pad should be placed under breast tissue

- Consider immediate cesarean delivery if no return of spontaneous circulation by 4 minutes

atropine is based on the hypothesis that vagal stimulation contributes to ventricular dysfunction. Other novel treatments include administration of C1 esterase inhibitor, which, besides inhibiting C1 esterase, also attenuates factor XIIa and complement activation and thus may improve symptoms of coagulopathy (19, 21).

OUTCOMES

In AFE patients who survive the initial stages of cardiovascular collapse, hypoxia, and coagulopathy, subsequent respiratory failure and lung injury patterns consistent with acute respiratory distress syndrome (ARDS) are often seen. ARDS and cardiogenic pulmonary edema may require lung protective mechanical ventilation and diuresis (1, 5, 19). Aggressive resuscitation with blood products may result in transfusion reactions. Hypoxia and impaired perfusion during the acute initial phases of AFE can result in end-organ injury and failure, including acute kidney injury that, in combination with possible electrolyte imbalances post-massive transfusion, may require renal replacement therapy. Patients may experience sepsis, contributing to hemodynamic instability, end-organ damage from hypoxia, and decreased perfusion, resulting in "shock liver" and exacerbating renal failure. Neurologic deficits are common, suffered by up to 85% of survivors (6), with severity of impairments correlating with incidence of cardiac arrest but are often out of proportion to the duration of cardiac arrest.

CONCLUSIONS

- AFE is a rare obstetric disorder presenting with a classic triad of respiratory distress, cardiovascular collapse, and DIC as a result of an abnormal maternal inflammatory response to amniotic/fetal material in the maternal circulation.

- Treatment of AFE is largely supportive and involves mechanical ventilation, invasive monitoring, treating pulmonary hypertension and heart failure with inotropes, vasopressors, and transfusion of blood products for DIC.

- Close monitoring of arterial blood gases and blood chemistry is imperative, and coagulation panels including ROTEM can help direct resuscitation.

- Cardiac arrest in AFE should be managed with standard ACLS using modifications for left lateral uterine displacement of the gravid uterus and consideration for perimortem cesarean delivery.

- Sequelae of AFE include respiratory failure from ARDS or cardiogenic pulmonary edema, sepsis, end-organ failure, and neurologic deficits.

REFERENCES

1. Fitzpatrick KE, Tuffnell D, Kurinczuk JJ, Knight M. Incidence, risk factors, management and outcomes of amniotic-fluid embolism: a population-based cohort and nested case-control study. BJOG. 2016 Jan;123(1):100–109.
2. Skolnik S, Ioscovich A, Eidelman LA, Davis A, Shmueli A et al. Anesthetic management of amniotic fluid embolism—a multi-center, retrospective, cohort study. J Matern Fetal Neonatal Med. 2019 Apr;32(8):1262–1266.
3. Bonnet MP, Zlotnik D, Saucedo M, Chassard D, Bouvier-Colle MH et al. Maternal Death Due to Amniotic Fluid Embolism: A National Study in France. Anesth Analg. 2018 Jan;126(1):175–182.
4. Shen F, Wang L, Yang W, Chen Y. From appearance to essence: 10 years review of atypical amniotic fluid embolism. Arch Gynecol Obstet. 2016 Feb;293(2):329–334.
5. Shamshirsaz AA, Clark SL. Amniotic fluid embolism. Obstet Gynecol Clin North Am. 2016 Dec;43(4):779–790.
6. Balinger KJ, Chu Lam MT, Hon HH, Stawicki SP, Anasti JN. Amniotic fluid embolism: despite progress, challenges remain. Curr Opin Obstet Gynecol. 2015 Dec;27(6):398–405.
7. Adamsons K, Mueller-Heubach E, Myers RE. The innocuousness of amniotic fluid infusion in the pregnant rhesus monkey. Am J Obstet Gynecol. 1971 Apr 1;109(7):977–984.
8. Pacheco LD, Saade G, Hankins GD, Clark SL. Amniotic fluid embolism: diagnosis and management. Am J Obstet Gynecol. 2016 Aug;215(2):B16–24.
9. Vasquez DN, Plante L, Basualdo MN, Plotnikow GG. Obstetric disorders in the ICU. Semin Respir Crit Care Med. 2017 Apr;38(2):218–234.
10. Fong A, Chau CT, Pan D, Ogunyemi DA. Amniotic fluid embolism: antepartum, intrapartum and demographic factors. J Matern Fetal Neonatal Med. 2015 May;28(7):793–798.
11. Erez O, Mastrolia SA, Thachil J. Disseminated intravascular coagulation in pregnancy: insights in pathophysiology, diagnosis and management. Am J Obstet Gynecol. 2015 Oct;213(4):452–463.
12. Butwick AJ, Goodnough LT. Transfusion and coagulation management in major obstetric hemorrhage. Curr Opin Anaesthesiol. 2015 Jun;28(3):275–284.
13. Pacheco LD, Saade GR, Costantine MM, Clark SL, Hankins GD. The role of massive transfusion protocols in obstetrics. Am J Perinatol. 2013 Jan;30(1):1–4.
14. Tanaka H, Katsuragi S, Osato K, Hasegawa J, Nakata M et al. Efficacy of transfusion with fresh-frozen plasma:red blood cell concentrate ratio of 1 or more for amniotic fluid embolism with coagulopathy: a case-control study. Transfusion. 2016 Dec;56(12):3042–3046.
15. Leighton BL, Wall MH, Lockhart EM, Phillips LE, Zatta AJ. Use of recombinant factor VIIa in patients with amniotic fluid embolism: a systematic review of case reports. Anesthesiology. 2011 Dec;115(6):1201–8.
16. Smith HM, Farrow SJ, Ackerman JD, Stubbs JR, Sprung J. Cardiac arrests associated with hyperkalemia during red blood cell transfusion: a case series. Anesth Analg. 2008 Apr;106(4):1062–1069.
17. Linko K, Saxelin I. Electrolyte and acid-base disturbances caused by blood transfusions. Acta Anaesthesiol Scand. 1986 Feb;30(2):139–144.
18. Jeejeebhoy FM, Zelop CM, Lipman S, Carvalho B, Joglar J et al. Cardiac arrest in pregnancy: a scientific statement from the American Heart Association. Circulation. 2015;132:1747–1773.
19. Sultan P, Seligman K, Carvalho B. Amniotic fluid embolism: update and review. Curr Opin Anaesthesiol. 2016 Jun;29(3):288–96.
20. Leanos OL, Hong E, Amezcua JL. Reflex circulatory collapse following intrapulmonary entrapment of activated platelets: mediation via 5-HT3 receptor stimulation. Br J Pharmacol. 1995 Oct;116(3):2048–2052.
21. Todo Y, Tamura N, Itoh H, Ikeda T, Kanayama N. Therapeutic application of C1 esterase inhibitor concentrate for clinical amniotic fluid embolism: a case report. Clin Case Rep. 2015 Jul;3(7):673–675.

REVIEW QUESTIONS

1. The classic triad of clinical symptoms see in patients experiencing amniotic fluid embolism include

   A. hypertension, coagulopathy, respiratory failure.
   B. hypoxia, right heart failure, coagulopathy.

C. change in mental status, hypoxia, circulatory collapse.
D. hypoxia, hyperthermia, left heart failure.

Answer: B. With the exception of hyperthermia (which has been suggested to be used a exclusionary factor in the diagnosis of AFE), each of the signs and symptoms listed may exist is a patient with AFE; however, the classic triad of signs and symptoms are hypoxia, right heart failure, and coagulopathy.

2. Diagnostic criteria for AFE include

A. sudden onset hypotension during labor.
B. hypoxia not responsive to administration of oxygen.
C. oozing from vascular access sites.
D. none of the above.

Answer: D. While A, B, and C are all possible symptoms of AFE, none of these are criteria for the diagnosis of AFE. In fact, there are no currently widely accepted criteria for the diagnosis of AFE, and the diagnosis should be by exclusion of more common diagnoses seen in the parturient.

3. The likely pathophysiological mechanism for AFE is best described as

A. abnormal maternal physiologic response to fetal material.
B. mechanical obstruction of blood flow within the right side of the heart.
C. translocation of fetal material into the maternal pulmonary circulation.
D. direct action of fetal material causing maternal pulmonary vasoconstriction.

Answer: A. While historically it was thought that AFE might be the result of embolic phenomenon or the presence of fetal material in the maternal circulation, more modern consideration of AFE has shown that if is due to an *abnormal maternal response* to fetal material in the maternal circulation.

4. When considering a diagnosis of amniotic fluid embolism, one must

A. confirm the diagnosis with a biomarker.
B. rule out other, more common diagnoses.
C. never begin treatment until the diagnosis is certain.
D. begin giving coagulation factors immediately.

Answer: B. Before settling on a diagnosis of AFE, especially if the symptoms are mild, one must rule out other, more common causes of the observed symptoms, including (but not limited to) sepsis, uterine atony, and pulmonary embolism. Even before the diagnosis is made, however, supportive care should be given. The choice to begin blood product transfusion should be guided by volume of blood loss and evaluation, either by clinical signs or laboratory value, of anemia or coagulopathy. While several biomarkers have been suggested for the diagnosis of AFE (zinc coproporphyrin, serum sialyl-Tn, Insulinlike-growth factor-binding protein-1), none are reliable or readily available.

5. Risk factors for AFE include all of the following *except*

A. artificial rupture of membranes.
B. polyhydramnios.

C. maternal age <25.
D. hypertensive disease of pregnancy.

Answer: C. Advanced maternal age (>35 years), not young maternal age, seems to be a risk factor for AFE.

6. All of the following lines or monitors may be useful in a patient experiencing AFE *except*

A. antecubital central venous catheter.
B. TEE.
C. arterial line.
D. central venous line.

Answer: A. In a patient experiencing AFE, TEE would be useful to evaluate the patient's volume status, as well as the contractility of her left and right ventricles. An arterial line would be useful to monitor potentially labile blood pressures and can be used for frequent blood sampling. A central venous line would be useful for transfusing large volumes of blood products as well as providing a conduit for potent vasopressors. An antecubital central venous catheter would be less useful than the other options listed. It could be used as a conduit for vasopressors, but due to its length and narrow gauge, it would not be useful for rapid blood transfusion.

7. ACLS in the pregnant patient is different than ACLS in the nonpregnant patient in the following way:

A. Epinephrine should be avoided due to effects on uterine blood flow.
B. Mask ventilation should be avoided in pregnant patients.
C. The mass effect of the gravid uterus should be counteracted in some way.
D. The rate of chest compressions should be at least 150/minute.

Answer: C. Under nonarrest circumstances, neither the administration of epinephrine nor mask ventilation would generally be recommended in pregnant patients, but, during an arrest, the primary consideration should be using proven techniques to aid in the return of spontaneous circulation. When doing CPR in the pregnant patient, either the patient should be put in a leftward tilt position or the gravid uterus should be manually laterally displaced.

8. Perimortem delivery of the fetus should be considered

A. never.
B. after 4 minutes of chest compressions.
C. after 10 minutes of chest compressions.
D. if fetal bradycardia is diagnosed through external fetal heart rate monitoring.

Answer: B. Perimortem delivery of the fetus should be considered after CPR has been ongoing without return of spontaneous circulation for 4 minutes.

9. Novel treatments for AFE include all of the following *except*

A. atropine.
B. ondansetron.

C. ketorolac.
D. metoclopromide.

Answer: D. Case reports have been published describing the use of atropine (to combat vagal tone), ondansetron (serotonin inhibitor), and ketorolac (thromboxane inhibitor) as novel treatments of AFE. There are no reports of metoclopromide being used to treat AFE.

10. Commonly seen outcomes of AFE include all of the following *except*

A. death.
B. long-term neurological deficit.
C. ARDS.
D. infertility.

Answer: D. Death following AFE occurs in up to 43% of patients. Neurological deficit is found in up to 85% of patients who have experienced AFE. Following AFE, the development if AFE is common. In patients who survive AFE who did not require hysterectomy as part of the surgical treatment of postpartum hemorrhage, infertility has not been described.

23.

OBSTRUCTIVE SLEEP APNEA WITH HYPERCARPNIA AND HYPOXIA AFTER LAPAROSCOPIC GASTRIC BYPASS SURGERY

Lauren Sutherland

STEM CASE AND KEY QUESTIONS

A 47-year-old male with morbid obesity and hypertension plans to undergo a laparoscopic gastric bypass surgery. He has a body mass index (BMI) of 55 and has failed dietary and lifestyle modifications to lose weight. He can walk about 1 block before becoming short of breath. His baseline blood pressure is 155/85. He does not smoke, but he has 2 alcoholic drinks daily before bed. His primary care physician suspects that he may have obstructive sleep apnea (OSA).

WHAT ARE THIS PATIENT'S RISK FACTORS FOR OSA? WHICH STOP-BANG CRITERIA DOES HE MEET?

On a further detailed history, the patient admits that he has been told by his wife that he snores heavily, and she has frequently seen him gasping for breath in his sleep. He works as an accountant and often finds it difficult to stay awake at work. On examination, his neck circumference is 50 cm.

HOW IS OSA DIAGNOSED?

The primary care physician sends the patient for a sleep study (i.e., polysomnography) to evaluate for OSA. The sleep study demonstrates an apnea-hypopnea index of 45 and a respiratory disturbance index of 60, and he desaturates as low as 75% during episodes of apnea. He is diagnosed with severe OSA.

HOW IS OSA MANAGED? HOW CAN THIS PATIENT BE OPTIMIZED FOR SURGERY?

Following the sleep study, the patient is prescribed continuous positive airway pressure (CPAP) at 15 cm H_2O. His insurance will not pay for the machine, so he does not receive it or start the therapy.

THE PATIENT PRESENTS FOR HIS GASTRIC BYPASS SURGERY. WHAT ARE SOME CONCERNS WITH ANESTHETIC MANAGEMENT OF A PATIENT WITH OSA? WHAT PRECAUTIONS CAN BE TAKEN IN AIRWAY MANAGEMENT?

One exam, he has a Mallampati score of 3 with a thyromental distance of 7 cm and significant redundant submental tissue. General anesthesia is induced, and the patient is bag-mask ventilated with 2 hands and an oral airway; he is intubated with a glidescope 4. During the procedure, the patient requires 80% inspired oxygen (FiO_2), frequent recruitment maneuvers, and positive end-expiratory pressure (PEEP) of 10 to maintain oxygen saturation (SpO_2) >95%. The surgery is otherwise uneventful; he is extubated to 6 L nasal cannula, and brought to the post-anesthesia care unit (PACU) without further monitoring.

WHAT ARE THE COMMON POSTOPERATIVE RESPIRATORY COMPLICATIONS IN PATIENTS WITH OSA?

On arrival to the PACU, he is noted to be somnolent and responsive only to painful stimuli, and an initial SpO_2 reads 88%. The patient is placed on a facemask nonrebreather at a flow of 15 L/minute. His oxygen saturation improves to 96%, but his respiratory rate decreases from 18 to 10; he remains somnolent with frequent apnea episodes observed. A right radial arterial line is placed, and the arterial blood gas (ABG) reads a pH of 7.16, pCO_2 of 70, and PaO_2 of 120.

WHAT IS THE DIFFERENTIAL DIAGNOSIS FOR THIS PATIENT'S SOMNOLENCE AND HYPOXEMIA?

The patient is diagnosed with hypercarbic respiratory failure, possibly due to excessive opioids or residual muscle weakness, and worsened by his underlying OSA. A dose of naloxone is administered with minimal improvement. The patient exhibits sustained tetanus on a train of 4 peripheral nerve stimulator.

HOW CAN HIS CONDITION BE MANAGED?

In hopes of avoiding reintubation, the patient is placed on a CPAP machine at a setting of 15 cm H_2O, and the FiO_2 is turned down to 40%. The patient's respiratory rate improves to 16 breaths per minute, and a follow-up ABG reads 7.32/50/108.

WHAT OTHER POSTOPERATIVE COMPLICATIONS MAY OCCUR IN PATIENTS WITH OSA?

Despite improvement of the ABG, the patient remains somnolent and is noted to have a right-sided facial droop with right-sided upper and lower extremity weakness. He is urgently intubated for airway protection, and he is taken for a noncontrast head CT scan. The scan reveals a large acute left middle cerebral artery stroke. He is taken to the neurological intensive care unit (ICU) for further management.

DISCUSSION

OSA is the most common type of sleep disordered breathing, and it is characterized by upper airway collapse resulting in episodes of apnea (complete cessation of breathing) and hypopnea (abnormal or shallow breathing) (1). These episodes are accompanied by oxygen desaturation, carbon dioxide retention, and sympathetic activation, resulting in daytime drowsiness and altered cardiopulmonary function (2, 3). Approximately 15% of the population of the United States is affected by OSA, a rising prevalence with the increasing rate of obesity (3). Undiagnosed and untreated OSA is extremely common, and with many recognized consequences of the disease, the health and cost burden of OSA is significant (1, 3). Patients who present for surgery should be screened for signs and symptoms of OSA, and caution should be taken with perioperative management.

ETIOLOGY AND PATHOGENESIS

During periods of sleep, especially rapid eye movement sleep, narrowing or closure of the upper airway may occur due to decreased neuromuscular tone or decreased upper airway muscle synchrony (4). Soft tissue compression (e.g., adipose tissue on the neck), tonsillar hypertrophy, or craniofacial skeletal abnormalities can predispose the airway to narrowing or collapse. Pharyngeal collapse leads to complete cessation of airflow despite breathing effort, leading to hypoxemia and hypercapnia. In normal sleep, peripheral chemoreceptors in the carotid body that mediate the response to hypercapnia and acidosis have a blunted response, resulting in a rise in carbon dioxide by 2 to 6 mmHg and fall in oxygen saturation by about 2% (4). Patients with OSA have increased sensitivity of these chemoreceptors, leading to an increased ventilatory effort in response to hypoxemia (4). Respiratory efforts against a narrowed or collapsed airway lead to profoundly negative intrathoracic pressure and a surge in sympathetic activity leading to hypertension and tachycardia. Eventual neurologic arousal restores upper airway patency and immediately suppresses this sympathetic activity.

Patients with OSA have overall increased sympathetic activation, both during sleep and wakefulness (4). Chronically increased sympathetic activity in patients with OSA results in baroreceptor dysfunction, leading to faster resting heart rate, decreased heart rate variability, and increased blood pressure variability (4, 5). These physiologic stresses lead to release of endogenous vasoactive substances such as endothelin, a potent vasoconstrictor, and decreased levels of nitric oxide, resulting in systemic and pulmonary vasoconstriction (5). There is evidence of increased levels of c-reactive protein (CRP), a marker of systemic inflammation, in patients with OSA with severity of OSA correlating to CRP level (6).

CLINICAL MANIFESTATIONS

Clinically, the OSA syndrome is defined by loud snoring, witnessed breathing interruptions, and awakenings gasping for breath, resulting in sleep fragmentation and daytime sleepiness. Additional symptoms include higher total amount of sleep, poor sleep quality, nocturia, insomnia, decreased concentration, morning headaches, memory loss, decreased libido, and irritability (7). Physical examination findings include central obesity, increased neck circumference, retrognathia, macroglossia, tonsillar hypertrophy, and nasal abnormalities.

Cardiovascular dysregulation from repeated episodes of apnea and hypopnea results in higher cardiovascular morbidity and a 2- to 3-fold risk of all-cause mortality (8). A causal relationship between OSA and hypertension, specifically resistant hypertension, has been demonstrated with more severe disease correlated with higher likelihood of hypertension (9). Severe OSA is independently correlated to increased risk of coronary artery disease (CAD) and mortality related to CAD (8). OSA is frequently observed in patients with congestive heart failure but may be underdiagnosed due to similar symptomatology; OSA is a risk factor for development of congestive heart failure, specifically in middle-age and older men (10). OSA is associated with nocturnal cardiac arrhythmias, and there is a strong association with atrial fibrillation, independent of other comorbid risk factors (11). There is a strong association between ischemic stroke and OSA, independent of other risk factors including hypertension (12, 13). Patients with OSA have impaired glucose tolerance and insulin resistance, and those with severe OSA have a 5-fold increase in risk of type 2 diabetes; the association of diabetes with OSA is independent of age, gender, BMI, and waist circumference (14). Daytime sleepiness caused by OSA can lead to decreased cognitive function, loss of work productivity, increased motor vehicle collisions, and poorer quality of life (15).

Obesity hypoventilation syndrome (OHS), a distinct disease defined by the triad of OSA, obesity, and daytime hypoventilation, has a prevalence of 10% to 20% in the OSA population (16). These patients demonstrate more significant upper airway obstruction (even in the supine position), reduced chest wall compliance, blunted central respiratory drive, and pulmonary hypertension. They exhibit a restrictive pattern on spirometry with a decreased forced expiratory volume (FEV1) and forced vital capacity (FVC) but normal FEV1/FVC ratio. Functional residual capacity, total lung capacity, and expiratory reserve volume are significantly reduced. The population of patients with OHS have a significantly higher rate of morbidity and mortality than patients who are similarly obese and have OSA (16).

RISK FACTORS

Male gender is a risk factor for OSA, with a prevalence of 24% in men 9% in women in the United States (3); however, women with OSA are less likely to be evaluated and diagnosed (1). Prevalence also increases with age, is highest in the 40 to 70 age range, and plateaus after age 65 (1). There is a steady increase in OSA risk with increasing BMI, specifically central obesity and increased neck circumference. Craniofacial abnormalities such as maxillary or mandibular dysmorphisms, narrow nasal cavities, and tonsillar hypertrophy place patients at higher risk. Additionally, there is likely a genetic component with increased risk in some nonobese families, specifically in the Asian population (1). Other suspected risk factors include smoking, hormonal changes due to menopause, acute alcohol use, and nasal congestion (1).

Several preoperative screening tools have been created to aid stratifying patients based on risk of OSA including the Berlin Questionnaire, the American Society of Anesthesiologists checklist, and the STOP-BANG questionnaire (17, 18). The STOP-BANG questionnaire has been validated in a surgical population; patients scoring less than 3 can be ruled out for OSA while a score of 5 to 8 places a patient at high probability of having moderate to severe OSA (17).

DIAGNOSTIC MODALITIES

Patients suspected to have OSA should undergo a comprehensive sleep history, evaluation of secondary conditions that may occur as a result of OSA, and a physical examination. Those deemed high risk should undergoing objective testing, either an in-laboratory polysomnography or home testing with portable monitors (7). Polysomnography involves recording of several physiologic measures, including heart rate, oxygen saturation, respiratory effort, airflow, electrocardiogram, electroencephalogram, electrooculogram, and chin electromyogram. The apnea-hypopnea index (AHI), or number of episodes of apnea or hypopnea per hour of sleep, and the respiratory disturbance index, which also includes respiratory effort related arousals, are ways to quantify the presence and grade the severity of OSA. An AHI of 5 in the presence of symptoms or an AHI of 15 without sleep-related symptoms is sufficient for diagnosis of OSA (7). Additionally, AHI can be used to categorize patients into mild (5 to 15), moderate (15 to 30) or severe (greater than 30) OSA. Portable monitors may be used for home-monitoring in patients with a high pretest probability of OSA.

TREATMENTS

Treatment of OSA aims to decrease apnea and hypopnea episodes as well as decrease sleep fragmentation. Interventions include behavioral modifications, devices for improved ventilation and oxygenation, and surgical interventions. Behavioral modification such as avoidance of alcohol or other sedating medications, proper sleep positioning (i.e., avoiding the supine position) and weight loss and exercise are recommended to all patients with OSA (7). Weight loss through lifestyle and dietary modification has been shown to significantly improve OSA severity, though not fully normalize symptoms (19). Bariatric surgery is a definitive treatment for OSA, with more invasive procedures (e.g., gastric bypass and biliopancreatic diversion) having the most profound effects on symptomatology (20). Positive airway pressure (PAP) devices including continuous mode (CPAP), bilevel (BiPAP), or autotitrating (APAP) may be applied through a nasal or full face mask to stent open the collapsing upper airways, and these devices are recommended to decrease apnea and hypopnea episodes in patients with OSA (7). Randomized controlled trials and meta-analyses have demonstrated reduction in apnea and hypopnea episodes, improvement in daytime sleepiness, improved quality of life, and a modest reduction systemic blood pressure with use of PAP devices (21), but there has not been a demonstrated reduction in cardiovascular events or a mortality benefit (22). Oral appliances that protrude the mandible or hold the tongue in a more anterior position can decrease upper airway collapsibility and may be utilized in patients with mild to moderate OSA who fail or decline CPAP therapy (7).

OPERATIVE MANAGEMENT

OSA is common in patients who present for general surgery and is present in up to 70% of patients who present for bariatric surgery (23). Patients with OSA are more susceptible to the respiratory depressant effects of sedatives and analgesics, and they are at risk for more cardiopulmonary complications perioperatively, including hypercapnia and hypoxemia, higher reintubation rates, cardiac arrhythmias, myocardial injury, delirium, unplanned ICU admissions, and longer hospital stays (24). The Society of Anesthesia and Sleep Medicine Guidelines on Preoperative Screening and Assessment of Adult Patients with OSA released recommendations in 2016 for preoperative management of this patient population (2). Patients should be risk stratified using the previously mentioned screening tools. While it is not recommended to delay surgery to perform more advance screening in patients at high risk for OSA, additional precautions may be taken such as allowing additional evaluation for comorbid uncontrolled systemic diseases and having positive airway pressure devices for perioperative use. Patients should continue to use positive airway pressure devices preoperatively through the time of surgery.

Anesthetic medications such as propofol, halogenated gases, opioids, and benzodiazepines cause an increased propensity for upper airway collapse and prevent the protective neurologic arousal and ventilatory response to hypercapnia and hypoxemia (23). The American Society of Anesthesiologists Practice Guidelines for the Perioperative Management of Patients with OSA recommend preferential selection of anesthetics and techniques such as local anesthetics, neuraxial anesthetics, or peripheral nerve blockade when possible (26). For moderate sedation, monitoring should include continuous capnography, and considering use of PAP devices, and there should be avoidance of deep sedation in favor of general anesthesia with a secure airway. Prior to induction of general anesthesia, sedatives for anxiolysis should be avoided when possible. Preoxygenation should occur with 100% oxygen and CPAP of 10 cm H_2O with the patient in a head-up position until an expired oxygen content of 90% is achieved. OSA is an independent risk factor for difficult mask ventilation and intubation but not supraglottic airway use (26); this patient population often has many predictors of difficult intubation including high Mallampati score, decreased thyromental distance, and increased neck circumference. Mask ventilation and endotracheal intubation should be undertaken by skilled practitioners with emergency airway equipment available and consideration of awake fiberoptic intubation in certain patients.

Intraoperative monitoring should be based on the type of surgery and patient comorbidities, but invasive arterial monitoring may be useful if noninvasive blood pressure measurements are unreliable or for ABG monitoring. Hypoxemia resulting from atelectasis and intrapulmonary shunt frequently occurs with mechanical ventilation intraoperatively may require higher PEEP and FiO_2. Ventilation may be more difficult due to increased extrathoracic pressure from adipose tissue. There should be a high index of suspicion for pulmonary hypertension related to obesity hypoventilation syndrome, and normal pH, PaO_2 and PCO_2 levels should be maintained to avoid pulmonary hypertensive crisis. Patients with OSA should be extubated on when fully awake, with verification of full muscle relaxation reversal, and in the non-supine position (26). Analgesia should be accomplished through regional techniques, nonsteroidal anti-inflammatory medications, and other methods with avoidance of opioid medications when possible.

POSTOPERATIVE MANAGEMENT AND INTENSIVE CARE

Postoperative management of patients with OSA or suspected OSA emphasizes appropriate monitoring for cardiopulmonary compromise and avoidance of medications that may result in respiratory depression. Continuous monitoring, specifically with pulse oximetry, should occur in a critical care or step-down unit by telemetry or an appropriately trained observer (26). There should be caution is usage of sedating medications such as opioids, benzodiazepines, or barbiturates. When systemic opioids are necessary, long-acting opioids or opioid infusions should be avoided in favor of patient-controlled analgesia delivery devices. Analgesic adjuvants with

less propensity for decreasing respiratory drive such as ketamine, dexmedetomidine may be useful for decreasing opioid requirements.

PAP devices should be used continuously in the postoperative period by patients who used them preoperatively as well as in those patients exhibiting frequent airway obstruction. Supplemental oxygen may be used when needed as patients are at risk of hypoxemia in the perioperative period; however, caution should be taken as supplemental oxygen may results in longer apneic episodes by suppression of hypoxic respiratory drive. Additionally, supplemental oxygen may delay detection of atelectasis, hypoventilation, or apnea on pulse oximetry. Specifically in patients with OHS, supplemental oxygen should be avoided whenever possible, and if necessary should be used concurrently with PAP. Patients with OSA may require longer stays in the recovery area and should not be discharged until demonstration of ability to maintain an adequate oxygen saturation while breathing room air in an unstimulated environment (26).

CONCLUSIONS

- OSA is a the most common type of sleep disordered breathing, and the prevalence is increasing with rising rates of obesity.

- Symptoms of OSA include snoring, daytime drowsiness, and observed apnea. Risk factors include male gender, increasing age, obesity, and high neck circumference.

- Diagnosis of OSA is made through polysomnography, and PAP is the mainstay of OSA management.

- Patients undergoing surgery should be screened for OSA through use of the STOP-BANG questionnaire, Berlin Questionnaire, or the American Society of Anesthesiologists checklist preoperatively. There should be a high index of suspicion for other comorbid conditions that are frequently associated with OSA.

- Patients with OSA or suspected OSA should be managed with special caution intraoperatively including prudent airway management, avoidance of long-acting sedating medications, and close hemodynamic monitoring. Postoperatively, patients require close monitoring for an extended period of time, and PAP devices should be utilized to prevent hypoventilation.

REFERENCES

1. Young, T., et al. (2004). "Risk factors for obstructive sleep apnea in adults." JAMA 291(16): 2013–2016.
2. Chung, F., et al. (2016). "Society of Anesthesia and Sleep Medicine guidelines on preoperative screening and assessment of adult patients with obstructive sleep apnea." Anesth Analg 123(2): 452–473.
3. Young, T., et al. (2009). "Burden of sleep apnea: rationale, design, and major findings of the Wisconsin Sleep Cohort study." WMJ 108(5): 246–249.

4. Caples, S. M., et al. (2005). "Obstructive sleep apnea." Ann Intern Med 142(3): 187–197.
5. Shamsuzzaman, A. S., et al. (2003). "Obstructive sleep apnea: implications for cardiac and vascular disease." JAMA 290(14): 1906–1914.
6. Shamsuzzaman, A. S., et al. (2002). "Elevated C-reactive protein in patients with obstructive sleep apnea." Circulation 105(21): 2462–2464.
7. Epstein, L. J., et al. (2009). "Clinical guideline for the evaluation, management and long-term care of obstructive sleep apnea in adults." J Clin Sleep Med 5(3): 263–276.
8. Punjabi, N. M., et al. (2009). "Sleep-disordered breathing and mortality: a prospective cohort study." PLoS Med 6(8): e1000132.
9. Peppard, P. E., et al. (2000). "Prospective study of the association between sleep-disordered breathing and hypertension." N Engl J Med 342(19): 1378–1384.
10. Gottlieb, D. J., et al. (2010). "Prospective study of obstructive sleep apnea and incident coronary heart disease and heart failure: the sleep heart health study." Circulation 122(4): 352–360.
11. Cadby, G., et al. (2015). "Severity of OSA is an independent predictor of incident atrial fibrillation hospitalization in a large sleep-clinic cohort." Chest 148(4): 945–952.
12. Redline, S., et al. (2010). "Obstructive sleep apnea-hypopnea and incident stroke: the sleep heart health study." Am J Respir Crit Care Med 182(2): 269–277.
13. Yaggi, H. K., et al. (2005). "Obstructive sleep apnea as a risk factor for stroke and death." N Engl J Med 353(19): 2034–2041.
14. Punjabi, N. M., et al. (2004). "Sleep-disordered breathing, glucose intolerance, and insulin resistance: the Sleep Heart Health Study." Am J Epidemiol 160(6): 521–530.
15. George, C. F. (2007). "Sleep apnea, alertness, and motor vehicle crashes." Am J Respir Crit Care Med 176(10): 954–956.
16. Chau, E. H., et al. (2012). "Obesity hypoventilation syndrome: a review of epidemiology, pathophysiology, and perioperative considerations." Anesthesiology 117(1): 188–205.
17. Chung, F., et al. (2012). "High STOP-BANG score indicates a high probability of obstructive sleep apnoea." Br J Anaesth 108(5): 768–775.
18. Chung, F., et al. (2008). "Validation of the Berlin questionnaire and American Society of Anesthesiologists checklist as screening tools for obstructive sleep apnea in surgical patients." Anesthesiology 108(5): 822–830.
19. Araghi, M. H., et al. (2013). "Effectiveness of lifestyle interventions on obstructive sleep apnea (OSA): systematic review and meta-analysis." Sleep 36(10): 1553–1562, 1562A–1562E.
20. Sarkhosh, K., et al. (2013). "The impact of bariatric surgery on obstructive sleep apnea: a systematic review." Obes Surg 23(3): 414–423.
21. Jonas, D. E., et al. (2017). "Screening for Obstructive sleep apnea in adults: evidence report and systematic review for the US Preventive Services Task Force." JAMA 317(4): 415–433.
22. McEvoy, R. D., et al. (2016). "CPAP for prevention of cardiovascular events in obstructive sleep apnea." N Engl J Med 375(10): 919–931.
23. Adesanya, A. O., et al. (2010). "Perioperative management of obstructive sleep apnea." Chest 138(6): 1489–1498.
24. Kaw, R., et al. (2012). "Postoperative complications in patients with obstructive sleep apnea." Chest 141(2): 436–441.
25. Leong, S. M., et al. (2018). "Obstructive sleep apnea as a risk factor associated with difficult airway management: a narrative review." J Clin Anesth 45: 63–68.
26. American Society of Anesthesiologists Task Force on Perioperative Management of Patients With Obstructive Sleep Apnea. (2014). "Practice guidelines for the perioperative management of patients with obstructive sleep apnea: an updated report by the American Society of Anesthesiologists Task Force on Perioperative Management of patients with obstructive sleep apnea." Anesthesiology 120(2): 268–286.

REVIEW QUESTIONS

1. A 50-year-old obese man presents for polysomnography to evaluate for OSA. His AHI is reported as 20. Based on this information, how severe is his OSA?

   A. He does not have OSA
   B. Mild OSA
   C. Moderate OSA
   D. Severe OSA

2. A 65-year old woman presents for a laparoscopic cholecystectomy. She is 153 cm tall and weighs 100 kg and has a neck circumference of 42 cm. Her blood pressure is 155/90. She admits to frequent daytime sleepiness and snoring loudly, but she has never been observed to have apnea episodes. What is her STOP-BANG score?

   A. 5
   B. 6
   C. 7
   D. 8

3. For the patient described in question 2, what is her risk of OSA?

   A. Low risk
   B. Intermediate risk
   C. High risk
   D. Cannot be determined

4. A patient is newly diagnosed with OSA and asks what other diseases and conditions he is at risk for. Which of the following is correct?

   A. OSA is a risk factor for development of hypertension, and he should periodically have his blood pressure checked.
   B. Patients with OSA always develop pulmonary hypertension, and they are at risk for cardiac arrest during surgical procedures.
   C. Patients with OSA have an increased risk of ischemic stroke, only because of the increased risk of hypertension.
   D. Ninety percent of patients with OSA also have type 2 diabetes.

5. A 66-year-old obese male with hypertension and an acute small bowel obstruction presents for small bowel resection. On your preanesthesia assessment, you discover that he has a STOP-BANG score of 7. He has never undergone a sleep study and does not have a diagnosis of OSA. How would you proceed?

   A. Cancel the procedure and obtain a sleep study.
   B. Delay the procedure and obtain a stress echocardiogram.
   C. Inform the patient that he has OSA and that he should use CPAP at home.
   D. Because this is an urgent procedure, proceed with extra caution due the high likelihood of OSA and associated perioperative risk.

6. A patient with severe OSA and hypertension, but a normal stress echocardiogram last month is scheduled to undergo a bilateral total knee replacement. How would you manage the anesthetic for the procedure?

A. Proceed with combined spinal epidural with light sedation for anesthesia during the procedure and utilize the epidural for postoperative pain control.

B. Proceed with spinal anesthesia with deep sedation using propofol.

C. Proceed with general endotracheal anesthesia with IV fentanyl and hydromorphone for postoperative pain.

D. Recommend that the patient undergo further cardiopulmonary evaluation prior to the procedure.

7. A patient with morbid obesity, severe OSA, and OHS presents for a laparoscopic colectomy for diverticulitis. What would be your anesthetic concerns for the procedure?

A. Difficulty ventilating the patient due to high extra-thoracic pressure from adipose tissue as well as high intra-abdominal pressure from insufflation for a laparoscopic procedure.

B. Hypercapnia from abdominal insufflation with carbon dioxide for a laparoscopic procedure.

C. Precipitation of pulmonary hypertensive crisis due to this patient's OHS and potential hypoxemia, hypercapnia, and acidosis during the procedure.

D. All of the above

8. A 35-year old woman with OSA arrives to the PACU following a salpingectomy for ectopic pregnancy. What extra precautions would you take in managing her in the postoperative period?

A. Administration of oxygen through a face mask non-rebreather to ensure she does not become hypoxic.

B. Administration CPAP through her home mask that she brought with her to the hospital.

C. Close monitoring with capnography and pulse oximetry to ensure adequate oxygenation and ventilation.

D. B and C

9. A 75-year-old man with OSA has been recovering in the ICU for 2 days following an aortic valve replacement. His postoperative issues have been hypoxia and hypercapnia requiring prolonged intubation. How would you optimize this patient for extubation?

A. Sit him upright, turn off all sedation, minimize the FiO_2 while maintaining an adequate SpO_2, and extubate to BiPAP as soon as can be done safely.

B. Sit him upright, place him on 100% FiO_2, and extubate him to high-flow nasal cannula as soon as can be done safely.

C. Place him in the supine position, administer low-dose sedation to ensure anxiolysis, and extubate to BiPAP as soon as can be done safely.

D. Keep him intubated for as long as possible to ensure adequate airway protection.

10. A patient with OSA and OHS is managed in the ICU 3 days following an exploratory laparotomy for perforated diverticulosis. In attempt to prepare the patient for extubation, you have discontinued all sedation and sat him in the upright position. He is placed on pressure support ventilation with an inspiratory pressure of 10 and a PEEP of 5. His respiratory rate is 8 breaths per minute. An ABG shows a pH of 7.2, PCO_2 70, PaO_2 104. What factors could explain the patient's respiratory acidosis?

A. Residual opioid effects from the fentanyl infusion that was discontinued 1 hour ago, causing hypoventilation.

B. Decreased central respiratory drive from OHS is causing hypoventilation.

C. With the inspiratory pressure of 10, he is taking tidal volumes of 25 cc due to reduced chest wall compliance.

D. All of the above

ANSWERS

1. Answer: C. Based on an AHI of 20, this patient has moderate OSA. Mild OSA is 5 to 15 episodes of apnea or hypopnea per hour, moderate is an AHI of 15 to 30, and severe is greater than 30.

2. Answer: B. This patient receives points for snoring, tired, pressure (hypertension), BMI greater than 35, age greater than 50, and neck circumference greater than 41 cm. She does not receive points for female gender or for observed apnea. This gives her a score of 6.

3. Answer: C. A STOP-BANG score of 6 gives the patient a high risk of having OSA.

4. Answer: A. Studies have demonstrated a causal relationship between OSA and hypertension. While a portion of patients with OSA develop OHS, not all patients with OSA have pulmonary hypertension. The risk of ischemic stroke in patients with OSA is independent of other factors such as hypertension. Patients with OSA have a 5-fold increase in risk of type 2 diabetes.

5. Answer: D. A small bowel obstruction requires urgent surgery and should not be delayed for further workup, even if there is high suspicion of OSA. While other comorbid conditions should be suspected in patients with OSA, having a stress echocardiogram is not appropriate for this patient who requires an urgent procedure. While the patient has a high likelihood of OSA, the patient should undergo polysomnography for official diagnosis of OSA and to guide recommendations on treatment.

6. Answer: A. This patient would benefit from avoidance of IV opioids during the perioperative period. Utilization of a combined spinal epidural would provide adequate anesthesia for the procedure as well as analgesia postoperatively. Deep sedation should be avoided in patients with OSA, as they are prone to airway obstruction intraoperatively.

7. Answer: D. Laparoscopic surgery may be extremely challenging in an obese patient with OSA and OHS, specifically because of high intra-abdominal pressure from insufflation, absorption of CO_2 through the peritoneum, and high risk of

pulmonary hypertension in this patient population. It may be advisable to recommend to the surgeon that the patient have an open procedure, rather than a laparoscopic one.

8. Answer: D. It is important to closely monitor patients with OSA in the postoperative period due to their propensity for airway obstruction related to anesthetic sensitivity and higher risk of cardiopulmonary complications. While ensuring patients do not become hypoxic is important, administration of excessive oxygen can hide hypoventilation or atelectasis and may result in longer apneic episodes by suppression of hypoxic respiratory drive.

9. Answer: A. Patients with OSA should be extubated in a timely manner to promote early mobilization, decrease atelectasis, and limit administration of sedative medications. To optimize a patient for extubation, he should be fully awake, placed in the upright position, FiO_2 limited to promote ventilation, and extubated to a PAP device.

10. Answer: D. Patients with OHS are highly sensitive to opioid-induced ventilatory impairment, and there may be residual effects from the fentanyl infusion. These patients also have decreased central respiratory drive, and ventilation may be more difficult due to decreased chest wall compliance.

24.

MESENTERIC ISCHEMIA WITH DEAD BOWEL AFTER MAJOR ABDOMINAL SURGERY

Robert Bowen and Liang Shen

STEM CASE AND KEY QUESTIONS

A 66-year-old woman with a history of diverticulitis and pancreatic cancer presents for Whipple procedure. Intraoperatively, dense adhesions were encountered which required prolonged dissection and operative time, with high blood loss and need for blood product transfusions and moderate-dose vasopressors. She was transferred to the surgical intensive care unit (ICU) intubated and sedated and requiring norepinephrine infusion to maintain blood pressure.

WHAT ARE RISK FACTORS FOR MESENTERIC ISCHEMIA? WHAT ARE THE SIGNS AND SYMPTOMS OF MESENTERIC ISCHEMIA, AND WHAT STUDIES CAN HELP WITH ITS DIAGNOSIS?

Over the next 8 hours, she is increasingly hypotensive, requires increasing doses of norepinephrine despite several liters of crystalloid fluid as well as pack red blood cell transfusions. Over this time period, her white blood cell and serum lactate level trend upward, and she experiences increasing abdominal distension and agitation requiring escalating doses of sedatives. The ICU team is concerned about acute abdomen and bowel ischemia.

WHAT ARE THE TYPES OF MESENTERIC ISCHEMIA, AND HOW DO THEY DIFFER IN PRESENTATION AND DIAGNOSIS?

An abdominal computed tomography (CT) scan with intravenous (IV) contrast is ordered to evaluate for acute abdominal process, which demonstrated distended, thin-walled small bowel loops with mesenteric pneumatosis and poorly visualized superior mesenteric artery (SMA) branches without clear evidence of vascular occlusion.

WHAT IS THE INITIAL TREATMENT OF MESENTERIC ISCHEMIA?

The patient is started on broad-spectrum antibiotics and taken to the operating room emergently. Intraoperatively, a portion of small bowel is noted to be ischemic and resected.

DO ALL PATIENTS WITH MESENTERIC ISCHEMIA REQUIRE EMERGENT SURGERY? WHAT OTHER TREATMENT OPTIONS ARE THERE, AND WHEN ARE THEY APPROPRIATE?

The patient returns to the ICU on a lower dose of norepinephrine. Over the next several hours, the patient is fluid-resuscitated, and norepinephrine is able to be titrated off. Her lactate level normalizes with IV fluids (Table 24.1).

Table 24.1 DISTINGUISHING CHARACTERISTICS OF TYPES OF MESENTERIC ISCHEMIA[1,7]

SUBTYPE	MOST COMMON ETIOLOGY	COMMON COMORBIDITIES	MOST COMMON VESSELS AFFECTED	PREFERRED IMAGING FOR DIAGNOSIS
Acute	Embolism	Atrial fibrillation or tachyarrhythmia, coronary artery disease, previous myocardial infarction	Superior mesenteric artery	Dual phase CT with angiography
Chronic	Atherosclerosis	Peripheral vascular disease, coronary artery disease	Diffuse	Dual phase CT with angiography
Nonocclusive	Decreased cardiac output	Shock, postoperative state, digitalis use, vasopressor use, long term hemodialysis	Diffuse	Angiography
Venous	Thrombosis	Hypercoagulability, previous deep vein thrombosis, hepatocellular carcinoma, paraneoplastic syndrome	Diffuse	Dual phase CT with angiography

Sources: Carver TW, Vora RS, Taneja A. Mesenteric ischemia. Critical Care Clinics. 2016;32(2):155–171; Klar E, Rahmanian PB, Bücker A. Acute mesenteric ischemia: a vascular emergency. Dtsch Arztebl Int. 2012;109(14):249–256.

FINDING	SENSITIVITY	SPECIFICITY
Pneumatosis, portal venous gas	5–60%	100%
Bowel wall thinning	40%	88%
Bowel wall thickening	85–88%	61–72%
Bowel dilatation	39–67%	29–81%
Absent bowel wall enhancement	88–100%	18–60%
Mesenteric fat stranding	96%	28–68%
Ascites	71%	31–83%
Bowel wall hyperattenuation (on non-contrast CT scan)	90–98%	10–18%

Source: Copin P, Zins M, Nuzzo A, et al. Acute mesenteric ischemia: a critical role for the radiologist. Diagnostic and Interventional Imaging. 2018;99:123–134.

WHAT IS THE PROGNOSIS OF PATIENTS WITH MESENTERIC ISCHEMIA?

After a prolonged ICU course complicated by delirium, hospital-acquired pneumonia, and surgical wound infection, the patient is able to be transferred to a subacute rehabilitation center on postoperative day 32 (Table 24.2).

DISCUSSION

Mesenteric ischemia results from decreased perfusion to the mesenteric blood vessels, leading to tissue hypoxia supplied by these vessels. This decreased perfusion can occur by several etiologies and, if left untreated, ultimately leads to tissue death, bowel necrosis, sepsis, and, commonly, death.

PRESENTATION

Patients with compromised mesentery can present in several fashions, and the presentation can vary based on the etiology and the chronicity of the condition. It is not a common condition, with prevalence estimated to be between 0.1 to 1 cases per 1000 hospital admissions.[1,2] Restricted to patients with acute abdomen, acute mesenteric ischemia represents approximately 1% of cases, and 10% when evaluating acute abdomen in patients greater than 70 years of age. This condition is slightly more common in women.[1,3] Patients with chronic mesenteric ischemia will generally present with symptoms of food avoidance ("food fear") because of post-prandial pain. Patients with acute mesenteric ischemia, typically aged in their 60s or 70s, will present with abdominal pain, typically out of proportion to exam. They also commonly complain of nausea, vomiting, and diarrhea. Fecal occult blood testing is frequent but not universally positive. Clinical symptoms include tachycardia. It is only very late in the disease process that patients may display peritoneal signs, such as distention, rigidity, guarding, and rebound tenderness. Peritoneal signs are only reported in 16% of patients.[1] The patient may present with sepsis or shock if left untreated for a long period of time.

ETIOLOGY

Historically, the most common cause of acute mesenteric ischemia is cardioembolic in origin. The SMA, due to its angle of origin, is preferentially impaired by the embolus. The cause of the embolus is generally related to atrial tachyarrhythmias such as atrial fibrillation but may also be from heart failure or cardiomyopathy. More recently, mesenteric ischemia from an arterial thrombotic etiology has been considered approximately equivalent to mesenteric ischemia from arterial embolic origin.[1] Approximately one-third of all patients with SMA embolus have a history of previous embolic event.[1] Dissection or inflammation is associated with a small minority of cases—less than 5%.[3]

The condition can also present in a chronic form, in which patients have had borderline oxygen delivery over the long term and have grown reliant on collateral circulation. Chronic mesenteric ischemia is overwhelmingly associated with arterial atherosclerosis, and when patients ultimately occlude a large vessel, they frequently do not present with the same acute symptomatology.[1,3]

Low cardiac output states are considered responsible for 20% to 30% of cases of mesenteric ischemia, referred to as nonocclusive mesenteric ischemia (NOMI).[2] In these cases, there can be decreased forward flow or increased resistance to flow, whether from intravascular/vascular causes (arterial vasoconstriction) or extravascular causes (increased intra-abdominal pressure). This etiology tends to be more common in older patients with pre-existing liver or kidney disease, major abdominal surgery, cardiac surgery, or cardiac conditions that would result in low forward-flow, like congestive heart failure, aortic insufficiency, or myocardial infarction. High postoperative vasopressor utilization, transfusion requirement, and surgical reexploration were most closely associated with the occurrence of NOMI after cardiac surgery. There is also an association with the utilization of intra-aortic balloon pump, likely related to potential malpositioning of the balloon, which can occlude mesenteric vessels. The alterations in microcirculation during vasopressor administration, resulting from α-receptor agonism and increased intestinal metabolism from β-receptor agonism, are theorized as culprits for mesenteric ischemia. Enteral feeding in situations of high vasopressor use is thought to worsen the imbalance between oxygen supply and demand and can precipitate ischemia. In NOMI, the entire intestine can suffer damage, as blood supply is universally decreased. The right colon, distal jejunum, and ileum tend to be more affected than other regions.

Impaired venous drainage accounts for approximately 10% of cases of mesenteric ischemia.[2] In these cases, symptoms tend to be less acute. Acute occlusion of the superior mesenteric vein leads to gradual venous engorgement, swelling, and hemorrhage. Factor V Leiden is the most common cause of venous thrombosis in these patients.[2]

ANATOMY

The celiac artery supplies the foregut—the esophagus through the second portion of the duodenum. Collateral circulation exists to the SMA via the pancreaticoduodenal arteries and, rarely, the arc of Buhler. The SMA supplies the midgut—the third portion of the duodenum through the splenic flexure of the colon. Superior to inferior mesenteric arterial collateral circulation exists via the arc of Riolan and the marginal artery of Drummond. The inferior mesenteric artery supplies the hindgut—the distal colon to the distal sigmoid colon, with hemorrhoidal arteries providing collateral circulation to the iliac arteries. Perfusion is tightly controlled on a local level, with 70% of post-prandial blood flow shunting to relevant mucosa.[1,2]

In half of patients with embolic SMA occlusion, the occlusion takes place distal to the takeoff of the middle colic, sparing the proximal jejunum via the inferior pancreaticoduodenal arteries but ultimately causing ischemia to the rest of the small bowel. In 15% of patients with embolic disease, the occlusion occurs at the origin of the SMA, causing ischemia from duodenum through transverse colon. For patients with thrombotic disease, the occlusion most commonly occurs at the origin of the SMA.[1]

For patients with venous thrombosis, varied patterns exist. There can either be micro-thrombi resulting from inflammatory states or large vessel thrombi affecting larger areas. NOMI appears similarly to small vessel venous thrombosis, with differential perfusion and ischemia on a microscopic and macroscopic level.[6]

RADIOLOGIC EVALUATION

Multiphasic CT with angiography is typically the imaging of choice in mesenteric ischemia, with approximate sensitivity of 94% and specificity of 95%.[6,7] Early in the disease process, thrombus or embolus may be detected in the arterial blood vessels, with contracted loops of small intestine in the affected area. Later in the disease process, the bowel walls will appear thin and gas filled, and ascites may be present. Eventually parietal, mesenteric, and portal pneumatosis may develop. Ultimately perforation will demonstrate pneumoperitoneum or retro-pneumoperitoneum.[1] NOMI is more difficult to detect on CT scan, but findings are similar to occlusive mesenteric ischemia except for lack of thrombus or embolus. Findings previously described in NOMI include diffuse narrowing of the SMA with poor visualization of secondary branches.[6] As compared to that of acute arterial ischemia, imaging of venous mesenteric ischemia will demonstrate more prominent edema and swelling of the affected tissues, with free fluid noted in the peritoneal cavity on CT scan in some instances. On surgical exploration the bowel tends to appear edematous and red.[5]

Magnetic resonance angiography (MRA) is not typically preferred for the diagnosis of mesenteric ischemia as it overestimates arterial stenosis, prolongs time to diagnosis, and thus is less cost-effective. Ultrasound can detect vessel occlusion, but it is difficult to obtain adequate imaging, particularly given the dilated loops of bowel and body habitus that may prevent adequate visualization of mesenteric vasculature.[3]

Selective mesenteric angiography is not considered the gold standard for mesenteric ischemia overall, as it is unable to discern alternative sources of abdominal pain in patients for whom mesenteric ischemia is not the sole suspicion. However, it can be used to confirm and treat suspected cases of NOMI.[1–3] Angiography in these patients will demonstrate mesenteric vasospasm, contrast reflux into the aorta, and delayed portal vein filling.[8] Additionally, angiography can offer a means for immediate treatment with selective administration of vasodilators.[2,4]

LABORATORY TESTING

White blood cell count, lactate, and d-dimer are commonly elevated in acute mesenteric ischemia. Due to the elevated lactate, patients also typically demonstrate a metabolic acidosis on arterial blood gas analysis. Concomitant conditions (e.g. infection causing elevated lactate, vomiting causing metabolic alkalosis) can confound laboratory values.[2,9,10] More dedicated testing utilizing intestinal fatty acid binding protein levels in the urine has demonstrated some promise for distinguishing acute mesenteric ischemia from other causes of abdominal pain, but the studies are limited by small sample size. The pooled sensitivity for this test was noted to be 0.80, while pooled specificity was noted to be 0.85.[11]

For chronic mesenteric ischemia, tests for nutritional status, such as albumin, transthyretin, transferrin, and c-reactive protein are typically utilized, as these patients tend to present after long courses and significant weight loss.[3]

INITIAL MANAGEMENT

Fluid resuscitation, broad spectrum antibiotics, and anticoagulation are the mainstays of initial management of patients with acute mesenteric ischemia.[1,2,12] These patients are commonly hypovolemic due to diarrhea and vomiting and should be adequately fluid-resuscitated while avoiding use of vasopressors given the likelihood of worsening splanchnic vasoconstriction and ischemia. Patients should not be permitted to eat or drink, given that it may both delay potential surgery and exacerbate ischemia from increasing mucosal oxygen demand.[3] Antibiotics are used to prevent or treat sepsis and septic shock related to bacterial translocation across ischemic intestinal mucosa, though no specific studies have examined the role of prophylactic antibiotics.[1,2,12]

A surgical team should be consulted emergently, as a delay in consultation and operation has a significant impact on mortality.[1,2] For embolic or thrombotic mesenteric ischemia, after discussion with the consultant surgical team regarding acceptability of bleeding risk, the patient should be started on treatment-dose heparin or other anticoagulant to prevent further clot propagation and decrease clot burden.[1,2,7,12–14]

For mesenteric ischemia resulting from venous thrombosis, operative management is generally not required, though endovascular procedures may be offered. The patient should similarly be started on anticoagulation.[2]

For NOMI, the use of selective mesenteric angiography can permit direct injections of vasodilators into the SMA to improve blood flow. Alprostadil, papaverine, or other prostacyclin analogues have all been used for this purpose.[2,3,7] There have been some studies that have evaluated the usage of ACE inhibitors in animal models to attempt to allay the vasoconstriction that results from activation of the renin-angiotensin-aldosterone pathway, but there have been no specific recommendations made to date.[1,12,15]

Early utilization of invasive hemodynamic monitors is advised,[3] as lactic acidosis and electrolyte derangements can develop. In hemodynamically unstable individuals, fluid balance must be carefully considered, and pressors reserved as a last option, given risk of worsening splanchnic vasoconstriction.[1-3]

SURGICAL MANAGEMENT

Mesenteric ischemia secondary to arterial embolism or thrombus is a surgical emergency, typically leading to laparotomy. There are 3 operative goals: to assess perfusion, to assess tissue viability, and to resect nonviable tissue. For patients suffering from nonocclusive or venous disease, operative management is generally reserved for cases with tissue necrosis. Anticoagulation is preferable, with decreased length of stay, greater viable bowel, and decreased mortality when compared to open thrombectomy.[1,2]

Although open procedures are commonly utilized for the treatment of mesenteric ischemia, endovascular treatment is possible for both arterial and venous sources of acute mesenteric ischemia.[7] Angioplasty, stenting, mechanical thrombectomy, and thrombolysis can all be utilized. The use of endovascular therapy has become more common over the past 10 years and is in fact preferable for patients with chronic mesenteric ischemia given the commonly atherosclerotic etiology.[13] Studies have demonstrated a mortality benefit, but this may be secondary to patient selection—patients who require open resection of bowel are not candidates for the endovascular procedures.[16] A combined procedure can be utilized, in which revascularization followed by evaluation and resection occurs, but is infrequent.[3,12]

POSTOPERATIVE MANAGEMENT

Patients should start anticoagulation as soon as is feasible after discussions with the surgical team, and unless there is a resolution to the conditions predisposing the patient to mesenteric ischemia, oral anticoagulants should continue indefinitely.[3] Serial evaluation for wound healing and gut integrity is essential, given the high likelihood of significant comorbidities such as atherosclerosis or diabetes. Frequent lab draws should be used to monitor electrolytes, and aggressive measures are often taken to ensure adequate nutritional status. Patients with chronic mesenteric ischemia are often malnourished given the "food fear" that develops, and patients can have lengthy bowel resections, leading to prolonged ileus and malabsorption

("short gut syndrome").[2,3] Total parenteral nutrition (TPN) can be utilized until enteral nutrition is possible.

PROGNOSIS

Mortality rates range between 60% and 80% for acute mesenteric ischemia, in part due to comorbid conditions and the advanced age typically associated with the condition.[1,2,10] The prognosis is heavily dependent on the length of time from insult to diagnosis—diagnosis within 12 hours is associated with 14% mortality; diagnosis after 24 hours is associated with mortality as high as 70%.[1] Thus, a high index of suspicion is crucial to the correct and timely diagnosis of mesenteric ischemia and will maximize chances of favorable outcomes.

CONCLUSIONS

- Mesenteric ischemia is an uncommon but concerning disease process with high mortality.

- There are 4 subtypes of mesenteric ischemia: acute mesenteric ischemia, chronic mesenteric ischemia, venous mesenteric ischemia, and nonocclusive mesenteric ischemia.

- Acute embolic mesenteric ischemia is most often secondary to atrial tachyarrhythmias and most often occludes the SMA.

- Chronic mesenteric ischemia is most often associated with atherosclerotic disease, and patients will often present with longstanding abdominal pain and food avoidance.

- Nonocclusive mesenteric ischemia requires angiography for diagnosis and management; all other forms are best evaluated with dual phase CT with angiography.

- In most cases, emergent surgery is necessary to ensure survival.

- Postoperative management include antibiotic therapy, anticoagulation, fluid resuscitation, and nutrition (often including TPN).

REFERENCES

1. Carver TW, Vora RS, Taneja A. Mesenteric ischemia. Critical Care Clinics. 2016;32(2):155–171.
2. Tilsed JVT, Casamassima A, Kurihara H, et al. ESTES guidelines: acute mesenteric ischaemia. Eur J Trauma Emerg Surg. 2016;42:253–270.
3. Clair DG, Beach JM. Mesenteric ischemia. N Engl J Med. 2016;374:959–968.
4. Groesdonk HV, Klingele M, Schlempp S, et al. Risk factors for nonocclusive mesenteric ischemia after elective cardiac surgery. J Thorac Cardiovasc Surg. 2013;145:1603–1610.
5. Reginelli A, Iacobellis F, Berritto D, et al. BMC Surgery. 2013;13(Suppl 2):S51.
6. Copin P, Zins M, Nuzzo A, et al. Acute mesenteric ischemia: a critical role for the radiologist. Diagnostic and Interventional Imaging. 2018;99,123–134.

7. Klar E, Rahmanian PB, Bücker A. Acute mesenteric ischemia: a vascular emergency. Dtsch Arztebl Int. 2012;109(14):249–256.

8. Minko P, Stroeder J, Groesdonk HV. A scoring-system for angiographic findings in nonocclusive mesenteric ischemia (NOMI): correlation with clinical risk factors and its predictive value. Cardiovasc Intervent Radiol. 2014;37:657–663.

9. Cakir M, Yildirim D, Sarac F, et al. In the experimental model of acute mesenteric ischemia, the correlation of blood diagnostic parameters with the duration of ischemia and their effects on choice of treatment. Journal of Investigative Surgery. 2019;32:507–514. doi:10.1080/08941939.2018.1437486

10. Leone M, Bechis C, Baumstarck C, et al. Outcome of acute mesenteric ischemia in the intensive care unit: a retrospective, multicenter study of 780 cases. Intensive Care Med. 2015;41:667–676

11. Sun DL, Cen YY, Li SM, et al. Accuracy of the serum intestinal fatty-acid-binding protein for diagnosis of acute intestinal ischemia: a meta-analysis. Sci. Rep. 2016;6:34371; doi: 10.1038/srep34371.

12. Corcos O, Castier Y, Sibert A. Effects of a multimodal management strategy for acute mesenteric ischemia on survival and intestinal failure. Clin Gastroenterol Hepatol. 2013;11:158–165.

13. Babaev A, Lee DW, Razzouk L. Management of Mesenteric Ischemia. Intervent Cardiol Clin. 2014;3:493–500.

14. Freitas B, Bausback Y, Schuster J, et al. Thrombectomy devices in the treatment of acute mesenteric ischemia: initial single center experience. Ann Vasc Surg. 2018;51:124–131. doi:10.1016/j.avsg.2017.11.041.

15. Tabriziani H, Ahmad A, Bergamaschi R, et al. A nonsurgical approach to mesenteric vascular disease. Cardiol Rev. 2018;2:99–106.

16. Erben Y, Protack CD, Jean RA, et al. Endovascular interventions decrease length of hospitalization and are cost-effective in acute mesenteric ischemia. J Vasc Surg. 2018;62:459–469.

REVIEW QUESTIONS

1. Which of the following patient comorbidities is a risk factor for acute arterial mesenteric ischemia?

    A. Atherosclerotic disease
    B. Atrial tachyarrhythmias
    C. Coagulopathy
    D. Pancreatitis

Answer: B. Acute mesenteric ischemia is primarily an embolic phenomenon, associated with atrial tachyarrhythmias, such as atrial fibrillation. Chronic mesenteric ischemia is associated with atherosclerotic disease, whereas coagulopathy and pancreatitis are not known to be risk factors for mesenteric ischemia.

2. Which artery is the *most* common source of embolic mesenteric ischemia?

    A. Celiac
    B. Superior mesenteric
    C. Middle colic
    D. Inferior mesenteric

Answer: B. The SMA is the artery primarily implicated in cases of acute arterial mesenteric ischemia, both embolic as well as thrombotic. The majority of embolic SMA occlusion takes place distal to the origin of the middle colic artery, which spares the proximal jejunum from ischemia, though some will occur at the origin of the SMA, leading to more extensive bowel ischemia. Thrombotic SMA occlusion primarily occurs at the origin of the SMA.

3. A 75-year-old woman with a history of atrial fibrillation presents to the emergency department with abdominal pain for 10 hours, associated with nausea and vomiting. Which diagnostic study is *most* likely to differentiate between acute mesenteric ischemia and other causes of her abdominal pain?

    A. Serum lactate level
    B. Abdominal magnetic resonance imaging (MRI)
    C. Serum d-dimer
    D. Abdominal CT angiogram

Answer: D. Acute mesenteric ischemia, typically presenting in patients in their 60s to 70s, will manifest commonly as abdominal pain, typically out of proportion to exam. Patients will often also experience nausea, vomiting, or diarrhea. Fecal occult blood testing is frequent but not universally positive. Late in the disease, patients may display peritoneal signs, such as distention, rigidity, guarding, and rebound tenderness. Abdominal CT angiography is the gold standard for diagnosis, which can demonstrate vascular occlusion as well as bowel distension, pneumatosis, or pneumoperitoneum later in the disease. Laboratory tests such as lactate and d-dimer are frequently elevated in patients with mesenteric ischemia but are also elevated in numerous other pathologies such as infection. Abdominal MRI without IV contrast will not be able to diagnose occlusive mesenteric ischemia, and while an MRA can, it is a slower modality than CT and therefore utilized less frequently.

4. Which disease is *least* likely to be associated with nonocclusive mesenteric ischemia?

    A. Congestive heart failure
    B. Atrial fibrillation
    C. Septic shock
    D. Hypovolemic shock

Answer: B. The etiology of NOMI is not well understood but believed to be a mismatch between oxygen delivery and demand to the mesenteric vessels. This can occur in a variety of scenarios, including congestive heart failure and low cardiac output; shock states resulting in poor splanchnic blood flow, with or without vasopressor use; and major abdominal or cardiovascular surgery. Atrial fibrillation or other atrial tachyarrhythmias are more associated with acute embolic mesenteric ischemia.

5. A 62-year-old man with a history of embolic stroke presents to the emergency department with acute abdominal pain and diarrhea. His heart rate is 112 and blood pressure 87/50. His abdomen is moderately tender on exam, without rebound tenderness or rigidity. An abdominal CT angiogram demonstrates occlusion of the distal superior mesenteric artery and dilated bowel loops without evidence of pneumatosis or pneumoperitoneum. What is the *most* appropriate next step in treatment of this patient?

    A. Emergent laparotomy
    B. Emergent endovascular thrombectomy

C. Fluid resuscitation

D. Norepinephrine infusion

Answer: C. The treatment of acute arterial mesenteric ischemia depends on presence of peritoneal signs or bowel integrity compromise. If either is present, emergent laparotomy to resect necrotic bowel is the treatment of choice. In situations of demonstrated superior mesenteric artery thrombosis on imaging without evidence of peritonitis or compromised bowel, endovascular treatments such as thrombectomy or local injection of thrombolytics and vasodilators may be a reasonable option. However, the initial treatment of acute arterial mesenteric ischemia especially in hemodynamically unstable patients, is to normalize blood pressure with IV fluids, consider broad spectrum antibiotics to prevent sepsis from bacterial translocation, and consider systemic anticoagulation to prevent further clot propagation. Vasopressor infusion, such as norepinephrine, should be considered only if hypotension is refractory to fluid resuscitation, as it can worsen splanchnic vasoconstriction and gut ischemia.

6. A 50-year-old woman is currently admitted to the gynecologic oncology service with ovarian cancer. She has significant metastases to the liver and mesentery and has been complaining of gradually worsening abdominal discomfort. CT angiography does not demonstrate significant perfusion defects to the intestines, although the bowel appears edematous. What is the *most* appropriate next step in management?

A. Reassure the patient that this is most likely related to disease progression

B. Evaluate the imaging for intestinal perforation

C. Evaluate the venous phase imaging

D. Evaluate the patient's medication regimen

Answer: C. Edematous bowel may be a sign of intestinal ischemia due to decreased venous drainage, particularly in a patient in whom these areas may be occluded by thrombus or tumor. Further evaluation of the CT angiography and the venous runoff phase may assist in making the diagnosis. Endovascular treatments such as stenting, shunting, or thrombolysis (if applicable) can assist in improving venous drainage. There are no signs of peritonitis or pneumoperitoneum noted, making perforation less likely in this case.

7. A 68-year-old man is in the ICU after undergoing bowel resection for mesenteric ischemia. His surgery was several days ago, and he has been advanced to a regular diet, but he is having large-volume diarrhea. He is requiring IV fluid boluses to remain normotensive. What is the most likely cause?

A. Iatrogenic infection

B. Short gut syndrome

C. Recurrence of occlusion

D. Sepsis

Answer: B. One risk of extensive bowel resection is the development of short gut syndrome, in which patients lack the bowel surface area to absorb adequate nutrients. It manifests typically with diarrhea and weight loss and is associated with significant morbidity and mortality. Patients will often require parenteral nutrition to maintain adequate nutritional status. The risk of this postoperative problem may even be predicted intraoperatively, based on the length of bowel resected.

8. A 65-year-old man presents to the emergency department with complaints of sharp abdominal pain. He has a history of atrial fibrillation and chronic obstructive pulmonary disease related to smoking. On examination, his abdomen demonstrates rebound tenderness. A CT scan is performed that shows inflammation of the bowel wall, fat-stranding, and free fluid in the abdomen. What is the most likely diagnosis?

A. Perforated diverticulitis

B. Ruptured appendix

C. Acute mesenteric ischemia

D. Cholecystitis

Answer: B. Although he demonstrates several risk factors for acute mesenteric ischemia, the most common cause of an acute abdomen in adults in this age range remains appendicitis. For adults over the age of 70, diverticulitis, small bowel obstruction, and large bowel obstruction are similarly more common causes of abdominal pain than mesenteric ischemia.

9. Which of the following arterial blood gases may be found in a patient with acute presentation of mesenteric ischemia?

A.

pH	7.33
pO_2	95
pCO_2	32
HCO_3	12
O_2 saturation	100
Na	146
Cl	110

B.

pH	7.45
pO_2	86
pCO_2	43
HCO_3	29
O_2 Saturation	96
Na	145
Cl	100

C.

pH	7.23
pO_2	64
pCO_2	48
HCO_3	20
O_2 Saturation	91
Na	143
Cl	107

D. All of the above

Answer: D. All of these can be arterial blood gases associated with mesenteric ischemia. Answer choice A demonstrates an anion gap metabolic acidosis, possibly from lactatemia, with adequate compensation. Answer choice B demonstrates a hypochloremic metabolic alkalosis, possibly from vomiting. In early stages of mesenteric ischemia, the lactate may remain normal, and the patient may not exhibit acidemia. Answer choice C demonstrates a metabolic acidosis with concurrent respiratory acidosis, resulting from lack of respiratory compensation—possibly from obstructive pulmonary disease or respiratory depression.

10. Which feature is *not* seen on CT for a patient with mesenteric ischemia?

A. Bowel wall thickening
B. Bowel wall thinning
C. Bowel wall hypoattenuation
D. Bowel wall hyperattenuation

Answer: C. Bowel wall hypoattenuation is a normal finding on non-contrast CT imaging. Bowel wall hyperattenuation (sensitivity 5%–18%, specificity 90%–98%), on the other hand, has been described in cases of mesenteric ischemia on unenhanced CT and is thought to be secondary either to intramural hemorrhage or increased wall pressure due to venous occlusion. Both bowel wall thickening (sensitivity 85%–88%, specificity 61%–72%), due to edema, and bowel wall thinning (sensitivity 40%, sensitivity 88%), due to arterial occlusion, can be seen in mesenteric ischemia. Altogether absent bowel wall enhancement is highly specific (88%–100%) but is not necessarily sensitive (18%–60%), for mesenteric ischemia.

25.

COMPLICATIONS OF BARIATRIC SURGERY INCLUDING RHABDOMYOLYSIS WITH ACIDOSIS AND ACUTE KIDNEY INJURY

Floria E. Chae and S. Veena Satyapriya

STEM CASE AND KEY QUESTIONS

A 45-year-old male with obesity (body mass index [BMI] 41), hypertension, hyperlipidemia, obstructive sleep apnea, and type 2 diabetes mellitus underwent laparoscopic Roux-en-Y. Intraoperative course was uneventful, surgical time was 3 hr. There was minimal blood loss <50 mL, urine output (UOP) was 200 mL, and 2 L of lactated Ringer's (LR) was given. The patient was extubated in the operating room (OR) and admitted to the medical/surgical stepdown unit. Postoperative day (POD) 0 labs that evening were as follows: white blood cells (WBC) 10, hemoglobin (Hgb) 14, platelets (PLT) 250, CO_2 26, creatine (Crt) 1.6, lactate 2, and creatine kinase (CK) 800.

On POD 1, he became tachypneic with 42 respiratory rate (RR), tachycardic to 123 bpm in sinus rhythm that did not respond to pain medications, saturation 95% on 5 L/min nasal cannula (NC). On exam, the patient has conversational dyspnea but is awake and answering questions; clear distant breath sounds, abdomen soft, obese, thrombotic thrombocytopenic purpura around the incision site, no drainage noted from the incision site. UOP declined to 350 mL since surgery despite multiple fluid boluses overnight. The decision is made to transfer the patient to the surgical intensive care unit (SICU) postoperatively for further monitoring and care. Labs in the SICU are as follows: WBC 17; Hgb 9; PLT 150; chemistry: Na 132, CO_2 22, Cl 108, blood urea nitrogen 55, Crt 2.1, CK 3400, arterial blood gas (ABG) 7.28/50/67/21, lactate 3.4; chest X-ray: bilateral basilar atelectasis, poor inspiratory effort, enlarged heart; blood pressure 100/60, heart rate 130, RR 40, 90% 5 L/min NC.

Due to clinical instability, the decision is made to send the patient to the OR for diagnostic laparoscopy, intraoperative esophagogastroduodenoscopy (EGD), and possible laparotomy. Intraoperatively, the gastrojejunal anastomosis was submerged under saline, and EGD identified an anastomotic breakdown and bleeding along the staple line. The leak was repaired and hemostasis achieved. A Blake drain was placed at the anastomosis. Estimated blood loss was 500 mL, UOP 50 mL, intravenous fluid (IVF) 3 L of LR. The patient remained intubated and was transferred to the SICU on 0.06 of norepinephrine. The patient was put on pressure-regulated volume control, with fraction of inspired oxygen (FiO_2) of 60% and positive end-expiratory pressure (PEEP) 10. Antibiotics were ertapenem and diflucan. Due to intraoperative bleeding, primary service did not want to start anticoagulation.

At POD 2–4 the patient remained intubated for hypoxia and increased vent requirements. On POD 4 the patient became acutely hypoxic, and vent requirements suddenly increased to PEEP 18, FiO_2 80%, ABG 7.25/40/55 Lactate 6, CK 12,000, Crt 3.2, UOP 100 in 24 hr.

BMI equals patient's weight in kilograms divided by height in meters squared[1].

$$BMI = kg/(m^2)$$

WHAT ARE THE INDICATIONS FOR BARIATRIC SURGERY?

Those patients with BMI ≥40 without comorbidities and bariatric surgery would not be associated with excessive risk should be eligible. Patients with BMI ≥35 and with one or more severe obesity-related comorbidities, such as type 2 diabetes, hypertension, hyperlipidemia, obstructive sleep apnea, obesity-hypoventilation syndrome, Pickwickian syndrome, nonalcoholic fatty liver disease or nonalcoholic steatohepatitis, pseudotumor cerebri, gastroesophageal reflux disease (GERD), asthma, venous stasis disease, severe urinary incontinence, debilitating arthritis, or considerably impaired quality

Table 25.1. **WORLD HEALTH ORGANIZATION'S GLOBAL DATABASE ON BMI[1]**

CLASS		BMI (KG/M²)
Underweight		>18.5
Normal		≥18.5–<25
Overweight		≥25–<30
Obese		
	Class 1	≥30–<35
	Class 2	≥35–<40
	Class 3	≥40

of life, may also be offered a bariatric procedure. Patients with BMI of 30–34.9 with diabetes or metabolic syndrome may also be offered a bariatric procedure; however, current evidence is limited as there are few studies and no net benefit has been demonstrated.[2]

WHAT ARE THE DIFFERENT TYPES OF BARIATRIC SURGERIES?

Bariatric surgery can be divided into restrictive and malabsorptive procedures. These procedures reduce caloric intake by modifying the upper gastrointestinal tract and can be performed open or laparoscopically. However, this classification is incomplete as there are other mechanisms aside from restriction and absorption that are involved including visceral signals.[3] Restrictive procedures include gastric banding and sleeve gastrectomy—these surgeries alter gastric anatomy. Malabsorptive procedures include Roux-en-Y bariatric bypass and biliopancreatic diversion and duodenal switch (BPD/DS), which alters both gastric and intestinal anatomy; the latter is reserved for patients with BMI >50 and is associated with greater nutritional risk due to increased length of the small intestine that is bypassed.[2,4]

WHAT PREOPERATIVE WORKUP SHOULD BE COMPLETED PRIOR TO BARIATRIC SURGERY?

Preoperative evaluation must include comprehensive medical history, psychosocial–behavioral exam, physical exam, and appropriate labs. Medical necessity for bariatric surgery should be documented. All patients should undergo appropriate nutritional evaluation before any bariatric surgery. Patients with known heart disease may require formal cardiology consultation and be evaluated for perioperative β-adrenergic blockade. Chest radiograph and standardized screening for obstructive sleep apnea should be considered. Routine screening for *Helicobacter pylori* should be considered in high-prevalence areas. Fasting lipid panel should be obtained in all patients with obesity and treatment initiated if indicated. Preoperative glycemic control should be optimized. Patients with a history of venous thromboembolism (VTE) or cor pulmonale should undergo appropriate diagnostic evaluation for deep venous thrombosis (DVT). Patients should stop using tobacco at least 6 weeks prior to surgery and should not use tobacco postoperatively at all. Routine screening of hypothyroidism or assessment of bone mineral density with dual-energy X-ray absorptiometry is not recommended.[2]

WHAT ARE THE INTRAOPERATIVE, PERIOPERATIVE, AND LATE COMPLICATIONS FROM BARIATRIC SURGERY?

Intraoperative complications include injuries to organs and blood vessel injuries requiring repair.[5] Perioperative complications include anastomotic leak, gastrointestinal bleeding, trocar injury, DVT, pulmonary embolism (PE), bowel obstruction, wound infection, pneumonia, acute kidney injury, and acute cardiac event. Late complications include anatomic stricture, marginal ulcer, bowel obstruction, incisional hernia, internal hernia, dumping syndrome, nutritional deficiencies, and cholecystitis.[6]

WHAT IS THE SIGNIFICANCE OF THIS PATIENT'S TACHYCARDIA, ELEVATED LACTATE, AND SOFT ABDOMEN?

Postoperative tachycardia can be due to many factors, such as hypoxia, pain, hypovolemia, fever, infection, etc. In post–bariatric surgical patients, postoperative tachycardia should be taken seriously. The most common cause is dehydration. However, diagnoses that must be considered are PE and surgical complications such as anastomotic fistula. Unlike non-obese patients, obese patients do not exhibit the classic signs of peritoneal irritation such as guarding or rigidity. Instead, non-specific signs such as fever, abdominal heaviness, hiccups, tachycardia, and acute urinary retention should raise suspicion and prompt a surgical consult. If anastomotic fistula goes undiagnosed, this can result in sepsis and cause acute renal failure, respiratory failure, and death.[6]

WHAT IS THE INCIDENCE OF VTE? WHAT ARE SOME RISK FACTORS? HOW CAN ONE PREVENT VTE?

VTE is a major cause of postoperative complications in the bariatric surgery population. It is generally reported at 1%–3% for DVT and 0.3%–2% for PE. Patient risk factors include history of VTE, increasing age, high BMI, and smoking. Surgical risk factors include anastomotic leak and prolonged immobilization. Methods to decrease VTE include use of appropriately dosed pharmacologic prophylaxis therapy, use of lower extremity compression device, and early postoperative mobilization.[7]

WHAT RENAL COMPLICATIONS IS THIS PATIENT AT RISK FOR?

Obese patients are at higher risk for renal complications such as acute kidney injury, rhabdomyolysis, and nephrolithiasis. Rhabdomyolysis, which is the breakdown of skeletal muscle, can result in electrolyte imbalance, hypovolemia, and acute kidney injury. Patients undergoing bariatric surgery are at increased risk due to intraoperative immobilization.[8] Obese patients have increased urinary urate and oxalate excretion, promoting calcium-oxalate stone formation.[9]

DISCUSSION

BACKGROUND

An estimated 1.7 billion people in the world are overweight and obese, and 25 million deaths per year worldwide are due to obesity-related complications.[10] Bariatric surgery may help weight loss and thereby have positive health impacts on diabetes, hypertension, dyslipidemia, obstructive sleep apnea, nonalcoholic steatohepatitis, GERD, arthritis and back pain, gout, subfertility, asthma, and others.[11] The most common bariatric surgical procedures include gastric banding, sleeve gastrectomy, Roux en Y gastric bypass (RYGB), and BPD/DS. Gastric banding is well tolerated and involves using a silicone ring around the stomach to induce delaying emptying and create a smaller gastric pouch. A sleeve gastrectomy removes two-thirds of the gastric volume by stapling along the greater curvature of the stomach. RYGB involves stapling the stomach to create a small upper gastric pouch and a distal pouch. The jejunum is divided and a gastrointestinal and jejuno-intestinal anastomosis is performed. Jejunal absorption is decreased as the Roux limb length increases. BPD/DS is comprised of sleeve gastrectomy and a short duodenal–ileal circuit with duodeno-ileal and ileo-ileal anastomoses.[4]

EPIDEMIOLOGY OF SURGICAL COMPLICATIONS

Surgical complications during the first days or weeks include septic complications (fistula and anatomic leak) and non-septic complications (hemorrhage). The most common cause of death is anastomotic leaks, followed by PE.

Although gastric banding is relatively safe and often preformed as same-day surgery, complications can occur. A meta-analysis by Chang et al. reported complication rates of gastric banding to be 13% in randomized control trials (RCTs) and 7.8% in observation studies (OS).[12] Gastric or esophageal perforation is rare; the French National Agency for Accreditation and Evaluation in Healthcare reported 0.3%.[13] Early band erosion and perforation can occur during the first few weeks. This may be due to a technical problem and unrecognized intra-operative gastric perforation, early postoperative infection, or gastric wall ischemia due to a tight band. The ring or port may become infected, which may lead to pus at the port site. Ring malposition and band slippage are rare but can be seen in the early postoperative course.

The sleeve gastrectomy complication rate is around 13% in RCTs and 8.9% in OS.[12] The most common complications are fistula and bleeding.

Complications of malabsorptive procedures are higher than those of restrictive procedures, at 21% in RCTs and 12% in OS.[12] For RYGB, anastomotic leaks are the most common, followed by bleeding. Bleeding risk is significantly higher in RYGB than other procedures; sources of bleeding include intraabdominal (along staple line) and intraluminal (gastric or intestinal).[14]

Complications for BPD/DS include all of the above-mentioned complications, and single-center studies have reported varying complication rates, with either similar rates or overall higher complication rates, with an overall trend in increased bleeding rates.[15]

DIAGNOSIS OF SURGICAL COMPLICATIONS

Anastomotic fistula causing peritonitis is the most common complication after surgery, typically occurring within the first 10 days postoperatively. Incidence after gastric bypass is 1%–3% and after sleeve gastrectomy 3%–7%.[6]

Identifying peritonitis is based on traditional clinical signs such as abdominal pain, guarding, and firmness, making the diagnosis difficult. Tachycardia is the most frequent sign. Polypnea or respiratory distress can also be a non-specific but concerning sign of gastrointestinal leak. Approximately half of non-ICU patients have no clinical signs at the time of diagnosis of peritonitis.[4] This could be related to a large amount of subcutaneous tissue, a subphrenic site, or an impaired inflammatory response. In ICU patients, fever, dyspnea, and tachycardia were reported in 74%, 98%, and 100% of cases, respectively.[16]

Radiological studies are recommended, but no consensus has been reached on the optimal imaging technique. Typically, computed tomography scans or upper gastrointestinal (UGI) studies are recommended to aid in the diagnosis of surgical complications. Madan et al. reported a positive predictive value of UGI studies of 67% and a negative predictive value of 99%. They observed that routine UGI studies were more predictive of early leak diagnosis than clinical signs.[17]

MANAGEMENT OF SURGICAL COMPLICATIONS

General principles in surgical management apply, such as identifying the infectious source, obtaining appropriate cultures, administering appropriate antibiotics, and source control. For clinically active bleeding, surgery is required to identify the source of bleeding and control blood loss. Fistula treatment depends on stability of the patient. If clinically unstable, then treatment is reoperation. If the patient is clinically stable and if there is no collection, then treat with conservative management. Consider percutaneous drainage if there is a limited fluid collection or reoperation if there is a generalized fluid collection.

Treatment for gastric or esophageal perforation after gastric banding includes copious lavage and effective drainage of the peritoneal cavity. The perforation must be sutured together with drainage in contact with the perforation. Infection of the ring or port necessitates removal of the infection device. Once infection is eradicated, one may place a new device. Band malposition needs urgent reoperation and removal or repositioning of the gastric band to prevent gastric ischemia.[4]

Montravers et al.[4] looked at patients undergoing reoperation for septic complicated abdomen, 49 patients who previously had bariatric surgery and 134 patients who had conventional surgery. Patients who previously had bariatric surgery had a 37% higher rate of Gram-positive cocci, a 33% lower rate of Gram-negative bacilli, and a 50% lower rate of anaerobes and multidrug-resistant strains. Rebibo reported higher rates of candida infections in patients who had gastric fistulas after laparoscopic sleeve gastrectomy.

MEDICAL COMPLICATIONS

Medical management entails supportive ICU care, adequate nutrition, early mobility as able, appropriate antibiotic therapy, and management of associated complications. Overall, clinical management does not differ significantly from other complicated abdominal surgery cases. Most of the strategies of ICU care are extrapolated from non-obese patients. VTE, nephrolithiasis, and rhabdomyolysis will be discussed.

Nutritional support (tube feeds or parenteral nutrition) should be considered in patients who are at high nutritional risk.[2] Montravers et al.[4] will place a feeding tube in the gastric remnant or at the jejunum to continue enteral nutrition distal to the site of anastomotic leak.

VTE

Epidemiology

Incidence of VTE varies but is generally reported at 1%–3% for DVT and 0.3%–2% for PE. Morino et al. reported that cause of death in 13- 38.2% was due to thromboembolic complication.[18] Superior mesenteric vein thrombosis should be considered in patients with postoperative abdominal pain.[9]

Pathophysiology

Risk factors include history of DVT/PE, increasing age, high BMI, and smoking. Anastomotic leak and prolonged immobilization can trigger VTE.[7]

Management

DVT prophylaxis is recommended for bariatric surgical patients within 24 hr after surgery.[2] Low–molecular weight heparin is adjusted to patient body weight, but data regarding the safety of weight-based doses is limited. As weight increases, the dose needs to be adjusted for unfractionated heparin, and monitoring therapeutic effect is required.[4]

The American Society for Metabolic and Bariatric Surgery's Bariatric Surgery Center of Excellence program requires all bariatric programs to devise and implement a detailed pathway for prevention of VTE. The Bariatric Outcomes Longitudinal Database (BOLD) is used to track anticoagulation and various methods of VTE prophylaxis. These methods include stockings, a foot pump, an intermittent venous compression device, and inferior vena cava (IVC) filter use. Greater than 93% of patients in BOLD received at least one form of prophylaxis, with most receiving two or more. Prophylactic use of IVC filters have been recommended for high-risk patients (extreme obesity, history of VTE, and immobility); however, strong evidence supporting efficacy at preventing VTE is lacking.[7] IVC filter for adjustable gastric band and RYGB was associated with increased incidence of postoperative VTE; however, this may be a reflection of the patient's high risk or that patients with IVC filters were less likely to receive other methods of VTE prophylaxis.[19–21]

NEPHROLITHIASIS

Epidemiology

Bariatric surgery, especially RYGB, is associated with increased lithogenicity. Fat malabsorption in these patients enhances the saponification of calcium in the gastrointestinal tract and limits the amount of available calcium to bind oxalate in the colon. Increased concentration of bile salt in the colon increases the colonic permeability to oxalate, increasing oxalate absorption and thus renal excretion.

Pathophysiology

In obese patients, proinflammatory mediators are upregulated, and this is thought to interact with the renal system, enhancing renal fibrosis via transforming growth factor beta 1 signaling. Accumulation of intracellular nonesterified free fatty acids and triglycerides is thought to contribute to organ dysfunction, including renal disease. In obese mouse models, overexpression of the gene which increases transcription of lipogenic genes led to significant proteinuria and glomerulosclerosis. Mice that lacked the gene which increases the transcription of lipogenic genes appear to be resistant to lipotoxic damage when given a high-fat diet. Oxidized low-density protein stimulates excess secretion of extracellular matrix and proinflammatory cytokines, which appear to contribute to glomerular injury. Hypertension leads to renal injury by stimulation of the renin–angiotensin system by sympathetic activation and possibly increased adipose tissue, leading to increased renal sodium and water retention, which leads to hyperfiltration, glomerulomegaly, and focal glomerulosclerosis.

Management

Management of kidney stones in bariatric patients is standard practice of removal and prevention.[9] Taking calcium supplements and having a low-oxalate diet have been shown to be effective at decreasing kidney stones in a retrospective study.[22]

RHABDOMYOLYSIS

Epidemiology

There has been an increasing awareness of rhabdomyolysis in bariatric patients. Patients undergoing bariatric surgery are at increased risk of rhabdomyolysis due to intraoperative immobilization. Chakravartty et al.[8] found that 14% of patients following bariatric surgery with rhabdomyolysis developed renal failure, and the mortality rate after renal failure was 25%.

Pathophysiology

The pathophysiology of rhabdomyolysis is muscle destruction by direct cell membrane destruction or energy depletion. Muscle cell necrosis releases cytotoxins that cause capillary edema and leads to extravasation and third spacing of fluids. Edema and ischemia cause additional metabolic acidosis and electrolyte abnormalities, perpetuating cell death. Rhabdomyolysis-associated acute kidney injury may be induced by hypovolemia, myoglobinuria, and metabolic acidosis.[23] Risk factors for rhabdomyolysis identified in the literature include high BMI, long duration of surgery, male gender, presence of hypertension, diabetes, and American Society of Anesthesiologists physical status >2. The most consistent risk factors are high BMI and duration of surgery.

Diagnosis

Generally, the biochemical definition of rhabdomyolysis is CK level 5 times normal or >1000 IU/L. Patients with muscle pain after bariatric surgery are at high risk for rhabdomyolysis causing renal injury, and prompt treatment should be started. Often, symptoms of myalgia are present in the postoperative recovery room, and rhabdomyolysis should considered. An epidural may mask muscle pain and prohibit early diagnosis. Chakravartty et al. propose, for patients without an epidural, that if they have myalgia or BMI >50 and/or operative time >4 hr, then CK should be measured daily for 72 hr. If the patient has a postoperative epidural, then CK levels should be measured daily for 72 hr. CK levels >5000 indicate that they are at high risk for renal failure, and CK <5000 suggests low risk for renal failure.[8]

Management

Management includes intravenous hydration to maintain high urine output of 200–300 mL/hr.[23] Increasing intraoperative fluid resuscitation does not seem to prevent rhabdomyolysis or progression to acute kidney injury.[24] However, early fluid resuscitation within 6 hr resulting in forced diuresis may prevent acute kidney injury and mortality. Bariatric patients often have cardiac and renal disease, and aggressive fluid resuscitation should be done with caution. Hyperkalemia needs to be treated in order to reduce risk of cardiac dysrhythmias. Bicarbonate therapy has been suggested but may produce paradoxical intracellular acidosis and volume overload.[25] There is no consensus regarding use of mannitol as side effects include volume depletion and potential worsening pre-renal azotemia.[26] Continuous renal replacement therapy can clear myoglobin from the bloodstream, but mortality rates remain unchanged.

CONCLUSION

- Bariatric surgical patients do not have typical signs of peritonitis. In the presence of prolonged tachycardia <120 bpm, tachypnea, hypoxia, or fever, an anastomotic leak must be considered. VTE should also be considered.

- Bariatric surgical patients are at increased risk of VTE. These patients should have pharmacologic and non-pharmacologic prophylaxis. High-risk patients may require extended chemoprophylaxis after hospital discharge.

- Bariatric surgical patients are at increased risk for rhabdomyolysis and nephrolithiasis. Myalgia in the postoperative recovery area should increase suspicion of rhabdomyolysis.

REFERENCES

1. National Institutes of Health. Clinical guidelines on the identification, evaluation, and treatment of overweight and obesity in adults—The evidence report. *Obes Res.* 1998;6(Suppl 2):51S–209S. Erratum in: Obes Res 1998;6(6):464.
2. Mechanick, JI, Youdim A, Jones DB, et al. Clinical practice guidelines for the perioperative nutritional, metabolic, and nonsurgical support of the bariatric surgery patient—2013 update: Cosponsored by American Association of Clinical Endocrinologists, The Obesity Society, and American Society for Metabolic & Bariatric Surgery. *Obesity (Silver Spring).* 2013;21(1):S1–27.
3. Pournaras DJ, Le Roux CW. The effect of bariatric surgery on gut hormones that alter appetite. *Diabetes Metab.* 2009;35:508–12.
4. Montravers P, Augustin P, Zappella N, et al. Diagnosis and management of the postoperative surgical and medical complications of bariatric surgery. *Anaesth Crit Care Pain Med.* 2015;34(1):45–52.
5. Greenstein AJ, Wahed AS, Adeniji A, et al. Prevalence of adverse intraoperative events during obesity surgery and their sequelae. *J Am Coll Surg.* 2012;215(2):271–7.e3.
6. Kassir R, Debs T, Blanc P, et al. Complications of bariatric surgery: Presentation and emergency management. *Int J Surg.* 2016;27:77–8.
7. Winegar DA, Sherif B, Pate V, DeMaria EJ. Venous thromboembolism after bariatric surgery performed by Bariatric Surgery Center of Excellence participants: Analysis of the Bariatric Outcomes Longitudinal Database. *Surg Obes Relat Dis.* 2011;7(2):181–8.
8. Chakravartty S, Sarma DR, Patel AG. Rhabdomyolysis in bariatric surgery: A systematic review. *Obes Surg.* 2013;23(8):1333–40.
9. Currie A, Chetwood A, Ahmed AR. Bariatric surgery and renal function. *Obes Surg.* 2011;21(4):528–39.
10. Deitel M. Overweight and obesity worldwide now estimated to involve 1.7 billion people. *Obes Surg.* 2003;13:329–30.
11. le Roux CW, Heneghan HM. Bariatric surgery for obesity. *Med Clin North Am.* 2018;102(1):165–82.
12. Chang SH, Stoll CR, Song J, Varela JE, Eagon CJ, Colditz GA. The effectiveness and risks of bariatric surgery: An updated systematic review and meta-analysis, 2003–2012. *JAMA Surg.* 2014;149(3):275–87.
13. Msika S. Surgery for morbid obesity: 2. Complications. Results of a technologic evaluation by the ANAES. *J Chir.* 2003;140:4–21.
14. Griffith PS, Birch DW, Sharma AM, Karmali S. Managing complications associated with laparoscopic Roux-en-Y gastric bypass for morbid obesity. *Can J Surg.* 2012;55:329–36.
15. Topart P, Becouarn G, Ritz P. Comparative early outcomes of three laparoscopic bariatric procedures: Sleeve gastrectomy, Roux-en-Y gastric bypass, and bilio-pancreatic diversion with duodenal switch. *Surg Obes Relat Dis.* 2012;8:250–4.
16. Kermarrec N, Marmuse JP, Faivre J, et al. High mortality rate for patients requiring intensive care after surgical revision following bariatric surgery. *Obes Surg.* 2008;18(2):171–8.
17. Madan AK, Stoecklein HH, Ternovits CA, Tichansky DS, Phillips JC. Predictive value of upper gastrointestinal studies versus clinical signs for gastrointestinal leaks after laparoscopic gastric bypass. *Surg Endosc.* 2007;21(2):194–6..
18. Morino M, Toppino M, Forestieri P, Angrisani L, Allaix ME, Scopinaro N. Mortality after bariatric surgery: analysis of 13,871 morbidly obese patients from a national registry. *Ann Surg.* 2007;246:1002–9.
19. Hamad GG, Bergqvist D. Venous thromboembolism in bariatric surgery patients: An update of risk and prevention. *Surg Obes Relat Dis.* 2007;3:97–102.
20. Barba CA, Harrington C, Loewen M. Status of venous thromboembolism prophylaxis among bariatric surgeons: Have we changed our practice during the past decade? *Surg Obes Relat Dis.* 2009;5:352–6.
21. Carmody BJ, Sugerman HJ, Kellum JM, et al. Pulmonary embolism complicating bariatric surgery: Detailed analysis of a single institution's 24-year experience. *J Am Coll Surg.* 2006;203:831–7.
22. Whitson JM, Stackhouse GB, Stoller ML. Hyperoxaluria after modern bariatric surgery: Case series and literature review. *Int Urol Nephrol.* 2010;42(2):369–74.
23. Chavez LO, Leon M, Einav S, Varon J. Beyond muscle destruction: A systematic review of rhabdomyolysis for clinical practice. *Crit Care.* 2016;20:135. doi: 10.1186/s13054-016-1314-5.

24. Wool DB, Lemmens HJ, Brodsky JB, Solomon H, Chong KP, Morton JM. Intraoperative fluid replacement and postoperative creatine phosphokinase levels in laparoscopic bariatric patients. *Obes Surg.* 2010;20(6):698–701.
25. Berend K, de Vries AP, Gans RO. Physiological approach to assessment of acid-base disturbances. *N Engl J Med.* 2015;372(2):195.
26. Bosch X, Poch E, Grau JM. Rhabdomyolysis and acute kidney injury. *N Engl J Med.* 2009;361(1):62–72.

REVIEW QUESTIONS

1. Risk factors for venous thromboembolism (VTE) in the bariatric surgery population include all of the following *except*

    A. Family history of VTE.
    B. High body mass index (BMI).
    C. Female gender.
    D. Smoking.

2. A 44-year-old man on postoperative day 7 from a laparoscopic Roux-en-Y gastric bypass (RYGB) is admitted to the intensive care unit (ICU) for observation with a sustained heart rate >120 beats per minute (bpm) and tachypnea with an increased work of breathing. His blood pressure is 140/75 and oxygen saturation is 90%. He is diaphoretic but alert and oriented × 3. Chest X-ray on admission to ICU shows bibasilar atelectasis. What is the most appropriate next step in diagnosis?

    A. Contrast-enhanced computed tomography (CT)
    B. Close monitoring and serial chest X-rays
    C. Exploratory laparotomy
    D. Stat echocardiogram

3. The most common surgical complication in post-bariatric surgery is

    A. gastrointestinal hemorrhage.
    B. anastomotic leak.
    C. development of fistula.
    D. gastric perforation.

4. A 47-year-old female is recovering from an uneventful laparoscopic gastric sleeve procedure. On postoperative day 1 she developed tachycardia and fevers and was transferred to the ICU for further monitoring. On arrival to the ICU, her heart rate is 140, her blood pressure is 60/50 and her initial arterial blood gas reveals a lactate of 3. What is the most appropriate next step in management for this patient?

    A. STAT echocardiogram, serial troponins
    B. CT angiogram
    C. Return to operating room for surgical reexploration
    D. Start systemic anticoagulation for presumed pulmonary embolism

5. A 54-year-old female is recovering in the post-anesthesia care unit (PACU) following an uncomplicated laparoscopic RYGB. She is not compliant with her prescribed CPAP at home. She complains of 10 out of 10 pain and is given 0.5 mg of intravenous (IV) hydromorphone after which she becomes apneic and obtunded. An arterial blood gas is drawn, which shows an acute on chronic respiratory acidosis. Her vitals are stable. Which of the following diagnoses in her PMH is the mostly likely cause of her acute change in clinical status in the PACU?

    A. Obstructive sleep apnea
    B. BMI >40
    C. Acute coronary syndrome
    D. Obesity hypoventilation syndrome

6. All of the following are part of the STOP-BANG screening questionnaire to evaluate individuals with multiple risk factors for obstructive sleep apnea *except*

    A. BMI >30.
    B. observed apnea.
    C. age older than 50.
    D. neck circumference greater than 40 cm.

7. Which of the following is true with regards to the diagnosis of bariatric patients who develop postoperative rhabdomyolysis?

    A. The shorter the length of the surgery, the greater the likelihood of developing rhabdoymyolysis.
    B. The biochemical definition of rhabdomyolysis includes creatine kinase level 10 times normal.
    C. High BMI is not a risk factor for development of rhabdomyolysis.
    D. There is a correlation between the duration of surgery and development of rhabdomyolysis.

8. Increasing intraoperative fluid resuscitation will prevent development of rhabdomyolysis.

    A. True
    B. False

9. All of the following are true statements regarding management of rhabdomyolysis *except*

    A. mannitol is considered first-line therapy in all patients that develop rhabdomyolysis.
    B. bicarbonate may cause paradoxical intracellular acidosis.
    C. rhabdomyolysis cannot be prevented by increasing intraoperative fluid resuscitation.
    D. hyperkalemia should be treated routinely and closely monitored to prevent cardiac dysrhythmias.

10. Bariatric surgery is associated with increased lithogenicity. Management includes decreasing calcium in diet.

    A. True
    B. False

ANSWERS

1. Answer: C. Among patient-related characteristics, evidence suggests that male gender is at a greater risk of VTE than women post bariatric surgery.

2. Answer: A. Anastomotic leaks are common complications of bariatric surgery. However, diagnosis is often difficult early on due to nonspecific clinical symptoms, which most commonly include sustained tachycardia and tachypnea. If the patient were stable to travel, CT imaging would allow for further investigation of thoracic or abdominal complications. Hemodynamic instability should prompt surgical reexploration. An echocardiogram could detect right ventricular strain that may accompany a pulmonary embolism. Sustained tachycardia (>120bpm) warrants exclusion of an anastomotic leak post RYGB.

3. Answer: B. Anastomotic leaks are common complications of bariatric surgery. While most occur intraoperatively or within the first few days after surgery, diagnosis and subsequent management are often delayed to the nonspecific clinical symptoms (tachycardia, dyspnea) that accompany this complication early on as described in question 2.

4. Answer: C. Sustained tachycardia with hemodynamic instability with an elevated lactate is concerning for anastomotic leak, thus surgical reexploration should not be delayed.

5. Answer: D. Obesity hypoventilation syndrome, also known as Pickwickian syndrome, exists when an obese individual has awake alveolar hypoventilation not attributed to other conditions. Patients with this syndrome are often more sensitive to the effects of alcohol and sedating medications such as narcotics in comparison to the general population. Ideally a multimodal analgesic plan that would minimize sedating meds would minimize postoperative respiratory complications in this patient.

6. Answer: A. The STOP-BANG questionnaire is frequently used as a preoperative evaluation tool to evaluate and manage patients in the perioperative period who have multiple risk factors for complications related to previously undiagnosed obstructive sleep apnea postoperatively. It requires "yes" or "no" responses, with each "yes" equivalent to 1 point in regards to:
Snoring
Tiredness
Observed apneas
Pressure: elevated blood pressure
BMI >35kg/m²
Age >50 years old
Neck circumference >40 cm
Gender: male

Scoring:
0–2: low risk
3–4: intermediate risk
≥5: high risk

7. Answer: D. The most consistent risk factors for development of rhabdomyolysis in the bariatric patient are duration of surgery and high BMI.

8. Answer: B. False. While management includes early IV hydration to induce a forced diuresis at time of diagnosis may prevent acute kidney injury and mortality, it does not appear that increased intraoperative resuscitation will actually prevent rhabdoymyolysis in the bariatric surgery patient.

9. Answer: A. There is no consensus regarding routine use of mannitol as the side effects include volume depletion and the possibility of worsening pre-renal azotemia.

10. Answer: B. False. Fat malabsorption in the post bariatric surgery patient enhances the saponification of calcium in the gastrointestinal tract—thus there is less available to bind oxalate in the colon. Additionally, increased bile sale in the colon increased the colonic permeability to oxalate. This leads to increased absorption and thus renal excretion, thereby increasing lithogenicity in bariatric surgery patients. Taking calcium supplements and a low oxalate diet have been shown to be effective in decreasing kidney stones in the post-bariatric surgery population.

26.

SEPSIS

LAPAROSCOPIC BOWEL SURGERY

Edward D. Foley and Manuel R. Castresana

STEM CASE AND KEY QUESTIONS

A 69-year-old male patient with a history of COPD and non-insulin dependent diabetes (type II) underwent a laparoscopic right hemicolectomy for adenocarcinoma of the colon 2 days ago. Today he is confused and complaining of abdominal pain. Blood pressure is 74/42 mmHg, heart rate 133 beats per minute (bpm) sinus, respiratory rate is 26 breaths per minute, and temperature is 38.7°C. A Foley urinary catheter, which has been in situ since surgery, has drained 30 cc per hour concentrated urine over the last 24 hours. SpO$_2$ on room air is 98%.

Despite initial improvement and continued resuscitation with intravenous (IV) fluids and antibiotics, tachycardia persists with heart rate at 120 bpm; he is febrile (39°C) and hypotensive 80/50 mmHg; and urine output decreases to 10 cc per hour. He is now somnolent and has cool extremities, with a central venous pressure (CVP) now reading 12 cmH$_2$0 and ScvO$_2$ 58% and an SpO$_2$ 91% with 50% supplemental oxygen via facemask.

He is now intubated and ventilated with FiO$_2$ of 0.6 with positive end-expiratory pressure 12 cmH$_2$0 and an arterial blood gas shows PaO$_2$ 80 mmHg. Lab values are Hb 14g/dL, white cell count 18, platelets 120,000, lactate 5, glucose 330mg/dL, creatinine 1.15mg/dL, bilirubin 1.2mg/dL. Computed tomography (CT) scan findings are consistent with diffuse purulent peritonitis likely due to dehiscence of his bowel anastomosis.

WHAT ARE YOUR IMMEDIATE PRIORITIES?

This elderly patient has classic signs of severe sepsis and likely septic shock. Rapid resuscitation is the first priority. You begin noninvasive hemodynamic monitoring and resuscitation ensuring peripheral IV access and infusion of a liter of crystalloid solution. As the fluid is being administered a central venous catheter and invasive arterial line should be inserted under sterile technique and a full set of blood tests including complete blood count, chemistries, and lactate with ScvO$_2$ ordered. The CVP reads 2 cmH$_2$0 and ScvO$_2$ is 52%. Blood glucose is normal. Two sets of blood cultures should be taken prior to, but must not delay, starting empiric

antimicrobial therapy. Following recognition of sepsis and septic shock, resuscitation should continue along with various measures aimed at effectively treating the underlying infection. Crystalloid or colloid IV fluids are acceptable, not starch-based fluid therapy. Source control should be achieved as soon as possible.

WHAT IS THE DIAGNOSIS, AND HOW WOULD YOU MANAGE THE PATIENT?

Most likely the diagnosis is anastomotic leak with diffuse peritonitis causing septic shock; less likely is intestinal ischemia or intraperitoneal bleed. Hospital-acquired pneumonia, myocardial infarction, and pulmonary embolus should also be considered. Severe sepsis is the most obvious diagnosis caused by fecal peritonitis; therefore, immediate treatment is mandatory. Septic shock with concurrent generalized tissue hypoperfusion is the major cause of multiorgan dysfunction in this critical care situation. Prompt correction of tissue hypoperfusion and improvement in tissue oxygenation with fluid resuscitation, vasopressors, and oxygen therapy is necessary in addition to rapid source control and empiric IV antibiotics, based on an assumption of the likely microorganisms causing the infection and local resistance patterns. If there is already dysfunction of several organ systems, continue aggressive resuscitation and draw blood for culture followed by systemic antibiotic therapy and if vasopressor support is required to aim for mean arterial pressure (MAP) >65mmHg, norepinephrine is the first-line therapy, followed by epinephrine inotropy and/or vasopressin. For patients refractory to these measures, consider adrenal insufficiency and start steroid therapy with hydrocortisone 200 mg/day.

WHAT IS THE FORMULA FOR SCVO$_2$, AND WHY IS THIS PATIENT'S SCVO$_2$ LOW?

$$ScvO_2 = SpO_2 - [VO_2/CO \times Hb \times 1.34]$$

(ScvO$_2$ central venous oxygen; SpO$_2$ oxygen saturation; VO$_2$ oxygen utilization; CO cardiac output; Hb hemoglobin concentration)

HOW WOULD YOU MANAGE THE PATIENT NOW?

First ensure that the patient is normovolemic. If hypoxemia with hypoperfusion of extremities and worsening mental status persist, more aggressive fluid resuscitation targeting a higher CVP with vasopressor and inotropic support may be necessary. Assessment of fluid status with echocardiography, pulse pressure variation, thoracic impedance, or pulmonary artery catheter placement should be considered. Invasive blood pressure monitoring should be initiated, and this patient should be transferred to a higher level of care in the intensive care unit (ICU). The arterial pressure waveform contributes a great deal of useful information—systolic and diastolic blood pressures are measured directly and heart rate is calculated from time between systolic peaks; waveform can now be used to derive further hemodynamic measures—area under the curve of the systolic part of the waveform is used for stroke volume assessment and hence cardiac output evaluation. Cardiac contractility can be derived from the upslope of the arterial pressure waveform, and the diastolic pressure decay and the position of the dicrotic notch (aortic valve closure) provides assessment of the systemic vascular resistance. Volume status may be estimated from changes in the pressure waveform over the respiratory cycle. Changes in intrathoracic pressure, particularly with an effect on venous return to the heart, can lead to periodic increases and decreases in arterial blood pressure. These changes are more marked in hypovolemia, so a measure of the degree of variability (pulse pressure or systolic pressure variability) is a reliable indicator of fluid responsiveness. Analysis of trends or response to interventions such as a fluid challenge or bedside leg-raise can yield very valuable information. This deterioration is likely septic in nature given the hypotension, secondary to vasodilatation, and rise in body temperature. Other possible causes to consider are myocardial infarction and adrenal insufficiency (AI). AI must be considered as it is not an uncommon complication of severe sepsis. After placement of an arterial catheter for dynamic blood pressure monitoring and arterial blood gas analysis, add norepinephrine infusion to improve MAP and consider an inodilator infusion such as dobutamine, if MAP allows, for improved cardiac output. Due to a falling SpO_2, a reduced level of consciousness, and the need for ongoing resuscitation, the patient is intubated and mechanical ventilation is initiated in the ICU. Thereafter, and once hemodynamically stable, in consultation with the primary surgical team, an abdominal CT scan should be ordered.

As ongoing intra-abdominal infection cannot be controlled with interventional radiology drain placement, he is taken back to the operating room for abdominal exploration, washout, and defunctioning ostomy formation. Thereafter, on transfer back to the ICU, lung protective ventilation strategies, glucose control, stress ulcer prophylaxis, deep vein thrombosis prophylaxis, and appropriate antibiotic therapy are initiated with consideration of early enteral feeding around day 3 ICU. In general, invasive procedures can be safely performed when platelet count is at least 50,000. If no antiplatelet drugs or significant uremia is present, then an operative procedure

can be safely performed. Other causes of thrombocytopenia are disseminated intravascular coagulopathy (DIC) and drug-induced thrombocytopenia such as heparin-induced thrombocytopenia. Sepsis is the most common cause of DIC. There is no difference in the incidence of DIC in patients with gram-negative and gram-positive sepsis. Systemic infection with other microorganisms (viruses/parasites) may also lead to DIC. Components of the cell membrane or bacterial exotoxins are the triggers for activation of the coagulation cascade. A scoring system devised by the subcommittee on DIC of the International Society of Thrombosis and Hemostasis has a sensitivity and specificity of 95% for the diagnosis. Lab tests show a progressive fall in platelet count and fibrinogen level and an increase in activated partial thromboplastin time and international normalized ratio. Fibrinogen also has a role as an acute phase protein so that a normal level does not exclude DIC and, therefore, a trend is more useful. Treatment is directed at correcting the underlying condition, but support for both thrombotic and hemorrhagic clinical features is required. A platelet count of 10,000 or lower requires transfusion to prevent spontaneous bleeding and <50,000 for a procedure. Fresh frozen plasma and cryoprecipitate are preferred for factor replacement and fibrinogen replacement, whereas coagulation factor concentrate may have traces of activated coagulation factors that may exacerbate the coagulopathy.

HOW DO YOU MANAGE HYPERGLYCEMIA IN THIS PATIENT?

It is likely to be an ongoing problem given the diabetes comorbidity and the initial hyperglycemia and the use of hydrocortisone. Confirm the elevated result and institute insulin treatment starting with an IV infusion of insulin and check glucose levels regularly. Control of glucose levels to 100 to 180 mg/dl reduces organ dysfunction and mortality based on Surviving Sepsis Campaign guidelines by preventing episodes of hypoglycemia.

WHAT CAN YOU DO TO PREVENT FURTHER DETERIORATION IN RENAL FUNCTION?

Maintain adequate renal perfusion pressure. Recognize that a MAP of 70 mmHg may be too low in chronically hypertensive patients to provide an adequate driving pressure and glomerular filtration rate (GFR). Norepinephrine (NE) is effective in raising blood pressure with little effect on cardiac output and often raises GFR. Renal dysfunction is largely prerenal in these patients. NE is titrated to a blood pressure level at which flow is reestablished with adequate urine output.

LAB RESULTS SHOW URINE OSMOLALITY 700 MOSM/L AND URINE NA CONCENTRATION 15 MMOL/L. HOW DO YOU INTERPRET THESE FINDINGS?

A low urine sodium concentration <20 mmol/l or a low fractional excretion of sodium <1% are indicative of avid sodium reabsorption and together with a high urine osmolality >500 mosm/kg/H$_2$0 indicates a preserved renal concentrating capacity. These findings represent an appropriate prerenal response to hypoperfusion; they are compatible with a reversible renal dysfunction upon achieving adequate flow and perfusion pressure, and a further increase in MAP may be indicated.

DISCUSSION

The Third International Consensus Definitions for Sepsis and Septic Shock (Sepsis-3) defines sepsis as life-threatening organ dysfunction caused by a dysregulated host response to infection.[1] Organ dysfunction can be represented by an increase in the Sequential Organ Failure Assessment (SOFA) score of 2 points or more, which is associated with an in-hospital mortality greater than 10%. Septic shock refers to profound circulatory, cellular, and metabolic abnormalities associated with a greater risk of mortality than with sepsis alone. Patients with septic shock can be clinically identified by a vasopressor requirement to maintain a MAP of 65 mmHg or greater and serum lactate level greater than 2 mmol/L (>18 mg/dL) in the absence of hypovolemia. Patients with at least 2 of the following clinical criteria on the quickSOFA score—respiratory rate of 22/min or greater, altered mentation, or systolic blood pressure ≤100 mmHg—are more likely to have a worse outcome. Recognizing the clinical signs of sepsis early in the course of the disease is important. The biochemical processes of sepsis are very complex and involve multiple host-derived mediator molecules including cytokines, complement and coagulation cascades, vasoactive mediators such as kinins, prostaglandins, and acute phase reactants as well as short-lived intermediates of oxygen and nitrogen. The effects of these molecules on oxygen delivery and blood flow are brought about by vasodilation, loss of endothelial barrier function, occlusion of capillaries, and impaired myocardial contractility. Multiple factors contribute to tissue hypoxia in sepsis. Vasodilation drastically increases the diameter of the vascular tree, reducing systemic vascular resistance and inducing relative hypovolemia and lowering effective blood pressure.[2] Inducible nitric oxide synthase enzyme is a potent smooth muscle relaxing agent and is expressed in the presence of cytokines and metabolites in septic shock where it catalyzes the conversion of the amino acid arginine to citrulline. Loss of the integrity of the endothelial barrier results in loss of protein and fluid into the interstitium. The resulting edema aggravates cellular hypoxia and impairs diffusion of oxygen similar to occlusion of capillaries by thrombi, activated leukocytes, and aggregates of erythrocytes. The combination of capillary occlusion and interstitial edema and loss of endothelial barrier function increases the local tissue oxygen deficit. Recognizing the perfusion defect in septic patients can be difficult as the clinical manifestations of sepsis and septic shock can be variable from one patient to the next. Tachycardia is a reflexive response to a relative intravascular volume deficit. Unresuscitated patients show signs of peripheral hypoperfusion, a rapid weak pulse, tissue pallor, and cyanosis. Serial measurement of serum lactate in conjunction with central or mixed venous oxygen monitoring allows evaluation of the adequacy of resuscitation, and rapid correction of these variables is critical. Early goal-directed therapy (EGDT) is comprised of early identification of high-risk patients, appropriate cultures, source control, and administration of appropriate antibiotics.[3] This is followed by early hemodynamic optimization of oxygen delivery, guided by preload (CVP), or surrogate, targeting with fluids, afterload (MAP) targeted with vasopressors, arterial oxygen content (packed red blood cells and/or oxygen supplementation), contractility (inotropic agents), and decreasing oxygen consumption (mechanical ventilation and sedation), and guided by ScvO$_2$. These principles are good practice recommendations for sepsis management in the ICU setting. The Surviving Sepsis Campaign recommends EGDT[2], which has become the standard of care worldwide, in the initial management of severe sepsis. However, three recent clinical trials ProCESS (Protocol-based Care for Early Septic Shock), ARiSE (Australasian Resuscitation in Sepsis Evaluation), and ProMiSe (Protocolized Management in Sepsis)[4,5,6] demonstrated that while EGDT did not cause harm, it did not improve outcome in patients with severe sepsis when compared with usual care. EGDT does not show improved survival for patients randomized to receive EGDT compared to usual care or to less invasive alternative hemodynamic resuscitation protocols. EGDT is, however, associated with increased admission to ICU. Also, there is no negative outcome associated with EGDT. Diagnosing infection in acutely ill patients is often enormously challenging. If sepsis is the most likely cause of acute deterioration, it is important to know the site from which the infection is arising as well as the infecting pathogen. Definitive identification of the microbial species and evaluation of the sensitivity profile and local antibiograms usually involves at least 48 hours. A gram stain (especially of the cerebrospinal fluid flow or urine) can provide information on the class of organism within an hour. Nosocomial infections are particularly challenging to diagnose and treat. Delays in initiating therapy increases the risk of death. Equally, failure to respond to initial antimicrobial therapy requires escalation of therapy and prompt deescalation when possible. Septic shock is a major cause of ICU admission and mortality. It leads to multiorgan dysfunction, failure, and death. Mortality rates can be in excess of 50%. The most common cause of sepsis is bacterial infection, but viral and fungal infections can also be a cause. Invading pathogens must evade host defenses, and then the number of organisms, various virulence factors, and ability of host defenses play a role in establishing infection and sepsis. The inflammatory response is the reason for the majority of the pathology seen in septic shock. Pathogen-released components or toxins such as lipopolysaccharide, peptidoglycan and bacterial DNA are recognized by toll-like receptors on cells of the immune system, such as monocytes. This recognition causes a positive feedback system and the release of pro-inflammatory interleukin (IL)-1, IL-6 and tumor necrosis factor-alpha, and the anti-inflammatory cytokines (IL-10 and IL-4), leading to complement activation, platelet aggregation, and the coagulation cascade. An exaggeration of this response as seen in severe sepsis and septic shock leads to organ dysfunction and cell and tissue death.

Neutrophils and lymphocytes undergo increased apoptosis; coagulation system activation leads to microvascular occlusion and DIC.[7] Increased capillary permeability, vasodilation, and micro-circulatory dysfunction lead to effective hypovolemia and cardiovascular compromise. Cardiac output is usually increased initially but sepsis-induced cardiac dysfunction can also be present. Severe sepsis shares some clinical features with other distributive shock states and also exhibits elements of hypovolemic and cardiogenic shock. Management should be goal-directed to deal with the shock syndrome and underlying condition. Emergency general surgery patients have among the highest mortality, morbidity, and complication rates of any patient group. Risk assessment should occur using a tool such the P-POSSUM score. A predicted mortality score $\geq$5% defines the high-risk surgical patient and $\geq$10% should have ICU level of care.[8]

CONCLUSIONS

- Sepsis is common cause of morbidity and mortality.

- Timely and targeted diagnosis and intervention can significantly alter outcome.

- Early and aggressive fluid resuscitation with balanced crystalloid solutions and maintenance of adequate blood pressure using norepinephrine as first line therapy are key goals.

- Early administration of antibiotics, with or without culture collection, as well as source control are crucial interventions.

- Biochemical and clinical markers of perfusion such as MAP, lactate, mixed/central venous oxygen saturation, urine output and mentation are relevant parameters to guide the adequacy of resuscitation.

- Maintaining blood glucose <180g/dl improves outcome.

- Hydrocortisone hastens resolution of shock without mortality benefit.

- The practitioner should be vigilant for the occurrence of acute kidney injury, coagulopathy, and sepsis-induced cardiomyopathy.

REFERENCES

1. Singer M, Deutschman CS, Seymour CW, et al. The Third International Consensus Definitions for Sepsis and Septic Shock (Sepsis-3). JAMA 2016;315(8):801–810.
2. Marik PE, Cavallazzi R, Vasu T, Hirani A. Dynamic changes in arterial waveform derived variables and fluid responsiveness in mechanically ventilated patients: a systematic review of the literature. Crit Care Med. 2009;37(9):2642–2647.
3. Dellinger RP, Levy MM, Carlet JM, et al. Surviving Sepsis Campaign: international guidelines for management of severe sepsis and septic shock. Crit Care Med. 2013;41:580–637.
4. Peake SL, Delaney A, Bailey M, et al.; ARISE Investigators, Anzics Clinical Trials Group. Goal-directed resuscitation for patients with early septic shock. N Engl J Med. 2014;371(16):1496–1506.
5. Yealy DM, Kellum JA, Huang DT, Barnato AE, Weissfeld LA, et al. PROCESS Investigators. A randomized trial of protocol-based care for early septic shock. N Engl J Med. 2014;370(18):1683–1693.
6. Mouncey PR, Osborn TM, Power GS, et al. Trial of early, goal-directed resuscitation for septic shock. N Engl J Med. 2015;372(14):1301–1311.
7. Levi M, Disseminated intravascular coagulation. Crit Care Med. 2007;35(9):2191–2195.
8. Saunders D, Murray D, AC Pichel, Varley S, Peden CJ; UK Emergency Laparotomy Network. Variations in mortality after emergency laparotomy: the first report of the UK Emergency Laparotomy Network Br J Anaes 2012;109:368–375.

REVIEW QUESTIONS

1. Management of septic shock due to colonic anastomotic breakdown includes

   A. Prompt administration of appropriate antibiotics.
   B. Targeting an ScvO$_2$ equal to 55%.
   C. Immediate administration of activated protein C.
   D. Low-dose hydrocortisone prior to administration of fluid resuscitation.

2. In adult patients, which of the following are clinical features of the early course of severe sepsis?

   A. Temperature 35.1°C
   B. Leucocyte count 10×10^9/L
   C. Respiratory rate of 8 breaths per minute
   D. Heart rate 72 beats per minute

3. The following are true regarding mechanisms responsible for tissue hypoxia in severe sepsis *except*

   A. Relative hypovolemia causing hypotension.
   B. Maldistribution of blood flow because of microvascular thrombosis.
   C. Maldistribution of blood flow because of arteriovenous shunting.
   D. Loss of intravascular fluid due to capillary leakage.
   E. Myocardial depression due to coronary vasospasm

4. Optimal timing for initial interventions after recognizing septic shock in a patient

   A. Within 1 hour to obtain adequate cultures.
   B. Within 1 hour for IV corticosteroids.
   C. Within 6 hours for aggressive fluid resuscitation.
   D. Within 12 hours for vasopressors after fluid resuscitation.

5. A known diabetic patient with a history of COPD and hypertension is in septic shock following abdominal aortic aneurysm repair in the ICU. She is intubated with the following invasive catheters—urinary Foley catheter, pulmonary artery catheter, peripheral IV catheter, and a nasogastric tube. List the common endemic causes of nosocomial infection that are possible causes of her sepsis

   A. Coagulase-negative staphylococci, enterococci, pseudomonas, E coli
   B. Anerobic organisms, mycoplasma, legionella, prions

C. Mycoplasma, enterococci, E coli, legionella

D. Zika virus, prions, methicillin-resistant *Staphylococcus aureus*, extended-spectrum beta lactamase organisms

6. Which of the following has been shown *not* to reduce the rate of contamination during the performance of blood cultures?

A. Skin preparation with chlorhexidine rather than povidone-iodine

B. Aspiration of blood through a central catheter using full sterile technique

C. Changing the needle prior to inoculating the specimen into a culture bottle

D. Disinfecting the stopper on the culture bottle prior to inoculation

7. Which 3 factors might improve cellular uptake of oxygen in sepsis?

A. Hypercarbia, pyrexia, acidemia

B. Tissue edema, shunting, alkalemia

C. Hypothermia, hypercarbia, tissue edema

D. Alkalemia, hypocarbia, pyrexia

8. What is the pathological basis for an increased mixed venous oxygen saturation in sepsis?

A. Shunting, capillary occlusion, tissue edema, increased blood flow rate

B. Vasospasm, venous thromboembolism, inhibition of apoptosis

C. Tissue edema, vasospasm, carotid baroreceptor reflex

D. IL-1, prostaglandins, nitric oxide

9. All of the following lab tests support a diagnosis of DIC *except*

A. Platelet count 50 × 109/L.

B. Prothrombin time 52 seconds.

C. Target cells on blood film.

D. Prolonged thrombin time.

10. What information can be derived from an arterial pressure waveform?

A. Stroke volume from the area under the entire waveform

B. Myocardial afterload from dP/dt

C. Hypovolemia from a high dicrotic notch

D. Vasodilation from a steep diastolic rate of decay

ANSWERS

1. A. Early volume resuscitation is a cornerstone of the treatment of septic shock and should take precedence over the other options presented. $ScvO_2$ is an appropriate parameter to determine the adequacy of resuscitation. Hydrocortisone may be useful in decreasing shock duration but should not be administered prior to volume resuscitation. Activated Protein C is no longer recommended for the treatment of septic shock.

2. A. Though less common than fever, hypothermia can occur in up to 35% of patients presenting with sepsis. Hypothermic sepsis predicts increased mortality over both normo- and hyperthermic patients. Tachypnoea is more frequently seen in the septic patient due to the presence of metabolic acidosis. Though sepsis can occur in the presence of a normal white blood cell count and heart rate, these parameters are more typically deranged.

3. E. Coronary arterial blood flow in sepsis has been shown to be increased rather than diminished. Myocardial depression due to changes at the microvascular level is the cause of cardiomyopathy, with endothelial dysfunction and tissue edema, mitochondrial dysfunction and changes in nitric oxide metabolism caused by systemic inflammation all playing a role.

4. A. Antibiotics should be administered within one hour of the clinical diagnosis of sepsis. Ideally cultures are obtained prior to this, but there should be no delay in the timely administration of antibiotics whether the patient has been cultured or not. Corticosteroids should only be administered after the patient has been appropriately resuscitated and source control/antibiotics instituted. The optimal timing of fluid resuscitation/vasopressors is as soon as the diagnosis of sepsis is made, and these can be administered concurrently.

5. A. Ventilator-associated pneumonia and catheter-related urinary tract infection in the ICU is most frequently associated with gram negative organisms, whereas central line-associated bloodstream infection is most often caused by gram positive, especially staphylococcal, organisms. However, there is certainly significant overlap, and candida species remain an important cause of infection related to invasive devices. Atypical organisms certainly cause infection requiring ICU admission, but are not common nosocomial infections. Zika virus requires an arthropod vector to transmit the disease. Nosocomial infection with prion disease is extremely rare and generally associated with contaminated surgical instruments.

6. D. Alcohol based chlorhexidine gluconate solution has been shown to be superior to povidone-iodine based solutions in preventing blood culture contamination. Blood cultures drawn from previously indwelling lines can be easily contaminated. This incidence can be reduced by using full sterile technique and drawing blood from a freshly placed line.

7. A. The oxyhemoglobin curve is shifted to the right in conditions of increased temperature, hydrogen ion concentration, and partial pressure of CO_2. This favors offloading of oxygen from hemoglobin.

8. A. Tissue edema causing mechanical impairment of tissue blood flow works in concert with the systemic inflammatory response to cause widespread dysfunction of the microcirculation. Microvascular thrombosis impairs tissue oxygen delivery as a result. In addition, alterations in nitric oxide metabolism cause pathological shunting at these vascular beds. Finally, oxygen utilization at the mitochondria level is impaired. Thus, despite elevated cardiac output, tissue oxygen delivery and utilization can lead to increased mixed venous oxygen saturation.

9. C. DIC is diagnosed combining both clinical presentation and laboratory tests demonstrating thrombosis and thrombolysis with consumptive coagulopathy. Prothrombin

and partial thromboplastin times are prolonged, with thrombocytopenia also prominent. In addition, fibrinogen is low, with d-dimer and fibrin degradation products being elevated. Target cells are erythrocytes with central and peripheral concentrations of hemoglobin with a colorless zone in between. They are characteristic of a variety of pathologic states. Hemoglobinopathies such as thalassemia, sickle cell disease and hemoglobin C disease demonstrate target cells, as does iron deficiency anemia, the post-splenectomy patient, and those with obstructive liver disease.

10. D. In arterial pressure waveform analysis, Stroke volume is calculated by integrating the area under the systolic portion of the wave. dP/dt reflects various components of systemic vascular resistance, left ventricular contractility, and intravascular volume status. It is not an accurate reflection of simply afterload. Similarly, though high dicrotic notch may be present in the hypovolemic patient, other hemodynamic variables affect the closing of the aortic valve such that this is non-diagnostic. In patients with a stable stroke volume, steep diastolic decay does indeed indicate vasodilation.

27.

ABDOMINAL COMPARTMENT SYNDROME

Brian Woods

STEM CASE AND KEY QUESTIONS

A 62-year-old man presents to the emergency department with abdominal pain. After initial evaluation, the admitting physician refers him for admission. The patient endorses nausea, vomiting, and abdominal pain for over 24 hours now. He has a history for prior admissions due to the same complaint related to his chronic alcohol abuse and admits to recent heavy drinking. His past medical history is significant for chronic obstructive pulmonary disease, continued tobacco dependence, essential hypertension, morbid obesity, obstructive sleep apnea, and atrial fibrillation. His procedural history includes a laparoscopic appendectomy and a failed catheter-based cardiac ablation several years ago. He does acknowledge having any drug allergies and does not take any medications routinely.

WHAT IS INTRA-ABDOMINAL HYPERTENSION?

On examination the patient appears uncomfortable and mildly toxic but cooperative and coherent. His blood pressure is 158/82 mmHg, pulse rate 108 beats per minute, respiratory rate 21 breaths per minute, and oral temperature 37.3°C. He weighs 119 kg and is 170 cm tall. He is oriented to person, place, time, and his reason for hospitalization. His skin is warm, dry, and without a frank rash. The mucous membranes are moist. His breath sounds are clear and somewhat distant. The heart tones are regular, with no adventitious sounds, and he has normal radial and pedal pulses. There is no ankle edema. His abdomen is frankly obese, diffusely tender without rebound, and without visible stigmata of liver disease. You cannot palpate the liver or spleen. He declines a rectal exam and examination of his groins and genitalia is unremarkable.

WHEN SHOULD INTRA-ABDOMINAL HYPERTENSION COME UNDER CONSIDERATION?

During conversation, he confirms that he has been drinking heavily for the past week after a period of prolonged abstinence. His current symptoms match prior episodes of admission, which upon review of his previous records you find were for acute pancreatitis. Previous episodes were managed conservatively with spontaneous resolution, but he insists his pain is worse than he remembers. He has not been able to eat for over a day and describes the pain as "all over my stomach" and without radiation to the back.

WHAT ARE COMMON CAUSES OF INTRA-ABDOMINAL HYPERTENSION?

He denies any recent surgeries. He feels this current admission is similar, although more painful, than his previous bouts of abdominal pain after "benders" and expresses confidence that it will resolve in a few days. Other than occasional diarrhea, he denies significant change in bowel habits.

Laboratory studies are largely unremarkable except for a somewhat elevated serum lipase. His electrocardiogram remains unchanged from previous admissions and consistent with history of atrial fibrillation. After review of his previous imaging including a computed tomography of the abdomen revealed nothing further than evidence of COPD but there are no significant pancreatic findings. It is decided not to obtain any new imaging at this time and to continue conservative management.

HOW DOES ONE DIAGNOSE INTRA-ABDOMINAL HYPERTENSION?

You recommend moderate intravenous hydration, antiemetics, analgesics, and restricted oral intake along with an alcohol withdrawal management protocol. Later that hospital day you are called to reevaluate him since he has become confused and his vitals now include a fever to 38.3°C, a pulse of 117 bpm, a respiratory rate of 30, and continued hypertension. On examination he is oriented only to name and only cooperates inconsistently. He appears to be in more pain, particularly upon abdominal palpation. He is pale, and his work of breathing is increased. You are concerned enough to transfer him to a higher acuity unit and to consult the surgical service. You request an abdominal computed tomography (CT) and further blood tests.

WHEN DOES INTRA-ABDOMINAL HYPERTENSION BECOME ABDOMINAL COMPARTMENT SYNDROME?

The surgeon recommends urinary catheter placement. A small amount of dark, non-bloody urine drains, and over the next several hours there is minimal output despite fluid boluses. The CT of the abdomen shows pancreatic inflammation without cysts or calcification, along with a distended stomach and extremely dilated loops of bowel consistent with an ileus. The bases of the lungs have new and significant atelectasis or consolidation. His liver is moderately enlarged and cirrhotic but his spleen appears normal. The rest of his anatomy is grossly normal with some mild atherosclerotic arterial changes.

HOW DO THE MANAGEMENT STRATEGIES FOR INTRA-ABDOMINAL HYPERTENSION AND ABDOMINAL COMPARTMENT SYNDROME OVERLAP AND DIFFER?

The patient's clinical status worsens overnight with increased confusion and work of breathing. He requires endotracheal intubation for airway protection and acute respiratory failure. An orogastric drain is placed for decompression with some initial air removal but scant return after that. He remains anuric and his blood pressure is continuing to drop; he is started on first one and then a second vasopressor. Crystalloid boluses are given without benefit, and his abdomen becomes more tense and distended and his respirator is alarming for elevated peak airway pressures. His skin is cool and mottled, and he has decreased peripheral pulses. Blood studies show a mixed metabolic and respiratory acidosis with a large alveolar to arterial (A-a) oxygen tension gradient, an elevated lactate, and a rapidly rising blood urea nitrogen and serum creatinine.

WHAT COMORBIDITIES CAN COMPLICATE THE DIAGNOSIS AND MANAGEMENT OF ABDOMINAL COMPARTMENT SYNDROME? HOW DO YOU CALCULATE THE ABDOMINAL PERFUSION PRESSURE?

You make adjustments to the ventilator settings but are unable to achieve an appropriately high minute ventilation in the face of decreasing tidal volumes (V_T) to try to reduce peak pressures less than 40 cm H_2O while increasing positive end expiration to allow for maintenance of oxygenation. Sedation is increased and cisatracurium is started for neuromuscular blockade and his peak inspiratory pressures improve slightly. Invasive hemodynamic monitoring shows a central venous pressure of 22 mmHg, a radial arterial pressure of 92/68 mmHg, and a bladder pressure of 24 mmHg. You obtain a transthoracic echocardiogram to further assess his status, which reveals tachycardia, normal valve function, mildly depressed biventricular function, and decreased filling volumes without any pericardial effusions.

WHAT ARE THE OUTCOMES FOR ABDOMINAL COMPARTMENT SYNDROME?

You discuss these findings with your surgical colleague, who recommends immediate laparotomy. Because the operating rooms are two floors below the patient's acute care unit, and because the patient has become hemodynamically tenuous, the operative team mobilizes to the bedside instead. The

laparotomy is performed uneventfully, and the intraoperative examination shows distended loops of bowel that is slightly dusky but without frank ischemia. The pancreas appears inflamed but is not manipulated in any way. Airway pressures improve dramatically upon opening of the fascia, and vasoactive infusion requirements decrease modestly. The abdominal contents are covered with a mesh and a vacuum type dressing.

Over the next 2 weeks the patient experiences acute kidney injury requiring dialysis, intolerance of enteral feeding, and slow resolution of vasodilatory shock and pancreatitis. He requires several operative examinations of the abdomen with eventual fascial closure performed serially. During this time he receives a tracheotomy and jejunal feeding tube. After nearly a month in the hospital, he transitions off mechanical ventilation but still requires continued physical and metabolic rehabilitation after his long acute illness, immobility, and deconditioning.

DISCUSSION

IAH and abdominal compartment syndrome (ACS) are devastating phenomena along a spectrum marked by abnormal pressure within the peritoneal cavity. Organ dysfunction results from intra-abdominal or extra-abdominal processes, causing reduced venous drainage compounded by direct mechanical effects. A commonly accepted definition of IAH is persistent intra-abdominal pressure (IAP) of 12 mmHg or greater; ACS occurs with persistent IAP >20 and new organ dysfunction (Box 27.1). The causes of abdominal hypertension are multiple, indicating different management strategies. Clinicians often fail to recognize IAH/ACS or to intervene promptly. Values for IAH are slightly lower in children, at 10 mmHg or greater (Kirkpatrick 2013).

ETIOLOGY AND PATHOGENESIS

IAH arises from pathology of the abdominal wall, within the abdomen, or outside the abdomen. Primary causes arise within the abdomen or pelvis and can be extra- or intraluminal to the gut. Secondary causes occur outside the abdominopelvic region; are often overlooked; and include sepsis, trauma, or positioning (Box 27.2).

Box 27.1 **INTRA-ABDOMINAL HYPERTENSION GRADES**

IAP is 5–7 mmHg in critically ill adults

IAH is defined as persistent or recurrent elevation of IAP
  ≥12 mmHg

IAH grades:
  Grade I 12-15 mmHg
  Grade II 16-20 mmHg
  Grade III 21-25 mmHg
  Grade IV > 25 mmHg

Note: ACS is sustained IAP >20 mmHg with new organ dysfunction.
Source: From Kirkpatrick (2013).

Box 27.2 COMMON INTRA-ABDOMINAL HYPERTENSION CAUSATIVE FACTORS

Abdominal surgery (intra-abdominal or abdominal wall)

Major trauma

Burns

Prone positioning

Gastroparesis, distension, or ileus

Bowel pseudo-obstruction

Volvulus

Acute pancreatitis

Peritonitis

Fluid collections

Pneumoperitoneum

Intra-abdominal infection or abscess

Tumors

Increased critical illness score

Age

Ascites

Acidosis

Coagulopathy

Hypothermia

Massive fluid resuscitation

Sepsis or shock

Pneumonia

Elevated head of bed

Positive end expiratory pressure >10 cm H_2O

Source: From Kirkpatrick (2013).

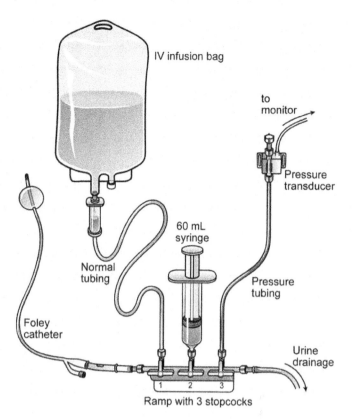

Figure 27.1 Measurement apparatus for abdominal pressure.
From Desie N, Willems A, De Laet I, et al. Intra-abdominal pressure measurement using the Foley Manometer does not increase the risk for urinary tract infection in critically ill patients. *Ann Intensive Care*. 2012;2012(Suppl 1):S10. doi:10.1186/2110-5820-2-S1-S10; Malbrain M. Different techniques to measure intra-abdominal pressure (IAP): Time for a critical re-appraisal. *Intensive Care Med*. 2004;30(3):357–371. doi:10.1007/s00134-003-2107-2 with permission.

DIAGNOSIS

Because IAH and ACS have major negative effects and are often overlooked, clinicians should maintain a high index of suspicion for patients at risk. Examples include patients with burns to the abdomen, major surgery of the abdominal wall, contents, or retroperitoneum, massive transfusion, and bowel obstruction. Physical examination has low sensitivity (Kirkpatrick 2000). Since early diagnosis and treatment likely improve outcomes, and because IAP measurement is relatively low risk and low cost, assessment can be undertaken with a reasonable index of suspicion.

There are multiple approaches to bladder pressure measurement (Box 27.3). The most common bedside method consists of bladder pressure measurement via a Foley catheter (Figure 27.1). These pressures are reproducible and reliable and correlate well with IAP in the absence of subcompartmental pressure phenomena, as with adhesions or localized abscess. (Gianini 2005). Bladder pressure measurements have

limitations including patient position, ventilation mode, the use of neuromuscular blocking drugs, and bladder or pelvic pathology.

TREATMENT

Root cause directs management of IAH/ACS. Intraluminal processes such as gastric distension or bowel obstruction indicate a need for suction decompression from above or below. Extraluminal pathology such as retroperitoneal bleed or abdominal aortic leak require surgical or catheter-based intervention as appropriate. Supportive care and source control treat secondary causes of IAH/ACS, including sepsis or massive volume overload (Figures 27.2 and 27.3). Competing concerns such as IAP, fluid balance, urine output, and oxygenation become difficult to navigate as physiologic reserve diminishes. Aggressive volume resuscitation even when appropriate can increase IAP and cause secondary ACS (Ball 2008). While invasive monitoring of central or pulmonary pressures require interpretation within the clinical context of respiratory and abdominal mechanics (Cheatham 2007), an echocardiogram or dynamic measures of hemodynamic function such as pulse pressure variation or global end diastolic volume potentially provide management indicators more resistant to the confounding effects of high IAP (Renner 2009).

Box 27.3 METHODS FOR INTRA-ABDOMINAL PRESSURE MEASUREMENT

Bladder or transvesical

Gastric

Rectal

Vaginal

Uterine

Intra-peritoneal

Inferior vena cava

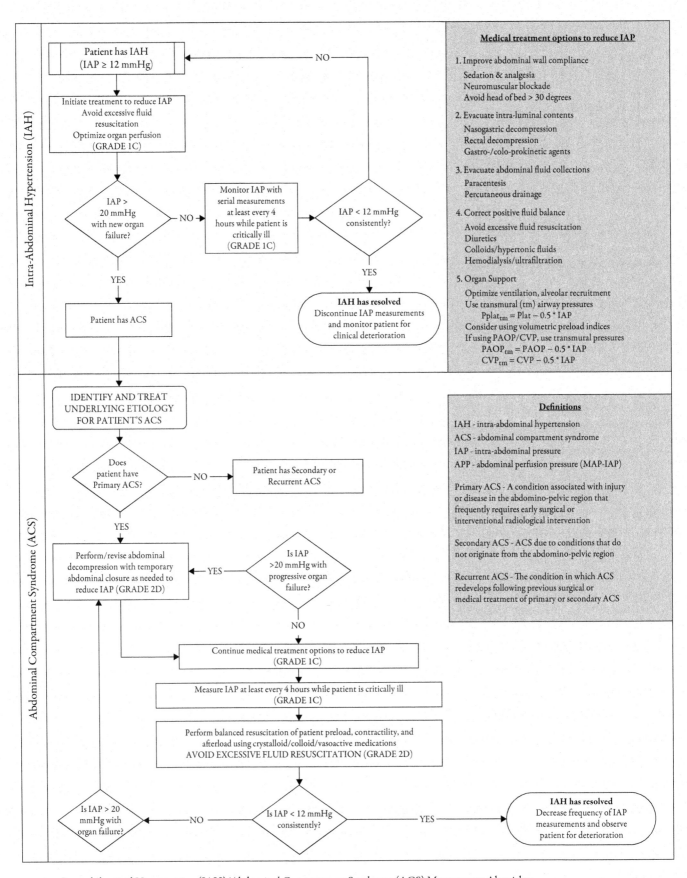

Figure 27.2 Intra-abdominal Hypertension (IAH)/Abdominal Compartment Syndrome (ACS) Management Algorithm.
From Kirkpatrick AW, Roberts DJ, De Waele J, et al. Intra-abdominal hypertension and the abdominal compartment syndrome: Updated consensus definitions and clinical practice guidelines from the World Society of the Abdominal Compartment Syndrome. *Intensive Care Med.* 2013;39(7):1190–1206.

IAH/ACS MEDICAL MANAGEMENT ALGORITHM

- *The choice (and success) of the medical management strategies listed below is strongly related to both the etiology of the patient's IAH/ACS and the patient's clinical situation. The appropriateness of each intervention should always be considered prior to implementing these interventions in any individual patient.*
- *The interventions should be applied in a stepwise fashion until the patient's intra-abdominal pressure (IAP) decreases.*
- *If there is no response to a particular intervention, therapy should be escalated to the next step in the algorithm.*

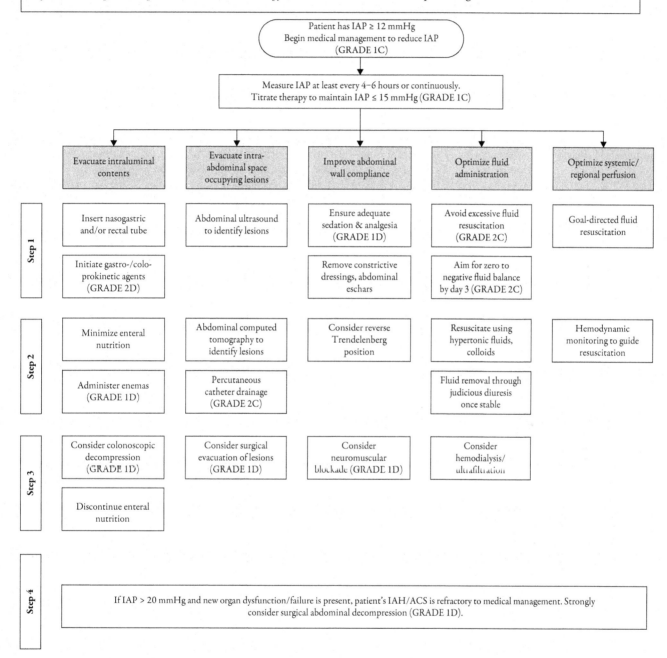

Patient has IAP ≥ 12 mmHg
Begin medical management to reduce IAP
(GRADE 1C)

Measure IAP at least every 4–6 hours or continuously.
Titrate therapy to maintain IAP ≤ 15 mmHg (GRADE 1C)

Evacuate intraluminal contents	Evacuate intra-abdominal space occupying lesions	Improve abdominal wall compliance	Optimize fluid administration	Optimize systemic/regional perfusion
Step 1 Insert nasogastric and/or rectal tube	Abdominal ultrasound to identify lesions	Ensure adequate sedation & analgesia (GRADE 1D)	Avoid excessive fluid resuscitation (GRADE 2C)	Goal-directed fluid resuscitation
Initiate gastro-/colo-prokinetic agents (GRADE 2D)		Remove constrictive dressings, abdominal eschars	Aim for zero to negative fluid balance by day 3 (GRADE 2C)	
Step 2 Minimize enteral nutrition	Abdominal computed tomography to identify lesions	Consider reverse Trendelenberg position	Resuscitate using hypertonic fluids, colloids	Hemodynamic monitoring to guide resuscitation
Administer enemas (GRADE 1D)	Percutaneous catheter drainage (GRADE 2C)		Fluid removal through judicious diuresis once stable	
Step 3 Consider colonoscopic decompression (GRADE 1D)	Consider surgical evacuation of lesions (GRADE 1D)	Consider neuromuscular blockade (GRADE 1D)	Consider hemodialysis/ultrafiltration	
Discontinue enteral nutrition				

Step 4 If IAP > 20 mmHg and new organ dysfunction/failure is present, patient's IAH/ACS is refractory to medical management. Strongly consider surgical abdominal decompression (GRADE 1D).

Figure 27.3 Alternative Medical Management Algorithm for IAH/ACS.
From Kirkpatrick AW, Roberts DJ, De Waele J, et al. Intra-abdominal hypertension and the abdominal compartment syndrome: Updated consensus definitions and clinical practice guidelines from the World Society of the Abdominal Compartment Syndrome. *Intensive Care Med.* 2013;39(7):1190–1206.

Monitoring of IAP is required until resolution of IAH/ACS; continuous or intermittent measurements can suffice with proper vigilance. Early intervention for IAH before development of ACS is recommended to reduce morbidity and mortality, and goals are directed toward organ function. Abdominal perfusion pressure (APP), calculated as the difference between mean arterial pressure and abdominal perfusion pressure, also helps guide monitoring and therapy. Guidelines suggest a target APP >60 mmHg. Analgesia and anxiolysis often improve IAP and should be employed before and continued during neuromuscular blockade, another effective treatment for IAH/ACS (Björk 2014).

If initial measures fail to improve APP or there are progressive signs of degrading organ function, surgical abdominal decompression should be considered. Earlier laparotomy to establish an open abdomen typically improves oxygenation and organ function rapidly and likely conveys improved outcomes (De Waele 2016). Laparotomy for open abdominal decompression should occur within 24 hours of ACS onset (Muresan 2017). Experts advocate different surgical approaches to decompression but most commonly favor a midline laparotomy approach (Box 27.4; Leppäniemi 2009).

Eventual closure of the open abdomen is a key goal. Even with serial laparotomies, stepwise closure of the fascia should be attempted. Various approaches to closure are advocated and often involve temporary mesh and vacuum packing (Figure 27.4). Gradual closure allows for avoidance of high airway pressures or worsened IAP and allow continued surveillance for exacerbation of offending intra-abdominal causes. A continued open abdominal cavity carries a high morbidity, given fluid and protein loss, fistula formation, unintentional exenteration, peritoneal infection, frozen bowel, pain, and care burden. Timing and degree of closure depends on the situation, often with reevaluation and progressive closure every 48 hours.

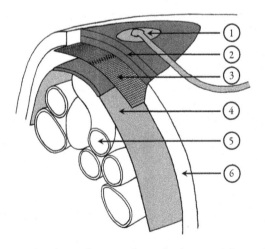

Figure 27.4 Mesh and wound vacuum closure for the open abdomen: (1) vacuum device; (2) foam; (3) mesh; (4) semipermeable sheet; (5) bowel; and (6) abdominal wall.
From Björck M, Wanhainen A. Management of abdominal compartment syndrome and the open abdomen. *Eur J Vasc Endovasc Surg.* 2014;47(3):279–287. doi:10.1016/j.ejvs.2013.12.014, with permission.

OUTCOMES

Improved results for IAH/ACS likely result from early recognition and intervention. Source control, rational fluid management, pain control, and organ support combined with proper timing and management of the open abdomen are the most effective means of treating ACS. The literature is limited in terms of describing outcomes, both by heterogeneity of cause (e.g., ruptured abdominal aortic aneurysm, blunt trauma, or intra-abdominal abscess) and treatment modality (Muresan 2017). However, both single-center and broader surveys suggest that judicious fluid resuscitation, damage control surgery, early surveillance, and rapid intervention have improved outcomes for IAH/ACS over the past few decades (Cheatham 2010). The open abdomen is no longer considered dire but a wise therapeutic maneuver with improved results. The collective experience for IAH/ACS should continue to expand, based on maintaining an index of suspicion for this phenomenon in patients at risk. Future directions for management include continued education and improved awareness, along with improving surgical materials and techniques that allow for complex abdominal wall reconstruction. Research proceeds into topics germane to IAH/ACS such as the microbiome and abdominal wall physiology (Kirkpatrick 2017).

CONCLUSIONS

- IAH/ACS are organ- and life-threatening phenomena.

- Published surveys of critical care and trauma care providers reveal that IAH/ACS are underrecognized and often mismanaged.

- Abdominal pressure should be measured recurrently or continuously in patients at risk for IAH/ACS; bladder pressure is facile, reproducible, and accurate.

- Interventions to reduce risk or ameliorate IAH/ACS should take place promptly.

- The open abdomen (OA) is appropriate in the management of ACS unresponsive to other measures and can occur in the operating room or the bedside with due consideration of resources and patient stability.

- IAH/ACS interact with the central nervous, respiratory, cardiovascular, hepatic, and renal systems in a multicompartment fashion.

- Evidence suggests that outcomes in IAH, ACS, and OA have improved over several decades but that continued education and improved techniques are necessary.

REFERENCES

Ball CG, Kirkpatrick AW, McBeth P. The secondary abdominal compartment syndrome: not just another post-traumatic complication. *Can J Surg.* 2008;51(5):399–405. doi:10.1017/S1446788700004638

Björck M, Wanhainen A. Management of abdominal compartment syndrome and the open abdomen. *Eur J Vasc Endovasc Surg.* 2014;47(3):279–287. doi:10.1016/j.ejvs.2013.12.014

Cheatham ML, Malbrain M. Cardiovascular implications of abdominal compartment syndrome. *Acta Clin Belg.* 2007;62(Suppl 1):98–112. doi:10.1179/acb.2007.62.s1.013

Cheatham ML, Safcsak K. Is the evolving management of intra-abdominal hypertension and abdominal compartment syndrome improving survival? *Crit Care Med.* 2010;38(2):402–407. doi:10.1097/CCM.0b013e3181b9e9b1

Chun R, Kirkpatrick AW. Intra-abdominal pressure, intra-abdominal hypertension, and pregnancy: a review. *Ann Intensive Care.* 2012;2012(Suppl 1):S5. doi:10.1186/2110-5820-2-S1-S5

Coccolini F, Montori G, Ceresoli M, et al. The role of open abdomen in non-trauma patient: WSES Consensus Paper. *World J Emerg Surg.* 2017;12(1):1–17. doi:10.1186/s13017-017-0146-1

De Laet I, Citerio G, Malbrain M. The influence of intra-abdominal hypertension on the central nervous system: current insights and clinical recommendations, is it all in the head? *Acta Clin Belg.* 2007;62(Suppl 1):89–97. doi:10.1179/acb.2007.62.s1.012

De Waele JJ, Kimball E, Malbrain M, et al. Decompressive laparotomy for abdominal compartment syndrome. *Br J Surg.* 2016;103(6):709–715. doi:10.1002/bjs.10097

Fowler J, Owens BD. Abdominal compartment syndrome after hip arthroscopy. *Arthrosc J Arthrosc Relat Surg.* 2010;26(1):128–130. doi:10.1016/j.arthro.2009.06.021

Fuchs F, Bruyere M, Senat MV, Purenne E, Benhamou D, Fernandez H. Are standard intra-abdominal pressure values different during pregnancy? PLoS ONE. 2013;8(10):8–11. doi:10.1371/journal.pone.0077324

Gianini F, De Cleva R, Beer I, Noritomi D, Gama-Rodrigues JJ. Subcompartmental intra-abdominal hypertension. *Intensive Care Med.* 2005;31(7):1005. doi:10.1007/s00134-005-2666-5

Hendrickson S, Chacko L, Wilson MH. Raised intracranial pressure following abdominal closure in a polytrauma patient. *JRSM Open.* 2015;6(1):2054270414565958. doi:10.1177/2054270414565958

Kirkpatrick AW, Brenneman FD, McLean RF, Rapanos T, Boulanger BR. Is clinical examination an accurate indicator of raised intra-abdominal pressure in critically injured patients? *Can J Surg.* 2000;43(3):207–211. doi:10.1109/TPEL.2008.2005192

Kirkpatrick AW, Roberts DJ, De Waele J, et al. Intra-abdominal hypertension and the abdominal compartment syndrome: updated consensus definitions and clinical practice guidelines from the World Society of the Abdominal Compartment Syndrome. *Intensive Care Med.* 2013;39(7):1190–1206. doi:10.1007/s00134-013-2906-z

Kirkpatrick AW, Sugrue M, Mckee JL, et al. Update from the Abdominal Compartment Society (WSACS) on intra-abdominal hypertension and abdominal compartment syndrome: past, present, and future beyond Banff 2017. *Anaesthesiol Intensive Ther.* 2017;49(2):83–87. doi:10.5603/AIT.a2017.0019

Leppäniemi A. Surgical management of abdominal compartment syndrome; indications and techniques. *Scand J Trauma Resusc Emerg Med.* 2009;17(1):17. doi:10.1186/1757-7241-17-17

Muresan M, Muresan S, Brinzaniuc K, et al. How much does decompressive laparotomy reduce the mortality rate in primary abdominal compartment syndrome? A single-center prospective study on 66 patients. *Medicine (Baltimore).* 2017;96(5):e6006. doi:10.1097/MD.0000000000006006

Papavasiliou A V., Bardakos N V. Complications of arthroscopic surgery of the hip. *Bone Joint Res.* 2012;1(7):131–144. doi:10.1302/2046-3758.17.2000108

Renner J, Gruenewald M, Quaden R, et al. Influence of increased intra-abdominal pressure on fluid responsiveness predicted by pulse pressure variation and stroke volume variation in a porcine model. *Crit Care Med.* 2009;37(2):650–658. doi:10.1097/CCM.0b013e3181959864

Rogers WK, Garcia L. Intraabdominal hypertension, abdominal compartment syndrome, and the open abdomen. *Chest.* 2018;153(1):238–250. doi:10.1016/j.chest.2017.07.023

Scalea TM, Bochicchio G V., Habashi N, et al. Increased intra-abdominal, intrathoracic, and intracranial pressure after severe brain injury: Multiple compartment syndrome. *J Trauma Inj Infect Crit Care.* 2007;62(3):647–656. doi:10.1097/TA.0b013e31802ee542

Sugrue M, De Waele JJ, De Keulenaer BL, Roberts DJ. A user's guide to intra-abdominal pressure measurement. Anaesthesiol Intensive Ther. 2015;47(3):241–251. doi:10.5603/AIT.a2015.0025

Wise R, Roberts DJ, Vandervelden S, et al. Awareness and knowledge of intra-abdominal hypertension and abdominal compartment syndrome: results of an international survey. Anaesthesiol Intensive Ther. 2015;47(1):14–29. doi:10.5603/AIT.a2014.0051

REVIEW QUESTIONS

1. You are caring for a 26-year-old parturient who was transferred from the operating room after delivery by cesarean section. Intraoperatively she experienced decreased uterine tone. The operative team transfused 1 unit of blood and several liters of crystalloid intraoperatively. She is alert and awake and develops abdominal pain as the spinal anesthetic diminishes. Her urine output is decreased, and the obstetrician recommends measurement of the urinary bladder pressure. What is your response?

   A. Peripartum IAP has no agreed upon normal value and no clinical value.

   B. Her recent surgery precludes accurate IAP measurement.

   C. The clinician can integrate bladder pressure measurements in this clinical context.

   D. Intrauterine pressure is superior to bladder pressure measurement.

   Answer: C. The normal parturient experiences physiologic, elevated IAP. Normal thresholds are not universally established, but elevated IAP in this setting suggests evolving IAH and should be followed. Because IAP decreases shortly after delivery, a rising IAP in this setting causes concern. Proper analgesia along with continued monitoring are indicated (Fuchs 2013). Prepartum bladder pressures are also elevated for reasons anatomic and physiologic; positioning the pregnant patient for IAP measurement can lead to varying results based on supine versus lateral tilt (Chun 2012). While elevated IAP in pregnancy can be considered IAH with physiologic compensation, pathologies specific (pre-eclampsia, eclampsia, ovarian hyperstimulation syndrome) and not specific to pregnancy can cause adverse IAH or ACS and should not be confused with normal pregnancy.

2. Which of the following hemodynamic parameters typically coincide with ACS?

   A. Low central venous pressure, low pulmonary artery systolic pressure, and low cardiac output

   B. High central venous pressure, low pulmonary artery systolic pressure, and low cardiac output

   C. Low central venous pressure, low pulmonary artery systolic pressure, and high cardiac output

   D. High central venous pressure, high pulmonary artery systolic pressure, and low cardiac output

Answer: D. High IAP causes organ dysfunction within and without of the abdominal cavity. Cardiac function is compromised by IAH in several ways. Preload decreases with less venous return from the abdomen, often in the setting of inferior vena cava (IVC) compression directly or by the diaphragm. For this reason, measurement of IVC respiratory collapse as a surrogate for volume status becomes unreliable (Rogers 2018). Contractility is compromised by external compression or rotation of the heart as the abdomen exerts pressure on the thorax; contractility can also be reduced by concomitant processes such as sepsis or ischemia. Afterload increases in IAH due to compensatory mechanisms and again the direct effects of IAH. Standard invasive hemodynamic monitors, since they are pressure-based, often reflect the pressure effects of IAH and must be interpreted in this light (Cheatham 2007).

3. You are called to evaluate a 32-year-old woman for severe abdominal pain after a hip arthroscopy. She is in distress, showing a great deal of discomfort, with a heart rate of 132 and blood pressure of 84/66. She is tachypneic. Her abdomen is notable for marked distension and diffuse pain on palpation, worse over the right flank and back. What is your leading diagnosis?

A. ACS after fluid extravasation
B. Retroperitoneal bleed
C. Postoperative ileus
D. Bowel perforation

Answer: A. ACS after hip arthroscopy is an unusual but reported event (Fowler 2010). Indeed, there is evidence that many hip arthroscopies lead to subclinical amounts of abdominal fluid. If the procedure is complicated or prolonged, the likelihood of large fluid shifts to the abdomen increases. Sudden decrease of intraoperative patient core temperature is suggestive of irrigant extravasation. Retroperitoneal bleeding, ileus, and bowel perforation are less likely complications of hip arthroscopy. Abdominal pain and distension after hip arthroscopy should raise suspicion for ACS (Papavasiliou 2012).

4. How should you manage this patient?

A. Expectant observation
B. Ultrasound or CT imaging with percutaneous drainage
C. Diuresis
D. Intravenous fluid bolus

Answer: B. Intervention after imaging is the best option of these choices. It is reasonable to proceed to exploratory laparotomy as well, depending on resource availability and patient condition.

5. In a survey published in 2015 by the World Society of the Abdominal Compartment Syndrome (WSACS), what percentage of respondents correctly identified the IAP that defines ACS?

A. 12%
B. 28%
C. 52%
D. 78%

Answer: B. As recently as 2015, a survey of concerned health professionals, the majority intensivists or surgical specialists, revealed marked knowledge deficiencies in awareness of IAH/ACS. The survey found that while decompression for ACS as well as the concept of abdominal perfusion pressure were consider by over 80%, key points such as the definition of ACS, how to measure IAP, frequency of measurement, and others were correctly identified by less than 30% (Wise 2015).

6. Which is optimal for temporary closure of the open abdomen?

A. Bogota bag
B. Temporary mesh with fascial traction
C. Negative pressure wound therapy with fascial traction
D. Skin closure with permissive hernia

Answer: B. Gradual closure with fascial traction, typically with a mesh, combined with negative pressure wound therapy, has the best recommendations due to greater closure rate and fewer complications such as fistulas. Gradual closure also allows for second-look surgery as well as a closure rate tailored to the patient's circumstance (Coccolini 2017).

7. Which of the following contraindicates open abdominal closure?

A. Ongoing coagulopathy
B. Refractory hypothermia
C. Abdominal infection
D. Hypoalbuminemia

Answer: C. While the others are undesirable and might initiate the decision to leave the abdomen open, they do not contraindicate second-look surgery or abdominal closure. Abdominal infection source control, however, is necessary before full closure of the open abdomen.

8. A multitrauma patient experiences recurrently high intracranial pressure (ICP) despite hypertonic saline, hyperventilation, and sedation. You recommend decompressive craniotomy; however, the family declines. What other maneuver can reduce ICP in multitrauma patients?

A. Albumin infusion
B. Decompressive laparotomy
C. Extracorporeal membrane oxygenation
D. Tranexamic acid

Answer: B. Subgroups of multitrauma patients with recurrently high ICP have been found to experience reduced ICP with decompressive laparotomy. Durability of the ICP reduction and patient outcomes are not certain; however, abdominal decompression is a viable option in such patients with limited options. IAP interacts with ICP through several proposed mechanisms, including elevated intrathoracic pressure, decreased venous return from the cranial vault (or elevated CVP), direct pressure transfer to the subarachnoid space, hypercapnea, and elevated catecholamine or more general stress levels. Abdominal insufflation also increases ICP. Intraabdominal pressure measurement should be considered in trauma patients with intracranial hypertension (Scalea 2007, De Laet 2007, Hendrickson 2015).

9. The WSACS recommends which of the following as a primary, reliable means to diagnose ACS?

   A. Physical examination including abdominal girth measurement
   B. Abdominal perfusion pressure calculation
   C. Oliguria
   D. Trans-bladder abdominal pressure measurement

Answer: D. The WSACS recommends serial or continuous IAP measurement in patients at risk for IAH. The other methods are nonspecific or unreliable (Kirkpatrick 2013).

10. According to WSACS, what is the proper volume of bladder instillation for IAP measurement?

   A. No fluid instillation is necessary.
   B. 10 mL
   C. 25 mL
   D. 100 mL

Answer: C. Various methods can measure the IAP; however, the most widely used, applicable, and studied is the trans-bladder. Authors describe different bladder instillation volumes; the WSACS recommends 25 mL as the best amount to maximize accuracy and reliability. Bladder pressure measurement apparati are commercially available or can be made with readily available equipment in different configurations. Clinical factors such as head elevation, the respiratory cycle, and muscle tone should be considered. While bladder pressure is more or less the gold standard for IAP measurement, other methods such as direct intra-abdominal, vaginal, rectal, uterine, or IVC are sometimes used (Kirkpatrick 2013, Sugrue 2015).

28.

CARDIAC TAMPONADE

Rachel Maldonado Freeman and Emily Anne Vail

STEM CASE AND KEY QUESTIONS

A 78-year-old male patient with a past medical history of hypertension, hyperlipidemia, diabetes mellitus, and symptomatic severe aortic valve stenosis presents to the cardiothoracic surgical intensive care unit (ICU) immediately after aortic valve replacement with a bioprosthetic valve. Intraoperative course was uneventful. Cardiopulmonary bypass (CPB) and aortic cross clamp times were 60 and 40 minutes, respectively. He received 2 liters of balanced crystalloid solution and 1 unit of packed red blood cells (PRBCs) during the procedure. The patient arrives in the ICU in sinus rhythm with a heart rate (HR) of 89 and systemic blood pressure (BP) of 107/80 mmHg. He is receiving 0.04 u/min of vasopressin and 0.4 mcg/kg/min of norepinephrine and sedated with dexmedetomidine and fentanyl. Approximately 4 hours after ICU admission, the patient develops acute onset tachycardia with HR 120 beats/minute and BP 90/67. Additional clinical data include:

- Central venous pressure (CVP) 7 mmHg

- Cardiac Index (CI) by thermodilution 1.8 L/min/m²

- Chest tube output 200 ml/hr, sanguineous

- Hemoglobin 6 g/dL (decreased from 8 g/dL immediately postop)

- Platelet count 60,000/mm²

- Arterial lactate 3.7 mmol/L

The patient is treated with 2 units of PRBCs. A blood sample for thromboelastogram (TEG) is drawn. Over the next hour, chest tube output decreases to 10 mL/hour. Despite this, vasopressor requirements increase and lactate rises to 4.8 mmol/L.

WHAT IS THE DIFFERENTIAL DIAGNOSIS OF LOW CARDIAC OUTPUT IN THE FIRST POSTOPERATIVE HOURS? WHAT IS CARDIAC TAMPONADE? WHAT ARE THE TYPICAL CAUSES OF TAMPONADE?

Max amplitude is decreased on the TEG. The patient receives a 6-pack of platelets and the CVP rises to 15 mmHg.

WHAT CVP VALUES ARE EXPECTED IN TAMPONADE? WHAT OTHER BEDSIDE DIAGNOSTIC TESTS CAN BE PERFORMED TO HELP DIAGNOSE POST-CARDIOTOMY CARDIAC TAMPONADE?

A bedside transthoracic echocardiogram (TTE) is available. Parasternal and subxiphoid views are prevented by the patient's body habitus, chest tubes, and dressings. An apical view is limited but does not demonstrate a clear pericardial effusion. Ventricular function appears hyperdynamic without evidence of right ventricular failure.

IF EVIDENCE OF PERICARDIAL EFFUSION OR TAMPONADE IS NOT DETECTED BY TTE, IS ADDITIONAL IMAGING NECESSARY? IF SO, WHAT?

The patient is too unstable for transport to computed tomography (CT) scan but a transesophageal echocardiogram (TEE) is available. TEE reveals intrapericardial thrombus posterior to the right ventricle with compression of the ventricle during diastole.

WHAT IS REGIONAL TAMPONADE? WHAT OTHER ECHOCARDIOGRAPHIC FINDINGS WOULD HELP MAKE THE DIAGNOSIS OF TAMPONADE? ONCE THE DIAGNOSIS OF TAMPONADE IS MADE, WHAT IS THE NEXT STEP IN MANAGEMENT?

Chest tube occlusion is suspected. Stripping of the chest tubes evacuates 100 mL of blood but the patient remains hypotensive. Repeat coagulation studies are normal. The cardiothoracic surgeon is notified and plans to perform emergent chest exploration and washout in the operating room.

WHILE WAITING FOR DEFINITIVE TREATMENT, WHAT STEPS SHOULD BE TAKEN TO TEMPORARILY STABILIZE THE PATIENT? IF IT BECOMES NECESSARY, HOW CAN ENDOTRACHEAL INTUBATION BE PERFORMED SAFELY?

After successful intubation and transfusion of an additional unit of PRBCs, the patient is transferred to the operating room. The patient's sternotomy is opened and the surgeons identify a large clot posterior to the heart and find bleeding from the atrial cannulation site. After successful clot evacuation and source control, the patient's hypotension resolves. The chest is closed and the rest of the hospital course is uneventful.

DISCUSSION

Post-cardiotomy tamponade is a difficult but crucial diagnosis to make. There are many potential etiologies of hypotension and shock in the immediate postoperative period, including post-bypass myocardial dysfunction, myocardial ischemia or infarction, hemorrhage, post CPB vasoplegia, and tamponade. A combination of hemodynamic disturbances may be present simultaneously, confusing the clinical presentation and potentially delaying diagnosis. Bleeding can be significant in up to 10% of cardiac surgeries and may lead to additional problems such as tamponade.[1] Risk factors for tamponade include preoperative or postoperative anticoagulation, surgery other than coronary artery bypass grafting (CABG), prolonged cardiopulmonary bypass, and red blood cell transfusion.[2]

ETIOLOGY AND PATHOGENESIS

Cardiac tamponade is a form of obstructive shock and is caused by compression of one or more cardiac chambers. As the noncompliant pericardium fills with fluid or blood, pericardial pressures increase, compressing cardiac chambers, impairing forward flow through the heart and great vessels thereby decreasing cardiac output. The right atrium and right ventricle, which have lower chamber pressures than the left-sided chambers, are affected first. In order to maintain an adequate cardiac output, the patient may compensate for decreases in stroke volume by increasing heart rate and contractility. As pericardial pressures increase, interventricular interdependence and respirophasic variation become exaggerated. Thus, with spontaneous inhalation, the filling of the right ventricle shifts the ventricular septum leftward, reducing left ventricular filling and decreasing stroke volume.

Common causes of cardiac tamponade include hemorrhage (post-cardiotomy, aortic dissection, chamber perforation during cardiac catheterization procedures, trauma), malignancy, uremia, inflammatory disease (rheumatoid arthritis, systemic lupus erythematous), hypothyroidism, and pneumopericardium.[3] Not all pericardial effusions lead to tamponade. Tamponade physiology occurs when accumulation of fluid is rapid or is organized enough to directly obstruct blood flow through the heart. Tamponade should be suspected in patients with hypotension and low cardiac output.[4]

As demonstrated in this case, postoperative tamponade most typically presents in the early postoperative period. Estimated incidence is between 0.2% and 8% and varies by type of procedure.[5] Early tamponade after cardiac surgery typically presents as regional tamponade or low pressure tamponade.[5] Regional tamponade occurs when one or more cardiac chamber is compressed by a clot or organized effusion of any size, impairing filling and forward flow.[5,6] Uneven clot distribution and regional compression may be more likely after cardiac surgery in which the pericardium is left open.[7] A common presentation of regional tamponade after cardiac surgery includes high chest tube output (greater than 200 mL/hr) with subsequent obstruction of the chest tubes, which impedes mediastinal drainage. Thus, high suspicion is warranted when chest tube output suddenly decreases or stops and is accompanied by significant hemodynamic changes. Low-pressure tamponade may occur in patients with coexisting hypovolemia, allowing small elevations in pericardial pressures to cause chamber compression and obstructive physiology.

Late or "delayed" tamponade typically presents 5 to 7 days after pericardiotomy and may be caused by initiation of anticoagulation therapy or pericarditis.[8,9] Late tamponade is a serious postoperative complication with an incidence of 0.8% to 4% and a higher mortality rate than early tamponade.[5,8] Diagnosis of late tamponade may be delayed when clinical symptoms are attributed to postoperative fatigue, deconditioning, congestive heart failure, or pulmonary embolism.[8]

CLINICAL FEATURES

In early post-cardiac surgery tamponade, presentation can be atypical and nonspecific. Classic signs of tamponade (pulsus paradoxus, elevated CVP, equalization of intracardiac pressures) are frequently not observed.[10] Instead, tamponade may be regional or low-pressure as described earlier. During this period, symptoms of tamponade may be masked by postoperative intubation, analgesia, or sedation or attributed to other causes. Awake patients may complain of chest pain or dizziness. In addition to tachycardia and hypotension, patients may demonstrate other signs of shock, including alterations in mental status, cool extremities, jugular venous distension, and/or muffled heart sounds. Electrocardiogram findings include decreased voltage or electrical alternans, caused by displacement of the heart within the large pericardial effusion. Pulsus paradoxus, defined as a decrease in systolic blood pressure by more than 10 mmHg during spontaneous inspiration, may also be observed. It results from exaggeration of respirophasic variation when intracardiac volume is fixed. In mechanically ventilated patients, additional intrathoracic pressure further decreases cardiac filling, which can further decrease cardiac output and eliminate pulsus paradoxus.

CVP tracings may demonstrate a disappearance of the y descent, which is representative of ventricular filling, and a prominent x descent. This results from the reduction of the pressure gradient between the atria and ventricle leading to less forward flow of blood during diastole. If a pulmonary artery catheter is in place, equalization of pulmonary diastolic pressures with atrial and ventricular diastolic pressures may be observed, usually between 15 and 30 mmHg.[11]

DIAGNOSTIC IMAGING

Though specificity is poor, chest radiographs may demonstrate enlargement of the cardio-mediastinal silhouette.

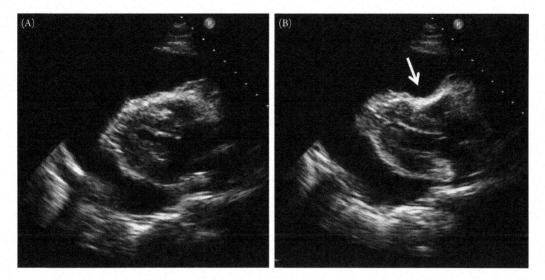

Figure 28.1 Demonstration of early diastolic collapse of the right ventricle. (A) Parasternal long axis view of the heart at end systole with a very large pericardial effusion. (B) In diastole, pericardial pressures exceed right ventricular pressures resulting in compression of right ventricular free wall. Reproduced with permission from Kearns M, Walley K. Tamponade: hemodynamic and echocardiographic diagnosis. Chest. 153(5);1266–1275, Figure 3.

Echocardiography remains the gold standard for diagnosis.[1,10] Echocardiography can be used to identify atrial and ventricular compression and determine the location and volume of pericardial fluid or clot. TTE is noninvasive and easy to obtain but windows may be limited immediately after cardiac surgery by habitus, pulmonary disease, positioning, surgical dressings, and chest tubes. TTE views may be insufficient to detect small or posterior clots.[10] In an observational study by Imren and colleagues, TTE evaluation resulted in false-negative diagnosis in 21% of 35 post-cardiac surgery patients with early tamponade.[12] Preferred TTE views are parasternal long and short axis, but subcostal views may be easier to obtain in critically ill patients.[1] If TTE does not demonstrate tamponade but high suspicion remains, TEE is recommended. On two-dimensional or M-mode imaging, tamponade can be diagnosed by diastolic collapse of the right ventricle, atrial collapse in more than one-third of the cardiac cycle, and inferior vena

cava (IVC) dilatation (Figures 28.1 and 28.2). Exaggerated respirophasic variation can be observed in transmitral and transtricuspid diastolic spectral doppler inflow velocities. Pulsus paradoxus is observed echocardiographically as respiratory variation in aortic outflow velocity. Of note, Doppler features of tamponade have only been validated in spontaneously breathing patients and may alternately be observed in patients with obesity, severe hypovolemia, chronic obstructive lung disease, pulmonary embolism, and right heart failure.[1] Although TTE and TEE methods are widely used, they are insufficiently sensitive to completely rule out tamponade. Absence of echocardiographic findings consistent with tamponade does not exclude the diagnosis. There are multiple case reports of tamponade not detected by either TTE and TEE. In these cases, missed diagnoses were attributed to inadequate views, incomplete imaging of pericardial sac, and hyperdense pericardial thrombi that are difficult to distinguish from adjacent soft tissue as demonstrated in Figures 28.3 and 28.4.[1,12] In stable patients, contrast chest CT may reveal pericardial effusion, enlargement of the vena cava, hepatic and renal vein enlargement, periportal edema, reflux of contrast material, bowing of the interventricular septum, pericardial thickening, and collapse of the right ventricle. Similarly, MRI may be diagnostic but is commonly not technically feasible or safe.[1] In cases where diagnostic testing is inconclusive and the patient is hemodynamically unstable, chest exploration and washout is indicated.

TREATMENT

Definitive treatment of tamponade requires evacuation of pericardial blood or fluid to relieve the compression of the heart chambers. Depending on the type of tamponade, drainage may be achieved by pericardiocentesis, pericardial window, or reopening of the surgical wound (sternotomy/thoracotomy). Pericardiocentesis is typically performed under ultrasound or

Figure 28.2 Subcostal view of the inferior vena cava showing a dilated IVC. Reproduced with permission from McCanny P, Colreavy F. Echocardiographic approach to cardiac tamponade in critically ill patients. J Crit Care. 2017 Jun;39:271–277, Image 15.

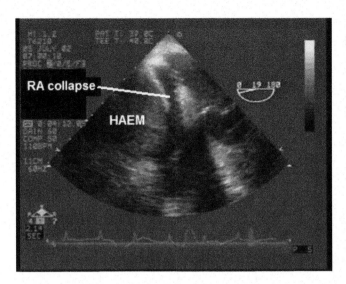

Figure 28.3 Transesophageal echocardiography midesophageal view showing a hematoma compressing the right chamber in a patient after cardiac surgery. Note the hyperdense thrombus is difficult to distinguish from adjacent soft tissue.
Reproduced with permission from McCanny P, Colreavy F. Echocardiographic approach to cardiac tamponade in critically ill patients. J Crit Care. 2017 Jun;39:271–277, Image 20.

fluoroscopic guidance but may not be effective if tamponade is caused by organized clot or fluid. A temporary drain may be placed if fluid reaccumulation is expected.[4]

If definitive treatment is not immediately available, measures to temporarily stabilize the patient attempt to compensate for impaired ventricular filling. Preload should be optimized to oppose increased pericardial pressure and sinus rhythm should be maintained. Avoidance of bradycardia will help maintain cardiac output when stroke volume is fixed. Correction of coexisting acidosis, hypoxemia, and hypercarbia

may be necessary. Vasopressors may temporarily increase systemic blood pressure but should only be administered if hypotension is life threatening as they also increase afterload.[3,5]

Increases in intrathoracic pressure during mechanical ventilation that further decrease cardiac filling are potentially life threatening and should be avoided by maintaining spontaneous ventilation. If endotracheal intubation becomes necessary, anesthetic induction should preserve spontaneous ventilation: inhalational anesthetics or ketamine are commonly used. After intubation, large tidal volumes and positive end expiratory pressure should be avoided.

In the event of cardiac arrest, return of spontaneous circulation (ROSC) is unlikely with chest compressions alone. In a study of baboons, chest compressions improved systolic blood pressure but could not achieve adequate diastolic or mean arterial pressures. Relief of tamponade is necessary to improve likelihood of ROSC.[13]

CONCLUSIONS

- Cardiac tamponade is caused by local or global compression of the cardiac chambers leading to reduced ventricular filling and hemodynamic compromise.

- Echocardiography may be the most sensitive method of diagnosis but cannot reliably rule out tamponade. In postoperative patients with a high index of suspicion, chest reexploration is recommended.

- Medical treatment of tamponade focuses on maintaining preload, afterload, and elevated heart rate until definitive treatment by pericardiocentesis, pericardial window, or surgical exploration may be performed.

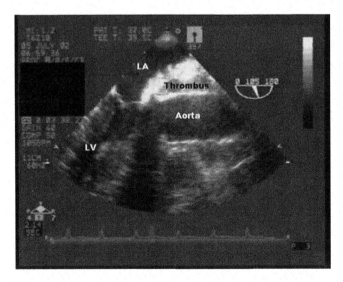

Figure 28.4 Transesophageal echocardiography long axis ascending aorta view, showing a hyperechoic thrombus adjacent to the ascending aorta and left atrium.
Reproduced with permission from McCanny P, Colreavy F. Echocardiographic approach to cardiac tamponade in critically ill patients. J Crit Care. 2017 Jun;39:271–277, Image 21.

REFERENCES

1. McCanny P, Colreavy F. Echocardiographic approach to cardiac tamponade in critically ill patients. J Crit Care. 2017 Jun;39:271–277.
2. Leiva EH, Carreno M, Bucheli FR, Bonfanti AC, Umana JP, Dennis RJ. Factors associated with delayed cardiac tamponade after cardiac surgery. Ann Card Anaesth. 2018 Apr-Jun;21(2):158–166.
3. Kearns M, Walley K. Tamponade: hemodynamic and echocardiographic diagnosis Chest. 2018 May;153(5):1266–1275.
4. Russo AM, O'Connor WH, Waxman HL. Atypical presentations and echocardiographic findings in patients with cardiac tamponade occurring early and late after cardiac surgery. Chest. 1993 Jul;104(1):71–78.
5. Carmona P, Casanovas I, Pena, JJ et al. Management of cardiac tamponade after cardiac surgery. J Cardiothorac Vasc Anesth. 2012 Apr;26(2):302–311.
6. Tusscher BL, Groeneveld JA, Kamp O, Jansen E, Beishuizen A, Girbes, A. Predicting outcome of thoracotomy for suspected pericardial tamponade following cardio-thoracic surgery in the intensive care unit. J Cardiothoracic Surg. 2011 May 30;6:79. doi:10.1186/1749-8090-6-79.
7. Grumann A, Baretto L, Dugard A, Morera P, Cornu E, Amiel JB, Vignon PP. Localized cardiac tamponade after open-heart surgery. Ann Thorac Cardiovasc Surg. 2012;18(6):524–529.
8. Meurin P, Weber H, Renaud N, Larrazet F, Tabet JY, Demolis P, Ben Driss A. Chest evolution of the postoperative pericardial effusion after day 15: the problem of the late tamponade. Chest. 2004 Jun;125(6):2182–2187.

9. King TE Jr, Stelzner TJ, Sahn SA. Cardiac Tamponade Complicating the Postpericardiotomy Syndrome. Chest. 1983 Mar;83(3):500–503.

10. Price S, Prout J, Jagger D, Gibson D, Pepper J. "Tamponade" following cardiac surgery: terminology and echocardiography may both mislead. Eur J Cardiothorac Surg. 2004 Dec;26(6):1156–1160.

11. Adler Y, Charron P, Imazio M et al.; The Task Force for the Diagnosis and Management of Pericardial Diseases of the European Society of Cardiology (ESC). ESC guidelines for the diagnosis and management of pericardial diseases. Euro Heart J. 2015 Nov 7;36(42):2921–2964.

12. Imren Y, Tasoglu I, Oktar GL, Benson A, Naseem T, Cheema FH, Unal Y. The importance of transesophageal echocardiography in diagnosis of pericardial tamponade after cardiac surgery. J Card Surg. 2008 Sep-Oct;23(5):450–453.

13. Luna GK, Pavlin EG, Kirkman T, Copass MK, Rice CL. Hemodynamic effects of external cardiac massage in trauma shock. J Trauma. 1989 Oct; 29(10):1430–1433.

REVIEW QUESTIONS

1. A 58-year-old man is recovering in the ICU 12 hours after coronary artery bypass surgery. He suddenly becomes hypotensive and requires supplemental vasopressor support. Cardiac tamponade is classified as what type of shock?

   A. Distributive
   B. Cardiogenic
   C. Obstructive
   D. Hypovolemic

2. Which of the following statements best defines pulsus paradoxus?

   A. A decrease in systolic blood pressure by more than 10 mmHg during spontaneous inspiration
   B. A decrease in systolic blood pressure by more than 10 mmHg during spontaneous expiration
   C. A decrease in heart rate by 10 beats per minute during inspiration
   D. A decrease in heart rate by 10 beats per minute during expiration

3. The ICU team is concerned that a patient is developing cardiac tamponade. The patient has a central line. What feature on a CVP tracing is consistent with cardiac tamponade?

   A. Exaggerated *x* descent and disappearance of the *y* descent
   B. Tall systolic *c-v* wave and loss of the *x* descent
   C. Cannon *a* waves
   D. Loss of *a* waves

4. Which method is most appropriate for diagnosis of cardiac tamponade in unstable patients?

   A. Chest X-ray
   B. Chest CT
   C. Echocardiography
   D. Cardiac magnetic resonance imaging (MRI)

5. An 83-year-old man immediately status post-aortic valve replacement becomes hypotensive in the ICU. Cardiac index is low and chest tube output has decreased. A bedside transthoracic echocardiogram demonstrates adequate images without evidence of tamponade. No transesophageal echocardiogram is immediately available. Which of the following would be the best next step in management?

   A. Transport the patient for a STAT CT scan
   B. Transport the patient to the operating room for chest exploration
   C. Repeat the echocardiogram in 6 hours
   D. Look for other diagnoses because tamponade has been ruled out

6. In a patient with tamponade, which of the following echocardiographic signs are *not* likely to be present?

   A. Diastolic collapse of the right ventricle
   B. Atrial collapse in more than one-third of the cardiac cycle
   C. IVC collapse with spontaneous inspiration
   D. Exaggerated respiratory variation of the aortic outflow velocity

7. A patient develops tamponade in the ICU. While waiting for surgical intervention, which of the following interventions may worsen the patient's clinical condition?

   A. Crystalloid fluid bolus
   B. Cardioversion to restore sinus rhythm
   C. Treatment of bradycardia
   D. Endotracheal intubation and positive pressure ventilation

8. A patient with suspected cardiac tamponade becomes progressively more unstable with altered mental status. She is tachypneic and unable to maintain her airway. What drug for anesthetic induction is most likely to allow the patient to maintain spontaneous ventilation after intubation?

   A. Ketamine
   B. Propofol
   C. Etomidate
   D. Fentanyl

9. All of the following statements about cardiac tamponade are true *except*

   A. All pericardial effusions lead to tamponade.
   B. Early tamponade after cardiac surgery is likely to be regional tamponade.
   C. Low-pressure tamponade may occur in post-cardiac surgery patients with coexisting hypovolemia.
   D. Late tamponade has a higher mortality rate than early tamponade.

10. Which of the following is *not* a risk factor for tamponade after cardiac surgery?

   A. Postoperative anticoagulation
   B. CABG surgery
   C. Intraoperative red blood cell transfusion
   D. Prolonged cardiopulmonary bypass

ANSWERS

1. Answer: C. There are 4 principle types of shock. Tamponade is a form of obstructive shock, in which blood flow into or out of the heart is restricted. Tension pneumothorax is another form of obstructive shock. Choice A is incorrect; distributive shock is caused by significant vasodilation. It is commonly caused by sepsis. Choice B is incorrect; cardiogenic shock is caused by myocardial or valvular dysfunction. Choice D is incorrect; hypovolemic shock results from significantly decreased intravascular fluid volume, such as hemorrhage.

2. Answer: A. Pulsus paradoxus is defined as a decrease in systolic pressure by more than 10 mmHg during spontaneous inspiration.[5] Under normal conditions, spontaneous inspiration increases venous return to the right heart and transiently reduces filling of the left heart, leading to a small decrease in left ventricular stroke volume and cardiac output. During exhalation, the opposite occurs. In pericardial disease, including cardiac tamponade, the observed variation in pulse pressure during spontaneous or mechanical ventilation is exaggerated. During right ventricular filling, outward expansion of the ventricular wall is limited by blood or fluid in the pericardial space. As the right ventricle fills, the interventricular septum bulges into the left ventricle, further reducing stroke volume. Choice B is incorrect; the decrease in blood pressure in pulsus paradoxus occurs during spontaneous inspiration. Choices C and D are incorrect; pulsus paradoxus does not describe a change in heart rate.

3. Answer: A. In cardiac tamponade, increased pericardial pressures decrease the pressure gradient between the right atrium and ventricle, reducing forward flow during early diastole. On the CVP tracing, altered atrial filling and drainage patterns are demonstrated by an exaggerated x descent and a reduced or eliminated y descent.[5] Choice B is incorrect; tall, fused c-v waves are observed in tricuspid regurgitation. Choice C is incorrect; cannon a waves are observed in atrioventricular dissociation. Choice D is incorrect; a waves are lost during atrial fibrillation.

4. Answer: C. Echocardiography is considered the gold standard diagnostic method for cardiac tamponade. Transthoracic or transesophageal echocardiography can be used at the bedside to identify chamber compression and determine the location and volume of pericardial fluid or thrombus.[1,10] Choice A is incorrect; although chest radiographs may demonstrate enlargement of the cardiomediastinal silhouette, the finding is nonspecific. Choices B and D are incorrect; although chest CT and cardiac MRI may be used to diagnose tamponade, practical challenges make these methods less feasible and potentially unsafe in unstable patients.[1]

5. Answer: B. Although tamponade is most often diagnosed using echocardiography, the diagnosis is a clinical one. Sensitivity of echocardiography is reduced when views are inadequate or when organized thrombus resembling adjacent viscera causes regional tamponade.[10] If there is high suspicion for tamponade, surgical exploration and evacuation of hematoma is the next best step.[11] Choice A is incorrect; CT imaging should not be performed on an unstable patient. Choice C is incorrect; unstable patients require immediate intervention. Choice D is incorrect; echocardiography is not perfectly sensitive and, if missed, tamponade can cause serious morbidity and mortality.

6. Answer: C. IVC collapse during spontaneous inhalation is not observed in tamponade. In normal subjects, IVC diameter decreases during spontaneous inhalation as blood flows out of the IVC and into the right atrium. In patients with tamponade, however, elevated cardiac chamber pressures impair IVC outflow, which dilates the IVC and prevents itscollapse.[1,3] Choices A, B, and D are true statements; all are echocardiographic findings that may be observed in patients with tamponade physiology.

7. Answer: D. If patients with tamponade require intubation, the additional positive intrathoracic pressure of mechanical ventilation will further decrease preload and may precipitate hemodynamic collapse. Therefore, positive pressure ventilation should be avoided whenever possible. Choices A, B, and C are true statements. To temporarily stabilize the patient, preload should be optimized with fluid boluses or blood transfusions to oppose increased pericardial pressure. Sinus rhythm should be maintained to maximize ventricular filling. Bradycardia will reduce cardiac output when stroke volume is fixed by extracardiac compression and should be treated when present.[5]

8. Answer: A. Ketamine is the anesthetic induction drug most likely to preserve a patient's spontaneous breathing. Choices B, C, and D are all more likely to abolish spontaneous ventilation than ketamine.[5]

9. Answer: A. Not all pericardial effusions cause tamponade. Tamponade physiology occurs when rapid accumulation of blood or fluid increases intrapericardial pressure or, in regional tamponade, when an organized fluid collection directly obstructs the flow of blood through the heart. Choices B, C, and D are true statements.[5,8]

10. Answer: B. Among adult cardiac surgical procedures, isolated CABG surgery carries the lowest risk of postoperative tamponade. Choices A, C, and D are all true statements. Both pre- and postoperative anticoagulation and prolonged cardiopulmonary bypass can increase the risk of bleeding; this blood may accumulate in the pericardium and lead to tamponade. Red blood cell transfusion has also been identified as a risk factor for postoperative tamponade, likely because it serves as a marker of clinically significant bleeding.[2]

29.

ATRIAL FIBRILLATION WITH RAPID VENTRICULAR RESPONSE POST MITRAL VALVE REPAIR

John Hance, Maggie Mechlin, and Erin S. Grawe

STEM CASE AND KEY QUESTIONS

A 76-year-old male is postoperative day 2 from a combined coronary artery bypass grafting (CABG) and mitral valve repair for ischemic mitral regurgitation. Past medical history includes coronary artery disease, hypertension, hyperlipidemia, insulin dependent diabetes mellitus, obstructive sleep apnea, hypothyroidism, and a history of spontaneous subdural hematoma 2 years ago, which was surgically evacuated. Current medications include dobutamine 5 mcg/kg/min and norepinephrine 3 mcg/min. The patient is extubated and receiving supplemental oxygen with 4 L nasal cannula. With these interventions, the patient's vital signs are stable. The patient is sitting up in bed, conversant, eating lunch, and has no complaints. However, acutely, the patient becomes tachycardic to 148 beats per minute (bpm) and blood pressures drops to 86/60 mmHg. Patient becomes agitated and tachypneic.

WHAT ARE THE NEXT STEPS TO DIAGNOSE THIS CHANGE IN HEMODYNAMICS?

A 12-lead electrocardiogram (ECG) is performed that shows atrial fibrillation (AF) with rapid ventricular response. Patient is laid supine and supplemental oxygen is increased. Norepinephrine infusion is increased due to low blood pressure. Labs are also drawn, which show potassium 3.8 mmol/L, bicarbonate 22 mmol/L, blood urea nitrogen 35 mg/dL, creatinine 1.2 mg/dL, and magnesium 1.8 mg/dL. Hemoglobin is 9.2 g/dL. Patient is given electrolyte replacement in the form of potassium chloride and magnesium sulfate.

WHAT RISK FACTORS DOES THIS PATIENT HAVE TO DEVELOP POSTOPERATIVE ATRIAL FIBRILLATION? WHAT IS THE INCIDENCE OF POSTOPERATIVE ATRIAL FIBRILLATION IN A CARDIAC SURGICAL PATIENT?

Patient complains he feels light-headed, then becomes increasingly agitated, he keeps pulling off his nasal cannula and trying to get out of bed and he is pulling at his chest tubes. His heart rate is now 156 bpm, irregular and blood pressure 89/64 mmHg despite increasing norepinephrine infusion, and SpO$_2$ 92% on 8 L NC. The patient has a pulmonary artery catheter in place. A thermodilution cardiac index was performed which showed a cardiac index (CI) = 1.8 L/min. This is a decrease from 2.6 L/min earlier that morning.

WHAT ARE THE TREATMENT OPTIONS FOR ACUTE ATRIAL FIBRILLATION WITH RAPID VENTRICULAR RESPONSE? IS THIS PATIENT STABLE OR UNSTABLE? WHEN DO YOU CONSIDER RATE CONTROL VERSUS RHYTHM CONTROL?

The patient is sedated with 2 mg midazolam and electrically cardioverted with 50 joules. The patient returns to normal sinus rhythm. Blood pressure increases to 126/84 mmHg and norepinephrine is discontinued. However, during the procedure the patient has an episode of emesis. The patient is turned to his side and his oropharynx is suctioned clear of gastric contents.

SHOULD YOU CONSIDER NPO GUIDELINES PRIOR TO ELECTRICAL CARDIOVERSION?

Despite emesis, the patient appears to be stable from a respiratory standpoint and there is no evidence of overt aspiration. After cardioversion, he is actually breathing more comfortably, his respiratory rate has decreased to 18 breaths/min, and his oxygen requirement is down to 4 L. The patient is calm and is interacting appropriately. He is no longer agitated and pulling at his lines and drains. A repeat cardiac index by thermodilution shows CI = 2.8 L/min. Dobutamine is decreased from 5 to 2.5 mcg/kg/min.

The patient remains in normal sinus rhythm for the next 3 hours but then again goes into AF with rapid ventricular response. This time, his heart rate is 132 bpm and blood pressure is 106/68. The patient is still alert and oriented and in no respiratory distress.

WHAT ARE TREATMENT OPTIONS FOR ATRIAL FIBRILLATION WHEN THE PATIENT IS HEMODYNAMICALLY STABLE? DOES THE PATIENT BEING ON DOBUTAMINE AFFECT WHICH MEDICATION IS GIVEN? SHOULD AMIODARONE HAVE BEEN ADDED AFTER THE FIRST EPISODE OF ATRIAL FIBRILLATION TO PREVENT THE RECURRENCE OF ATRIAL FIBRILLATION?

Amiodarone 150 mg is given over the next 15 minutes. Heart rate has decreased from 130 to 121 bpm. A second bolus of amiodarone 150 mg is given. The patient remains in AF but the heart rate now is in the 90s. Blood pressure is now 95/62.

WHY WOULD THE BLOOD PRESSURE DROP AFTER A BOLUS OF AMIODARONE? THE PATIENT'S HEART RATE IS CONTROLLED BUT THE PATIENT REMAINS IN ATRIAL FIBRILLATION. WHAT ARE THE CONSIDERATIONS FOR RATE VERSUS RHYTHM CONTROL IN POSTOPERATIVE ATRIAL FIBRILLATION?

The patient is maintained on an amiodarone infusion of 1 mg/min for the next 6 hours, then 0.5 mg/min thereafter. The next morning, the patient remains in AF. He had several brief episodes overnight in which he converted to sinus rhythm, but then back to AF. His heart rate ranges from 80 to the 90s, and his blood pressure is within normal limits on no vasopressors. His CI remains 2.8 L/min, central venous pressure (CVP) is 18 mmHg, and pulmonary artery pressure (PAP) 42/28 mmHg. Lasix 40 mg intravenous (IV) is given and dobutamine is discontinued.

WHEN SHOULD ANTICOAGULATION BE STARTED IN THIS PATIENT? WHAT ARE THE SPECIFIC RISK FACTORS FOR ANTICOAGULATION FOR THIS PATIENT?

The patient has had minimal bleeding from his chest tubes over the last 2 postoperative days. However, given his history of spontaneous subdural hematoma in the past, the decision was made to avoid anticoagulation in this patient. As such, the patient was made NPO and cardioversion was again attempted 6 hours after his last meal.

The patient was cardioverted again at 50 joules after 2 mg midazolam for sedation. He converted to normal sinus rhythm. Blood pressure remains stable. The patient remains in sinus rhythm for the remainder of his hospital course.

SHOULD THE PATIENT BE CONTINUED ON AMIODARONE DESPITE ACHIEVING SINUS RHYTHM? HOW LONG SHOULD THE AMIODARONE BE CONTINUED? WHY DO YOU THINK THE PATIENT REMAINED IN SINUS RHYTHM AFTER THE SECOND CARDIOVERSION BUT NOT THE FIRST? WHAT CONDITIONS WERE DIFFERENT?

The patient was converted from IV amiodarone to oral amiodarone, 400 mg BID. Metoprolol XL 50 mg was also started

the next day as blood pressure and cardiac output remained stable. He was continued on furosemide until his preadmission weight had been achieved. He was discharged on both amiodarone and metoprolol. At his 2-week post-discharge appointment with the cardiac surgeon, an electrocardiogram (ECG) was performed that showed persistence of normal sinus rhythm. Amiodarone was discontinued.

WHAT ARE THE TOXICITIES ASSOCIATED WITH SHORT-TERM AND LONG-TERM USE OF AMIODARONE? GIVEN THIS PATIENT'S MEDICAL HISTORY AND SURGICAL PROCEDURE, WOULD THIS PATIENT HAVE BENEFITED FROM ATRIAL FIBRILLATION PROPHYLAXIS PRIOR TO THE SURGERY?

DISCUSSION

INCIDENCE

Postoperative atrial fibrillation (POAF) occurs in 25% to 30% of cases after CABG and has been reported to be as high as 40% to 50% after valvular heart surgery.[1-3] The peak incidence of POAF occurs on the second postoperative day.

PATHOPHYSIOLOGY

Atrial fibrillation (AF) is characterized as paroxysmal, persistent, or permanent. AF is paroxysmal when the rhythm is terminated within 7 days and persistent when it is present for more than 7 days. Long-standing persistent is used to describe AF persisting for longer than 1 year. Permanent AF is a therapeutic mindset where the provider and patient accept AF and eliminate treatments that attempt to achieve sinus rhythm.

The cause of AF is multifactorial. Left atrial enlargement has been implicated as a result of myocyte hypertrophy, fibrosis, and altered protein distribution, which alters electrical conduction through atrial tissue.[1,4]

Three models have been postulated to explain the pathophysiology of AF. The "multiple-wavelet" hypothesis suggests that there are multiple impulse waves that are randomly conducted and maintained by an area of relative short refractory period resulting in discordant rhythm.[4] The second is based on a single or multiple driver model that postulates that there are rapidly conducting foci that form a closed reentry loop with a short refractory period that results in fibrillatory conduction. A single focus may fire rapidly to maintain the rhythm or multiple foci may fire at periodic intervals to sustain AF.[1,4] The third model suggests that AF is the result of rapidly conducting foci originating in 1 or more pulmonary veins, the inferior or superior vena cava, or the left atrial free wall.[1]

The response of AF to different medical and procedural therapies suggests that there is likely more than one pathophysiologic explanation. Each pathophysiologic mechanism mentioned earlier has merit clinically.

RISK FACTORS

The most potent risk factor for the development of AF is patient age. For every 10-year increase in patient age, the risk of having AF increase by 75%. Other factors include prior AF, obesity, male gender, COPD, pulmonary hypertension, and conditions predisposing to left atrial enlargement including structural heart disease, left ventricular hypertrophy, and reduced left ventricular systolic function.

POAF risk is highest immediately after surgery and subsequently on the second postoperative day.[1,5] POAF is likely triggered by the stress response to surgery from autonomic stimulation and neurohormonal activation, as well as atrial stretch due to large fluid shifts.[1] Indeed, risk factors for POAF include older age, obesity, longer cross clamp times, and mitral valve procedures.[5]

IMPLICATIONS/EFFECT ON OUTCOMES

POAF is associated with hemodynamic instability, myocardial infarction, congestive heart failure, stroke, increased length of stay, increased hospital cost, and even increased mortality.[2,3,6,7] Patients with POAF have a 5-fold increased risk of stroke, a 3-fold increased risk of heart failure, and a 2-fold increased mortality rate.[7,8] Length of stay increases by approximately 2 to 3 days.[2,9] A review of the STS database showed an increased intensive care unit cost of $3000 and an increase in total hospital cost of $9000.[8]

Stroke develops primarily from stasis of blood and thrombus formation in the left atrial appendage. This occurs as a consequence of inadequate propulsive contractions in AF. On an outpatient basis, the risk of stroke is calculated using the CHA2DS2-VASc score with anticoagulation being recommended with a score greater than or equal to 2 and corresponding to an adjusted annual stroke rate of at 2.2% or higher.[10] However, in the immediate postoperative setting, anticoagulation is frequently held due to increased risk of bleeding.

Hemodynamic compromise occurs due to loss of atrial kick leading to reduced stroke volume and cardiac output by as much as 20% to 30%. Rapid ventricular response further diminishes cardiac output due to decreased diastolic filling. Over a prolonged period of time, irregular ventricular contraction increases the risk of heart failure and volume overload further exacerbating AF.

TREATMENT

The management of POAF is managed similarly to AF with few exceptions. The unstable patient should undergo immediate direct current (DC) cardioversion. For the stable patient, initial treatment focuses on minimizing electrolyte abnormalities and hypoxemia, optimizing fluid status, and minimizing or stopping catecholaminergic inotropes.[11] Electrolyte correction enhances normal cardiomyocyte action potential propagation at the cellular level. Treating hypoxemia minimizes pulmonary vein vasoconstriction and subsequent increased in right ventricular and atrial pressure.[2] Fluid optimization similarly minimizes atrial stretch at the structural level.[2,12] Minimizing catecholaminergic support helps minimize propagation of irregular and erratic atrial signals through the atrioventricular (AV) node. After these measures, rate or rhythm control strategies are employed depending on clinician choice.[11] Due to the lack of strong evidence in favor of a rate versus rhythm control strategy, institutional protocols can vary significantly.[1]

Rate control is frequently achieved with beta blockade. The primary goal is to treat and prevent rapid ventricular response. Rate goals are not well established, but a rate less than 110 should be targeted to minimize palpitations and hypotension.[13] In patients with COPD or asthma, calcium channel blockers may be used. Diltiazem inhibits transient outward and delayed potassium currents in atrial myocytes diminishing action potential propagation. Its actions can worsen heart failure and cause ileus. One should be cautious adding diltiazem after beta blockade has been administered due to increased risk for heart block. This is exacerbated further if rhythm control with amiodarone is ultimately employed. Digoxin can be used for rate control in POAF and is considered when heart failure is also present. Digoxin inhibits the sodium potassium ATPase, which increases intracellular sodium and calcium concentrations, thereby improving contractility. Its vagomimetic effects treat rapid ventricular response. Digoxin has increased toxicity in the setting of low potassium, low magnesium, high calcium, and with concomitant use of amiodarone and calcium channel blockers. Toxicities include nausea, vision changes, accelerated junctional rhythms, and ventricular escape rhythms.[1]

Nearly 80% of patients will convert to sinus rhythm within 48 hours whether a rate or rhythm control strategy is implemented,[14] and virtually all patients will have normal sinus rhythm within 6 weeks postoperatively. An initial rate control strategy may be worthwhile in the immediate period after POAF develops since there is a reasonable chance for conversion. However, because anticoagulation is needed for patients who remain in POAF after 48 hours, one must weigh the risks of anticoagulation versus attempted rhythm control.

Rhythm control is considered when patients have ongoing symptoms despite rate controlled POAF, inability to achieve rate control, intolerance to rate control medications, or in asymptomatic patients with increased risk for bleeding. Early DC cardioversion (<48 hours) is therefore helpful to achieve sinus rhythm and prevent need for anticoagulation; preferably under transesophageal echocardiogram guidance to rule out thrombus in the left atrial appendage, which could dislodge and cause stroke.[11] DC cardioversion is highly effective and terminates 95% of POAF.[10] Scheduling DC cardioversion the day after diagnosis is beneficial to allow time for spontaneous conversion, to allow the patient to eat comfortably until midnight, and to consider and start chemical cardioversion adjuncts to improve the success of electrical cardioversion.

When chemical cardioversion is employed, it is generally for symptomatic patients or those who did not convert with rate control methods alone. Amiodarone is most commonly used. Amiodarone inhibits inward potassium current, increases the threshold for depolarization, and has anti-sympathetic effect on the AV node. Chronic use is associated with pulmonary, hepatic, thyroid, ocular, and neurologic toxicity.[11] Sotalol is an anti-arrhythmic drug with beta-blocking properties that also prolongs cardiac action potential duration by inhibition of potassium efflux. Recent studies have found sotalol to be as effective as amiodarone in conversion of POAF to sinus rhythm.[15,16] This may thus serve as a reasonable alternative in patients at risk for side effects from amiodarone use.

EFFICACY AND EVIDENCE FOR PROPHYLAXIS

Due to the burden of POAF, various studies have evaluated various medications thought to potentially be beneficial in the prevention of POAF. The medications studied are generally those that would logically target the proposed mechanisms of POAF.

Multiple studies have evaluated the benefit of various beta blockers as prevention for POAF. This is highlighted by a recent meta-analysis of 33 studies showing significant reduction in POAF rates after cardiac surgery (odds ratio [OR] 0.33, $p < 0.00001$).[17] Current guidelines suggest that beta blockers be initiated for at least 24 hours prior to CABG and reinstituted shortly after for the prevention of POAF.[18]

Amiodarone is similarly well studied and associated with an overall reduction in POAF (OR 0.43, $p < 0.00001$).[17] Its use is largely tempered by the risk for perioperative hypotension, bradycardia, and heart block. Similarly, sotalol has also been investigated and has been shown to reduce the risk of POAF after cardiac surgery.[1,17] However, its application is limited by QT prolongation, bradycardia, and ventricular arrhythmia.

Reducing inflammation and oxidative stress in the perioperative period has been studied using a multitude of agents. The use of corticosteroids was evaluated in a meta-analysis of 3323 patients. Low-dose preoperative corticosteroid use (total dose <1000 mg hydrocortisone) caused reduction in POAF (25.1% vs. 35.1%, $p < 0.01$) and was as effective as higher dosages. Corticosteroids increased the risk of hyperglycemia but not infection.[6]

Colchicine prophylaxis was found to reduce POAF (12.0% vs. 22.0%, $p = 0.021$) in a subset analysis of the Colchicine for the Prevention of the Postpericardiotomy Syndrome trial, which was primarily evaluating the effect of this drug on prevention of post-pericardiotomy syndrome.[19] However, when a dedicated trial was performed, there was no difference between colchicine and placebo in the prevention of POAF (33.9% vs. 41.7%, 95% CI, −2.2%–17.6%).[20]

Additional studies have evaluated the efficacy of drugs such as N-acetylcysteine, ascorbic acid, ACE-inhibitors, statins, and non-steroidal anti-inflammatory drugs in the prevention of POAF.[7,21-27] While some of the initial data is compelling, the studies overall lacked the power or reproducibility to support widespread implementation.

Despite a wealth of data on various medications aimed at the prevention of POAF, there has been an overall lack of generalizability in practice. This has led to wide variation in institutional practice patterns regarding prophylaxis.

SURGICAL TREATMENTS FOR ATRIAL FIBRILLATION

There are 2 broad interventional approaches to treat AF: catheter ablation and open surgery. Catheter ablation techniques are performed in an electrophysiology laboratory via a minimally invasive groin stick and fluoroscopy. Energy devices include radiofrequency ablation, cryoablation, and laser ablation and are similarly effective.[28-30] Catheter ablation is frequently used to perform pulmonary vein isolation (PVI), a technique that ablates the muscle sleeve of the pulmonary veins where nearly 90% of AF is initiated.[31] The success of PVI is greatest in patients with paroxysmal AF (70% to 80%).[32]

Dr. James Cox developed an open-heart approach to the ablation of AF in 1987. Through multiple iterations, it has evolved into a lesion set that resembles a maze-like pattern on the atria to permanently interrupt aberrant electrical impulses. The Cox Maze III is a cut-and-sew technique that has a 96% cure rate at 10 years and 99% freedom from stroke.[33] It is considered the gold standard for surgical AF treatment. Despite this, it is limited by procedural complexity, time required to perform the procedure, and complications.

In response to this, the cut-and-sew method has been replicated with open chest energy devices with >85% success at 6 months.[34-36] The mini Maze is a thoracoscopic method that allows small incisions to be made on each side of the chest without the need for sternotomy, particularly useful for patients with isolated AF. Success rates are best for paroxysmal AF (80% to 90%) versus persistent AF (50% to 75%).[37] An open Maze procedure has the benefit of added left atrial appendage ligation to limit clot formation and stroke risk.

INDICATIONS FOR ANTICOAGULATION

The decision to anticoagulate must be balanced with the risk of postoperative bleeding and stroke. Early use of warfarin is associated with tamponade.[1,38] The use of the CHA2DS2-VASc score is not well studied in patients developing AF after cardiac surgery. Nonetheless, the American Association for Thoracic Surgeon guidelines suggest that the CHA2DS2-VASc score is useful to guide anticoagulation decisions for POAF within 48 hours of onset.[11] Guidelines clearly recommend anticoagulation regardless of CHA2DS2-VASc score after 48 hours of POAF. International normalization ratio of 2 to 3 is recommended for at least 4 weeks after the return of sinus rhythm.[39] New oral anticoagulants (dabigatran, rivaroxiban, apixaban) are reasonable as an alternative to warfarin for some patients including those who do not have a prosthetic heart valve, hemodynamically significant valve disease, severe renal dysfunction, or risk of gastrointestinal bleeding.[11]

Cardioversion in the early (<48 hours) period after the onset of postoperative AF is frequently considered safe without confirmation of thrombus in the left atrial appendage. However, this should be individualized and performed with caution as there are reports of thrombus formation within this timeframe after the development of AF.[40]

In patients where there was pre-existing AF and anticoagulation was held for procedural reasons, it is most reasonable to start a heparin drip as a bridge to Coumadin when the bleeding risk diminishes. This allows the benefits of therapeutic anticoagulation while warfarin becomes therapeutic. It also diminishes the theoretical hypercoagulable state created by depletion of protein C and S with Coumadin therapy alone.

CONCLUSIONS

- AF is common after cardiac surgery with the highest incidence after valvular surgery, up to 40% to 50%.

- Risk factors for postoperative AF include advanced age, prior AF, obesity, male gender, COPD, pulmonary hypertension, and conditions predisposing to left atrial enlargement including structural heart disease, left ventricular hypertrophy, and reduced left ventricular systolic function.

- AF post-cardiac surgery significantly effects outcomes and increases the risk of hemodynamic instability, myocardial infarction, congestive heart failure, stroke, increased length of stay, increased hospital cost, and even increased mortality.

- Treatment for POAF focuses on minimizing electrolyte abnormalities and hypoxemia, optimizing fluid status, and minimizing or stopping catecholaminergic inotropes. DC cardioversion can be used if the patient is hemodynamically unstable. Selection of rate control versus rhythm control strategies are dependent on the specific patient as neither strategy has been shown to be superior in postoperative patients. Medical therapies include beta blockade, calcium-channel blockade, amiodarone, digoxin, and sotalol.

- Varying strategies have been used to prophylax against POAF in high-risk patients. Preoperative beta blockade seems to be the most used and widely accepted. Other medications have been studied with successful outcomes, but limited data exist.

REFERENCES

1. Raiten JM, Ghadimi K, Augoustides JG, et al. Atrial fibrillation after cardiac surgery: Clinical update on mechanisms and prophylactic strategies. J Cardiothorac Vasc Anesth. 2015;29(3):806–816.
2. Bessissow A, Khan J, Devereaux PJ, Alvarez-Garcia J, Alonso-Coello P. Postoperative atrial fibrillation in non-cardiac and cardiac surgery: An overview. J Thromb Haemost. 2015;13(Suppl 1):S304–S312.
3. Ishii Y, Schuessler RB, Gaynor SL, Hames K, Damiano RJ J. Postoperative atrial fibrillation: The role of the inflammatory response. J Thorac Cardiovasc Surg. 2017;153(6):1357–1365.
4. Waks JW, Josephson ME. Mechanisms of atrial fibrillation: Reentry, rotors and reality. Arrhythm Electrophysiol Rev. 2014;3(2):90–100.
5. Melby SJ, George JF, Picone DJ, et al. A time-related parametric risk factor analysis for postoperative atrial fibrillation after heart surgery. J Thorac Cardiovasc Surg. 2015;149(3):886–892.
6. Ho KM, Tan JA. Benefits and risks of corticosteroid prophylaxis in adult cardiac surgery: A dose-response meta-analysis. Circulation. 2009;119(14):1853–1866.
7. Chen WT, Krishnan GM, Sood N, Kluger J, Coleman CI. Effect of statins on atrial fibrillation after cardiac surgery: A duration- and dose-response meta-analysis. J Thorac Cardiovasc Surg. 2010;140(2):364–372.
8. LaPar DJ, Speir AM, Crosby IK, et al. Postoperative atrial fibrillation significantly increases mortality, hospital readmission, and hospital costs. Ann Thorac Surg. 2014;98(2):527–533; discussion 533.
9. Polanczyk CA, Goldman L, Marcantonio ER, Orav EJ, Lee TH. Supraventricular arrhythmia in patients having noncardiac surgery: Clinical correlates and effect on length of stay. Ann Intern Med. 1998;129(4):279–285.
10. January CT, Wann LS, Alpert JS, et al. 2014 AHA/ACC/HRS guideline for the management of patients with atrial fibrillation: A report of the American College of Cardiology/American Heart Association Task Force on Practice Guidelines and the Heart Rhythm Society. J Am Coll Cardiol. 2014;64(21):e1–e76.
11. Frendl G, Sodickson AC, Chung MK, et al. 2014 AATS guidelines for the prevention and management of perioperative atrial fibrillation and flutter for thoracic surgical procedures. J Thorac Cardiovasc Surg. 2014;148(3):e153–e193.
12. Danelich IM, Lose JM, Wright SS, et al. Practical management of postoperative atrial fibrillation after noncardiac surgery. J Am Coll Surg. 2014;219(4):831–841.
13. Gillinov AM, Bagiella E, Moskowitz AJ, et al. Rate control versus rhythm control for atrial fibrillation after cardiac surgery. N Engl J Med. 2016;374(20):1911–1921.
14. Biancari F, Mahar MA. Meta-analysis of randomized trials on the efficacy of posterior pericardiotomy in preventing atrial fibrillation after coronary artery bypass surgery. J Thorac Cardiovasc Surg. 2010;139(5):1158–1161.
15. Somberg J, Molnar J. Sotalol versus amiodarone in treatment of atrial fibrillation. J Atr Fibrillation. 2016;8(5):1359.
16. Milan DJ, Saul JP, Somberg JC, Molnar J. Efficacy of intravenous and oral sotalol in pharmacologic conversion of atrial fibrillation: A systematic review and meta-analysis. Cardiology. 2017;136(1):52–60.
17. Arsenault KA, Yusuf AM, Crystal E, et al. Interventions for preventing post-operative atrial fibrillation in patients undergoing heart surgery. Cochrane Database Syst Rev. 2013;(1):CD003611.
18. Hillis LD, Smith PK, Anderson JL, et al. 2011 ACCF/AHA guideline for coronary artery bypass graft surgery: Executive summary: A report of the American College of Cardiology Foundation/American Heart Association Task Force on Practice Guidelines. Circulation. 2011;124(23):2610–2642.
19. Imazio M, Brucato A, Ferrazzi P, et al. Colchicine reduces postoperative atrial fibrillation: Results of the Colchicine for the Prevention of the Postpericardiotomy Syndrome (COPPS) Atrial Fibrillation substudy. Circulation. 2011;124(21):2290–2295.
20. Imazio M, Brucato A, Ferrazzi P, et al. Colchicine for Prevention of Postpericardiotomy Syndrome and Postoperative Atrial Fibrillation: The COPPS-2 randomized clinical trial. JAMA. 2014;312(10):1016–1023.
21. Ozaydin M, Peker O, Erdogan D, et al. N-acetylcysteine for the Prevention of Postoperative Atrial Fibrillation: A prospective, randomized, placebo-controlled pilot study. Eur Heart J. 2008;29(5):625-631.
22. Liu XH, Xu CY, Fan GH. Efficacy of N-acetylcysteine in preventing atrial fibrillation after cardiac surgery: A meta-analysis of published randomized controlled trials. BMC Cardiovasc Disord. 2014;14:52.
23. Mathew JP, Fontes ML, Tudor IC, et al. A multicenter risk index for atrial fibrillation after cardiac surgery. JAMA. 2004;291(14):1720–1729.
24. Miceli A, Capoun R, Fino C, et al. Effects of angiotensin-converting enzyme inhibitor therapy on clinical outcome in patients undergoing coronary artery bypass grafting. J Am Coll Cardiol. 2009;54(19):1778–1784.
25. Cheruku KK, Ghani A, Ahmad F, et al. Efficacy of nonsteroidal anti-inflammatory medications for prevention of atrial

fibrillation following coronary artery bypass graft surgery. Prev Cardiol. 2004;7(1):13–18.

26. Horbach SJ, Lopes RD, da C Guaragna JC, et al. Naproxen as prophylaxis against atrial fibrillation after cardiac surgery: The NAFARM randomized trial. Am J Med. 2011;124(11):1036–1042.

27. Zheng Z, Jayaram R, Jiang L, et al. Perioperative rosuvastatin in cardiac surgery. N Engl J Med. 2016;374(18):1744–1753.

28. Schmidt M, Demoule A, Prochet R, et al. Dyspnea in mechanically ventilated critically ill patients. Crit Care Med. 2011;39:2059–2065.

29. Luik A, Radzewitz A, Kieser M, et al. Cryoballoon versus open irrigated radiofrequency ablation in patients with paroxysmal atrial fibrillation: The prospective, randomized, controlled, noninferiority FreezeAF study. Circulation. 2015;132(14):1311–1319.

30. Kuck KH, Brugada J, Furnkranz A, et al. Cryoballoon or radiofrequency ablation for paroxysmal atrial fibrillation. N Engl J Med. 2016;374(23):2235–2245.

31. Haissaguerre M, Jais P, Shah DC, et al. Spontaneous initiation of atrial fibrillation by ectopic beats originating in the pulmonary veins. N Engl J Med. 1998;339(10):659–666.

32. Oral H, Knight BP, Tada H, et al. Pulmonary vein isolation for paroxysmal and persistent atrial fibrillation. Circulation. 2002;105(9):1077–1081.

33. Damiano RJ, Jr. Alternative energy sources for atrial ablation: Judging the new technology. Ann Thorac Surg. 2003;75(2):329–330.

34. Gaynor SL, Diodato MD, Prasad SM, et al. A prospective, single-center clinical trial of a modified cox maze procedure with bipolar radiofrequency ablation. J Thorac Cardiovasc Surg. 2004;128(4):535–542.

35. Ninet J, Roques X, Seitelberger R, et al. Surgical ablation of atrial fibrillation with off-pump, epicardial, high-intensity focused ultrasound: Results of a multicenter trial. J Thorac Cardiovasc Surg. 2005;130(3):803–809.

36. Mack CA, Milla F, Ko W, et al. Surgical treatment of atrial fibrillation using argon-based cryoablation during concomitant cardiac procedures. Circulation. 2005;112(9 Suppl):I1–I6.

37. Wudel JH, Chaudhuri P, Hiller JJ. Video-assisted epicardial ablation and left atrial appendage exclusion for atrial fibrillation: Extended follow-up. Ann Thorac Surg. 2008;85(1):34–38.

38. Society of Thoracic Surgeons Task Force on Resuscitation After Cardiac Surgery. The society of thoracic surgeons expert consensus for the resuscitation of patients who arrest after cardiac surgery. Ann Thorac Surg. 2017;103(3):1005–1020.

39. Fernando HC, Jaklitsch MT, Walsh GL, et al. The Society of Thoracic Surgeons practice guideline on the prophylaxis and management of atrial fibrillation associated with general thoracic surgery: Executive summary. Ann Thorac Surg. 2011;92(3):1144–1152.

40. Verhaert D, Puwanant S, Gillinov AM, Klein AL. Atrial fibrillation after open heart surgery: How safe is early conversion without anticoagulation? J Am Soc Echocardiogr. 2009;22(2):212.e1–212.e3.

41. Auer J, Weber T, Berent R, Lamm G, Eber B. Serum potassium level and risk of postoperative atrial fibrillation in patients undergoing cardiac surgery. J Am Coll Cardiol. 2004;44(4):938–939; author reply 939.

42. Pillarisetti J, Patel A, Bommana S, et al. Atrial fibrillation following open heart surgery: Long-term incidence and prognosis. J Interv Card Electrophysiol. 2014;39(1):69–75.

43. Marik PE, Fromm R. The efficacy and dosage effect of corticosteroids for the prevention of atrial fibrillation after cardiac surgery: A systematic review. J Crit Care. 2009;24(3):458–463.

44. Davis EM, Packard KA, Hilleman DE. Pharmacologic prophylaxis of postoperative atrial fibrillation in patients undergoing cardiac surgery: Beyond beta-blockers. Pharmacotherapy. 2010;30(7):749, 274e–318e.

45. Pisters R, Lane DA, Nieuwlaat R, de Vos CB, Crijns HJ, Lip GY. A novel user-friendly score (HAS-BLED) to assess 1-year risk of major bleeding in patients with atrial fibrillation: The Euro Heart Survey. Chest. 2010;138(5):1093–1100.

REVIEW QUESTIONS

1. A 55-year-old woman is post-operative day 3 from a mitral valve replacement due to long-standing rheumatic heart disease and mitral stenosis. She becomes tachycardic and her rhythm changes to AF. Which feature of her history and surgery have *least* contributed to development of AF?

   A. Mitral valve replacement
   B. Age >55 years old
   C. Left atrial enlargement
   D. Perioperative inflammation

   Answer: B. Most studies cite age >65 as a risk factor for POAF. An enlarged left atrium, while not specifically mentioned, can be presumed in the setting of long-standing mitral stenosis and has been implicated in the development of postoperative AF. Mitral valve surgery has the highest risk of postoperative AF. Inflammation is known to contribute to the development of postoperative AF, many therapies are aimed at suppressing the postoperative inflammatory state.

2. Which of the following explains how intravascular hypervolemia may contribute to the development of postoperative AF?

   A. Retention of free water leads to electrolyte imbalance.
   B. Hypervolemia develops in patients with renal insufficiency; the actual risk factor is related to kidney dysfunction.
   C. Hypervolemia leads to stretch or dilation of the atria, which interferes with normal conduction.
   D. Hypervolemia is associated with pulmonary edema which is a risk factor for postoperative AF.

   Answer: C. The peak incidence of postoperative AF is on day 2, which is also when many patients start to mobilize fluids and increase their intravascular volume, which will lead to atrial stretch.

3. Which of the following can contribute to hemodynamic instability with AF?

   A. Loss of atrial contraction and its contribution to cardiac output
   B. Rapid ventricular response, which leads to shortened diastolic time and filling
   C. A and B
   D. None of the above

   Answer: C. Atrial contraction can account to up to 30% of the stroke volume and therefore 30% of the cardiac output. The absence of atrial contraction in AF therefore leads to a decrement in cardiac output. Since the left ventricle fills during diastole, by increasing the heart rate and decreasing diastolic time, the ventricle has a lower end diastolic volume to eject in systole. If a patient has diastolic dysfunction as well, the loss of atrial contraction and the shortened ventricular filling time may synergistically and dramatically decrease the stroke volume and therefore cardiac output.

4. Which of the following is true regarding perioperative beta blockers and AF?

    A. Prolonged withholding of a patient's home beta blocker can contribute to the development of AF.
    B. All patients should be given a beta blocker within 24 hours of surgery.
    C. Metoprolol is the most effective beta blocker for preventing postoperative AF.
    D. Metoprolol should be given to all cardiac surgery patients on postoperative day 1 to prevent AF.

Answer: A. Studies looking at preoperative beta blockers for postoperative AF prophylaxis have shown that in patients who continue their preoperative beta blocker until the time of surgery, they have a lower risk of developing postoperative AF. While it is recommended to begin beta blockers following cardiac surgery within 24 hours, this should only be done after looking at the whole clinical picture of the patient. For instance, in a patient who requires ongoing vasopressor or inotropic support it may not be appropriate to begin beta-blocker therapy. While metoprolol is one of the most commonly used beta blockers perioperatively, a recent meta-analysis demonstrated that carvedilol is superior to metoprolol for prevention of postoperative AF.

5. Which of the following is *not* a mechanism of pathophysiology of postoperative AF?

    A. Multiple foci in the atria generating electrical impulses that collide with each other
    B. Rapid firing foci near the pulmonary veins
    C. A re-entry loop develops in the atria (from one or multiple foci)
    D. Hyperkalemic cardioplegia alters the resting membrane potential

Answer: D. Choice A is called the "multiple wavelets" theory. Choice B does not have a specific title, but its existence is supported by the fact that successful interventional procedures often involve isolation of these foci from surrounding tissue. Choice C is the single-driver or multiple-driver model where rapidly firing foci generate a closed re-entry loop.[4] If the main cause were hyperkalemic cardioplegia, most AF would be in the intra and immediate postoperative phases, not in the biphasic immediately postoperative and 2 to 4 days postoperative timing.

6. A 67-year-old male is postoperative day 2 from CABG. He has been progressing as anticipated; he is not requiring inotropes or vasoactive infusions. He has been given 2 doses of intravenous furosemide to aid in diuresis with the goal of returning to his preoperative weight. Which of the following electrolyte abnormalities, commonly found in this phase of his recovery, has been shown to increase the development of postoperative AF?

    A. Hypokalemia
    B. Hypermagnesemia
    C. Hyponatremia
    D. Hyperphosphatemia

Answer: A. Patients with hypokalemia (serum potassium <3.9 mmol/l) develop AF following cardiac surgery at a significantly higher rate than those a serum potassium >4.4 mmol/L.[41] Hypomagnesemia has also been associated with postoperative AF (likely because of its impact on potassium absorption). Hyponatremia and hyperphosphatemia are not known to impact the likelihood of development of postoperative AF.

7. You are designing a clinical trial on postcardiac surgery new onset AF. In order to test your intervention most efficiently, which group of patients should be included?

    A. Off-pump CABG patients
    B. Mitral valve replacement patients
    C. CABG with intraoperative cardiopulmonary bypass patients
    D. Heart transplant patients

Answer: B. Mitral valve surgery has the highest incidence of postoperative AF. While rates of postoperative AF vary in different studies, AF after valvular surgery is always cited with a higher incidence.[42,43]

8. Which of the following patients is most likely to develop new-onset postoperative AF?

    A. A 72-year-old man who had a 2-vessel, off pump, coronary artery bypass who has been on long-term, high-intensity statins
    B. A 67-year-old woman who had a mitral and aortic valve repair for mitral regurgitation and aortic stenosis
    C. A 62-year-old man who had a 2-vessel coronary artery bypass and received intraoperative and postoperative corticosteroids
    D. A 32-year-old woman with tricuspid valve replacement for bacterial endocarditis

Answer: B. Valvluar surgery, especially mitral valvular surgery, has the highest risk of development of AF. There is a plethora of research on mechanisms for development of postoperative AF, among a myriad of other factors, inflammation comes up again and again. Strategies have been employed to alter the inflammatory response with the hope of altering the risk of postoperative AF. Statins, steroids, colchicine, and nonsteroidal anti-inflammatory medications are among the most studied for this, all of which have shown various degrees of decreasing the risk of postoperative AF.

9. A 78-year-old woman is scheduled to have a replacement of her aortic valve due to severe aortic stenosis as well as a 2-vessel CABG. She has a history of COPD, hypertension, diabetes mellitus, and obesity. Since she has multiple risk factors for the development of AF, you wish to begin preoperative prophylaxis to reduce the risk of postoperative AF. Which regimen would accomplish this most effectively with the least complications?

    A. IV amiodarone administered during cardiopulmonary bypass
    B. Oral metoprolol beginning 7 days prior to surgery and continued postoperatively

C. Anterior pericardiotomy

D. Oral digoxin beginning on postoperative day 2

Answer: B. A number of regimens have been investigated to prevent the development of postoperative AF. The preponderance of evidence supports the use of enteral beta-blockers starting at least 24 hours preoperatively. There are data to support the use of amiodarone for postoperative AF prophylaxis; however, studies have had a variety of approaches to the use of amiodarone (preoperative oral regimens continued postoperatively, intraoperative intravenous infusion continued postoperatively) without one clearly superior regimen. However, amiodarone has many systemic side effects and toxicities (pulmonary, hepatic, and thyroid problems are well established), and for that reason, it is not the regimen with the least amount of complications.

Paricardiotomy has been shown to decrease the risk of postoperative AF, likely due to less physical irritation of the heart if pericardial effusion develops (periocardiotomy facilitates drainage). This benefit is when the pericardiotomy is posterior to the heart.[1]

Digoxin has benefit for rate control but not for rhythm control; therefore, it is not beneficial to prevent AF as an arrhythmia. There have not been trials of digoxin alone as a prophylactic agent for postoperative AF, and therefore its use for this purpose alone cannot be recommended.[44]

10. A 78-year-old female with a history of hypertension and diabetes develops postoperative AF post-mitral valve replacement for ischemic mitral regurgitation. How long would you allow the patient to remain in AF before starting anticoagulation assuming minimal risk of bleeding?

A. 12 hours

B. 48 hours

C. 5 days

D. 2 weeks

Answer: B. The American Association for Thoracic Surgeons recommends starting anticoagulation within 48 hours of the development of postoperative AF.[11] The decision to initiate anticoagulation should be based on risk of stroke as guided by the CHA2DS2-VASc score (this patient has a score of 5, which corresponds to an annual stroke rate of 6%) and risk of bleeding, which is determined by a number of postsurgical factors. In the outpatient setting, bleeding risk can be estimated by using the HAS-BLED risk calculator.[45]

30.

VENTRICULAR FIBRILLATION/VENTRICULAR TACHYCARDIA AFTER CORONARY ARTERY BYPASS GRAFTING

Eric Feduska and Kristen Carey Rock

STEM AND KEY QUESTIONS

A 37-year-old female with a history of morbid obesity, hypertension, and unstable angina presents for an elective 2-vessel coronary artery bypass grafting (CABG). The procedure was uneventful with successful grafting of the left internal mammary artery to the left anterior descending artery and a saphenous vein graft to the left circumflex artery. Although initially stable on arrival to the intensive care unit (ICU), she begins to have wide variability in her heart rate and blood pressure and develops dynamic ST elevations on telemetry. Her serum electrolytes and hemoglobin on departure from the operating room were all within normal limits. Within an hour of arriving to the ICU, the patient develops ventricular tachycardia (VT) requiring advanced cardiac left support (ACLS).

WHAT CAUSES OF VENTRICULAR ARRHYTHMIAS SHOULD BE IN THE DIFFERENTIAL DIAGNOSIS IN THE IMMEDIATE POSTOPERATIVE PERIOD AFTER CABG?

After loading the patient with 300 mg of amiodarone and started on an amiodarone infusion at 1mg/min, ACLS is successful and there is successful return of spontaneous circulation (ROSC). Despite this intervention, the patient has 3 additional episodes of VT. A stat transthoracic echocardiogram is ordered.

IS AMIODARONE THE BEST PHARMACOLOGIC CHOICE FOR TREATMENT OF VT? WHAT ARE OTHER DRUG CHOICES? IS OVERDRIVE PACING A VIABLE OPTION FOR NONPHARMACOLOGIC THERAPY?

The echocardiogram does not suggest any focal regional wall motion abnormalities, and biventricular systolic function is normal. Despite her normal serum electrolytes, the patient is given intravenous boluses of potassium and magnesium and the cardiac surgeon is called to the bedside.

SHOULD THE PATIENT BE RETURNED URGENTLY TO THE OPERATING ROOM FOR REEXPLORATION? WHAT IS THE UTILITY OF TRANSTHORACIC ECHOCARDIOGRAPHY IN DETECTING POSTOPERATIVE GRAFT DYSFUNCTION? SHOULD THE PATIENT BE TAKEN TO THE CARDIAC CATHETERIZATION LAB INSTEAD OF THE OPERATING ROOM?

The cardiac surgeon decides to return to the operating room to place the patient on veno-arterial extracorporeal membrane oxygenation (VA ECMO) before transporting the patient to the cardiac catheterization lab for coronary angiography.

WHEN IS VA ECMO INDICATED FOR REFRACTORY VT/VF?

The patient is stabilized on VA ECMO and taken for coronary angiography, which reveals diffuse vasospasm of both her native coronary arteries and the newly placed grafts. Nicardipine is injected directly into all native vessels and grafts with some effect. The patient is also placed on intravenous nitroglycerin. She slowly recovers with no further episodes of malignant arrhythmias. She is decannulated from VA ECMO 2 days later and discharged from the hospital of postoperative day 10.

IS THE PATIENT A CANDIDATE FOR AN INTERNAL CARDIAC DEFIBRILLATOR FOR VT/VF? WITH WHAT MEDICATIONS SHOULD SHE BE DISCHARGED FROM THE HOSPITAL?

DISCUSSION

Heart disease remains the leading cause of death in the United States, and coronary heart disease at 43.8% is the largest contributor to mortality.[1] CABG is recommended for patients with obstructive coronary artery disease whose predicted survival would be improved compared to medical therapy or percutaneous coronary intervention. Although CABG is well tolerated by most patients with an unadjusted perioperative mortality of 2.3%,[2] major complications can occur in the immediate and longer term postoperative course of these patients. Postoperative arrhythmias are among the most commonly encountered postoperative complications associated with CABG. Their clinical significance ranges from benign to life-threatening.

Atrial tachyarrhythmias are the most common postoperative heart rhythm disorder. Ventricular arrhythmias are less frequent. Ventricular conduction disturbances most extreme forms, VT and VF, are rare but carry a high mortality rate. Basic evaluation and management principles are key to the initial approach to the patient with an arrhythmia. Given the unsatisfactory short- and long-term outcomes of VT/VF, prompt recognition and aggressive management of these potentially fatal arrhythmias should be pursued.

INCIDENCE, ETIOLOGY, AND RISK FACTORS

Simple ventricular premature beats (VPBs) are commonplace and occur in virtually every postoperative CABG patient. Complex VPBs such as nonsustained ventricular tachycardia (NSVT) are also common with incidences ranging from 17% to 97%.[3] Nonsustained ventricular tachycardia is thought to be reperfusion-induced and typically regarded as benign,[4,5] although some patients may be at increased risk of future life-threatening arrhythmias.[6]

Sustained VT and VF are less common and occur in approximately 1% to 3% of postoperative CABG patients.[1,7] Sustained VT/VF can occur anytime from the immediate postoperative period to several weeks later but most often manifests within the first few days postoperatively. Ominously, the mortality of postoperative cardiac surgery patients with VT/VF is 20% to 30%.[8]

Although difficult to predict, studies have found unifying risk factors for postoperative VT/VF. In the largest study to date regarding predictors of ventricular arrythmias after cardiac surgery, 4 independent factors were found to be associated with ventricular arrythmias (Box 30.1).[9]

The most concerning etiology of malignant ventricular arrhythmias post-CABG is due to ischemia. Myocardial ischemia is estimated to be present in 33% of CABG patients perioperatively, most of whom will exhibit this ischemia in the first 16 to 18 hours, and it carries increased morbidity and mortality for those who develop it.[10] Ischemia can result from a variety of pathologies not reviewed here but can be divided into a few main categories: acute infarction, reperfusion of previously ischemic tissues or myocardial stunning, supply demand mismatch, graft malfunction, or vasospasm.

Box 30.1. PREDICTORS OF PERIOPERATIVE VENTRICULAR ARRHYTHMIAS

Older age >65
Peripheral vascular disease
Depressed ejection fraction (<50%)Emergency surgery

In cases where previous areas of ischemic or infarcted myocardium are reperfused, ventricular arrhythmias can be particularly challenging to control. Suspicion for this phenomenon should arise in patient with history of prior infarction or unstable angina, reduced ejection fraction or preoperative advanced heart failure symptoms, pulmonary or systemic hypertension.[8]

PATHOGENESIS

Cardiac surgery creates unique conditions for the pathogenesis of malignant ventricular arrhythmias, given the hemodynamic fluctuations, inflammatory changes, and the use of cardioplegia and cardiopulmonary bypass that occur intraoperatively. The pathogenesis of post-CABG sustained VT/VF involves the complex interplay of both patient and surgical-related risk factors.

Coronary artery bypass graft surgery comes with all the same stresses seen with other major operations: tissue trauma, inflammation, and ischemia. Additionally, it is associated with wide swings in hemodynamics, electrolytes, fluid shifts, coagulation abnormalities, temperature, gas exchange, pain, and catecholamines. Superimpose these stressors on patients with baseline structural heart disease and often extracardiac comorbidities and one has the perfect substrate for a highly unstable electrical milieu.

The extent of left ventricular dysfunction is a major factor in the development of ventricular arrhythmias in patients with coronary artery disease. Myocardial fibrosis results in loss of cell-to-cell signaling and is thought to be responsible for most ventricular arrhythmias. These focal myocardial scars are not expected to be affected by revascularization and are primed for arrhythmogenesis in the postoperative period.

Ventricular tachycardia usually originates within the ventricular myocardium, outside of the normal conduction system, resulting in direct myocardial activation. In patients with previous myocardial infarction, the border zone between scar and normal tissues is a common place for a reentrant circuit to form a monomorphic VT (Figure 30.1).[8] Polymorphic VT not caused by torsades de pointe, can be caused by heterogenous repolarization in previous ischemic ventricular tissue, ongoing ischemia and hemodynamic instability, elevated synthetic or endogenous catecholamines, or metabolic derangements (Figure 30.2). Polymorphic VT with QT prolongation, otherwise known as torsades de pointes, is caused by early after polarizations and can be precipitated by a number of QT prolonging medications given in the postoperative setting including metoclopramide, ondansetron, haloperidol, and some antiarrhythmics.

Ventricular fibrillation results from multiple localized areas of micro-reentry without any organized electrical activity. As the duration of VF increases, progressive cellular ischemia and acidosis develop, resulting in an electrophysiologic deterioration, manifested by an increase in fibrillation cycle length and prolonged diastole duration between fibrillation action potentials.

Pacemaker-induced VT/VF is perhaps a less common cause but certainly should be included in the differential diagnosis of etiologies particularly as many surgeons elect to

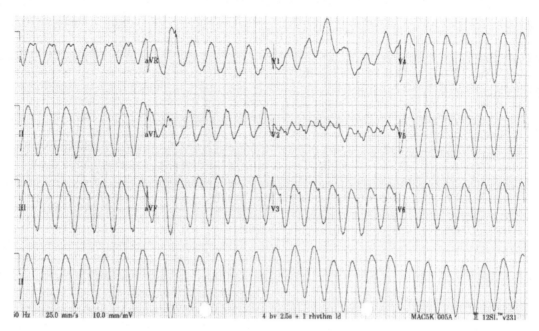

Figure 30.1 Monomorphic Ventricular Tachycardia.

place temporary epicardial pacing wires intraoperatively and an increasing number of patients have pre-existing implanted cardiac devices. Inappropriate sensing, or the use of an inappropriate pacing mode, can create an R-on-T phenomenon and thus induce a ventricular arrhythmia. For patients with pre-existing devices, intraoperative use of electrocautery can necessitate the conversion of the device to an asynchronous mode, which prevents the device from being inhibited by premature beats and predisposes to accidental pacing-on-T induced arrhythmias.

CLINICAL MANIFESTATION AND DIAGNOSIS

Randomized trials, technological advances, and better understanding of arrhythmia mechanisms using intracardiac recordings and programmed electrical stimulation and mapping techniques have resulted in improved approaches to rhythm disturbances. The diagnosis of VT/VF post-CABG is usually not difficult as most patients are on continuous telemetry monitoring. Sustained VT/VF in their most extreme forms manifest as a sudden loss of coordinated filling and ejection of the heart, resulting in hemodynamic collapse.

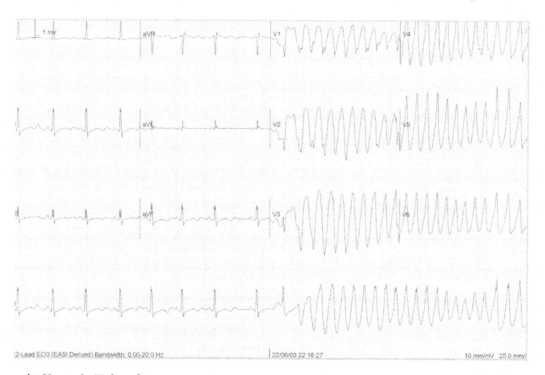

Figure 30.2 Polymorphic Ventricular Tachycardia.

Based on electrocardiogram (ECG) criteria, wide complex tachycardias may be either ventricular or supraventricular. In patients with significant coronary heart disease or other structural heart disease, a wide QRS complex tachycardia should be considered to be VT until proven otherwise.

Whenever possible, a 12-lead ECG should be obtained. If the patient has temporary epicardial pacing wires and the origins of the patient's arrhythmia remains elusive, an atrial ECG can be helpful in diagnosing complex dysrhythmias. This can be particularly useful in differentiating a supraventricular tachycardia with a rate-related bundle branch block from true VT. The hemodynamic instability of patients with ventricular arrhythmias is variable and depends upon the rate of the tachyarrhythmia and left ventricular systolic and diastolic function.

TREATMENT/MANAGEMENT

The postoperative CABG patient requires meticulous attention to the identification and treatment of electrolyte or other metabolic imbalances, myocardial ischemia, and potential mechanical complications of surgery. Given the potentially deadly consequences and rapid decompensation resulting from sustained ventricular arrhythmias, basic treatment along with advanced diagnosis and management should happen simultaneously. Asymptomatic and hemodynamically stable short runs of NSVT do not often need aggressive treatment. However, they may be a harbinger of VT/VF—therefore the differential of reversible causes of ventricular arrhythmias should be reviewed, including attention to serum electrolytes (Box 30.2). Postoperative sustained ventricular arrhythmias treatment follows the same principles outlined by ACLS with some important caveats.

Sustained ventricular tachyarrhythmias should be promptly cardioverted either by drug infusions or electrically. Symptomatic monomorphic VT is best addressed with immediate synchronized electrical cardioversion.[11] The most common symptoms are angina, pulmonary edema, hypotension, and altered mental status. Sustained, rapid monomorphic VT, or polymorphic VT, including torsades de pointes, present

Box 30.2. REVERSIBLE CAUSES OF VENTRICULAR ARRYTHMIAS

Hypoxia
Hypercarbia
Acidosis
Hypotension
Electrolyte imbalances
Mechanical complications

- Tamponade
- Pneumothorax
- Pulmonary artery catheter
- Tube thoracostomy

Hypothermia
Proarrhythmic drugs
Ischemia or graft failure

as pulselessness and should be treated with defibrillation, an unsynchronized electrical shock.

In the realm of pharmacological intervention, stable monomorphic VT can be treated with amiodarone, lidocaine, or procainamide (Table 30.1).[12] Simultaneously, preparations should be made for urgent electrical cardioversion or defibrillation should the patient deteriorate. In the event of recurrence, suppression of the arrhythmia by pharmacologic means should continue, and further evaluation should focus upon the presence of arrhythmia triggers. Among antiarrhythmic medications, amiodarone is the most effective for preventing recurrent sustained monomorphic ventricular tachycardia (SMVT), although sotalol and dronedarone are also very efficacious.[13]

Critical in the pharmacologic management of polymorphic VT is the identification of QT prolongation. Polymorphic VT in patients with a normal QT interval is treated in the same manner as monomorphic VT.[14] If, however, the patient's polymorphic VT is punctuated by sinus rhythm with QT prolongation or torsades de pointes, treatment is with magnesium sulfate, isoproterenol, overdrive pacing, or a combination of these options.[14] Administration of antiarrhythmics devoid of potassium-channel blocking properties (i.e., phenytoin or lidocaine) may also help by shortening the QT interval in this setting. Procainamide and amiodarone are, in general, contraindicated because of their QT-prolonging effects.[15]

In practice, it may be relatively unclear whether an observed episode of polymorphic VT is related to QT-interval prolongation. In such cases, magnesium and a sodium-channel blocking agents may be administered empirically.[16] Notably, among the antiarrhythmic agents that prolong the QT interval, the incidence of torsades de pointes is lowest with amiodarone.[16] Therefore, amiodarone is a rational alternative therapy for refractory polymorphic VT of unclear etiology; however, expert consultation is recommended.[17]

The most important interventions in the treatment of ventricular fibrillation are nonpharmacological and are nearly the same as unstable sustained VT and VT; these are immediate identification of the rhythm and rapid defibrillation along with simultaneous correction of reversible etiologies. When caught and intervened upon early, success rates are high.[17–20]

Initiation or resumption of beta blocker therapy is nearly universal in patients undergoing CABG surgery. The benefits of beta blocker therapy are numerous and include decreased oxygen demand, decreased risk of ventricular fibrillation, decreased automaticity, reductions in cardiac remodeling, improved left ventricular hemodynamic function, improved coronary diastolic perfusion, and inhibition of platelet aggregation.[21–27] Post-bypass cardiogenic shock, vasoplegia, heart block, or bradycardia may preclude the initiation of beta blockers in the immediate postoperative CABG patient. Their role in the prevention and treatment of sudden cardiac death in both patients with acute myocardial infarction (MI) and heart failure with reduced ejection fraction, however, is well established.[15–17]

After or during initial stabilization, simultaneous advanced diagnostics focusing on the cause of the malignant arrhythmia

Table 30.1 ANTIARRHYTHMICS

AGENT	VAUGHAN WILLIAMS CLASS	DOSING	SIDE EFFECTS / TOXICITY	NOTES
Procainamide	IA	Ventricular arrhythmias: IV Loading dose: 500 to 600 mg administered as a slow infusion over 25 to 30 minutes or 100 mg/dose at a rate not to exceed 50 mg/minute repeated every 5 minutes as needed to a maximum dose of 1,000 mg. Discontinue loading dose when arrhythmia is controlled, hypotension occurs, QRS complex widens by 50% of its original width, or total of 600 mg to 1,000 mg is given. Maintenance infusion: 2 to 6 mg/minute by continuous infusion.	Non-specific central nervous system and gastrointestinal symptoms Lupus-like syndrome (chronic use) - US Boxed Warning Severe bone marrow toxicity (pancytopenia or agranulocytosis - rare) - US Boxed Warning Watch for proarrhythmic effects; monitor and adjust dose to prevent QTc prolongation. Avoid use in patients with QT prolongation. Atrial Fibrillation / Atrial Flutter: procainamide may increase ventricular response rate in patients with atrial fibrillation or flutter; control AV conduction before initiating. Fever can be a manifestation of an allergic response to procainamide	An alternative intravenous dosing regimen is 20 to 50 mg/minute until the arrhythmia terminates or a maximum dose of 15 to 17 mg/kg is administered[12] Once VT terminates, it is usually not necessary to continue a maintenance infusion, although procainamide can be resumed or continued if VT recurs. Procainamide has the advantage of slowing VT even when it fails to terminate, usually resulting in greater hemodynamic stability
Lidocaine	IB	VF or pulseless VT (off-label use - alternative to amiodarone): IV/IO: Initial: 1 to 1.5 mg/kg bolus. If refractory VF or pulseless VT, repeat 0.5 to 0.75 mg/kg bolus every 5 to 10 minutes (maximum cumulative dose: 3 mg/kg)[11]. Follow with continuous infusion (1 to 4 mg/minute) after return of perfusion[11] Hemodynamically Stable Monomorphic VT: IV: 1 to 1.5 mg/kg; repeat with 0.5 to 0.75 mg/kg every 5 to 10 minutes as necessary (maximum cumulative dose: 3 mg/kg). Follow with continuous infusion of 1 to 4 mg/minute[15]	Central nervous system (CNS) toxicity, cardiovascular toxicity, and gastrointestinal toxicity	Reduce maintenance infusion in patients with CHF, shock, or hepatic disease; initiate infusion at 10 mcg/kg/minute (maximum dose: 1.5 mg/minute or 20 mcg/kg/minute).
Amiodarone	III	Pulseless VT or VF IV/IO push: Initial: 300 mg rapid bolus; administer supplemental dose of 150 mg if rhythm persists or recurs[11] Stable VT: IV: 150 mg over 10 minutes, then 1 mg/minute for 6 hours, followed by 0.5 mg/minute[12] Breakthrough Stable VT: 150 mg supplemental doses given over 10 minutes[11]	Amiodarone has a wide range of potential toxicities involving the lungs, thyroid, liver, eyes, and skin. Patients receiving amiodarone chronically should have baseline evaluations and regular follow-up of lung, liver, thyroid, skin and eyes Amiodarone can directly cause both sinus bradycardia and AV nodal block, due primarily to its calcium channel blocking activity. Amiodarone is highly protein bound and hepatically metabolized, as such, it has the potential to alter plasma concentrations of other protein bound and hepatically metabolized drugs including several antiarrhythmics. Hypotension: A major problem noted with the intravenous preparation is hypotension- particularly when given rapidly. The hypotension has been attributed to the solvents used in the preparation'''	Intravenous amiodarone has a different electrophysiologic and pharmacologic profile from oral amiodarone. Conversion from IV to oral therapy has not been formally evaluated. Some experts recommend a 1 to 2 day overlap when converting from IV to oral therapy especially when treating ventricular arrhythmias. Pulmonary and hepatic toxicity appears to correlate more closely with the total cumulative dose than with serum drug levels. However, severe liver toxicity has occurred shortly after initiation so close monitoring is recommended.

(continued)

Table 30.1 CONTINUED

AGENT	VAUGHAN WILLIAMS CLASS	DOSING	SIDE EFFECTS / TOXICITY	NOTES
Sotalol	III	**Ventricular Arrhythmias** Initial dose: 75 mg infused over 5 hours twice daily Dose range: Usual therapeutic dose: 75 to 150 mg twice daily **Monomorphic VT** (hemodynamically stable) (off-label use): IV: 1.5 mg/kg over 5 minutes[11]	Sotalol can cause life threatening ventricular tachycardia associated with QT interval prolongation - Do not initiate if the baseline QTc interval is longer than 450 msec. If CrCl ≤60 mL/minute, dosing interval adjustment is necessary. Bradycardia and reverse use dependence – sotalol exhibits the phenomenon of reverse use dependence where the heart rate and QT interval become inversely related (the QT interval is prolonged as the heart rate slows)	Sotalol has beta blocking and class III activities; d-sotalol is a pure class III agent. Commercially available sotalol is a racemic (equal part) mixture Sotalol is effective in patients with arrhythmogenic right ventricular cardiomyopathy who have non-life-threatening VT. Most other antiarrhythmics have little effect in this specific patient population***

11: Neumar RW, Shuster M, Callaway CW, et al. Part 1: Executive Summary: 2015 American Heart Association Guidelines Update for Cardiopulmonary Resuscitation and Emergency Cardiovascular Care. *Circulation.* 2015; 132:S315.

12: Al-Khatib SM, Stevenson WG, Ackerman MJ, et al. 2017 AHA/ACC/HRS Guideline for Management of Patients With Ventricular Arrhythmias and the Prevention of Sudden Cardiac Death: A Report of the American College of Cardiology/American Heart Association Task Force on Clinical Practice Guidelines and the Heart Rhythm Society. *J Am Coll Cardiol* 2017; S0735-1097(17)41306-4.

15: Zipes DP, Camm AJ, Borggrefe M, et al. ACC/AHA/ESC 2006 guidelines for management of patients with ventricular arrhythmias and the prevention of sudden cardiac death: a report of the American College of Cardiology/ American Heart Association Task Force and the European Society of Cardiology Committee for Practice Guidelines (Writing Committee to Develop Guidelines for Management of Patients With Ventricular Arrhythmias and the Prevention of Sudden Cardiac Death). *J Am Coll Cardiol.* 2006;48(5):e247-346.

*** Gallik DM, Singer I, Meissner MD, et al. Hemodynamic and surface electrocardiographic effects of a new aqueous formulation of intravenous amiodarone. *Am J Cardiol* 2002; 90:964.

••• Wichter T, Borggrefe M, Haverkamp W, et al. Efficacy of antiarrhythmic drugs in patients with arrhythmogenic right ventricular disease. Results in patients with inducible and noninducible ventricular tachycardia. *Circulation* 1992; 86:29.

should be a parallel focus of care. Emergent bedside ultrasound is a useful bedside tool to diagnose cardiac tamponade or pneumothorax. Tamponade causing hemodynamic instability is an indication for emergent bedside decompression and evacuation via open chest exploration. Transthoracic echocardiography (TTE) can diagnose regional wall motion abnormalities or acute systolic heart failure, which can signify acute coronary syndrome, whether de novo or secondary to graft failure. Such a diagnosis would dramatically improve the utility of cardiac catheterization or even a return to the operating room. Given the morbidity of urgent redo cardiac surgery, the cardiac catheterization lab seems to be a very reasonable first approach when the diagnosis is not clear. Additional causes of ventricular arrhythmias that can be diagnosed on TTE are left ventricular outflow tract (LVOT) obstruction and its related pathology, systolic anterior motion of the mitral valve (SAM). Initial treatments of SAM include minimizing the use of inotropes, optimizing ventricular preload, and increasing left ventricular afterload.

As in the case outlined here, vasospasm is a rare and under-recognized, but serious, complication of CABG surgery that can result in ischemia-induced VT or VF. Postoperative vasospasm may be more common in middle-aged women with single-vessel disease.[28] Additional inciting factors may include sympathetic or adrenergic stimulation, cold, local trauma, release of vasoconstricting substance by platelets, electrolyte imbalances, or histamine release.[29] While vasospasm can be suspected with an ECG suggestive of ST changes, it can only definitively be diagnosed by coronary angiogram. Treatments for vasospasm include systemic versus intracoronary delivery of either nitroglycerin or a calcium channel blocker (i.e., nicardipine or diltiazem).[30] Patients who are definitively diagnosed with coronary spasm should be discharged with a calcium channel blocker as part of their postoperative medication regimen.

Although generally not first-line treatment, if epicardial pacing wires, permanent pacemaker, or automatic internal cardiac defibrillator (AICD) are present, these devices may be used to break VT. The first manner in which this may be done is called resetting. For this method to work, an exogenous electrical stimulus must occur antidromically to the VT circuit and be timed such that the reentrant circuit encounters refractory tissue but the artificial stimulus can conduct orthodromically. Entrainment is similar: an artificial electrical wavefront continuously and consistently enters the VT circuit when the circuit is excitable and allows the paced beat to conduct orthodromically to the myocardium and antidromically to arrest the VT circuit.[31] Expert consultation is advised, and not all VT will be responsive to these methods, depending on the type of VT and the site of the pacing wires in relation to the VT circuit.

In situations where ventricular arrhythmias are refractory to ACLS and initial pharmacological treatments, VA ECMO may be a way to stabilize the patient until additional interventions such as pharmacological termination of the arrhythmia, cardiac catheterization for ischemia, or operative revision of grafts can be accomplished. In a recent retrospective case control study comparing patients with refractory VT and VF who received ECMO support ($n = 320$) with those who did not ($n = 640$), the odds ratio of death was 0.59 for ECMO use of 1 day or less. However, for patients on ECMO for more than 1 day, the odds ratio was 2.88.[32] Further prospective studies are required.

For patients that survive persistent episodes of VT or VF after CABG, electrophysiologic ablation and/or AICD may be considered. The MADIT II trial established a survival benefit for patients post-MI with ejection fractions less than 30%.[33] The 2012 American College of Cardiology guidelines for AICD therapy suggest that patients with NSVT due to MI with left ventricular ejection fraction (LVEF) less than or equal to 40% who have inducible VF or sustained VT on electrophysiological study have a class 1 indication for device placement.[34]

PROGNOSIS

With an increasingly older and medically complex patient population, morbidity and mortality after CABG surgery is expected to increase despite procedural advances. Since CABG became a recognized standard treatment of coronary artery disease, it remains the best hope for survival in patients with the most advanced forms. The improvements in patient longevity and quality of life, however, do not come without risk. Operative mortality for even the lowest risk elective patients is around 1%. Mortality only rises when the procedure is performed at low-volume centers or on patients with multiple comorbidities.[35,36]

Risk predictive models such as the STS database used to predict operative mortality include variables that have dominated this chapter's discussion—namely ischemia as evidenced by new Q waves after CABG, increasing patient age, and poor left ventricular dysfunction.[37] With VT and VF being the most common arrhythmic causes of sudden cardiac death, it comes as no surprise that these rhythms are associated with higher hospital mortality.[5,7,9]

CONCLUSIONS

- Patient factors and surgery-related factors place postoperative CABG patients at higher risk for malignant ventricular arrhythmias.

- Distinguishing the type of VT as monomorphic, polymorphic, or polymorphic with QT- prolongation guides pharmacologic treatment options.

- If a patient develops VT/VF, treatment and advanced diagnostics must occur simultaneously. Reversible causes of VT/VF must be considered.

- Development of VT/VF connotes a higher mortality postoperatively. Patients may be candidates for electrophysiologic ablation or implantable cardioverter-defibrillator (ICD) therapy.

REFERENCES

1. Benjamin EJ, Virani SS, Callaway CW, et al.; American Heart Association Statistics Committee and Stroke Statistics Subcommittee. Heart disease and stroke statistics-2018 update: a report from the American Heart Association. Circulation. 2018;137(12):e67–e492.

2. Society of Thoracic Surgeons. Adult Cardiac Surgery Database: executive summary 10 years. 2017. https://wwww.sts.org/sites/default/files/documents/ACSD2017Harvest3_ExecutiveSummary.pdf. Accessed May 22, 2018.

3. Pires LA, Wagshal AB, Lancey R, Huang SK. Arrhythmias and conduction disturbances after coronary artery bypass graft surgery: epidemiology, management, and prognosis. Am Heart J. 1995;129:799.

4. Huikuri HV, Yli-Mayry S, Korhonenetal UR. Prevalence and prognostic significance of complex ventricular arrhythmias after coronary arterial bypass graft surgery. Int J Cardiol. 1990;27(3):333–339.

5. Smith RC, Leung JM, Keith FM, Merrick S, Mangano DT. Ventricular dysrhythmias in patients undergoing coronary artery bypass graft surgery: incidence, characteristics, and prognostic importance. Am. Heart J. 1992;123(1):73–81

6. Ascione R, Reeves BC, Santo K, et al. Predictors of new malignant ventricular arrhythmias after coronary surgery: a case-control study. J Am Coll Cardiol. 2004;43:1630.

7. Steinberg JS, Gaur A, Sciacca R, Tan E. New-onset sustained ventricular tachycardia after cardiac surgery. Circulation. 1999;99:903.

8. Bojar RM. Cardiovascular management: Cardiac Arrhythmias. In Manual of perioperative Care in Adult Cardiac Surgery, 5th ed. Oxford, UK: Wiley-Blackwell; 2011:529–554.

9. El-Chami MF, Sawaya FJ, Kilgo P, et al. Ventricular arrhythmia after cardiac surgery: incidence, predictors, and outcomes. J Am Coll Cardiol 2012;60(25):2664–2671.

10. Hirsch WS, Ledley GS, Morries NK. Acute ischemic syndromes following coronary artery bypass graftin. Clin Cardiol. 1998;21:625–632.

11. Neumar RW, Shuster M, Callaway CW, et al. Part 1: executive summary: 2015 American Heart Association guidelines update for cardiopulmonary resuscitation and emergency cardiovascular care. Circulation. 2015;132:S315.

12. Al-Khatib SM, Stevenson WG, Ackerman MJ, et al. 2017 AHA/ACC/HRS guideline for management of patients with ventricular arrhythmias and the prevention of sudden cardiac death: a report of the American College of Cardiology/American Heart Association Task Force on Clinical Practice Guidelines and the Heart Rhythm Society. Circulation. 2017;138(13): e210–e271.

13. Link MS, Atkins DL, Passman RS, et al. Part 6: electrical therapies: automated external defibrillators, defibrillation, cardioversion, and pacing: 2010 American Heart Association guidelines for cardiopulmonary resuscitation and emergency cardiovascular care. Circulation 2010;122:S706.

14. Tilz RR, Lenarczyk R, Scherr D, et al. Management of ventricular tachycardia in the ablation era: results of the European Heart Rhythm Association Survey. Europace. 2017;20(1):209–213.

15. Zipes DP, Camm AJ, Borggrefe M, et al. ACC/AHA/ESC 2006 guidelines for management of patients with ventricular arrhythmias and the prevention of sudden cardiac death: a report of the American College of Cardiology/American Heart Association Task Force and the European Society of Cardiology Committee for Practice Guidelines (Writing Committee to Develop Guidelines for Management of Patients With Ventricular Arrhythmias and the Prevention of Sudden Cardiac Death). J Am Coll Cardiol. 2006;48(5):e247–e346.

16. Mattioni TA, Zheutlin TA, Dunnington C, Kehoe RF. The proarrhythmic effects of amiodarone. Prog Cardiovasc Dis. 1989;31:439–446.

17. Faddy SC, Powell J, Craig JC. Biphasic and monophasic shocks for transthoracic defibrillation: a meta-analysis of randomized controlled trials. Resuscitation. 2003;58(1):9–16.

18. Morrison LJ, Dorian P, Long J, et al. Out-of-hospital cardiac arrest rectilinear biphasic to monophasic damped sine defibrillation waveforms with advanced life support intervention trial (ORBIT). Resuscitation. 2005;66(2):149–157.

19. Martens PR, Russell JK, Wolcke B, et al. Optimal response to cardiac arrest study: defibrillation waveform effects. Resuscitation. 2001;49(3):233–243.

20. Stothert JC, Hatcher TS, Gupton CL, et al. Rectilinear biphasic waveform defibrillation of out-of-hospital cardiac arrest. Prehosp Emerg Care. 2004;8:388–392.

21. Anderson JL, Morrow DA. Acute myocardial infarction. N Engl J Med. 2017;376:2053–2064.

22. Anderson JL, Morrow Nuttall SL, Toescu V, Kendall MJ. beta Blockade after myocardial infarction: beta blockers have key role in reducing morbidity and mortality after infarction. BMJ. 2000;320:581.

23. Friedman LM, Byington RP, Capone RJ, et al. Effect of propranolol in patients with myocardial infarction and ventricular arrhythmia. J Am Coll Cardiol. 1986;7(1):1–8.

24. Rydén L, Ariniego R, Arnman K, et al. A double-blind trial of metoprolol in acute myocardial infarction. Effects on ventricular tachyarrhythmias. N Engl J Med. 1983;308:614–618.

25. Hu K, Gaudron P, Ertl G. Long-term effects of beta-adrenergic blocking agent treatment on hemodynamic function and left ventricular remodeling in rats with experimental myocardial infarction: importance of timing of treatment and infarct size. J Am Coll Cardiol. 1998;31:692–700.

26. Galcerá-Tomás J, Castillo-Soria FJ, Villegas-García MM, et al. Effects of early use of atenolol or captopril on infarct size and ventricular volume: a double-blind comparison in patients with anterior acute myocardial infarction. Circulation. 2001;103:813–819.

27. Doughty RN, Whalley GA, Walsh HA, et al. Effects of carvedilol on left ventricular remodeling after acute myocardial infarction: the CAPRICORN Echo substudy. Circulation. 2004;109(2):201–206.

28. Paterson HS, Jones MW, Baird DK, Hughes CF. Lethal postoperative coronary artery spasm. Ann Thorac Surg. 1998;65:1571–1573.

29. Shafei H, Bennett JG. Coronary artery spasm during mitral valve replacement. Eur J Cardiothorac Surg. 1990;4:398–400.

30. Ahmad T, Kishore KS, Maheshwarappa NN, Pasarad AK. Postoperative diffuse coronary spasm after two valve surgery: a rare phenomenon. Indian Heart J. 2015;67(5):465–468.

31. Josephson ME, Almendral J, Callans DJ. Resetting and entrainment of reentrant ventricular tachycardia associated with myocardial infarction. Heart Rhythm 2014;11(7):1239-49.

32. Chen CY, Tsai J, Hsu TY et al. ECMO used in a refractory ventricular tachycardia and ventricular fibrillation patient: a national case-control study. Medicine. 2016;95(13):e3204.

33. Moss AJ, Zareba W, Hall WJ, Klein H, et al. Prophylactic implantation of a defibrillator in patients with myocardial infarction and reduced ejection fraction. N Engl J Med. 2002;346(12):877–883.

34. Epstein AE, DiMarco JP, Ellenbogen KA, Estes NA, et al. 2012 ACCF/AHA/HRS focused update incorporated into the ACCF/AHA/HRS 2008 guidelines for device-based therapy of cardiac rhythm abnormalities: a report of the American College of Cardiology Foundation/American Heart Association Task Force on Practice Guidelines and the Heart Rhythm Society. J Am Coll Cardiol. 2013;61:e6–e75.

35. Hannan EL, Racz MJ, Walford G, et al. Long-term outcomes of coronary-artery bypass grafting versus stent implantation. N Engl J Med. 2005;352:2174.

36. Peterson ED, Coombs LP, DeLong ER, et al. Procedural volume as a marker of quality for CABG surgery. JAMA. 2004;291:195.

37. Hattler BG, Madia C, Johnson C, et al. Risk stratification using the Society of Thoracic Surgeons Program. Ann Thorac Surg. 1994;58:1348.

REVIEW QUESTIONS

1. A 68-year-old man with a history of hypertension, ischemic cardiomyopathy (Ef 15% to 20%), and an ICD is postop from cardiac surgery. His ICD was inactivated prior to the

operating room. Three hours after presenting to the ICU, the patient develops atrial fibrillation with rapid ventricular response and a heart rate of 140 to 150 beats/min. His blood pressure decreases to 68/42, and the patient who was previously oriented is not responsive to painful stimuli.

Which of the following is the best next step in the management of this patient?

A. Place a magnet over his ICD
B. Bolus amiodarone 300 mg rapid IV push
C. External synchronized cardioversion
D. External defibrillation

Answer: C. The patient is exhibiting unstable sustained VT due to atrial fibrillation with a rapid ventricular response. Treatment involves immediate electrical synchronized cardioversion. The patient's ICD has been inactivated and the placement of a magnet is unlikely to reactivate it. Medical management of unstable sustained VT is not the first line intervention for unstable sustained VT. External defibrillation is not recommended for unstable sustained VT.

Link MS. Clinical practice. Evaluation and initial treatment of supraventricular tachycardia. N Engl J Med. 2012;367:1438.
Page RL, Joglar JA, Caldwell MA, et al. 2015 ACC/AHA/HRS guideline for the management of adult patients with supraventricular tachycardia: a report of the American College of Cardiology/American Heart Association Task Force on Clinical Practice Guidelines and the Heart Rhythm Society. J Am Coll Cardiol 2016;67:e27.

2. A 31-year-old male arrives to your ICU after having undergone a laparoscopic converted to open small bowel resection and anastomosis for an incarcerated hernia. During the case the surgeon requested 40mg of IV furosemide to decrease bowel edema. The anesthesiologist reports that the case was otherwise uneventful except for one episode of hemodynamically significant sustained VT that responded to a one-time dose of esmolol. The estimated blood loss and urine output is recorded as 100 mL and 2 L, respectively.

You are called emergently to the patient's bedside after an episode of cardiac arrest with ROSC achieved after 1 minute of CPR. The nurse reports that just prior to his arrest the patient was complaining of incisional site pain and his heart rate increased from 80 to 130 beats/min at which time he lost consciousness.

His current vital signs are pulse 116, blood pressure 62/38, respiratory rate 16, SpO$_2$ 92% on 4 L NC.

Which of the following is the most appropriate immediate intervention?

A. Immediate unsynchronized cardioversion for unstable sustained VT
B. 1 mg of epinephrine
C. Intravenous fluids, phenylephrine, and beta blockade
D. Isoproterenol bolus and infusion

Answer : C. The patient is demonstrating SAM likely due to undiagnosed hypertrophic cardiomyopathy (HCM). HCM patients frequently have SAM, which positions the mitral valve within the LVOT. Mechanical impedance of flow due to mitral valve contact of the ventricular septum can lead to acute hemodynamic collapse. Hemodynamic collapse is often preceded by reductions in preload, afterload, or supraventricular tachyarrhythmias, which contribute to LVOT obstruction. Management involves increasing preload by rapid intravenous fluid bolus or passive leg raised, intravenous phenylephrine, and intravenous beta blockade.

Maron BJ. Hypertrophic cardiomyopathy: a systematic review. JAMA. 2002;287:1308.
Spirito P, Seidman CE, McKenna WJ, Maron BJ. The management of hypertrophic cardiomyopathy. N Engl J Med. 1997;336:775.

3. A 56-year-old female with a history of Wolf-Parkinson-White syndrome currently on procainamide is now recovering in the ICU after having undergone a video-assisted thoracoscopic surgery for adenocarcinoma of the lung. While in the ICU her heart rate increases to 160. An ECG is obtained and shows a wide complex QRS tachycardia. Her preoperative ECG showed normal sinus rhythm with a right bundle branch block.

Which of the following is *not* a potential cause of her wide complex QRS tachycardia?

A. Atrial flutter with right bundle branch block (RBBB)
B. Atrial tachycardia with concomitant procainamide use
C. Orthodromic atrioventricular reentrant tachycardia
D. Ventricular tachycardia

Answer: B. Major causes of wide QRS complex tachycardias can be broadly divided into intrinsic intraventricular conduction delays: left bundle branch block, RBBB, and intraventricular conduction delays conduction patterns; extrinsic intraventricular conduction delays: electrolyte abnormalities (hyperkalemia) or drug-induced type I antiarrhythmic drugs and sodium channel blocking agents; supraventricular tachyarrhythmias with associated conduction delay; and VT.

Atrioventricular reentrant tachycardia (AVRT) associated with an accessory pathway (Wolff-Parkinson-White syndrome) can prove to be a diagnostic challenge. In general, AVRT is divided into 2 types with respect to its accessory pathway: orthodromic and antidromic AVRT. The width of the QRS complex can usually distinguish between these arrhythmias with orthodromic AVRT having a narrow complex QRS and antidromic AVRT having a wide complex QRS. This patient's confounding past medical history of Wolff-Parkinson-White and right bundle branch block along with her use of a type I antiarrhythmic makes her ECG diagnosis especially dubious; however, the question highlights the differential for wide QRS complex tachycardia.

Ceresnak SR, Tanel RE, Pass RH, et al. Clinical and electrophysiologic characteristics of antidromic tachycardia in children with Wolff-Parkinson-White syndrome. Pacing Clin Electrophysiol 2012;35:480.
Wellens HJ. The wide QRS tachycardia. Ann Intern Med 1986;104:879.

4. A 66-year-old patient with a left ventricular assist device (LVAD) implanted 1 year earlier presents to your ICU after

having undergone a laparoscopic cholecystectomy. The patient has a history of ischemic cardiomyopathy with severely reduced LVEF (20%) and moderately reduced right ventricular function.

The case was uneventful except for a few episodes of NSVT that self-resolved. In the ICU you are called to the bedside to evaluate a rhythm irregularity. The monitor shows sustained monomorphic ventricular tachycardia (SMVT).

The patient's MAP by radial arterial line reads 78, and he is otherwise asymptomatic.

The patient's nurse believes that he has been going in and out of this rhythm throughout the day, but because of his stable hemodynamics it was not reported.

Which of the following is the most appropriate initial intervention?

  A. Immediate and repeated unsynchronized defibrillations until resolution of VT
  B. No immediate interventions given the patient's stable hemodynamics
  C. Increasing the LVADs pump speed to better augment his cardiac output
  D. Initiation amiodarone and propranolol

Answer: D. In stable patients with sustained monomorphic VT, IV pharmacologic therapy may be attempted prior to electrical cardioversion. Repeated shocks from defibrillation can result in myocardial injury. Hemodynamically tolerated ventricular arrythmias can progress to a malignant arrythmia at any time and should be urgently addressed.

Amiodarone is recommended as a first-line therapy given its superior efficacy for terminating most ventricular arrhythmias. In patients with frequent recurrences of VT, adjunctive use of beta blockers can help ablate sympathetic facilitation and reduce SMVT.

Al-Khatib SM, Stevenson WG, Ackerman MJ, et al. 2017 AHA/ACC/HRS guideline for management of patients with ventricular arrhythmias and the prevention of sudden cardiac death: a report of the American College of Cardiology/American Heart Association Task Force on Clinical Practice Guidelines and the Heart Rhythm Society. Circulation. 2017;138(13):e210–e271.
Hirsowitz G, Podrid PJ, Lampert S, et al. The role of beta blocking agents as adjunct therapy to membrane stabilizing drugs in malignant ventricular arrhythmia. Am Heart J 1986; 111:852.

5. A 66-year-old women with severe ischemic cardiomyopathy (EF 10%) is in your cardiac ICU after having undergone catheter ablation for electrical storm. Initially the ablation appeared to have been a success, but several hours after the procedure her VT reoccurs.

Which of the following is *not* regarded as a salvage therapy for patients with refractory electrical storm?

  A. Thoracic epidural anesthesia
  B. Cardiac transplantation
  C. Insertion of an intra-aortic balloon pump (IABP) or a left ventricular assist device (VAD)
  D. Deep cervical plexus block

Answer: B. In cases of refractory VT and electrical storm, catheter ablation is recommended for the elimination of recurrent VT. Rarely will VT or electrical storm recur after catheter ablation. In these challenging cases, several salvage therapies have proven to be successful when used in combination with standard medical therapies; these are: thoracic epidural anesthesia, cardiac transplantation, IABP/VAD insertion, cardiac sympathetic denervation, stellate ganglion block, and others.

Bourke T, Vaseghi M, Michowitz Y, et al. Neuraxial modulation for refractory ventricular arrhythmias: value of thoracic epidural anesthesia and surgical left cardiac sympathetic denervation. Circulation. 2010;121:2255.
Meng L, Tseng CH, Shivkumar K, Ajijola O. Efficacy of stellate ganglion blockade in managing electrical storm: a systematic review. JACC Clin Electrophysiol 2017;3:942.
Schwartz PJ, Priori SG, Cerrone M, et al. Left cardiac sympathetic denervation in the management of high-risk patients affected by the long-QT syndrome. Circulation 2004;109:1826.

31.

LVAD COMPLICATED BY RV FAILURE

Aaron M. Mittel and Gebhard Wagener

STEM CASE AND KEY QUESTIONS

A 63-year-old, 70-kg male has been admitted to the intensive care unit (ICU) following insertion of a left ventricular assist device (LVAD) with the hope of eventually receiving a heart transplant. Preoperatively, he had been admitted to the hospital with an acute heart failure exacerbation and has required inotropes to maintain cardiac output. He has known ischemic cardiomyopathy and a preoperative left ventricular (LV) ejection fraction of 15%. Intraoperative transesophageal echocardiography (TEE) identified a moderate to severe reduction in right ventricular (RV) function. Since his arrival in the ICU, he has remained sedated and has been hemodynamically supported with dobutamine, milrinone, and moderate dose norepinephrine.

Additionally, he has had ongoing, slow, serosanguinous output from his chest tubes and has required occasional transfusion.

WHY IS RV FAILURE AN IMPORTANT CONSIDERATION FOLLOWING LVAD PLACEMENT? WHAT IS YOUR DIFFERENTIAL DIAGNOSIS OF OLIGURIA IN THIS PATIENT?

On the afternoon of postoperative day 1, he develops progressive oliguria and is now only producing 15 mL per hour of urine output. He has a stable mean arterial pressure (MAP) of 70 mmHg, pulmonary artery pressures of 45/20 mmHg, and a central venous pressure (CVP) of 18 mmHg. Mixed venous oxygen saturation (SvO_2) is 58%. LVAD speed and power indices are within normal limits, with a low-normal pulsatility index (PI). Pulmonary capillary wedge pressure (PCWP) is 14 mmHg. Forty milligrams of intravenous (IV) furosemide is administered, with minimal effect.

WHAT IS THE ROLE OF CVP IN DIAGNOSING RV FAILURE? WHAT IS THE LVAD PULSATILITY INDEX, AND HOW IS THIS AFFECTED BY RV FAILURE? HOW SHOULD YOU APPROACH FLUID MANAGEMENT OF THIS PATIENT? SHOULD YOU ADD AN INHALED PULMONARY VASODILATOR TO THIS PATIENT'S DRUG REGIMEN?

More aggressive diuresis is undertaken with boluses of IV furosemide and IV chlorothiazide and the initiation of a furosemide infusion. There is a moderate increase in urine output—however, CVP remains elevated with no change in PI. Bedside TTE at this time shows a dilated and globally hypokinetic RV. The decision is taken to start inhaled nitric oxide (iNO).

WHAT IS A SUCTION EVENT? HOW IS IT DIAGNOSED? WHAT ARE THE POTENTIAL REMEDIES? WHEN SHOULD YOU CONSIDER MECHANICAL SUPPORT DEVICES FOR RV FAILURE?

For several hours after the implementation of iNO, there is a marked improvement. CVP decreases, PI, SvO_2, and urine output all increase. However, intermittent ectopy progresses into longer runs of nonsustained ventricular tachycardia accompanied by drops in PI and MAP and a rise in CVP. The arrhythmia is initially treated with amiodarone, and bedside TTE at this time shows a decrease in LV end diastolic diameter with bowing of the interventricular septum into the LV cavity. LVAD speed is decreased, with echocardiographic improvement and a decrease in ventricular tachycardia. However, the patient continues to have a high vasopressor requirement, elevated CVP, and oliguria. Discussion is initiated with the surgical and cardiology teams regarding the placement of right-sided mechanical circulatory support.

DISCUSSION

Durable LVAD insertion is an increasingly used option for long-term management of advanced heart failure. Historically, LVAD implantation was restricted to those patients who were candidates for eventual heart transplantation ("bridge to transplant"), with the goal of maintaining end-organ function while awaiting transplantation. More recently, durable LVADs have also been used as "destination therapy," in which transplantation is not an option for a given patient. Destination therapy devices can improve quality of life and extend lifespan for these patients and are increasingly utilized options for heart failure patients.[1] Additionally, some patients will initially anticipate using an LVAD as a bridge to transplantation but may be removed from consideration as a transplant candidate due to advancing comorbidities or other reasons.

In addition to long-term, durable device options, a multitude of comparatively short-term LVADs exist for temporary management of LV failure. These devices are generally restricted for use in situations in which relatively rapid improvement in LV function is anticipated (e.g., viral myocarditis) or when additional time is necessary to support end organs while evaluating the patient for durable device candidacy ("bridge to recovery" or "bridge to decision").[2] These various support options and the decision to choose one specific device over another are outside the scope of this chapter. However, they all share some common physiologic constructs and are associated with a unique risk of perioperative RV failure (RVF).[3] This chapter focuses on the risks associated with RVF and treatment options in the immediate perioperative period.

BIVENTRICULAR PHYSIOLOGY FOLLOWING CONTINUOUS FLOW LVAD

Contemporary LVADs deliver continuous, nonpulsatile, arterial flow to end organs. Following LVAD implantation and activation, a geometric change occurs in which the interventricular septum (IVS) is shifted leftward as LV volume is ejected through the LVAD outflow tract. The IVS is crucial for normal RV contractility; this shift leads to a deterioration in RV function.[3] However, this impairment is offset by a decrease in left atrio-ventricular pressure and thus a reduction in RV afterload. Simultaneously, the increased LV outflow yields an increase in venous return to the right heart; this is usually well tolerated by a compliant RV.[3,4] The patient with underlying RV systolic dysfunction, a noncompliant RV, significant pulmonary hypertension, or likely to experience dramatic variations in preload (e.g., active hemorrhage) is thus at risk of experiencing RVF after LVAD placement.[5]

DEFINITION OF RVF FOLLOWING LVAD PLACEMENT

RVF following LVAD insertion is challenging to diagnose, in part due to the absence of consensus on its formal definition. Ultimately, post-LVAD RVF is a clinical diagnosis rather than one defined by explicit criteria. However, many researchers choose to follow the RVF definition proposed by the Interagency Registry for Mechanically Assisted Circulatory Support (INTERMACS). Per the INTERMACS definition, post-LVAD RVF is present when there is a cardiac index <2.2 L/min/m^2, CVP is at least 17 mmHg without other cause for acute cardiac dysfunction (including left-sided heart failure with elevated pulmonary capillary wedge pressure greater than 18 mmHg, tamponade, or pneumothorax), and there are clinical sequale associated with high venous pressure.[6]

The INTERMACS criteria further grades the severity of RVF based on a combination of hemodynamic and symptomatic features. Severe RVF is based on the need for an right ventricular assist device (RVAD) or prolonged use of inotropes or pulmonary vasodilators beyond 14 days after surgery, while moderate RVF is defined by the need for pharmacologic support with inotropes or pulmonary vasodilators for 7 to 14

days. Mild RVF is defined by an ability to wean from pharmacologic support within 7 days of surgery.[6] Table 31.1 outlines the INTERMACS definition and severity scaling of post-LVAD RVF.

EPIDEMIOLOGY AND PREOPERATIVE RISK FACTORS FOR RVF

The commonality of RVF following LVAD insertion is uncertain, in part due to the inherent challenges of its recognition. Various citations report an incidence ranging from 9% to 44% post-LVAD. Despite lack of consensus on its prevalence, development of RVF is universally recognized to be associated with poor outcomes.[7,8] It has been associated with significant increases in end-organ failure rates, longer hospital lengths of stay, increases in mortality rates, and other undesirable complications.[9] In one analysis, only 70% of patients who developed RVF following LVAD implantation survived at 180 days, compared to 90% of those without RVF.[10]

A number of broad-based demographic factors are associated with post-LVAD RVF. For instance, increased age at time of surgery, prior cardiac surgery, female gender, and nonischemic heart failure etiology increase the risk of RVF.[7,11] Additionally, patients who are receiving LVADs as destination therapy as opposed to a bridge-to-recovery/transplant are more likely to develop RVF.[8] Many of these destination therapy patients are older or have very long-standing heart failure and thus tend to have more significant preoperative organ dysfunction (e.g., the need for mechanical ventilation or dialysis) or the need for preoperative mechanical circulatory support (e.g., use of an intra-aortic balloon pump).[10,12]

In addition to demographic risk factors, certain physiologic patterns are associated with post-LVAD RVF. In general, patients with baseline RV dysfunction (i.e., dilatation, poor contractility, and/or non-compliance), pulmonary hypertension, or dynamic changes in RV loading conditions are mechanistically at high risk for post-LVAD RVF.[5] These patients are sometimes classified more discretely based on hemodynamic and imaging variables attributed to RV function. Specifically, patients with elevated CVP values, CVP greater than two-thirds the PCWP, abnormal RV function on echocardiography, or high pulmonary vascular resistance are more likely to develop RVF.[8,13-15] However, it is important to note that these risk factors have largely been identified in single-center, retrospective analyses, and no one single risk factor has been found to be common to RVF in all studies.

Ultimately, the risk factors associated with post-RVF are relatively diverse and often not easily conceptualized for a given patient. However, as proposed by Patlolla et al., these factors can consolidated into unifying concepts of baseline "frailty" and RV "vulnerability."[5] Frailty is present in those patients who have a high risk of RVF due to comorbid illnesses. These patients are typically advanced in age, have a larger extra-cardiac disease burden, and are often destination-therapy candidates only. Similarly, patients with a "vulnerable" RV represent those who have semi-objective documentation of RV dysfunction as well as those with significant pulmonary hypertension, as they may have difficulty meeting cardiac performance demands despite an otherwise low burden of comorbidities. This conceptual model of frailty plus vulnerability provides a useful framework to understand the likelihood of post-LVAD RVF in a given patient.

INTRAOPERATIVE CONSIDERATIONS FOR RVF

In addition to preoperative risk factors, intraoperative events may increase the risk of post-LVAD RVF. These are perhaps globally defined as events that increase the likelihood of RV ischemia or require additional cardiac performance to meet high systemic cardiac output demands. In the former, RV ischemia may occur as a consequence of intraoperative hypotension or poor myocardial preservation during cardiopulmonary bypass.[16,17] Additionally, patients undergoing highly complex cardiac surgery are at particularly high risk of perioperative vasoplegic shock, which is often associated with a need for supra-normal cardiac output and may begin in the operating room.[18] The at-risk RV may be unable to keep up with demand, and RVF may thus develop despite absence of change in RV performance. The concepts of frailty, baseline RV vulnerability, and associated perioperative risk factors are summarized in Figure 31.1.

POSTOPERATIVE DIAGNOSIS OF RVF

RVF is a difficult diagnosis to make, and thus the clinician managing patients following LVAD insertion must maintain a high level of suspicion for its presence. Generally, RVF presents with hypotension and cardiogenic shock. However, this may not be immediately recognizable in the postoperative period; several factors may be concomitant with RVF, or even

lead to its development. These include hypotension and shock due to hypovolemia, severe vasoplegia, pneumothorax, and/or tamponade. As these are life-threatening and often rapidly correctable, they should be ruled out before RVF is settled upon as a definitive diagnosis.

MONITORING OF LVAD PARAMETERS

Contemporary LVADs display some proprietary performance indices that may be useful to help diagnose acute RVF. These are displayed and adjusted in methods unique to each device. For the purposes of simplicity, this discussion revolves around parameters displayed on the HeartMate II system: pump speed, estimated flow, power, and PI. To accurately interpret them together, the clinician must understand that LVADs are valve-less continuous flow devices that are extraordinarily sensitive to preload, afterload, and native cardiac function.[19] Thus, the cardiac cycle creates cyclical variation in both native cardiac output and also in LVAD flow, which can be interpreted in real time.

Pump speed is the only parameter set by clinicians. Proper speed is that which effectively unloads the LV, allows for stable cardiac output, and minimizes interventricular shift. Power, on the other hand, is not a set parameter but is directly measured by the LVAD system. Increasing power requirements represent an increase in the amount of blood flowing through the LVAD, a decrease in afterload, increasing blood viscosity, or thrombus on the LVAD rotor (and vice versa for decreased power). Unlike power, flow is not directly measured but is indirectly estimated based on measured power and set speed. This is an important concept, as an increase in reported flow may represent genuine increases in blood flowing through the device (e.g., low afterload) or inaccurate estimates of blood

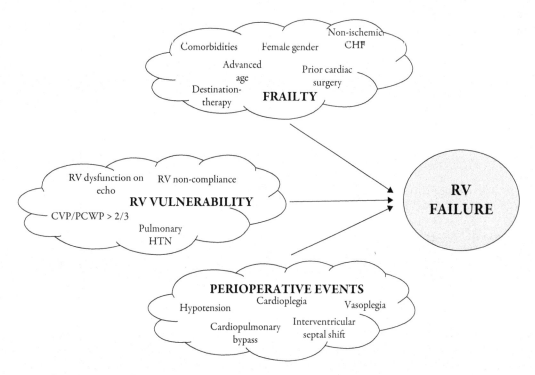

Figure 31.1 Determinants of right ventricular failure.

flow (e.g., thrombus on rotor and high-power requirements). Finally, the pump's PI is perhaps the most commonly used parameter to identify dynamic changes in biventricular filling and function. The PI measures the amplitude of flow pulses through the device, which generally are caused by systolic and diastolic changes in ventricular pressure. The magnitude of these pulses is averaged over 15-second intervals and displayed as a unitless value. PI is significantly influenced by underlying cardiac function and volume status.[19]

RVF is associated with reduced LV filling and therefore a reduction in both native and LVAD cardiac output; it usually presents with low power, low flows, and low PI at a given speed. It is important to recognize that each of these aberrations can be due to alternative conditions. Thus it is important to perform a comprehensive evaluation to rule out alternative etiologies.

TREATMENT OF RVF FOLLOWING LVAD

RVF is associated with poor clinical outcomes. For post-LVAD transplant candidates, RVF management is crucial to ensure adequate end-organ functioning such that they may eventually receiving curative therapy. In destination therapy patients, the end goal of RVF management is discharge from the hospital and an acceptable quality of life. With timely recognition and treatment of RVF, these are achievable goals.

FLUID AND VOLUME MANAGEMENT

Traditionally, the management of RVF has focused on fluid loading to ensure adequate RV preload and cardiac output. However, overaggressive volume administration may be associated with harm, putatively due to the effects of venous hypertension.[20] This is especially important in the post-LVAD population, where ventricular interdependence is reduced. Thus clinicians caring for patients at high risk of post-LVAD RVF should target RV euvolemia. This is generally accomplished by targeting a CVP less than 15 mmHg. This requires a delicate balance of volume administration and removal. Indeed, many patients who have evidence of post-LVAD RVF need significant diuresis. Patients who exhibit concomitant renal failure may need early dialysis for volume removal.

PHARMACOLOGIC MANAGEMENT

The need for vasoactive drugs is common during all cardiac surgical procedures and is especially common in patients receiving LVADs.[18] They are frequently initiated in the operating room in response to observed or expected echocardiographic and physiologic indices of cardiovascular dysfunction. Generally speaking, most patients require administration of inotropes (e.g., dobutamine, milrinone) to augment cardiac performance, based on the assumption that a frail and/or vulnerable RV will be harmed by intraoperative events.[19,21] There are no notable studies comparing the use versus non-use of these agents on long-term outcomes, nor on one agent versus another. Indeed, long-term use of these agents following LVAD implantation is associated with poor outcomes.

This is probably most reflective of the fact that patients with long-term needs for inotropes are those with the most severe RV dysfunction.[22] Nevertheless, use of short-term inotropes is in keeping with current guidelines for management of cardiogenic shock,[23] and clinicians should tailor their choices to individualized cardiac function.

MAP targets vary based on individual patient needs and institutional preferences. However, it is important to realize that diastolic and mean arterial hypotension will result in potential RV ischemia, and thus potential exacerbations of RV dysfunction. Furthermore, following LVAD placement, significant systemic hypotension will result in increased LV unloading, subsequent leftward shift of the interventricular septum, and potential compromise of RV systolic function. Thus vasopressors and/or vasodilators may be necessary to keep MAP ranges tightly controlled.[19]

PULMONARY HYPERTENSION AND PULMONARY VASODILATORS

Patients with pulmonary hypertension are particularly challenging; LVAD-induced unloading of the LV may not dramatically decrease RV afterload, depending on the etiology and severity of pulmonary hypertension. Certainly, following LVAD insertion, classic triggers of pulmonary hypertensive crises should be avoided, including hypoxia, hypercarbia, acidemia, hypothermia, and others.[24] However, additional pharmacologic support may be necessary in some patients, particularly those deemed to have pulmonary hypertension not caused by chronic LV failure.

Pharmacologic support for pulmonary hypertension post-LVAD usually begins with IV inodilators, (e.g., milrinone, dobutamine).[19,21] However, these are insufficient in some patients, and thus several studies have investigated the use of inhaled pulmonary vasodilators to reduce RV afterload. Commonly used agents include iNO and epoprostenol. Trials of these agents have generally shown improvement in hemodynamics and a possible reduction in the need for mechanical circulatory support but have not shown statistical significance in reduction of rates of RVF.[25,26] Weaning from these agents is complex and requires optimization of fluid status as well as alternative support strategies for the vulnerable RV. Frequently, alternative pulmonary vasodilators with reduced dosing frequency, such as iloprost and/or sildenafil, are substituted for continuous inhalations and may be continued in the post-ICU setting.[27,28]

MECHANICAL CIRCULATORY SUPPORT

In some patients, the combination of careful fluid management, IV vasoactive support, and inhaled pulmonary vasodilator therapy may be insufficient to avoid RVF. In these patients, prevention of progressive cardiogenic shock is ameliorated with the use of short-term mechanical circulatory support in the form of RVADs. Currently, there are no long-term RVADs approved for use, and thus mechanical therapy is employed in situations where support of end organs is necessary while awaiting improvement in native RV function.

Specific discussion regarding the choice of RVAD is often surgeon, cardiologist, patient, and institution specific and is therefore outside the scope of this chapter. Generally speaking, options for support include the use of veno-arterial extracorporeal membrane oxygenation, which can provide gas exchange as well as perfusion to end organs.[29] Alternatively, several percutaneous and/or paracorporeal pumps exist in which blood is drained from the right atrium and directed into the pulmonary arteries, reducing RV volume overload while ensuring LV filling.[30,31] Rarely, if prolonged RVAD support is required, surgeons may implant a "durable" RVAD in the RV anterior wall. This is usually accomplished with low-profile centrifugal-flow pumps, such as the HeartWare VAD.[32]

Ultimately, the need for RVAD insertion is associated with poor clinical outcomes. It is unclear whether empiric insertion of an RVAD at the same time as LVAD insertion in high-risk patients may reduce the sequelae of post-LVAD RVF. In one retrospective analysis, early placement of RVAD (i.e., before the development of RVF) did not affect overall survival, suggesting that the underlying cardiac dysfunction is the primary determinant of long-term survival rather than the use or non-use of mechanical support.[33]

CONCLUSION

RVF following LVAD insertion is an extraordinarily complex physiologic problem. Ultimately, RV performance almost always is impaired after LVAD implantation due to the loss of interventricular dependence associated with LVAD-induced decompression of the LV and the leftward shift of the interventricular septum. Fortunately, as the LV is unloaded, PCWP is generally reduced, and increased venous return to the RV ensures both adequate RV preload and comparably low afterload. However, post-LVAD RVF occurs with alarming frequency in patients with extra-cardiac frailty or RV vulnerability. Ultimately, treatment of RVF is largely targeted at optimizing RV preload and afterload. Use of inotropic agents, inhaled pulmonary vasodilators, and mechanical circulatory support devices may all be necessary. However, it is important to realize that outcomes following development of RVF are generally poor, and thus avoidance of RVF remains the ultimate perioperative goal when caring for the patient who has undergone LVAD insertion.

REFERENCES

1. Kirklin JK, Naftel DC, Pagani FD, et al. Seventh INTERMACS annual report: 15,000 patients and counting. Journal of Heart and Lung Transplantation. 2015;34(12):1495–1504.
2. Takayama H, Soni L, Kalesan B, et al. Bridge-to-decision therapy with a continuous-flow external ventricular assist device in refractory cardiogenic shock of various causes. Circulation Heart Failure. 2014;7(5):799–806.
3. Tchoukina I, Smallfield MC, Shah KB. Device management and flow optimization on left ventricular assist device support. Critical Care Clinics. 2018;34(3):453–463.
4. Sladen RN. New innovations in circulatory support with ventricular assist device and extracorporeal membrane oxygenation therapy. Anesthesia and Analgesia. 2017;124(4):1071–1086.
5. Patlolla B, Beygui R, Haddad F. Right-ventricular failure following left ventricle assist device implantation. Current Opinion in Cardiology. 2013;28(2):223–233.
6. intermacs/appendices-4-0/appendix-a-4-0. Accessed August 27, 2018. IRfMACSIAAAedaappAahwuem. 2018.
7. Ochiai Y, McCarthy PM, Smedira NG, et al. Predictors of severe right ventricular failure after implantable left ventricular assist device insertion: analysis of 245 patients. Circulation. 2002;106(12 Suppl 1):I198–I202.
8. Drakos SG, Janicki L, Horne BD, et al. Risk factors predictive of right ventricular failure after left ventricular assist device implantation. American Journal of Cardiology. 2010;105(7):1030–1035.
9. Dang NC, Topkara VK, Mercando M, et al. Right heart failure after left ventricular assist device implantation in patients with chronic congestive heart failure. Journal of Heart and Lung Transplantation. 2006;25(1):1–6.
10. Kormos RL, Teuteberg JJ, Pagani FD, et al. Right ventricular failure in patients with the HeartMate II continuous-flow left ventricular assist device: incidence, risk factors, and effect on outcomes. Journal of Thoracic and Cardiovascular Surgery. 2010;139(5):1316–1324.
11. Frazier OH, Rose EA, Oz MC, et al. Multicenter clinical evaluation of the HeartMate vented electric left ventricular assist system in patients awaiting heart transplantation. Journal of Thoracic and Cardiovascular Surgery. 2001;122(6):1186–1195.
12. Patel ND, Weiss ES, Schaffer J, et al. Right heart dysfunction after left ventricular assist device implantation: a comparison of the pulsatile HeartMate I and axial-flow HeartMate II devices. Annals of Thoracic Surgery. 2008;86(3):832–840; discussion 832–840.
13. Kato TS, Farr M, Schulze PC, et al. Usefulness of two-dimensional echocardiographic parameters of the left side of the heart to predict right ventricular failure after left ventricular assist device implantation. American Journal of Cardiology. 2012;109(2):246–251.
14. Grant AD, Smedira NG, Starling RC, Marwick TH. Independent and incremental role of quantitative right ventricular evaluation for the prediction of right ventricular failure after left ventricular assist device implantation. Journal of the American College of Cardiology. 2012;60(6):521–528.
15. Wang Y, Simon MA, Bonde P, et al. Decision tree for adjuvant right ventricular support in patients receiving a left ventricular assist device. Journal of Heart and Lung Transplantation. 2012;31(2):140–149.
16. Mets B. Anesthesia for left ventricular assist device placement. Journal of Cardiothoracic and Vascular Anesthesia. 2000;14(3):316–326.
17. Gudejko MD, Gebhardt BR, Zahedi F, et al. Intraoperative hemodynamic and echocardiographic measurements associated with severe right ventricular failure after left ventricular assist device implantation. Anesthesia and Analgesia. 2019;128(1):25–32.
18. Shaefi S, Mittel A, Klick J, et al. Vasoplegia after cardiovascular procedures-pathophysiology and targeted therapy. Journal of Cardiothoracic and Vascular Anesthesia. 2018;32(2):1013–1022.
19. Slaughter MS, Pagani FD, Rogers JG, et al. Clinical management of continuous-flow left ventricular assist devices in advanced heart failure. Journal of Heart and Lung Transplantation. 2010;29(4 Suppl):S1–S39.
20. Damman K, van Deursen VM, Navis G, Voors AA, van Veldhuisen DJ, Hillege HL. Increased central venous pressure is associated with impaired renal function and mortality in a broad spectrum of patients with cardiovascular disease. Journal of the American College of Cardiology. 2009;53(7):582–588.
21. Lampert BC, Teuteberg JJ. Right ventricular failure after left ventricular assist devices. Journal of Heart and Lung Transplantation. 2015;34(9):1123–1130.
22. Schenk S, McCarthy PM, Blackstone EH, et al. Duration of inotropic support after left ventricular assist device implantation: risk factors and impact on outcome. Journal of Thoracic and Cardiovascular Surgery. 2006;131(2):447–454.

23. Yancy CW, Jessup M, Bozkurt B, et al. 2013 ACCF/AHA guideline for the management of heart failure: executive summary: a report of the American College of Cardiology Foundation/American Heart Association Task Force on Practice Guidelines. Circulation. 2013;128(16):1810–1852.

24. Pilkington SA, Taboada D, Martinez G. Pulmonary hypertension and its management in patients undergoing non-cardiac surgery. Anaesthesia. 2015;70(1):56–70.

25. Potapov E, Meyer D, Swaminathan M, et al. Inhaled nitric oxide after left ventricular assist device implantation: a prospective, randomized, double-blind, multicenter, placebo-controlled trial. Journal of Heart and Lung Transplantation. 2011;30(8):870–878.

26. Groves DS, Blum FE, Huffmyer JL, et al. Effects of early inhaled epoprostenol therapy on pulmonary artery pressure and blood loss during LVAD placement. Journal of Cardiothoracic and Vascular Anesthesia. 2014;28(3):652–660.

27. Antoniou T, Prokakis C, Athanasopoulos G, et al. Inhaled nitric oxide plus iloprost in the setting of post-left assist device right heart dysfunction. Annals of Thoracic Surgery. 2012;94(3):792–798.

28. Critoph C, Green G, Hayes H, et al. Clinical outcomes of patients treated with pulmonary vasodilators early and in high dose after left ventricular assist device implantation. Artificial Organs. 2016;40(1):106–114.

29. Tramm R, Ilic D, Davies AR, Pellegrino VA, Romero L, Hodgson C. Extracorporeal membrane oxygenation for critically ill adults. Cochrane Database of Systematic Reviews. 2015;1:CD010381.

30. Fujita K, Takeda K, Li B, et al. Combined therapy of ventricular assist device and membrane oxygenator for profound acute cardiopulmonary failure. ASAIO Journal. 2017;63(6):713–719.

31. Takeda K, Garan AR, Ando M, et al. Minimally invasive CentriMag ventricular assist device support integrated with extracorporeal membrane oxygenation in cardiogenic shock patients: a comparison with conventional CentriMag biventricular support configuration. European Journal of Cardio-Thoracic Surgery. 2017;52(6):1055–1061.

32. Bernhardt AM, De By TM, Reichenspurner H, Deuse T. Isolated permanent right ventricular assist device implantation with the HeartWare continuous-flow ventricular assist device: first results from the European Registry for Patients with Mechanical Circulatory Support. European Journal of Cardio-Thoracic Surgery. 2015;48(1):158–162.

33. Takeda K, Naka Y, Yang JA, et al. Timing of temporary right ventricular assist device insertion for severe right heart failure after left ventricular assist device implantation. ASAIO Journal. 2013;59(6):564–569.

REVIEW QUESTIONS

1. Following insertion and activation of a durable LVAD, RV function may deteriorate due to which of the following mechanisms?

   A. Non-pulsatile flow through the right coronary artery
   B. Loss of interventricular dependence after leftward shift of the interventricular septum
   C. Overabundant venous return and right ventricular congestion
   D. All of the above

2. A 34 year-old patient is admitted with malaise, fevers, and new-onset heart failure. He is diagnosed with viral myocarditis. As his condition deteriorates, an LVAD is surgically inserted with hopes of rapid recovery over the next few days to weeks. Which of the following terms describe this approach to his mechanical circulatory support?

   A. Bridge to recovery
   B. Destination therapy
   C. Bridge to transplant
   D. Bridge to nowhere

3. According to INTERMACS criteria, RV failure is clinically diagnosed when CVP is greater than which of the following values?

   A. 10 mmHg
   B. 15 mmHg
   C. 17 mmHg
   D. 18 mmHg

4. Which of the following preoperative characteristics increase the risk of RV failure after LVAD insertion?

   A. Male gender
   B. Diagnosis of ischemic cardiomyopathy
   C. Presence of pulmonary hypertension
   D. LVAD indicated as destination therapy, rather than as a bridge to transplant

5. Which of the following accurately describes LVAD physiology?

   A. LVADs are valveless devices which are exquisitely sensitive to afterload.
   B. LVADs are valveless devices which dynamically adjust their function to ensure a stable cardiac output
   C. LVADs are valveless devices which can produce both anterograde and retrograde flow depending on loading conditions
   D. LVADs are valved devices which rely on native cardiac function to optimize intra-device flow patterns

6. 2 weeks following insertion of an LVAD, a 68 year-old female develops profound vasodilatory shock secondary to infection. Her mean arterial pressure falls to 50 mmHg for several hours before vasopressor therapy is initiated. She is subsequently diagnosed with new onset RV failure in the setting of a high CVP. Which of the following mechanisms explain the development of RV failure in this patient?

   A. Coronary hypoperfusion in the setting of poor coronary perfusion pressure
   B. Leftward shift of the interventricular septum due to afterload reduction and continuous flow via the LVAD
   C. Insufficient volume loading of the RV
   D. Both A and B

7. Which of the following LVAD settings is the only parameter set by clinicians?

   A. Pump speed
   B. Pump power
   C. Pump pulsatility index
   D. Pump flow

8. The LVAD pulsatility index is a measure of which of the following?

   A. Amplitude of flow pulses through the device
   B. Power usage over time

C. Fluctuations in viscosity over time
D. Flow compared to the patient's body surface area

9. 10 days after insertion of a destination therapy LVAD, a 62 year old male with non-ischemic cardiomyopathy continues to require continuous milrinone to support his cardiac output. He has been weaned off other pharmacologic vasoactive agents. Based on INTERMACS criteria, how should his RV function be described?

A. Normal, as expected, RV performance and reliance on pharmacologic support
B. Mild RV failure
C. Moderate RV failure
D. Severe RV failure

10. True or false: failure to wean effectively from vasoactive drugs 4 weeks after LVAD implantation is an indication for durable RVAD insertion.

A. True. This is indicative of severe RV failure and requires aggressive mechanical circulatory support.
B. False. Durable RVAD support is not indicated until 8 weeks after LVAD insertion and inability to wean off other support agents.

A. False. Durable RVAD support is not indicated until other mechanical support options have been tried first.
D. False. There are no definitive durable RVAD mechanical support options.

ANSWERS

1.   B. Loss of interventricular dependence after leftward shift of the interventricular September
2.   A. Bridge to recovery
3.   C. 17 mmHg
4.   C. Presence of pulmonary hypertension
5.   A. LVADs are valveless devices which are exquisitely sensitive to afterload
6.   D. Both A and B
7.   A. Pump speed
8.   A. Amplitude of flow pulses through the device
9.   C. Moderate RV failure
10.   D. There are no definitive durable RVAD mechanical support options References

32.

AN LVAD PATIENT PRESENTING WITH INTRACRANIAL HEMORRHAGE

Haley Goucher Miranda

STEM CASE AND KEY QUESTIONS

A 60-year-old gentleman presents to the emergency department with a chief complaint of headaches and left leg weakness for the past 3 hours. He has a past medical history of atrial fibrillation, hypertension, and ischemic cardiomyopathy for which he underwent HeartMate II (HMII) left ventricular assist device (LVAD) implantation 15 months ago. LVAD interrogation demonstrates no recent alarms, although recorded flows and pump pulsatility index (PI) values have been lower than baseline over the past 2 days. Mean arterial pressure (MAP) is 115 mmHg on noninvasive blood pressure (NIBP) cuff. Labs are notable for an international normalized ratio (INR) of 2.1, platelets of 86, alanine aminotransferease of 290, aspartate transaminase of 321, serum creatinine (Cr) of 2.1 (baseline Cr 1.5), and lactate dehydrogenase (LDH) of 553. Blood and urine cultures are sent as well to assess for an infectious etiology.

WHAT ARE TYPICAL LVAD SETTINGS AND PARAMETERS, AND HOW ARE THE DEVICE READINGS INTERPRETED BY THE CARE TEAM?

On cycling through his controller, it is noted that his HMII has an RPM of 9400, a PI of 7.6, and a power of 6.1 W. He states he has had intermittent headaches and difficulty sleeping over the last 3 days that progressed to his current left leg weakness today, prompting his activation of emergency medical services. Basic laboratories are ordered along with a noncontrast and cerebral angiography head computed tomographies (CTs). This image (Figure 32.1) prompted his emergent admission to the intensive care unit (ICU).

WHAT IS THE SIGNIFICANCE OF THE CHANGES IN THIS PATIENT'S LVAD PARAMETERS? WHAT ARE THE COMMON CLINICAL SCENARIOS THAT MAY BE SUGGESTED BY ALTERATIONS IN LVAD FLOW, PULSATILITY INDEX, AND PUMP POWER? HOW ARE THESE CONFIRMED AND MANAGED?

On arrival to the ICU, the patient is mildly lethargic and confused but can be roused by voice easily and follows freely while complaining about his continued headache pain. This first assessment places him at a Glasgow Coma Scale (GCS) of 13, and on further exam he has problems following a finger with eyes and is complaining of light sensitivity. All of this is consistent with the right occipital intraparenchymal hemorrhage that was seen on his CT scan, but there is no sign of aneurysm on the CT angiography.

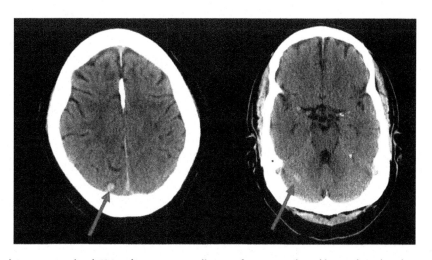

Figure 32.1 The patient's initial non-contrast head CT evidencing two small areas of intraparenchymal hemorrhage (IPH).

WHAT FURTHER HISTORY, PHYSICAL
EXAM, AND DIAGNOSTIC TESTING
SHOULD BE CONSIDERED? TO WHAT UNIT
SHOULD THIS PATIENT BE ADMITTED?
WHAT SHOULD THIS PATIENT'S
HEMODYNAMIC GOALS BE FOLLOWING
HIS ACUTE STROKE?

With an LVAD, magnetic resonance imaging is absolutely contraindicated and therefore is not an option. Neurosurgery is called to aid in his assessment and to be prepared for an intervention in case his bleed worsens and surgical treatment of intracranial hypertension is needed. An emergent transthoracic echocardiogram (TTE) is obtained and confirms that his left ventricular end diastolic diameter (LVEDD) is increased and overall left ventricular ejection fraction (LVEF) is <10%, consistent with decreased LVAD ejection secondary to afterload. A nicardipine infusion is started with a goal of intense blood pressure reduction to MAP 85 to 90 to reduce the extension of his hemorrhagic stroke and improve LVAD outflow.

INDEPENDENTLY OF THE NEED FOR ANTICOAGULATION, WHAT IS THE MECHANISM BY WHICH LVADS PREDISPOSE PATIENTS TO AN INCREASED RISK OF BLEEDING? SHOULD THIS PATIENT'S ANTICOAGULATION BE REVERSED? IF SO, WHAT OPTIONS SHOULD BE CONSIDERED?

Given his thrombocytopenia, platelets are ordered for emergent transfusion and DDAVP 0.3 mcg/kg is ordered as well to help improve his native platelet dysfunction. The decision is also made to reverse his coumadin-induced coagulopathy to minimize complications from his hemorrhagic stroke. Given his hypertension and concern for volume overload, the decision is made to use a 4-factor prothrombin complex concentrate. With his elevated INR, the decision is to use 25 units/kg of 4-factor prothrombin complex concentrate and accept the increased risk of LVAD thrombosis to help maximize his neurologic recovery.

WHAT DEVICE CHANGES MAY BE CONSIDERED GIVEN THAT THE PATIENT IS NOW OFF ANTICOAGULATION?

Over the next 12 hours, there is no degradation in his neurologic status and a repeat CT scan shows no significant interval change in the size of his stroke or any midline shift. He is slightly less lethargic, and his confusion is much improved overall. Over the next several days he is segued back to oral antihypertensives and tolerates gentle diuresis. With a MAP of 84 by NIBP and continued RPMs of 9400 his PI has risen back to 6.3 and his power has decreased down to 5.2 W, very near to his pre-stroke baseline. A third non-contrast head CT shows a decrease in the size of his hemorrhage, and a repeat TTE reveals a decrease in LVEDD with an increase in LVEF to ~25%.

WHEN SHOULD RESTARTING ANTICOAGULATION BE CONSIDERED FOR THIS PATIENT?

Ten days after his initial presentation, he is convalescing well and been progressively improving with physical and occupational therapy. Another repeat non-contrast CT of his head reveals continued improvement, and the decision is made to start back his anticoagulation regimen slowly. He is started on half his previous warfarin dose and aspirin 81 mg. After 3 days his INR has risen to 1.6 without any waning of his neurologic status, and his warfarin is increased back to his original home dose with a goal of 2 to 2.5. The rest of his recovery is proceeding well, and on day 22 post-admission he is transferred to an acute rehabilitation center.

DISCUSSION

UNDERSTANDING LVAD PARAMETERS

There are a multitude of LVAD types currently available, but for the purposes of this review, only the 3 most commonly implanted pumps in the United States are discussed: the HeartWare (HVAD), HMII, and HeartMate III (HMIII) devices. There are 3 device parameters for the HVAD device: pump speed, pump flow, and pump power. In addition to these values, the HMII and HMIII devices also display a PI. In all three of these devices, the only device parameter that can be directly adjusted by the treatment team is the pump speed. Typical clinical parameter ranges for these devices are displayed in Table 32.1. Pump flow, power, and pulsatility index are dependent on both the pump speed and the physiology of the individual patient.[1]

Pump flow is expressed in liters per minute and represents estimated output through the LVAD. Flows generally increase in a linear fashion with increases in pump speed. However, pump flow is simply a calculated value based on pump power requirements. Increases in pump power requirements not reflective of true increases in device throughput, such as thrombosis, will thus result in falsely elevated pump flows. Values are mainly useful to follow as a trend over time; they should not be used to guide inotropic therapy, and pulmonary artery catheterization will be required if accurate assessment of cardiac output is indicated.

Pump power is the energy necessary to power the LVAD at the set pump speed and is measured in watts (W). It is a direct measurement of pump motor voltage and current. Acute or sustained changes in pump power greater than 2 W above baseline require investigation, and elevations in power >10 W may be indicative of pump thrombus.

PI is a measurement reflective of intrinsic cardiac pulsatility and is a dimensionless number that ranges from 1 to 10. Higher PI levels indicate greater pulsatility and increased left

DEVICE	SPEED (RPM)	FLOW (LPM)	POWER (WATTS)	PULSATILITY INDEX
HeartWare (HVAD—Medtronic)	2500–2900	4–7	3–7	*n/a
HeartMate II (HMII—Thoratec)	8600–9800	4–8	6–7	4–6
HeartMate III (HMIII—Thoratec)	5000–6000	3–6	3–7	1–4

*HVAD does not report PI, but allows for a graphic waveform analysis. Normal peak-to trough variability of flow waveform is 2–4 L/min.

ventricular filling. Lower PI levels signify that the device is providing greater support and offloading of the left ventricle. PI levels tend to be fairly stable for an individual patient. Decreases in PI tend to be reflective of low-output states, though the differential for this is quite wide (i.e., hypovolemia, tamponade, right ventricle [RV] failure).

It is important to note that LVAD parameters are not sensitive or specific for any given clinical diagnosis. Parameter trends are perhaps most useful, as significant changes from baseline warrant further investigation. Common clinical scenarios and their associated changes in pump parameters are summarized in Table 32.2 and are briefly discussed later. There is not enough information provided in the case stem to clinically determine the cause of the new end-organ dysfunction and elevated LDH, but pump thrombosis and RV failure should both be ruled out.

COMMON CLINICAL COMPLICATIONS

Pump Thrombosis

LVAD thrombosis is one of the most feared postoperative complications and occurs in 2% to 13% of adult patients.[2]

Thrombosis refers to the development of clot in any component of the device, including the inflow cannula, the rotor, or the outflow graft. Thrombosis may form in the pump itself or from clot migration from the left atrium or left ventricle. Thrombosis may result in reduced LVAD function and impaired systemic perfusion that may deteriorate into cardiogenic shock or even death. In addition, clot embolization into the splanchnic, peripheral, or cerebral circulations are risks that carries a high degree of morbidity and mortality.[3]

Suspected pump thrombosis is often associated with increased pump power readings >2W above baseline or >10 watts total; flows may be artificially increased. An elevated serum lactate dehydrogenase more than 2.5 times the upper limit of normal and a plasma free-hemoglobin >20 mg/dL are consistent with hemolysis, which is required for the diagnosis of suspected pump thrombosis; worsening heart failure symptoms should also be present.[4]

Management of pump thrombosis is challenging, especially in a patient with a history of bleeding complications in whom further anticoagulation or thrombolytic therapy would be absolutely contraindicated. Failing medical therapy, surgical intervention with pump exchange or heart

Table 32.2 COMMON PATHOLOGIC CONDITIONS AND ASSOCIATED LVAD PARAMETER CHANGES

DIAGNOSIS	FLOW	PUMP POWER	PULASTILITY INDEX	CONFIRMATORY TESTING	SUGGESTED MANAGEMENT
Right ventricular failure	↓	↑	↓	2D-echocardiogram, pulmonary artery catheterization	Diuresis, inotropes, consider increasing pump speed
Cardiac tamponade	↓	↑	↓	2D echocardiogram with doppler confirming RV collapse or pericardial effusion	Fluid resuscitation, emergent surgical exploration
Systemic hypertension	↓	↑	↑	Non-invasive or arterial blood pressure monitoring	Antihypertensives as needed to maintain MAP < 90 mmHg
Hypovolemia	↓	↑	↓	History and physical exam; stool guaiac; GI consultation if GIB suspected	Judicious fluid resuscitation and supportive transfusions as necessary
Pump thrombosis	↑	↑	↓	Elevated LDH (>2.5 serum upper limit of normal), increased plasma free hemoglobin (>20 mg/dL); reduced diastolic velocities or increased S/D flow velocity ratios of the inflow or outflow grafts on doppler echocardiogram[27]	Increasing anticoagulation goals, consideration of thrombolysis (when not contraindicated); pump exchange or heart transplantation

transplantation may be required. Pump exchange has, however, been associated with increased risk of stroke and infectious complications in addition to significantly decreased survival rates at two years (56% for pump exchange vs. 69% for primary implant).[2]

Right Ventricular Failure

RV failure is discussed extensively in another chapter of this book. Briefly, in the setting of RV failure, LVAD parameters will generally demonstrate decreased flow, reduced pulsatility index, and increased pump power requirements. Depending on the chronicity of the insult, end-organ dysfunction from venous congestion and reduced systemic flows may be present.

Tamponade

Cardiac tamponade will present with reduced pump flow and PI but increased power readings.[5] In the absence of any recent procedural or surgical intervention, tamponade is extremely unlikely to be seen in the patient in the case study here.

Systemic Hypertension

Systemic hypertension will result in reduced pump flows and increased pump power and pulsatility index. Power requirements increase in response to increased afterload. HVAD flows are particularly sensitive to elevated MAP. PI increases as the heart must contribute more myocardial work in the setting of reduced pump flows.

Hypovolemia

Hypovolemia will result in decreased pump flows and PI but increased pump power requirements. If severe, the left ventricle can become overly decompressed and the inflow cannula may "suck down" against the interventricular septum. Ventricular arrhythmias may result from the subsequent myocardial irritability. The LVAD alarm interrogation may also demonstrate "suction events" where pump flows and power may drop precipitously.

LVAD ASSESSMENT

Initial Management

LVAD patients presenting with a stroke should be treated in accordance with current stroke guidelines, with notable exceptions discussed later. Activation of the acute stroke team is indicated for this patient based on the onset and timing of his symptoms.[6] The GCS and National Institutes of Health Stroke Scale should be assessed and documented. Non-contrast head CT should be emergently performed. Importantly, the LVAD team should be made immediately aware of the patient's presentation. If no LVAD team is available, emergent transfer to an appropriate tertiary care center should be arranged.

Neuroimaging Considerations

This patient's initial non-contrast head CT (Figure 32.1) demonstrates 2 small areas of intraparenchymal hemorrhage (IPH). For hemorrhagic stroke in the LVAD patient, repeat head CT should be performed at 12 and then at 24 hours to evaluate for hemorrhagic expansion.[7,8]

For intraparenchymal or subarachnoid hemorrhage with suspected bacteremia, CT angiography can be considered, as it has demonstrated nearly 100% sensitivity and specificity for detecting aneurysmal lesions >3 mm.[9] However, if CT angiography is negative and mycotic aneurysms continue to be suspected, digital subtraction angiography (DSA) is recommended, as this modality is more sensitive for aneurysms <3 mm and for more distal intraparenchymal lesions often seen with septic emboli.[8,9]

Magnetic resonance imaging is contraindicated given the presence of the LVAD device components.

Other Diagnostic Considerations

The possibility of septic emboli should also be entertained, as there is evidence that bloodstream infections increase the risk of both hemorrhagic and ischemic cerebrovascular accidents in the LVAD population by a factor of 8- to 20-fold.[8,10] Two sets of blood cultures should thus be obtained upon admission.

Neurosurgery should be consulted, as intracranial hemorrhage in the anticoagulated LVAD patient may precipitously worsen. Decompressive hemicraniectomy or evacuation of hemorrhage may be indicated, though the need for this intervention carries an extremely poor prognosis in the few studies that report outcomes (80% 30-day mortality per Wilson et al.).[11]

An echocardiogram should be performed to evaluate biventricular size and function. If increasing pump speed is considered as a strategy to reduce thrombosis risk while off of anticoagulation, a ramp study should also be performed to assess for intermittent opening of the aortic valve.[1]

Level and Location of Care

Although driven by breadth and duration of individual institutional experience with LVADs, continuing care will likely be best managed in the cardiothoracic ICU. However, if critical care nursing staff, mid-level providers, and intensivists have been adequately cross-trained on both LVAD devices and post-stroke assessment and care, neurological ICU admission may be most appropriate when endovascular interventions are required.

Hemodynamic Goals for LVAD Patients Post-Acute Stroke

Though there are no current official guidelines for blood pressure goals for LVAD patients with hemorrhagic CVA (HCVA).[7] Maintaining the systolic blood pressure <140 mmHg (as in the general hemorrhagic stroke population) is not useful for the LVAD patient, as this goal in the setting of the reduced pulse pressure of the LVAD would still allow for severe systemic hypertension as reflected by MAP. A MAP <90 mmHg is generally accepted as a reasonable target. This goal is based on data from the ADVANCE trial, which demonstrated a MAP of >90 mmHg was strongly associated with increased risk of HCVA.[12] In that trial, implementation of an improved blood pressure management (IBPM) protocol was shown to significantly reduce the primary incidence of hemorrhagic stroke in HVAD patients by more than 3-fold (8.4% without IBPM vs. 2.6% with IBPM; p-value 0.03).[8,12]

LVAD ANTICOAGULATION AND SECONDARY BLEEDING DIATHESIS

Though there have been advances in the hemocompatibility and design of these devices, LVAD pumps consist of foreign material that is highly thrombogenic when exposed to blood components, thus providing the need for systemic anticoagulation after pump implantation. Both primary platelet activation and stimulation of the intrinsic clotting cascade can occur with direct exposure to the pump material. Pump surface irregularities act as a site of platelet adhesion, which can then drive further platelet aggregation and deposition of fibrin cross-linking material.[13] If left unchecked, these processes result in device thrombus, which carries a host of subsequent complications that may require pump exchange, which is associated with significantly reduced patient survival.

Coagulopathy may also result from acquired von Willebrand syndrome (AVWS).[14] Functionally, the loss of high-molecular weight (HMW) multimers of von Willebrand factor due to mechanical shear stresses associated with the LVAD results in a syndrome consistent with type 2A von Willebrand's disease. The loss of HMW multimers impairs the binding of von Willebrand factor (vWF) to both platelets and collagen, which quantitatively results in decreased vWF collagen-binding (CB) capacity and ristocetin cofactor assays.[15] Notably, however, the aforementioned quantitative tests are not predictive of bleeding risk.[14] Nevertheless, if major bleeding occurs, treatment with desmopressin or Factor VIII:vWF concentrates (derived from fresh frozen plasma [FFP]) should be considered as part of the anticoagulation reversal strategy.[8]

Angiodysplasia of the microvasculature has long been implicated as a potential etiology of the coagulopathy associated with continuous-flow devices. The etiology of the angiodysplasia is likely multifactorial.[14] Venous congestion of the gastrointestinal (GI) tract due to heart failure may increase intracapillary hydrostatic pressure and lead to excessive oozing. In addition, as with patients with aortic stenosis, the decreased pulse pressure seen with continuous-flow LVADs may lead to hypoperfusion of the gut mucosa and subsequent activation of hypoxia-inducible factors that stimulate angiogenesis. Furthermore, studies have also demonstrated that vWF deficiency itself may have a role in regulating angiogenesis. In mice models, vWF deficiency increased the expression of vascular endothelial growth factor receptor-2, resulting in increased vascularization.[16] In combination, all of these mechanisms contribute to the pathologic angiodysplasia seen in the LVAD patient.

EMERGENT REVERSAL OF ANTICOAGULATION

Given that the patient has presented with a HCVA, anticoagulation should at minimum be held upon admission. The 2013 International Society for Heart and Lung Transplantation Guidelines for Mechanical Circulatory Support recommend either discontinuation or reversal of anticoagulation in the setting of hemorrhagic stroke (Class 1 Recommendation, Level of evidence: B).[17] Current practices vary by center. The decision to reverse anticoagulation will be dependent on individual patient history and severity of the patient's neurological deficits. Patients with mild neurological deficits and postoperative courses complicated by concerns for pump thrombus will likely be considered poor candidates for full anticoagulation reversal. However, American Stroke Association guidelines for hemorrhagic stroke in the general population recommend reversal of warfarin pharmacotherapy if INR is >1.4 upon presentation, as the risk of hematoma expansion within the first 24 hours is considerable.[7]

Prospective studies of acute intracranial hemorrhage (ICH) in the LVAD patient population are lacking, and no formal guidelines currently exist. Willey et al. described their center's general approach to anticoagulation reversal in the setting of acute hemorrhagic stroke in the LVAD population.[8] Their treatment algorithm for patients on warfarin (with INR >1.4) and antiplatelet agents calls for the administration of 10 mg of intravenous (IV) vitamin K in addition to prothrombin complex concentrates (PCCs) or 6 units of FFP. Furthermore, in patients who demonstrate >30 mL of ICH on neuroimaging, desmopressin acetate 0.3 mcg/kg and six units of platelets are administered to combat the possibility of AVWS and antiplatelet agents, respectively. Any heparinoid therapy is managed with discontinuation of treatment and administration of IV protamine. Recombinant factor VIIa is avoided due to the potential for device-related thrombotic complications.[8]

Serum LDH is monitored daily after reversal, and plasma-free hemoglobin testing is performed if LDH is suggestive of hemolysis. Unless indicated sooner for a change in neurological exam, routine repeat CT scan is performed at 12 and then 24 hours to monitor for stability. Notably, however, if neuroimaging is concerning for hemorrhagic transformation of an ischemic stroke, anticoagulation reversal is only considered if bleeding worsens or results in cerebral edema, since reversal may precipitate additional thrombotic events.

It is important to assess the intravascular volume status of an LVAD patient upon presentation. The average LVAD patient may not be able to hemodynamically tolerate the precipitous increase in preload associated with the transfusion of six to twelve units of blood components. When necessary, minimizing the preload increases associated with reversal of anticoagulation with PCCs should be considered to prevent right ventricular volume overload and the induction of acute, dynamic tricuspid regurgitation and right ventricular failure.

When holding anticoagulation, there is concern for increasing the risk of device thrombosis. The PREVENT trial suggested that in the three months post-device implantation, maintaining pump speeds > 9000 rpm for the HeartMate II device significantly reduced the risk of pump thrombosis.[18] If clinically tolerated, increasing this patient's pump speed may thus be somewhat protective. An echocardiographic ramp study at the increased pump speed should ideally confirm at least intermittent aortic valve opening to further reduce the risk of thrombosis.[1]

Following any cerebrovascular accident, the patient's status will need to be reevaluated by the advanced heart failure team if they were previously a candidate for heart transplantation. An acute neurologic insult may preclude them from further consideration for transplant.

ANTICOAGULATION AFTER BLEEDING COMPLICATION

As with anticoagulation reversal upon presentation, there are no clear consensus guidelines on restarting pharmacotherapy after an ischemic or hemorrhagic stroke in the LVAD patient population. Most of the data comes from single-center retrospective studies, and current practices are largely derived from studies in the general stroke population for patients whom possess an indication for anticoagulation. A meta-analysis of patients with ICH in whom anticoagulation with warfarin was reinitiated demonstrated no significant increase in the risk of ICH recurrence but a reduction in thromboembolic complications.[19] It should, however, be noted that atrial fibrillation was the indication for anticoagulation in the majority of these patients, and the timing of resumption of anticoagulation was quite variable (10 days to 2 months). Generalizing this data to an LVAD population with multiple mechanisms of coagulopathy—and perhaps a more urgent indication for reinitiating therapy—is thus problematic.

A single-center retrospective review of 36 LVAD patients with ICH demonstrated no episodes of pump thrombosis or recurrent hemorrhage when aspirin was held for 1 week and warfarin for 10 days.[11] Of note, IPH was the ICH subtype associated with the highest mortality (59% 30-day mortality rate), and a GCS score of less than 11 upon presentation was most predictive of 30-day mortality (100%). A retrospective analysis of 14 HMII LVAD patients in whom warfarin and/or aspirin was held after episodes of severe GI bleeding found 1 pump thrombosis event that required pump exchange. Importantly, however, these patients were off warfarin for a mean duration of more than a year (range 21 to 1980 days), and no other adverse thromboembolic or hemorrhagic events were noted.[20]

Ultimately, timing of anticoagulation initiation after ICH will need to be individualized depending on severity of the ICH and risk of thrombosis. However, resuming aspirin is reasonable if head CT remains stable at 5 to 7 days. If tolerated and imaging remains stable, restarting warfarin at 10 to 14 days may subsequently be considered.[8]

Patients with LVADs are becoming increasingly prevalent in the general population. According to the most recent publicly available INTERMACS database report, more than 21,000 patients in the United States have received a durable LVAD, and more than 2600 implantations were performed in 2016 alone at a total of more than 170 registered INTERMACS centers.[21] It thus behooves the general critical care physician to have an intimate knowledge of common postoperative complications associated with LVAD therapy.

Perhaps the most feared postoperative complication LVAD patients are at risk of experiencing is a hemorrhagic or ischemic cerebral vascular accident, with a reported cumulative incidence ranging between 7% and 17% depending on length of follow-up and device type.[12,21,22] HCVAs have been demonstrated to carry a particularly poor prognosis according to the INTERMACS database, with a 30-day survival rate of only 45.3% (vs 80.7% for ischemic cerebrovascular accident).[12,22] Stroke has also been demonstrated to be the most common cause of death in patients after 6 months post-device implantation.[21]

Future generations of devices may allow for less aggressive anticoagulation of the LVAD patient, theoretically reducing the risk of hemorrhagic stroke. There is already some evidence that suggests the HMIII may require less anticoagulation and may induce AVWS to a lesser degree than the HMII.[15,23] Like the HVAD, the HMIII is a centrifugal flow pump design that is smaller than the HMII and allows for intrapericardial device placement. The completely magnetically levitated pump rotor of the HMIII reduces device contact and mechanical stress, which may improve device durability and reduce the risk of pump thrombosis when compared to the axial-flow HMII.[24] Additionally, the HMIII incorporates an artificial pulse feature in which small fluctuations in pump speed result in enhanced pulsatility, with the goal of potentially reducing the higher stroke rates associated with the HVAD.[25]

Until primary prevention is improved, however, the intensivist should be aware of differences in the acute management of hemorrhagic stroke in the LVAD patient compared to the general population. Strict control of blood pressure is required, with a recommended MAP goal of <90 mmHg. Blood cultures and digital subtraction angiography should be performed to rule out mycotic aneurysm if infection is suspected. Reversal of anticoagulation should be strongly considered, though the regimen should be titrated to the circumstances of the individual patient. While off anticoagulation, the ICU team should monitor the patient daily for increases in serum LDH and/or plasma-free hemoglobin, as elevations in these values provide an early indication of pump thrombosis.

CONCLUSIONS

- Patients with LVADs are at an increased risk of bleeding complications due to chronic anticoagulation, the potential for mechanical trauma to blood components, and the effects of continuous blood flow on the microcirculation.

- Both hemorrhagic and ischemic stroke remain a major cause of morbidity and mortality after LVAD implantation.

- Acute reversal of anticoagulation after hemorrhagic stroke must be carefully considered on a case-by-case basis given the potential risk of pump thrombosis or thromboembolism.

- Recommended management of hemodynamics post-hemorrhagic stroke include maintaining a MAP <90 mmHg.

- Blood cultures and digital subtraction angiography should be performed to rule out mycotic aneurysms if systemic infection is suspected.

REFERENCES

1. Slaughter MS, Pagani FD, Rogers JG, et al. Clinical management of continuous-flow left ventricular assist devices in advanced heart failure. Journal of Heart and Lung Transplantation. Apr 2010;29(4 Suppl):S1–S39.
2. Mehra MR, Stewart GC, Uber PA. The vexing problem of thrombosis in long-term mechanical circulatory support. Journal of Heart and Lung Transplantation. Jan 2014;33(1):1–11.
3. Bartoli CR, Ailawadi G, Kern JA. Diagnosis, nonsurgical management, and prevention of LVAD thrombosis. Journal of Cardiac Surgery. Jan 2014;29(1):83–94.
4. John R, Holley CT, Eckman P, et al. A decade of experience with continuous-flow left ventricular assist devices. Seminars in Thoracic and Cardiovascular surgery. Summer 2016;28(2):363–375.
5. Devore AD, Mentz RJ, Patel CB. Medical management of patients with continuous-flow left ventricular assist devices. Current Treatment Options in Cardiovascular Medicine. Feb 2014;16(2):283.
6. Powers WJ, Rabinstein AA, Ackerson T, et al. 2018 guidelines for the early management of patients with acute ischemic stroke: a guideline for healthcare professionals from the American Heart Association/American Stroke Association. Stroke. Mar 2018;49(3):e46–e110.
7. Hemphill JC, 3rd, Greenberg SM, Anderson CS, et al. Guidelines for the management of spontaneous intracerebral hemorrhage: a guideline for healthcare professionals from the American Heart Association/American Stroke Association. Stroke. Jul 2015;46(7):2032–2060.
8. Willey JZ, Demmer RT, Takayama H, Colombo PC, Lazar RM. Cerebrovascular disease in the era of left ventricular assist devices with continuous flow: risk factors, diagnosis, and treatment. Journal of Heart and Lung Transplantation. Sep 2014;33(9):878–887.
9. de Oliveira Manoel AL, Mansur A, Murphy A, et al. Aneurysmal subarachnoid haemorrhage from a neuroimaging perspective. Critical Care. Nov 13 2014;18(6):557.
10. Aggarwal A, Gupta A, Kumar S, et al. Are blood stream infections associated with an increased risk of hemorrhagic stroke in patients with a left ventricular assist device? ASAIO Journal. Sep-Oct 2012;58(5):509–513.
11. Wilson TJ, Stetler WR, Jr., Al-Holou WN, Sullivan SE, Fletcher JJ. Management of intracranial hemorrhage in patients with left ventricular assist devices. Journal of Neurosurgery. May 2013;118(5):1063–1068.
12. Teuteberg JJ, Slaughter MS, Rogers JG, et al. The HVAD left ventricular assist device: risk factors for neurological events and risk mitigation strategies. JACC: Heart Failure. Oct 2015;3(10):818–828.
13. Koliopoulou A, McKellar SH, Rondina M, Selzman CH. Bleeding and thrombosis in chronic ventricular assist device therapy: focus on platelets. Current Opinion in Cardiology. May 2016;31(3):299–307.
14. Connors JM. Anticoagulation management of left ventricular assist devices. American Journal of Hematology. Feb 2015;90(2):175–178.
15. Geisen U, Brehm K, Trummer G, et al. Platelet secretion defects and acquired von Willebrand syndrome in patients with ventricular

assist devices. Journal of the American Heart Association. Jan 13 2018;7(2).
16. Starke RD, Ferraro F, Paschalaki KE, et al. Endothelial von Willebrand factor regulates angiogenesis. Blood. Jan 20 2011;117(3):1071–1080.
17. Feldman D, Pamboukian SV, Teuteberg JJ, et al. The 2013 International Society for Heart and Lung Transplantation Guidelines for mechanical circulatory support: executive summary. Journal of Heart and Lung Transplantation. Feb 2013;32(2):157–187.
18. Maltais S, Kilic A, Nathan S, et al. PREVENtion of HeartMate II Pump Thrombosis Through Clinical Management: the PREVENT multi-center study. Journal of Heart and Lung Transplantation. Jan 2017;36(1):1–12.
19. Murthy SB, Gupta A, Merkler AE, et al. Restarting anticoagulant therapy after intracranial hemorrhage: a systematic review and meta-analysis. Stroke. Jun 2017;48(6):1594–1600.
20. Kamdar F, Eckman P, John R. Safety of discontinuation of anti-coagulation in patients with continuous-flow left ventricular assist devices. Journal of Heart and Lung Transplantation. Mar 2014;33(3):316–318.
21. Kirklin JK, Pagani FD, Kormos RL, et al. Eighth annual INTERMACS report: special focus on framing the impact of adverse events. Journal of Heart and Lung Transplantation. Oct 2017;36(10):1080–1086.
22. Acharya D, Loyaga-Rendon R, Morgan CJ, et al. INTERMACS analysis of stroke during support with continuous-flow left ventricular assist devices: risk factors and outcomes. JACC: Heart Failure. Oct 2017;5(10):703–711.
23. Netuka I, Ivak P, Tucanova Z, et al. Evaluation of low-intensity anticoagulation with a fully magnetically levitated centrifugal-flow circulatory pump-the MAGENTUM 1 study. Journal of Heart and Lung Transplantation. May 2018;37(5):579–586.
24. Schroder JN, Milano CA. A tale of two centrifugal left ventricular assist devices. Journal of Thoracic and Cardiovascular Surgery. Sep 2017;154(3):850–852.
25. Bourque K, Cotter C, Dague C, et al. Design rationale and preclinical evaluation of the HeartMate 3 left ventricular assist system for hemocompatibility. ASAIO Journal. Jul–Aug 2016;62(4):375–383.
26. Dang G, Epperla N, Muppidi V, et al. Medical management of pump-related thrombosis in patients with continuous-flow left ventricular assist devices: a systematic review and meta-analysis. ASAIO Journal. Jul–Aug 2017;63(4):373–385.

REVIEW QUESTIONS

1. Which of the following LVAD parameters would be most suggestive of a thromboembolic etiology of stroke?

   A. Increased pump power with power elevation events
   B. Decreased pump flow
   C. Decreased pulsatility index
   D. Decreased pump power
   E. Increased pump flow

2. What characteristic changes are seen in hemostatic assays of patients implanted with continuous-flow LVADs?

   A. Decrease in high molecular weight multimers of von Willebrand factor
   B. Thrombocytopenia
   C. Schistocytosis
   D. Increased vWF CB capacity (vWF:CB).

3. Diagnosis of major hemolysis as defined by the INTERMACS registry would be consistent with which of the following:

   A. Plasma-free hemoglobin >20 mg/dL and serum lactate dehydrogenase >3x the upper limit of normal range

B. Plasma-free hemoglobin >40 mg/dL and LDH > 3x the upper limit of normal range

C. Plasma-free hemoglobin >20 mg/dL, LDH > 2.5x upper limit of normal range, and hemoglobinuria

D. Plasma-free hemoglobin >20 mg/dL, LDH > 2.5x the upper limit of normal range, and hematochezia

4. Recommended management of LVAD patients presenting with HCVA consists of all the following except

A. Maintaining MAP <90 mmHg
B. Repeat head CT within 24 hours
C. Rapid reversal of warfarin with FFP if INR >1.4
D. Obtaining 2 sets of blood cultures

5. What clinical scenario would not be consistent with the following HMII LVAD parameters: Pump flow 3.4 L/min, Power 6.8, PI 2.1?

A. Systemic hypertension
B. RV failure
C. Hypovolemia
D. Cardiac tamponade

6. Which of the following is the diagnostic neuroimaging modality of choice if mycotic aneurysm is suspected in an LVAD patient?

A. Magnetic resonance angiography
B. CT angiography
C. Conventional angiography
D. Digital subtraction angiography

7. An LVAD patient on warfarin and aspirin 325 mg presents with an acute hemorrhagic stroke with a National Institutes of Health Stroke Scale (NIHSS) of 8, GCS of 14, and an INR of 2. Lower extremity edema is present. What anticoagulation reversal strategy is most recommended?

A. Desmopressin 0.4 mcg/kg in addition to holding aspirin and coumadin

B. Holding aspirin and warfarin; administering appropriate weight-based dose of PCCs, desmopressin 0.4 mcg/kg, and 2 units of platelets

C. Holding aspirin, warfarin, administering IV vitamin K 10 mg, and repeating CT in 24 hours

D. Holding aspirin and warfarin and administering 2 units of FFP

8. Of the design features and clinical characteristics listed here, which is least likely to be associated with the HeartWare LVAD versus the HeartMate II device?

A. Higher rate of stroke
B. Centrifugal-flow design
C. Intrapericardial implantation
D. Higher rate of pump thrombosis

9. Which of the following therapies would be least recommended as part of a treatment strategy for suspected LVAD thrombosis in a patient with a remote history of hemorrhagic stroke?

A. Increase INR goal to 2.5 to 3.5

B. IV unfractionated heparin
C. IV tirofaban
D. IV alteplase

10. The PREVENT trial in HeartMate II patients demonstrated that following certain guidelines could reduce the risk of pump thrombosis. Which of the following was not part of their recommendations?

A. Maintain MAP <90 mmHg
B. Initiate heparin bridging within 48 hours with an initial goal PTT of 40 to 45 sec
C. Maintain pump speeds >9000 RPM, and avoid pump speeds <8600 RPM
D. Initiate aspirin 81 to 325 mg postoperative day 1

ANSWERS

1. A. Of all the answers provided, only increased pump power with power elevation events are suggestive of pump thrombosis, a complication which increases the risk of thromboembolic stroke.

2. A. As per the discussion in question 4, mechanical shear stress associated with the continuous-flow LVADs results in loss of high-molecular weight multimers of vWF. This results in decreased vWF:CB capacity.[14] Thrombocytopenia may or may not be present. Schistocytosis may be present in cases of severe hemolysis.

3. C. INTERMACS defines major hemolysis as plasma-free hemoglobin >20 mg/dL or a serum lactate dehydrogenase >2.5x the upper limit of normal in addition to clinical signs of hemolysis or abnormal pump function. Hemoglobinuria, anemia out of proportion to chronic illness, or pump malfunction with abnormal pump parameters meet criteria for major hemolysis.

4. C. Although no formal guidelines exist for the LVAD patient, current practices recommend maintaining MAP <90 mmHg.[18] Blood cultures should be obtained as systemic infection strongly increases the risk of mycotic aneurysms and hemorrhagic CVA.[8] Repeat non-contrast head CT should be performed within 24 hours to evaluate for ICH stability, or sooner if indicated by a change in neurologic exam.

5. A. All the answers provided can reduce pump flows and increase pump power requirements, but only systemic hypertension is not associated with a low PI. PI will typically be higher than baseline in cases of systemic hypertension, as the native myocardium will contribute more to total output in cases of increased afterload. Anticoagulation reversal with FFP may or may not be advised even if INR is >1.4, as PCCs may be preferred if the patient appears to be hypervolemic.

6. D. Digital subtraction angiography (DSA) is the modality of choice if septic emboli are suspected, as it is most sensitive for small (<3 mm) or distal intracerebral aneurysms. CT angiography or conventional angiography may be appropriate modalities if DSA is not available. Magnetic resonance imaging is contraindicated for patients with LVADs.

7. B. When NIHSS is >6 or patients present with altered level of consciousness, reversal of warfarin therapy is prudent.[8]

Of the options described, answer B is most appropriate, as PCCs will provide the most rapid reversal of warfarin with less associated volume than FFP. Desmopressin administration is performed to improve the expression of vWF from endothelial cells, combating the AVWS present in the majority of LVAD patients.[14] Platelet administration should be considered if the patient is on ASA or clopidogrel. ASA and warfarin should be held in the acute period after hemorrhagic stroke.

8. D. The HeartWare (HVAD) device is a centrifugal design continuous-flow LVAD that is compact enough to allow for intrapericardial implantation. The HVAD has been associated with a lower rate of pump thrombosis or pump failure when compared to the HMII. It, however, has an increased incidence of both hemorrhagic and ischemic stroke.[24]

9. D. Thrombolytic therapy with IV tPA (i.e., IV alteplase) is relatively contraindicated in patients with a history of intracranial hemorrhage according to the most recent stroke guidelines. It would be absolutely contraindicated in the setting of an acute ICH. The other anticoagulation strategies listed have all demonstrated some efficacy with less relative risk of provoking bleeding complications.[26]

10. D. The goal of the PREVENT trial was to assess the risk of early pump thrombosis in HMII patients. An increased incidence of pump thrombosis in HMII patients started in 2011, and the investigators developed a broad set of standardized recommendations to help reduce the occurrence of this complication. Multiple surgical recommendations were included that are not addressed here. Anticoagulation and antiplatelet management recommendations included initiation of IV unfractionated heparin (with an initial aPTT goal of 40 to 45 sec) or low molecular weight heparin (LMWH) within 48 hours if surgical bleeding was acceptable. In addition, they recommended initiating warfarin therapy within 48 hours, with a goal of reaching an INR of 2.0 to 2.5 by postoperative days 5 to 7. Aspirin therapy of 81 to 325 mg was recommended to start between postoperative days 2 and 5. Maintaining a pump speed of >9000 RPMs with a low limit of 8600 RPMs was also recommended, as was maintaining a MAP <90 mmHg.[18]

33.

VASOPLEGIA SYNDROME MANAGEMENT POST CARDIAC SURGERY

Christopher Tam

STEM CASE AND KEY QUESTIONS

A 78-year-old male with past medical history significant for hypertension, hyperlipidemia, diabetes mellitus type 2, carotid stenosis, end-stage renal disease on hemodialysis presents to the hospital with substernal chest pain, shortness of breath, and diaphoresis. ST segment elevations are noted in the anterior and inferior leads on his electrocardiogram. The patient is emergently transported to the cardiac catheterization lab where he is intubated for flash pulmonary edema. Cardiac catherization demonstrates triple vessel coronary artery disease; 70% left main, 90% mid-LAD, 90% mid-circumflex artery, and 90% right coronary artery with a left ventricular ejection fraction of 30% and severe mitral regurgitation. An intra-aortic balloon pump (IABP) is placed, and the patient is transferred to the operating room for an emergent surgery. He receives a 3-vessel bypass and a bioprosthetic mitral valve replacement. The total cardiopulmonary bypass (CPB) time is 150 minutes, and the aortic cross clamp time is 120 minutes. The patient separates from CPB using inotropic support including epinephrine at 2 mcg/min and milrinone at 0.25 mcg/kg/min. The IABP is set at 1:1 to provide maximum augmentation and vasopressor support of vasopressin 4 units/hr, and norepinephrine 25 mcg/min is started. On post-bypass transesophageal echocardiogram (TEE), the patient's left ventricle ejection fraction (LVEF) had normalized to 55% with revascularization. Cardiac output and cardiac index by thermodilution are 5.5 L/min and 3.0 L/min/m^2 respectively. The patient's blood pressure remains 85/60 mmHg with a low surgical ventricular restoration (SVR) on the aforementioned medications despite adequate fluid resuscitation. Vasodilatory shock from vasoplegia syndrome post-CPB is suspected.

WHAT IS VASOPLEGIA SYNDROME? WHAT ARE SOME DIFFERENTIAL DIAGNOSIS TO EXCLUDE?

Surgical hemostasis is achieved and the patient is transferred to the cardiothoracic intensive care unit. His cardiac index has increased to 4.0 L/min/m2, and he remains borderline hypotensive with a low SVR on 6 units/hr of vasopressin and 25 mcg/min of norepinephrine. Laboratories reveal a normal arterial blood gas, normal serum electrolytes, and a mildly elevated white blood cell count of 14,000. Hemoglobin is 9 grams/dL. On physical exam his extremities are warm and well perfused and his temperature is 37.8°C. Blood cultures are drawn and sent to the lab.

WHAT ARE SOME CLINICAL SIGNS OF VASOPLEGIA SYNDROME?

Renal replacement therapy is resumed in the next 24 hours and a follow-up TEE reveals hyperdynamic ventricular function consistent with an elevated cardiac index (CI) by thermodilution. The patient continues to be tachycardic with a heart rate of 110 to 120 beats per minute, and his central venous pressure (CVP) is 5 mmHg. Milrinone therapy is discontinued without a change in pressor requirement. SVR is 600 dyn/s/cm^5.

WHAT ARE SOME TREATMENT OPTIONS FOR VASOPLEGIA SYNDROME? IS THERE A ROLE OF STEROIDS?

Over the next 2 days the patient continues to require high-dose pressor therapy for hypotension and low SVR with a high cardiac output. Initial blood cultures fail to grow any organism, and his hemoglobin levels remain stable at 9 grams/dL. Serum electrolytes are monitored and repleted as necessary. After discussion with the surgical team, methylene blue infusion at 1 mg/kg and high-dose steroid therapy are administered.

WHAT IS THE PROGNOSIS OF VASOPLEGIA SYNDROME FOLLOWING CARDIAC SURGERY WITH CPB?

Gradually over the next 4 days the patient's blood pressure improves and his pressor medication is tapered off. His SVR normalizes with a cardiac index of 2.4 L/min/m2. On postoperative day 8 he receives tracheostomy for prolonged respiratory failure and pulmonary toilet for increased respiratory secretions. Eventually the patient is transferred to a long-term acute care hospital.

DISCUSSION

Vasoplegia syndrome was initially described by Gomes et al. in 1994 in *The Journal of Thoracic and Cardiovascular Surgery* and is a severe form of vasodilatory shock that occurs shortly after separation from CPB.[1] It occurs in 9% to 44% of patients following cardiopulmonary bypass surgery.[2] The incidence of vasoplegia syndrome in the literature varies significantly due to variations in definition and cardiovascular procedures. It is a clinical diagnosis of exclusion that typically manifests with increased CI (>2.2 L/min/m^2) and decreased SVR, resulting in hypotension despite high doses of vasopressor infusion and adequate fluid resuscitation (mean arterial pressure [MAP] <50 mmHg, Systemic Vascular Resistance Index [SVRI] <1600 dyn/s/cm^5). The differential diagnosis includes sepsis, anaphylaxis, acute heart failure, protamine reaction, pulmonary emboli, hypocalcemia, anemia, hypovolemia, arterial line reading error, or medication error.[2,3] Capillary refill and partial pressure of oxygen are unchanged.[3] Oliguria is often seen due to vasoconstriction of the efferent arteriole leading to hypoperfusion of the kidneys.[3]

ETIOLOGY AND PATHOGENESIS

Although the exact etiology of this syndrome in unclear, it is theorized that vasoplegia syndrome is caused by multiple mechanisms related to a systemic inflammatory response following CPB leading to vasodilatation resistant to vasopressor therapy.[4,5] It is associated with significant morbidity and mortality including prolonged intensive care unit (ICU) stay, prolonged time on the ventilator, and increased risk of sternal wound infections.[4,5] Norepinephrine resistant vasoplegia is associated with a worse prognosis, and patients who remain vasoplegic greater than 36 to 48 hours have mortality rate $>25\%$.[2]

With the initiation of CPB, inflammatory mechanisms are activated: contact activation, extrinsic coagulation pathway, intrinsic coagulation pathway, complement, fibrinolysis, and ischemic-reperfusion injury (see Figure 33.1).[2]

Plasma contact with the foreign surface of CPB triggers the activation of Hagemann Factor (Factor XII), which simultaneously activates the intrinsic pathway of coagulation, fibrinolysis, and the complement system.[2,6] The intrinsic coagulation pathway triggers thrombogenesis, hence the need for systemic anticoagulation prior to CPB to prevent macro-clots.[2,6] However, despite heparinization, micro-clots occur, leading to obstruction of microcirculation and overall a consumptive coagulopathy picture (i.e., disseminated intravascular coagulation, which can cause bleeding and end organ injury.[2,6]

The activation of the kallikrein system breaks down kinins from kininogen, especially bradykinin that can lead to systemic vasodilatation. Kallikrein also has a role in in cleaving plasminogen into plasmin, leading to fibrinolysis, which can cause bleeding, hence the use of antifibrinolytics (i.e., epsilon-aminocaproic acid or tranexamic acid) during CPB.[2,6]

Complement system activation leads to the release of anaphylatoxins; C¢3a and C¢5a, which triggers vasodilation and

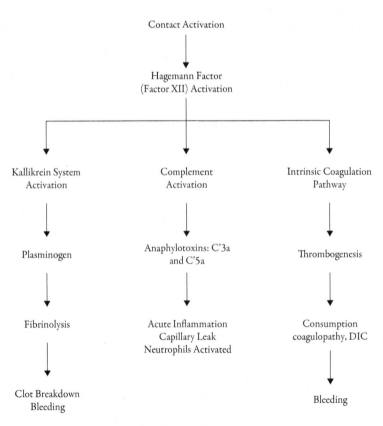

Figure 33.1 Inflammatory cascade following a "trigger" such as cardiopulmonary bypass.

leukocyte activation. Leukocytes may also be activated by shear stress and contact with the CPB circuit.[2,6] Consequences of leukocyte activation include degranulation, adhesion, aggregation, and release of toxic oxygen free radicals and proteolytic enzymes.[2,6] Furthermore, leukocytes also trigger the activation of cytokines; tumor necrosis factor (TNF)-alpha, interleukin (IL)-6, and IL-8, which exacerbate the inflammatory response by increasing neutrophil adhesion and activation.[2,6] The net result is diffuse capillary leak with interstitial edema, multiorgan dysfunction, and abnormal vascular response (i.e., vasodilatory shock). IL-6 and IL-8 have negative inotropic effects, which can lead to poor cardiac outcomes.[2,6]

Further inflammatory response occurs following the release of the aortic cross-clamp, causing ischemia-reperfusion injury. Reperfusion of the lung and heart stimulates the release of proinflammatory mediators, which adds to further inflammatory insult.[6]

PHYSIOLOGY OF VASCULAR SMOOTH-MUSCLE TONE

Regulation of vascular smooth muscle tone is dependent on the function of ligand gated channels that regulate actin and myosin activity (see Figure 33.2). Adequate vasoconstriction requires hormonal and neuronal ligands such as angiotensin II and norepinephrine to bind onto vascular smooth muscles, thereby triggering an increase flux in intracellular calcium flux.[5] Increased intracellular calcium leads to complex formation with calmodulin, which activates kinase to phosphorylate myosin to stimulate actin and myosin activity hence vasoconstriction (see Figure 33.3).[5] Resting membrane potential ranges from –30 mV to –60 mV[5]. With depolarization, a positive potential energy leads to a secondary influx of calcium into the smooth muscle cytoplasm, resulting in vasoconstriction. Hyperpolarization or vasodilatation involves opening of K-adenosine triphosphate (ATP) channels that leads to an efflux of potassium and membrane hyperpolarization (see Figure 33.4).[5]

Membrane hyperpolarization prevents the influx of calcium by inactivating the voltage gated channel. It can be triggered by decreased ATP or acidosis or by other potential neurohormonal activators of K-ATP channels including atrial natriuretic peptide, calcitonin-gene related peptide, and adenosine.[3,5] All of the aforementioned can be markedly increased in septic shock.

PATHOPHYSIOLOGY OF VASOPLEGIA SYNDROME

It is hypothesized that the vasoplegia syndrome can be caused by one of three mechanisms: increased nitric oxide (NO) synthesis, acute vasopressin deficiency, and opening of K+–ATP channels.[4] NO production is increased as a result of increased expression of NO synthase in vascular smooth muscle cells and endothelial cells.[4,5] During vasodilatory shock, the levels of NO are markedly elevated and contribute to systemic hypotension and resistance to vasopressor drugs.[4,5] The mechanism of increased expression has not been fully identified but likely involves cytokines including IL-1, IL-6, and TNF-alpha.[2] NO causes vasodilation through activation of K+–Ca2+ channels by direct nitrosylation and/or activation of cyclic guanosine monophosphate (GMP)-dependent kinase, which activates myosin phosphatase and dephosphorylates myosin causing vasodilatation and vasopressor resistance.[5]

Vasopressin has 2 physiologic functions. Secreted from the posterior pituitary antidiuretic hormone regulates permeability of renal collecting ducts to water based on plasma osmolality, and it also plays a vital role in cardiovascular homeostasis.[5] For osmolality regulation the plasma concentration of vasopressin is 1 to 7 pg/dL. Cardiovascular hemostasis requires a plasma concentration 10 to 200 pg/dL.[5] Vasopressin is a potent regulator of arterial pressure in response to hypotension occurring with acute hemorrhage or sepsis.[5] During the initial phase of shock, vasopressin levels are extremely high; however, as cardiovascular collapse progresses, vasopressin

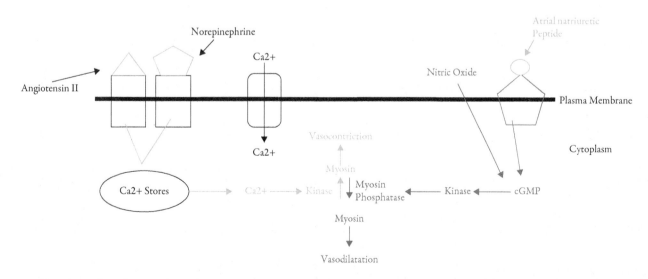

Figure 33.2 Physiology of vascular smooth muscle tone.

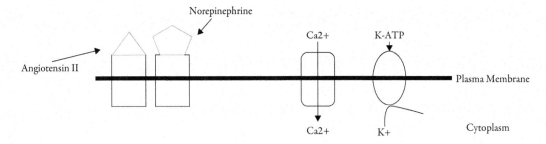

Figure 33.3 Resting potential: vasoconstriction physiology.

concentration decreases.[5] Although the exact mechanism is not known, it is believed that after profound sustained baroreceptor stimulation, vasopressin concentrations in the neurohypophysis become depleted.[5] Morales et al., in 1999, demonstrated that during hemorrhagic shock, vasopressin levels were >300 pg/ml during the acute phase of hypotensive hemorrhage but decreased to less than 30 pg/ml after 1 hour of hypotension.[7] Similarly, Landry et al. in 1999 demonstrated that patients with septic shock, late-phase hemorrhagic shock, or vasodilatory shock following CPB or left ventricular assist device (VAD) placement had inappropriately low plasma vasopressin concentrations.[8,9]

The exogenous administration of vasopressin has been shown to have efficacy in improving the blood pressure in patients with refractory shock who are unresponsive to volume resuscitation and catecholamine administration. Patients may respond to vasopressin and not catecholamines for several reasons: vasopressin plasma levels are low, therefore vascular receptors are available; catecholamine receptors may be saturated and therefore desensitized to further exogenous supply; vasopressin potentiates vasoconstrictor effects of catecholamines; vasopressin can blunt the increase in cGMP induced by NO and vasopressin inactivates K^+–ATP channels.[5] The K^+–ATP channels under physiologic conditions are generally closed; however, during states of shock, intracellular ATP decreases and leads to the opening of those channels.[5]

Opening of the channels causes hyperpolarization and subsequently vasodilatation.[5]

RISK FACTORS FOR VASOPLEGIA SYNDROME

There are multiple risk factors that predispose patients to vasoplegia syndrome following cardiac surgery. These risk factors have been published extensively in the literature:

Byrne et al. published in the *European Journal of Cardiothoracic Surgery* in 2004 a retrospective study for risk factors of vasoplegia syndrome following orthotopic heart transplantation (OHT) at Brigham and Women's Hospital between 1992 and 2001.[11] A total of 187 patients underwent OHT; 147 were included in the study. Twenty-eight of 147 (19%) developed vasoplegia syndrome, that is, defined as SVR <800 dynes with serum bicarb <20 mEq/L.[10] They identified that preoperative intravenous (IV) heparin and body surface area (BSA) >1.9 m² are independent risk factors for the development of postoperative vasoplegia.[10] However, preoperative heparin use and vasoplegia may be confounded by the fact that patients needing heparin preoperatively possessed more comorbidities and required VAD, extracorporeal membrane oxygenation, and/or IABP.[10] Increased BSA may place increased strain on a newly transplanted heart that cannot be overcome in some patients, leading to the development of vasoplegia.[10] The study did not demonstrate an

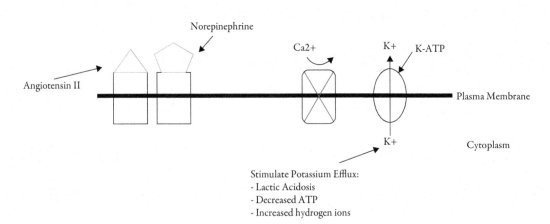

Figure 33.4 Hyperpolarization: vasodilatation physiology.

increased risk of vasoplegia among patients using angiotensin-converting enzyme inhibitors (ACEi).[10]

Levin et al. published in *Circulation* in 2009 a retrospective study that analyzed 2823 adult cardiac surgery patients. Five hundred seventy-seven of 2823 (20.4%) were vasoplegic defined according to vasopressor dose requirement; epinephrine/norepinephrine ≥150 ng/kg/min, dopamine ≥10 mcg/kg/min, or vasopressin ≥4 units/hr (maximum infusion rates).[11] Of these vasoplegic patients, 58.3% had a clinically significant decline in MAP (>20%) within the first 5 minutes of initiating CPB that lasted >2 minutes.[11] These patients also had increased mortality or increased length of hospital stay >10 days (p = 0.005). Additional risk factors for developing vasoplegia include EuroScore, procedure type (valve surgery, aortic surgery, patients undergoing surgery with preoperative heart failure), prebypass MAP, preoperative use of beta blocker and ACEi, preoperative vasopressor use, and pre- and post-bypass hematocrit.[11] The authors also noted that longer perfusion time was associated with increased risk of vasoplegia, whereas lower CPB temperature was protective.[11]

Sun et al. published in *Cardiovascular Revascularization Medicine* in 2011 the incidence of vasoplegic syndrome following coronary artery bypass grafting (CABG) versus open heart surgery (CABG ± valves, valve replacement/repair, aorta surgery, cardiac tumor resection).[12] Vasoplegia syndrome was defined as MAP ≤70 mmHg, SVRI ≤1400 dynes-s cm^{-5} m^{-2}, CI ≥2.5 min^{-1} m^{-2}, and CVP ≥10 mmHg.[12] The study included only patients who met these criteria within 24 hours postoperatively (N = 632; CABG = 334, open heart surgery = 295).[12] They found that patients undergoing open heart surgery had increased risk for vasoplegia syndrome (17%) over CABG patients (6.9%).[12] Preoperative LVEF <35% was identified as an independent predictor of vasoplegia syndrome.[12] Female gender had a protective effect for vasoplegia syndrome (P = 0.01).[12]

Patarroyo et al. published in *The Journal of Heart and Lung Transplantation* in 2012 preoperative risk factors and clinical outcomes of vasoplegia in patients following orthotopic heart transplantation.[13] This retrospective study looked at 311 patients. They defined vasoplegia as low SVR <800 dyne/s/cm^5 for more than 2 consecutive readings despite multiple (≥2) IV pressor drugs at high dose (epinephrine ≥4 mcg/min, norepinephrine ≥4 mcg/min, dopamine ≥5 mcg/kg/min, vasopressin ≥1 unit/hr) with preserved cardiac index (>2.5 min^{-1} m^{-2}) between 6 and 48 hours after surgery.[13] Thirty-five out of 311 (11%) developed vasoplegia syndrome.[13] These patients were most likely to be UNOS status 1a; have a higher BSA (P = 0.0007), a history of hypothyroidism (P = 0.0075), or previous cardiothoracic surgery (P = 0.0006), or prolonged CPB time (118 ± 37 minutes vs. 142 ± 39 minutes; p = 0.0002); or a donor heart ischemic time (191 ± 46 minutes vs. 219 ± 51 minutes; p = 0.002).[13] Preoperatively, the vasoplegic cohort was more likely to have VADs (P <0.0001) and total artificial hearts (P <0.0001).[13] The association of higher BSA and vasoplegia may be due to a persistent inflammatory state with increased inflammatory cytokines, IL-6, IL-8, TNF-alpha.[13]

This study did not find an association between ACEi or angiotensin II receptor blockers and increased risk of vasoplegia.[13]

Carrell et al. published in *The Journal of Cardiothoracic Surgery* in 2000 a prospective study looking at potential risk factors preoperatively and intraoperatively associated with vasoplegia syndrome.[14] They also evaluated the morbidity and mortality of vasoplegia syndrome during a 1-year period in a single hospital center in Switzerland.[14] They included 800 patients who underwent CABG and/or valve replacement. One hundred seventy-five of 800 (21.9%) patients developed vasoplegia.[14] They determined that the patient's temperature, duration of CPB, total cardioplegia volume, reduced left ventrical function, and preoperative treatment with ACEi predicted early development of postoperative vasoplegia syndrome.[14] Although there was not an increase in mortality, the vasoplegia group had prolonged ICU stays with higher morbidity.[14]

In summary, the risks for vasoplegia syndrome are multifactorial, including prolonged bypass and cross-clamp time, poor preoperative left ventricular function, preoperative vasodilatory and cardiogenic shock, and complex cardiac surgical repair. Unfortunately, many of the risk factors that lead to vasoplegia syndrome are not amenable to modification, and the overall morbidity and mortality in this patient population is higher.

MARKERS FOR VASOPLEGIA SYNDROME

Copeptin is a peptide in the c-terminal part of pro-arginine vasopressin (AVP), which is the precursor to vasopressin.[15] Copeptin and AVP are secreted from the neurohypophysis with hemodynamic or osmotic stimulation (see Figure 33.5).[15] Elevated preoperative levels of copeptin have been associated with an increased incidence of perioperative vasoplegia syndrome.[15] In contrast to AVP, copeptin is stable both in serum and plasma at room temperature and can be measured as a fragment of AVP that is in circulation.[15]

Colson et al. published in *Critical Care* in 2011 a potential marker prebypass for vasoplegia syndrome that may prelude to an earlier diagnosis of vasoplegia syndrome.[15] Colson et al. studied 64 patients who underwent CPB surgery; 10 out of 64 (15%) developed vasoplegia syndrome.[16] The authors found a higher concentration of copeptin (a precursor of AVP) in plasma pre-CPB (P <0.001) but lower AVP concentrations (p <0.01) in vasoplegic patients than in those who did not have vasoplegia.[16] They defined vasoplegia as MAP <60 mmHg and CI ≥2.2 l/min/m^2.[16] The patients in the vasoplegia group had preoperative hyponatremia and decreased left ventricular function and were more likely to be New York Heart Association class IV heart failure patients. They also received more complex cardiac surgical procedures.[16] This study suggests that high preoperative copeptin (30.1 vs. 4.8; p <0.001) may be predictive of postoperative vasoplegia and suggests that activation of the arginine vasopressin system before surgery may lead to depletion of endogenous stores of vasopressin and produce a vasopressin deficit during surgery.[16]

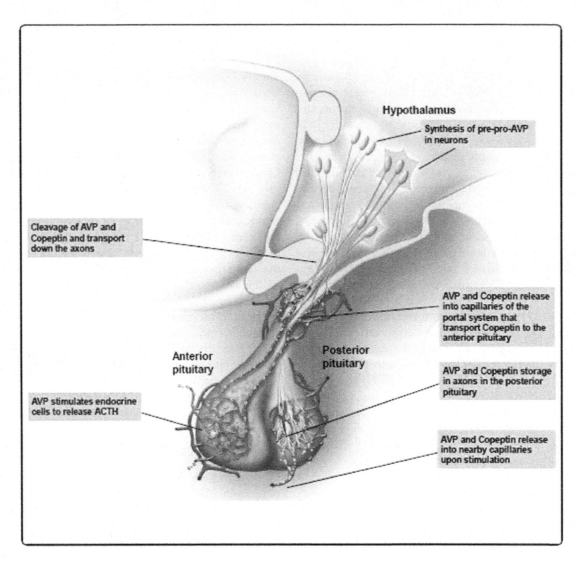

Figure 33.5 Synthesis of AVP and copeptin in the hypothalamus and pituitary.

MANAGEMENT

Management of patients with vasoplegia syndrome focuses on utilizing agents to reverse the mechanisms responsible. First-line therapy includes adequate fluid resuscitation in conjunction with catecholamines such as norepinephrine and epinephrine.[4] If the patient remains vasoplegic, vasopressin may be added. Methylene blue and hydroxocobalamin are used as salvage therapies when vasoplegic shock is refractory to the aforementioned therapies.[4]

Vasopressin at a physiologic infusion dosage of 0.04 units/min can replete endogenous vasopressin in patients who may be vasopressin deficient. Vasopressin has several mechanisms of action to stimulate vasoconstriction including activation of V1 vascular receptors, modulation of ATP sensitive K-ATP channels, modulation of NO, and potentiation of adrenergic agents leading to vasoconstriction.[5] Prophylactic VP infusion 20 minutes prior to CPB may reduce post-CPB vasopressor support. Papadopoulos et al. published in the *Journal of Cardiothoracic Surgery* in 2010 a study evaluating perioperative low-dose vasopressin infusion in reducing the incidence of vasoplegia.[17] The study was a prospective randomized trial,

following two cohorts: vasopressin or normal saline group.[17] They looked at a total of 50 patients in the study (including patients on ACEi and impaired LVEF 30% to 40%); 25 in the vasopressin group (1 out of 25), and 25 in normal saline group (6 out of 25).[17] The authors found that low-dose infusion during CPB and for the next 4 hours reduced catecholamine requirements and prevented vasoplegia.[17] Noto et al. published a retrospective study in *Interactive Cardiovascular and Thoracic Surgery* in 2009 regarding the use of terlipressin in the management of refractory vasoplegic hypotension following cardiac surgery.[18] Terlipressin is a synthetic analogue of vasopressin currently unavailable in the United States. It is used in the management of hepatorenal syndrome, esophageal varices, and catecholamine resistant vasoplegia syndrome.[18] It binds to and has greater selectivity for V1 receptors than vasopressin with stronger vasopressor effect with a longer half-life of 6 hours versus vasopressin's half-life of 24 minutes.[18] Although Noto et al. showed that terlipressin was successful in raising SVR and MAP, other studies comparing terlipressin and norepinephrine showed that they were both equally effective in increasing MAP.[19] Furthermore, raising SVR alone may increase myocardial work and therefore myocardial stress, which may lead to decreased cardiac output.[20] Terlipressin also causes time-dependent thrombocytopenia when given as an infusion.[19]

As previously mentioned, much of the vasoplegia pathophysiology is related to an inflammatory immune response, which leads to vasodilatation. Corticosteroids have been studied as a potential treatment for catecholamine refractory vasoplegia. They reduce IL-6, IL-8, TNF-alpha, leukotrienes, and other cytokines. However, 2 large randomized controlled trials published in recent years failed to demonstrate improvement in vasoplegia syndrome outcomes. The Dexamethasone for Cardiac Surgery trial was a large multicenter (8 cardiac surgical centers), randomized, placebo control study conducted in the Netherlands. It compared a single high dose IV (1 mg/kg) dose of dexamethasone with a placebo in patients undergoing cardiac surgery with CPB.[21] The primary end points included death, myocardial infarction, stroke, renal failure, and respiratory failure occurring within 30 days of randomization.[21] Secondary end points included postoperative infection, postoperative a-fib, highest serum glucose concentration in the ICU, highest body temperature in the ICU, postoperative delirium, postoperative mechanical ventilation duration, time to discharge from ICU, and time to hospital discharge.[21] The study looked at a total of 4494 patients: 2239 randomized to steroids and 2255 randomized to placebo.[21] The authors found that dexamethasone reduced postoperative infection, duration of postoperative mechanical ventilation, and lengths of ICU and hospital stays.[21] In contrast, dexamethasone was associated with higher postoperative glucose levels.[21] However, dexamethasone did not affect primary outcomes.[21]

Another high-powered study titled "Steroids in Cardiac Surgery" was a randomized, double-blinded study published in the *Lancet* in 2015.[22] The authors enrolled 7507 patients from 80 hospitals and/or cardiac surgery centers in 18 countries. Methylprednisolone was dosed twice; once pre-CPB and once during CPB compared with a placebo group.[22] The primary outcomes were 30-day mortality in high-risk patients (defined by Euro-SCORE >6) and a composite of death with major morbidity (i.e., myocardial injury, stroke, renal failure, or respiratory failure) in 30 days.[22] The authors found that methylprednisolone did not reduce risk of death or major morbidity.[22]

Methylene blue has been increasingly used as a rescue drug for the treatment of catecholamine refractory vasoplegia. Methylene blue interferes with NO metabolism in endothelial and vascular smooth muscle cells (see Figure 33.6).[23] It binds to and inhibits NO synthase and guanylate cyclase, thereby blocking the vasodilatory effects of NO.[23] It is also likely that methylene blue binds plasma NO, creating a "scavenging" effect.[23] An initial bolus dose of 1.5 mg/kg to 2 mg/kg and/or a continuous infusion of 0.25 mg/kg/hr to 2 mg/kg/hr over 8 hours is recommended.[23,24] Methylene blue is metabolized in erythrocytes by nicotinamide adenine dinucleotide phosphate.[23] The efficacy of methylene blue is controversial, with potential serious side effects including methemoglobinemia, serotonin syndrome, and end organ failure with associated decreased, renal blood flow, mesenteric blood flow, hemolytic anemia, hyperbilirubinemia, and transient transaminitis.[25]

Levin et al. published in the *Annals of Thoracic Surgery* in 2004 a randomized control study evaluating the efficacy of prophylactic methylene blue to reduce morbidity and mortality following cardiac surgery.[26] The authors demonstrated

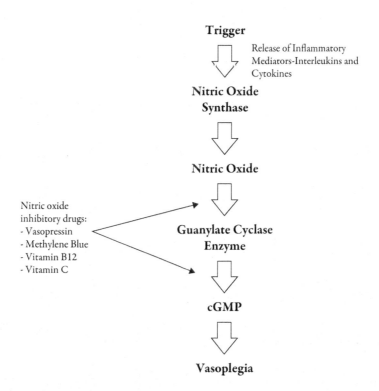

Figure 33.6 Synthesis of nitric oxide and mechanism of action of various treatment.

reduced mortality, renal failure, respiratory failure, encephalopathy, arrhythmia, sepsis, and multiorgan failure (all *p* <0.05) in the treatment group.[26] Those treated with methylene blue experienced an earlier resolution of vasoplegia compared with the placebo group.[26] However, another study by Weiner et al., demonstrated methylene blue was associated with poor outcomes. This was a retrospective study published in the *Journal of Cardiothoracic and Vascular Anesthesia* in 2013. The results of the study showed that patients who received methylene blue had higher total morbidity, pulmonary complications (pneumonia, tracheostomy, prolonged mechanical ventilation), hyperbilirubinemia, and days of inotropic support (*p* <0.05 for all aforementioned complications).[27] The authors speculated that methylene blue inhibition of NO and subsequent vasoconstriction had deleterious effects on end organ microvasculature.[27]

High-dose vitamin B12 has also reportedly been used in patients with vasoplegia syndrome after cardiac surgery. Roderique et al. published a case report in the *Annals of Thoracic Surgery* in 2014 describing the successful use of vitamin B12 during cardiopulmonary bypass in a patient undergoing CABG, double valve replacement, and patent foramen ovale closure with a prolonged period of time on CPB.[28] The authors infused 5g IV of hydroxocobalamin over 10 minutes with significant improvement in blood pressure and reduction in dosage of catecholamine infusion.[28] The putative mechanism of action is the direct binding to NO and inhibition of NO synthase as well as guanylate cyclase thereby preventing vasodilatation.[28] There are no known side effects with vitamin B12.[28]

Interestingly, vitamin C has also been studied as a noncatecholamine adjunct drug to treat patients with decompensated septic shock. The study was conducted as a pilot where patients received 1.5 grams of vitamin C every 6 hours in addition to 50 mg hydrocortisone IV every 6 hours for 4 days and 200 mg IV thiamine every 12 hours for 4 days.[29] The authors found a significant reduction in catecholamine dosage and an overall decreased mortality in the treatment group.[29] The study has not been replicated, and the use of vitamin C has not been studied in the postoperative cardiac surgery population. Further research is needed to demonstrate a true efficacy of vitamin C in the treatment of vasoplegia syndrome.

CONCLUSION

Vasoplegia syndrome is a form of vasodilatory shock that is a complication of cardiopulmonary bypass. Cardiopulmonary bypass causes a systemic inflammatory response that activates K-ATP channels and increases NO levels, causing vasodilation. There are multiple risk factors. Treatment includes catecholamines, vasopressin, and adequate fluid resuscitation. Ironically, corticosteroid administration has not demonstrated improvement in the overall outcomes for patients with vasoplegia syndrome. Methylene blue and vitamin B12 are rescue drugs that may be utilized; however, further research and clinical trials are warranted.

REFERENCES

1. Evora PR. Twenty years of vasoplegic syndrome treatment in heart surgery: methylene blue revised. Rev Bras Cir Cardiovasc. 2015;30(1):84–92.
2. Omar S, Zedan A, Nugent K. Cardiac vasoplegia syndrome: pathophysiology, risks factors and treatment. Am J Med Sci. 2015;349(1):80–88.
3. Liu H et al. Vasoplegic syndrome: an update on perioperative considerations. J Clin Anesth. 2017;40:63–71.
4. Shaefi S et al. Vasoplegia after cardiovascular procedures: pathophysiology and targeted therapy. J Cardiothorac Vasc Anesth. 2018;32:1013–1022.
5. Landry DW, Oliver JA. The pathogenesis of vasodilatory shock. New Engl J Med. 2001;345(8):588–595.
6. Kozik DJ. Characterizing the inflammatory response to cardiopulmonary bypass in children. Ann Thorac Surg. 2006;81(6):S2347–2354.
7. Morales D et al. Reversal by vasopressin of intractable hypotension in the late phase of hemorrhagic shock. Circulation. 1999;100: 226–229.
8. Argenziano M et al. A prospective randomized trial of arginine vasopressin in the treatment of vasodilatory shock after left ventricular assist device placement. Circulation. 1997;96(Suppl 2)286–290.
9. Landry DW et al. Vasopressin deficiency contributes to the vasodilation of septic shock. Circulation. 1997;95:1122–1125.
10. Byrne JG et al. Risk factors and outcomes for "vasoplegia syndrome" following cardiac transplantation. Euro J Cardio-Thorac Surg. 2004(25):327–332.
11. Levin MA. Early on-cardiopulmonary bypass hypotension and other factors associated with vasoplegic syndrome. Circulation. 2009;120:1664–1671.
12. Sun X et al. Is vasoplegic syndrome more prevalent with open-heart procedures compared with isolated on-pump CABG surgery? Cardiovasc Revasc Med. 2011;12(4):203–209.
13. Patarroyo M et al. Pre-operative risk factors and clinical outcomes associated with vasoplegia in recipients of orthotopic heart transplantation in the contemporary era. J Heart Lung Transplant. 2012;31:282–287.
14. Carrel T et al. Low systemic vascular resistance after cardiopulmonary bypass: incidence, etiology and clinical importance. J Card Surg. 2000;15:347–353.
15. Nickel CH et al. The role of copeptin as a diagnostic and prognostic biomarker for risks stratification in the emergency department. BMC Med. 2012;10:7.
16. Colson PH et al. Post cardiac surgery vasoplegia is associated with high preoperative copeptin plasma concentration. Critical Care. 2011;15:R255.
17. Papadopoulos G et al. Perioperative infusion of low-dose of vasopressin for prevention and management of vasodilatory vasoplegic syndrome in patients undergoing coronary artery bypass grafting: a double blind randomized study. J Cardiothorac Surg. 2010;5:17.
18. Noto A et al. A retrospective analysis of terlipressin in bolus for the management of refractory vasoplegic hypotension after cardiac surgery. Interact Cardiovasc Thorac Surg. 2009;(9):588–592.
19. Morelli A et al. Continuous terlipressin versus vasopressin infusion in septic shock (TERLIVAP): a randomized, controlled pilot study. Critical Care. 2009;13:R130.
20. Morelli A et al. Effects of short-term simultaneous infusion of dobutamine and terlipressin in patients with septic shock: the DOBUPRESS study. Brit J Anaesth. 2008;100(4):494–503.
21. Dieleman JM et al. Intraoperative high-dose dexamethasone for cardiac surgery. JAMA. 2012;308(17):1761–1767.
22. Whitlock RP et al. Methylprednisolone in patients undergoing cardiopulmonary bypass (SIRS): a randomized, double-blind, placebo-controlled trial. Lancet. 2015;386:1243–1253.
23. Riha H and Augoustides JGT. Pro: methylene blue as a rescue therapy for vasoplegia after cardiac surgery. J Cardiothorac Vasc Anesthes. 2011;25(4):736–738.

24. Ginimuge PR and Jyothi SD. Methylene blue: revisited. J Anaesthesiol Clin Pharmacol. 2010;26(4):517–520.
25. Leyh RG. Methylene Blue: the drug of choice for catecholamine-refractory vasoplegia after cardiopulmonary bypass? J Thorac Cardiovasc Surg. 2003;125:1426–1431.
26. Levin RL et al. Methylene blue reduces mortality and morbidity in vasoplegic patients after cardiac surgery. Ann Thorac Surg. 2004;77:496–499.
27. Weiner MM et al. Methylene blue is associated with poor outcomes in vasoplegic shock. J Cardiothorac Vasc Anesthes. 2013;27(6):1233–1238.
28. Roderique JD et al. The use of high-dose hydroxocobalamin for vasoplegic syndrome. Ann Thorac Surg. 2014;97:1785–1786.
29. Marik PE et al. Hydrocortisone, vitamin C and thiamine for the treatment of severe sepsis and septic shock: a retrospective before-after study. Chest. 2017;151:1229–1238.

REVIEW QUESTIONS

1. A 75-year-old male underwent an aortic valve replacement, mitral valve replacement, and 2-vessel CABG with CPB time 150 minutes and aortic cross clamp time 140 minutes. Immediately post-bypass the patient has required high vasopressor dosages to maintain MAP >60 mmHg. Cardiac output and cardiac index is 4.5 LPM and 2.64 L/min/m². He is currently on norepinephrine at 28 mcg/min, vasopressin at 4 units/hr, and epinephrine 2 mcg/min infusions. Upregulation of which of the following can lead to such hypotension seen after cardiopulmonary bypass?

A. NO synthase
B. G protein coupled receptors
C. Ca2+ voltage gated channels
D. Adenylate cyclase

Answer: A. NO synthase has been theorized as one of the potential mechanisms of vasodilatation, secondary to the inflammatory response from CPB. Increased NO synthase promotes the hyperpolarization cascade in the vasculature, causing vasodilation. Some treatment options target the reduction of NO synthesis intravascularly.

2. A 54-year-old male status post coronary artery bypass grafting × 4 vessel, aortic valve replacement, and mitral valve repair is on postoperative day 0 on high-dose vasopressor infusions, including norepinephrine at 25 mcg/min and vasopressin at 4 units/hr, with preserved biventricular function. The ICU attending starts the patient on high-dose steroid therapy: hydrocortisone 50 mg IV every 8 hours as adjunctive therapy to lower vasopressor requirements. What effects do high dose steroids have in vasoplegic patients?

A. Decreased vasopressor requirements
B. Compromised healing
C. Longer ICU stay
D. Decreased ventilator days

Answer: D. Two large randomized controlled trials published in *JAMA* and *The Lancet* in the utility of high-dose steroids for postoperative vasoplegia syndrome did not show any decreased vasopressor requirements or overall change in morbidity and mortality of these patients. The studies also did not demonstrate increased risk for sternal wound infection or longer ICU days. The outcomes did demonstrate decreased ventilator days and ICU length of stay.

3. A 36-year-old female post ascending aortic and aortic arch repair for an aneurysm is on high doses of vasopressor infusions: norepinephrine at 22 mcg/min and vasopressin at 3 units/hr. A methylene blue bolus dose and then an infusion was started by the intraoperative cardiac anesthesiologist. Which of the following matches the correct bolus and infusion dosage of methylene blue, respectively?

A. 4 mg/kg, 0.25 mg/kg/hr over 24 hrs
B. 1.5 mg/kg, 1 mg/kg/hr over 8 hrs
C. 0.5 mg/kg, 3.5 mg/kg/hr over 12 hrs
D. 0.75 mg/kg, 1.5 mg/kg/hr over 24 hrs

Answer: B. According to the literature, 1.5 mg/kg to 2 mg/kg was used as the bolus dose and a continuous infusion of 0.25 mg/kg/hr to 2 mg/kg/hr over 8 hours was used.

4. Using the case scenario in question 3, what are the potential side effects of methylene blue use?

A. Methemoglobinemia
B. Serotonin syndrome
C. Gut ischemia
D. All of the above

Answer: D. Repeated doses of methylene blue can cause methemoglobinemia, serotonin syndrome, especially patients on selective serotonin reuptake inhibitors, and decreased vascular perfusion to the gut.

5. The patient is a 58-year-old female s/p CABG × 5 vessel with postoperative vasoplegia syndrome on norepinephrine 22 mcg/min and vasopressin 5 units/hr. A bolus dose of methylene blue was given in the operating room by the cardiac anesthesiologist with no significant improvement in vasopressor requirements. The critical care intensivist decides to give a dose of vitamin B12 for the vasoplegia syndrome. Which of the following is a potential side effect of vitamin B12?

A. Seizures
B. Hyperglycemia
C. Anemia
D. No known side effects

Answer: D. No known side effects have been reported for Vitamin B12 use. Common to see is discoloration in blood and urine; however, there is no known side effect to its use.

6. The patient is a 68-year-old male status post aoritc valve replacement, mitral valve repair, and ascending aortic aneurysm repair postoperative day 0 on high-dose vasopressor infusion support of norepinephrine at 26 mcg/min, vasopressin 5 units/hr, and epi at 3 mcg/min, with the following vitals: arterial blood pressure: 95/40, pulmonary artery pressure: 40/20, central venous pressure: 15, cardiac output/cardiac index: 3.5/2.1 and mixed venous saturation of 54%. What is the likely diagnosis?

A. Vasoplegia syndrome
B. Cardiac tamponade

C. Right heart failure

D. Left heart failure

Answer: B. Immediately postoperatively, cardiac tamponade is one of the top differential diagnosis in the event there are any hemodynamic perturbations. The patient in this scenario is in vasodilatory shock with borderline cardiac output as well as elevated pulmonary artery pressures and central venous pressure. Although high vasopressor requirements are seen in vasoplegia syndrome, elevated pulmonary artery and central venous pressures with a borderline cardiac output are not. These clinical findings can be seen also in left and right heart failure; however, the initial differential to rule out has to be cardiac tamponade.

34

DIAGNOSIS OF BRAIN DEATH AND MANAGEMENT OF THE BRAIN DEAD PATIENT

J. David Bacon and Kevin W. Hatton

STEM CASE AND KEY QUESTIONS

A 35-year-old male is admitted to the intensive care unit following a self-inflicted gunshot wound to the head. He is intubated and placed on mechanical ventilation. A computed tomography (CT) scan demonstrates penetrating injury with cranial fracture along the right temporal bone and blood, air, and metallic foreign bodies within the cranial vault. On presentation to the intensive care unit (ICU), he has no spontaneous respiratory effort, he does not respond to verbal or painful stimuli, and his pupils are maximally dilated and do not respond to bright light.

IS THIS PATIENT DEAD?

Death is a complicated medicolegal diagnosis that is specifically defined by national, state, and/or local laws. Clinical examination for cardiac death evidences a heart rate and blood pressure currently within normal limits, while the electrocardiogram demonstrates sinus rhythm without evidence of ischemia. Loss of cardiac function (cardiac death) has not occurred, and circulatory function is providing adequate blood flow to maintain distal organ function. Given the patient's head injuries and lack of responsiveness, a diagnosis of brain death (the irreversible cessation of all brain function) is considered.

HOW IS BRAIN DEATH DETERMINED?

Two days after admission to the ICU, no change in the patient's hemodynamics have occurred and no change in his Glasgow Coma Scale (GCS) has been noted despite a lack of sedation, normothermia, and a negative urine toxicology report. The attending intensivist proceeds to evaluate the patient for brain death. The radiographic findings demonstrating severe head trauma are reviewed. A neurologic exam demonstrates loss of voluntary responses (LOVR) and a loss of involuntary responses (LOIR). GCS is determined to be 3. When the physician initiates an apnea test, the patient becomes hemodynamically unstable and the test is terminated.

WITH THIS PATIENT UNABLE TO COMPLETE THE APNEA TEST DUE TO HEMODYNAMIC INSTABILITY AFTER SEPARATION FROM MECHANICAL VENTILATION, ARE THERE ADDITIONAL TESTS THAT ARE USED TO CONFIRM THE DIAGNOSIS IN THIS CASE?

A neurology consult is requested, and the neurologist repeats the intensivist's examination, resulting in the same findings. After a discussion with the critical care team, a decision is made to perform ancillary testing to evaluate the patient's intracranial blood flow and electrical activity. Nuclear-based cerebral scintigraphy and transcranial doppler (TCD) ultrasonography both demonstrate no intracranial blood flow. A full-montage electroencephalography (EEG) is also performed and records electrocerebral silence. Based on the results of clinical brain death testing and ancillary testing, the patient is declared brain dead.

WHAT IS THE MAIN GOAL OF CONTINUED INTENSIVE CARE SUPPORT?

Following the diagnosis of brain death, the organ donation network is contacted by the patient's physicians. It is determined that the patient has no documentation concerning his wishes with respect to organ donation, and the donation team approaches the patient's family and initiates a discussion concerning brain death and organ donation. After several family meetings with physicians and donation counselors, the family agrees to consent the patient for organ donation. Potential recipient candidates are evaluated. Meanwhile, the focus of the ICU team shifts to optimizing organ function by preserving hemodynamic stability, replacing lost endocrine system function, reversing coagulopathy, and preventing nosocomial infections (pneumonia, bacteremia, or urinary tract infections).

A few hours later, the patient develops severe polyuria (>500 mL/hr urine output) with hypotension.

WHAT IS THE MOST LIKELY EXPLANATION FOR THE INCREASED URINE OUTPUT AND HYPOTENSION? HOW IS IT TREATED?

The medical team suspects the patient most likely has central Diabetes insipidus from antidiuretic hormone (ADH) no longer being released from the posterior pituitary. This causes reduced free water uptake in the renal distal tubule. Laboratory testing reveals a low urine sodium concentration, low urine specific gravity, low urine osmolarity, and serum hypernatremia. Intravenous fluid boluses are used to restore adequate intravascular volume decreased from polyuria, and a vasopressin infusion is initiated to restore free water resorption from the urine. Once intravascular fluid volume is corrected, serum hypernatremia is treated with enteral free water administration. After initiation of vasopressin infusion and restoration of intravascular fluid volume, the patient remains hypotensive.

WHAT IS THE MOST LIKELY CAUSE OF CONTINUED HEMODYNAMIC INSTABILITY IN THIS PATIENT?

With the diagnosis of diabetes insipidus, it is likely the patient has loss of anterior pituitary gland function. Exogenous thyroid hormone and corticosteroid therapy is started empirically. Invasive blood pressure monitoring is started to manage hypotension, and an echocardiogram is ordered to assess cardiac function. While awaiting organ harvest, the patient develops ventricular fibrillation and has no pulse.

WHAT ACTIONS SHOULD BE TAKEN IN THE BRAIN DEAD PATIENT AWAITING ORGAN HARVEST IF CARDIAC ARREST OCCURS?

Advanced Cardiac Life Support (ACLS) is initiated as per guidelines. Chest compressions and vasopressor boluses are initiated, and spontaneous circulation is rapidly restored. The organ donor network is apprised of the donor's deteriorating condition, and the patient is transported to the operating room for urgent organ harvest.

DISCUSSION

Death is a complicated medicolegal concept. For the majority of history, the diagnosis of death has been made based on clinical evaluation of an unconscious patient, sometimes for extended periods that may last days after the initial loss of consciousness (LOC). Improvements in physical examination and ancillary testing, including laboratory, radiographic, and ultrasonographic techniques, have made some aspects of the diagnosis easier while causing additional controversy in others. Unfortunately, as a result of real or perceived errors in diagnosis, public skepticism remains high about the medical community's ability to accurately diagnose death. Nevertheless, most legal scholars, medical experts, and legal statutes recognize two forms of death: cardiac death, the irreversible cessation

of cardiac function, and brain death, the irreversible cessation of brain function. In this discussion, we focus primarily on the diagnosis and physiologic ramifications of brain death.

As previously described, brain death is defined as the irreversible cessation of all brain function. Brain death is a difficult diagnosis primarily based on the results of physical examination findings and central reflex testing. While physical examination and central reflex testing themselves are easily performed, interpreting the results can be challenging, even for experienced clinicians. Guidelines published by the American Academy of Neurology attempt to reduce confusion and codify a practical approach to this challenging diagnosis.[1] The diagnosis of brain death is further complicated by a number of confounding factors, including hypotension, hypothermia, electrolyte abnormalities, metabolic disturbances, and the presence of drugs that depress the central nervous system (CNS) or cause neuromuscular blockade. These confounders must be ruled out prior to performing brain death testing.[1,2] Once these confounding factors have been treated or eliminated, clinical brain death testing primarily revolves around 4 central tenants: identification of neurologic injury, determination of LOC, determination of LOVR, and determination of LOIR, including the demonstration of loss of central reflexes and inappropriate apnea (Figure 34.1). In addition, typically 2 (and sometimes more) different physicians should separately complete brain death testing at different times to ensure that the patient's condition is fully evaluated for permanence.

In the diagnosis of brain death, clinicians must first identify a severe neurologic injury that could result in prolonged and persistent LOC, LOVR, and LOIR. Though it lends additional validity to the diagnosis of brain death, it is not necessary to identify the underlying disease process that led to the neurologic injury. For example, while CT scan may demonstrate massive intracranial hemorrhage and midline shift as the neurologic injury that has produced the findings of LOC, LOVR, and LOIR, it is not necessary to define the cause of the intracranial hemorrhage to diagnose brain death. This determination of neurologic injury may be discovered through a comprehensive medical and surgical history and a detailed clinical examination, as well as a review of available laboratory and radiographic testing. In most cases, the neurologic injury diagnosis should be supported by neuroimaging, which may also be required by local laws.

After identification of a severe neurologic injury, the diagnosis of brain death is further supported by evaluation and documentation of prolonged and persistent LOC, LOVR, and LOIR. As described earlier, these features should be evaluated only after confounding factors have been treated or ruled out, using the specific history, physical exam, and diagnostic features described in Table 34.1. LOC should then be observed over a period of time (although the time frame for this initial observation is not well defined), and observation for a minimum of 4 hours, and longer in certain instances, seems advisable. During this period, the patient should have a GCS of 3 with every evaluation. After prolonged LOC has been defined, LOVR should be established to visual, verbal, and painful stimuli applied to multiple locations, including all four extremities. In some patients, spinal reflexes may

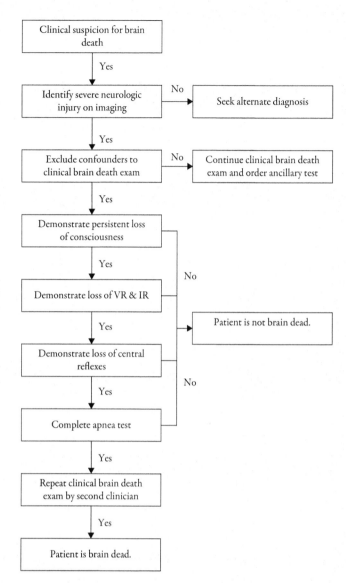

Figure 34.1 Algorithm for clinical brain death examination. VR = voluntary responses. IR = involuntary response.

Table 34.1 CLINICAL FEATURES TO DEFINE ABSENCE OF CONFOUNDING FACTORS FOR CLINICAL DIAGNOSIS OF BRAIN DEATH. CNS = CENTRAL NERVOUS SYSTEM. NMB = NEUROMUSCULAR BLOCKING.

CONFOUNDING FACTOR	CLINICAL FEATURES THAT EXCLUDE CONFOUNDING FACTOR
Hypothermia	Core body temperature ≥ 36 C
Hypotension	Systolic blood pressure ≥ 100 mmHg with or without vasopressor support
Electrolyte or metabolic disturbance	pH > 7.20 [Na] = 120-160 mEq/dL Serum blood glucose = 70-300 gm/dL
CNS depressing drugs	Medical history Urine drug screen
NMB drugs	Medical history Peripheral nerve stimulation

occur, particularly when painful stimuli are applied the lower extremities.[3,4] Spinal reflexes themselves do not contribute to or refute the diagnosis of brain death, but voluntary movement or involuntary posturing to any of these stimuli is incompatible with the diagnosis of brain death.

If no voluntary or involuntary motor response occurs from visual, verbal, or painful stimuli, central reflex testing and inappropriate apnea testing should be completed. Central reflex testing is performed for each of the 7 brainstem reflexes described in Table 34.2. When applicable, this testing should be performed bilaterally to ensure that there is no reflex response from either side of the patient. Once central reflex testing is complete, inappropriate apnea testing should be evaluated by removing the patient from mechanical ventilation, supplying supplemental oxygen, and observing the patient for spontaneous respiratory effort. While supplemental oxygen can be supplied in several ways, a T-Piece setup as described in Box 34.1 and shown in Figure 34.2 can be easily and safely used for most patients.[5,6] After approximately 10 minutes, an arterial blood gas sample should be drawn, and after this sample has been obtained, the patient can be returned to normal mechanical ventilation. The apnea test confirms brain death if there was no spontaneous respiratory effort and the arterial blood gas sample demonstrated a partial pressure of carbon dioxide ($PaCO2$) $\geq$60mm Hg, assuming a normal baseline $PaCO2$ value, or a $PaCO2$ rise of $\geq$20mm Hg above baseline when this baseline value is significantly elevated ($PaCO2$ >50 mmHg). If the rise in $PaCO2$ does not meet either of levels, the apnea test should be repeated with a longer period of observation.

Some specific medical conditions may mimic brain death, including the so-called locked-in syndrome and Guillain-Barre syndrome. Locked-in syndrome results from injury at the level of the pons when other portions of the midbrain remain intact. This most commonly results from a basilar artery embolic stroke. Patients are unable to move their limbs, grimace, or swallow.[7] In these patients, radiographic evaluation demonstrates only subtle neurologic injury within the brainstem; they may retain the ability to blink and/or move their eyes, and they do not have loss of consciousness. In Guillain-Barre syndrome and other acute or chronic inflammatory demyelinating polyneuropathies, patients have decreased conduction along peripheral and/or cranial nerves. This may result in profound weakness with loss of all voluntary and involuntary muscle movements.[8]

The growing popularity of illicit, designer street drugs has added another complexity to the determination of brain death. New synthetic intoxicants are not routinely tested via commercially available blood or urine drug screens. In some cases, there may be no option for drug testing, and patients may be profoundly intoxicated with a CNS depressant drug despite the absence of a positive medical history and no objective laboratory data. For this reason, the first step in brain death testing is frequently an evaluation and determination of a brain injury. When diagnostic testing, including CT scans and magnetic resonance imaging, does not match the clinical picture, an unknown intoxication may be present. In such cases, continued supportive care to allow for drug

Table 34.2 CENTRAL REFLEXES TO BE TESTED FOR EVALUATION OF BRAIN DEATH, INSTRUCTIONS TO ELICIT EACH REFLEX AND RESPONSE THAT IS CONSISTENT WITH BRAIN DEATH.

REFLEX	TEST	RESPONSE
Pupillary light reflex	Shine bright light in each eye	Pupil remains dilated and fixed at mid-position.
Corneal reflex	Touch patient cornea with tip of cotton applicator	No blink or eye motion.
Oculo-cephalic reflex	Rapidly turn head left and right from a neutral midline position	Eye follows the movement of the head and doesn't move within socket.
Vestibulo-ocular reflex	Cold water irrigated into auditory canal of each ear	No eye movement noted.
Facial grimace	Painful stimulus to supraorbital ridge and temporomandibular joint	No facial muscle movement.
Gag reflex	Stimulate posterior pharynx, typically with tip of suction catheter	No gag.
Cough reflex	Stimulate trachea, typically with endotracheal suctioning	No cough.

clearance and a possible change in clinical status is prudent. Unfortunately, there is no way to know the exact waiting period for the clearance of an unknown drug. Therefore, if no clinical improvement has occurred after a given period of time, additional testing may be necessary.

In clinical situations where brain death testing is ambiguous, testing cannot be fully completed, or there is some controversy with the underlying diagnosis of severe neurologic injury, ancillary testing will be needed to confirm the diagnosis of brain death. These additional tests evaluate either intracranial blood flow or electrical activity. Such tests include 4-vessel cerebral angiography, single-photon emission computed tomography (SPECT) scan, or cerebral scintigraphy, computed tomography angiography (CTA), magnetic resonance angiography (MRA), or TCD ultrasonography to evaluate blood flow or EEG, bispectral index (BIS) monitoring, and somatosensory evoked potentials (SSEP) to evaluate cerebral electrical activity[9,10] (Figure 34.3). Typically, only 1 additional test is required to confirm a diagnosis of brain death. The SPECT scan, 4-vessel cerebral angiography, and EEG are the most commonly used ancillary tests to confirm the diagnosis of brain death.

POST-BRAIN DEATH ORGAN PRESERVATION

After establishing the diagnosis of brain death, the patient is declared legally "dead" and the goals of care for the patient's body typically continue in one of two ways. If the patient's body is considered a poor candidate for organ donation, if the family refuses consent for organ donation, or if no family exists, the focus of care turns to protecting the patient's dignity

Box 34.1 STEPS TO CONDUCT APNEA TEST WITH A T-PIECE. FIO2=FRACTION OF INSPIRED OXYGEN. PEEP=POSITIVE END-EXPIRATORY PRESSURE. ETT=ENDOTRACHEAL TUBE.

- Evaluate for contraindications to apnea test, including significant hypoxemia, hypotension or cardiac arrhythmia.

- Adjust ventilator respiratory rate to achieve normocarbia.

- Pre-oxygenate the patient with 100% FiO2 and PEEP of 5 cm H20 for 10-15 minutes.

- Separate patient from mechanical ventilation.

- Attach a T-piece with a PEEP valve to the ETT. Set PEEP to 5-10 cm H20. Set oxygen flow to 15 LPM.

- Observe patient chest and abdomen for spontaneous respiratory effort for 10-15 minutes.

- If no spontaneous respiratory effort has occurred during the apnea period, draw arterial blood gas and re-connect patient to mechanical ventilation. Titrate respiratory rate to normocarbia.

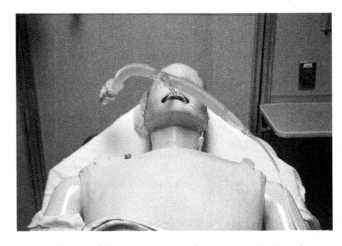

Figure 34.2 Picture of T-piece setup in simulator mannequin. Note the positive end-expiratory pressure valve placed on the distal end of the setup.

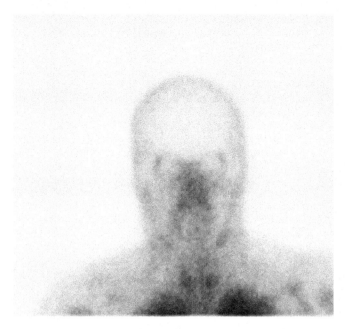

Figure 34.3 Cerebral scintigraphy scan demonstrating absence of intracranial blood flow.

and maximizing family comfort. Supporting therapies, including mechanical ventilation and medications, are withdrawn and the patient's body, after a grieving period, is moved to the morgue. If, on the other hand, the patient's body is deemed a good candidate for organ donation and the patient's family provides consent for organ donation, continued critical care for the brain dead patient's body will continue until the time of organ donation. Critical care for the brain dead patient centers around optimizing organ function until transplantation. Common goals for this phase of care include maintenance of hemodynamic stability, optimization of organ perfusion, replacement of lost endocrine function, correction of coagulopathy, and prevention of nosocomial infections.[11–14]

Hemodynamic instability frequently begins in the moments just before brain death. Many patients will experience a "sympathetic storm" during brain death and brainstem herniation.[15] This sympathetic storm typically manifests as severe hypertension with tachycardia that can lead to profound myocardial dysfunction and neurogenic pulmonary edema in the early post-brain death period.[16] Following this sympathetic storm, hypotension is common and is multifactorial, resulting from hypovolemia, left ventricular dysfunction, and loss of systemic vascular resistance.[17] Individualized patient management to optimize fluid balance, stabilize vasomotor tone through vasopressor infusions, and restore inotropic function through pharmacologic or mechanical cardiac support may require use of invasive hemodynamic monitoring techniques including echocardiography or pulmonary artery catheterization.[18-20] In addition, thyroid hormone and corticosteroid replacement therapy are commonly needed to improve hemodynamic status.

Following herniation and brain death, pituitary and hypothalamic function stops, resulting in 3 important endocrinological pathologies. First, most patients will develop diabetes insipidus (DI) from the loss of ADH secreted by the posterior pituitary and hypothalamus. DI causes severe polyuria (>300–500 mL/hr urine), hypernatremia ([Na] >160 mEq/dL), low urine specific gravity (<1.020), and very low urine osmolarity (<150 mOsm/kg). DI treatment includes fluid resuscitation, free water administration, and vasopressin infusion. The second endocrinopathy that most brain dead patients will develop is an acute corticosteroid insufficiency due to loss of adrenocorticotropic hormone release from the anterior pituitary. Steroid replacement with hydrocortisone bolus or infusion is commonly administered to donors empirically. Finally, hypothyroidism occurs from loss of thyroid stimulating hormone. Thyroid replacement with levothyroxine infusion is occasionally used, especially in patients with reduced cardiac output. Other hormones are also affected by brain death, including testosterone and estrogen; however, replacement or treatment of side effects is rarely needed.

Coagulopathy, disseminated intravascular coagulopathy (DIC), thrombocytopenia, and anemia are also regularly present in the brain dead patient. Ongoing laboratory assessment of coagulation status and transfusion of clotting factors, fibrinogen, and platelets may be required throughout the post-brain death period prior to organ donation. The benefits of blood component therapy should be balanced against their risk of inflammatory and infectious complications, as well as the potential for inducing new or additional antibodies that could limit organ transplantation. In patients with DIC, treatment with antifibrinolytic agents, including tranexamic acid or aminocaproic acid, may be used. Coagulopathy may be complicated by hypothermia that can frequently be treated with forced-air warming blankets and by increasing the room temperature.

Finally, healthcare associated infections (HAI) should be meticulously avoided and, if they are suspected or diagnosed, they should be aggressively treated to prevent additional organ system dysfunction and inflammatory injury. Pneumonia, bloodstream infections, and urinary tract infections are all common complications following brain death. Many neurologic injuries, including blunt and penetrating brain injuries, carry an additional risk of aspiration at the time of injury and secondary pneumonia that may develop during the period after brain death. Since these patients all have endotracheal tubes and require mechanical ventilation, their risk of ventilator-associated pneumonia is significant. Invasive bloodstream and urinary catheters are also frequently used in these patients and contribute to the risk of non-pneumonia HAI. Sinusitis, ventriculitis, meningitis, and wound infections are also important contributors to HAI during this period. Infections should be treated aggressively with empiric widespread antibiotics and, when possible, removal of infected catheters and foreign bodies. Significant or uncontrolled infection may make future organ transplantation impossible.

Despite appropriate critical care, some brain dead patients will continue to deteriorate and may develop cardiac arrest prior to organ harvest. Although controversial, most patients should undergo cardiopulmonary resuscitation with ACLS protocols to facilitate return of spontaneous circulation (ROSC). If ROSC is not rapidly achieved, extracorporeal life support (ECLS) may be necessary to restore perfusion to transplantable organs.[21] If ECLS is not available, patient transport to the operating room may be necessary for emergent organ harvest. Organs removed in this fashion may have reduced viability in transplanted patients.

The diagnosis of brain death has become significantly more sophisticated but remains a challenge for physicians, healthcare workers and affected family and friends. Published guidelines have attempted to provide a framework for the diagnosis and management of brain death; however, significant variation in brain death exams and interpretation, as well as disagreement concerning the use of ancillary testing, has created additional controversy. Nonetheless, a standard step-wise approach based on medical history and physical examination demonstrating the permanent loss of consciousness, voluntary responses, involuntary responses, and central reflexes is critical to the diagnosis of brain death. Following this diagnosis, the critical care management goals shift to optimizing organ function for future organ transplantation through the restoring hemodynamic stability, replacement of lost endocrine function, reversal of severe coagulopathy, and prevention of secondary healthcare-associated infections.

CONCLUSIONS

- Death is a complicated medicolegal concept that is defined by national and state laws. Brain death, the irreversible cessation of all brain function, and cardiac death, the irreversible cessation of cardiac function, are both recognized forms of death in the United States.

- Brain death is determined, primarily through clinical evaluation, after confounding factors have been excluded. The clinical evaluation of brain death includes the demonstration of a severe neurologic injury resulting in the permanent loss of consciousness (coma), voluntary responses, involuntary response, and central reflexes (including respiratory drive).

- Patients who cannot undergo full clinical evaluation for brain death or have equivocal results in their evaluation should undergo additional or ancillary testing to confirm the diagnosis of brain death. These tests including, 4-vessel cerebral angiography, SPECT scan or cerebral scintigraphy, CTA, MRA, and TCD ultrasonography to evaluate intracranial blood flow or EEG, BIS monitoring, and SSEP to evaluate the electrical activity of the brain.

- Following the diagnosis of brain death, patients who will undergo organ harvest procedures require ongoing critical care to optimize organ perfusion and viability during transplant. Common goals for this phase of care include hemodynamic stabilization and optimization, replacement of lost endocrine function, correction of coagulopathy, and prevention of nosocomial systemic infectious diseases.

REFERENCES

1. Wijdicks EF, Varelas PN, Gronseth GS, Greer DM; American Academy of Neurology. Evidence-based guideline update: determining brain death in adults: report of the Quality Standards Subcommittee of the American Academy of Neurology. Neurology. 2010;74(23):1911–1918.

2. Molina DK, McCutcheon JR, Rulon JJ. Head injuries, pentobarbital, and the determination of death. Am J Forensic Med Pathol. 2009;30(1):75–77.

3. Saposnik G, Maurino J, Saizar R, Bueri JA. Spontaneous and reflex movements in 107 patients with brain death. Am J Med. 2005;118(3):311–314.

4. Jain S, DeGeorgia M. Brain death-associated reflexes and automatisms. Neurocrit Care. 2005;3(2):122–126.

5. Levesque S, Lessard MR, Nicole PC, et al. Efficacy of a T-piece system and a continuous positive airway pressure system for apnea testing in the diagnosis of brain death. Crit Care Med. 2006;34(8):2213–2216.

6. Kramer AH, Couillard P, Bader R, Dhillon P, Kutsogiannis DJ, Doig CJ. Prevention of hypoxemia during apnea testing: a comparison of oxygen insufflation and continuous positive airway pressure. Neurocrit Care. 2017;27(1):60–67.

7. Virgile RS. Locked-in syndrome: case and literature review. Clin Neurol Neurosurg. 1984;86(4):275–279.

8. Bernard V, Van Pesch V, Hantson P. Guillain-Barre syndrome mimicking brain death pattern: a poorly reversible condition. Acta Neurol Belg. 2010;110(1):93–96.

9. Heran MK, Heran NS, Shemie SD. A review of ancillary tests in evaluating brain death. Can J Neurol Sci. 2008;35(4):409–419.

10. Munari M, Zucchetta P, Carollo C, et al. Confirmatory tests in the diagnosis of brain death: comparison between SPECT and contrast angiography. Crit Care Med. 2005;33(9):2068–2073.

11. McKeown DW, Bonser RS, Kellum JA. Management of the heartbeating brain-dead organ donor. Br J Anaesth. 2012;108(Suppl 1):i96–i107.

12. Kotloff RM, Blosser S, Fulda GJ, et al. Management of the potential organ donor in the ICU: Society of Critical Care Medicine/American College of Chest Physicians/Association of Organ Procurement Organizations consensus statement. Crit Care Med. 2015;43(6):1291–1325.

13. Malinoski DJ, Daly MC, Patel MS, Oley-Graybill C, Foster CE, 3rd, Salim A. Achieving donor management goals before deceased donor procurement is associated with more organs transplanted per donor. J Trauma. 2011;71(4):990–995; discussion: 996.

14. Salim A, Velmahos GC, Brown C, Belzberg H, Demetriades D. Aggressive organ donor management significantly increases the number of organs available for transplantation. J Trauma. 2005;58(5):991–994.

15. Smith M. Physiologic changes during brain stem death--lessons for management of the organ donor. J Heart Lung Transplant. 2004;23(9 Suppl):S217–S222.

16. Audibert G, Charpentier C, Seguin-Devaux C, et al. Improvement of donor myocardial function after treatment of autonomic storm during brain death. Transplantation. 2006;82(8):1031–1036.

17. Mohamedali B, Bhat G, Tatooles A, Zelinger A. Neurogenic stress cardiomyopathy in heart donors. J Card Fail. 2014;20(3):207–211.

18. Casartelli M, Bombardini T, Simion D, Gaspari MG, Procaccio F. Wait, treat and see: echocardiographic monitoring of brain-dead potential donors with stunned heart. Cardiovasc Ultrasound. 2012;10:25.

19. Venkateswaran RV, Townend JN, Wilson IC, Mascaro JG, Bonser RS, Steeds RP. Echocardiography in the potential heart donor. Transplantation. 2010;89(7):894–901.

20. Dujardin KS, McCully RB, Wijdicks EF, et al. Myocardial dysfunction associated with brain death: clinical, echocardiographic, and pathologic features. J Heart Lung Transplant. 2001;20(3):350–357.

21. Fan X, Chen Z, Nasralla D, et al. The organ preservation and enhancement of donation success ratio effect of extracorporeal membrane oxygenation in circulatory unstable brain death donor. Clin Transplant. 2016;30(10):1306–1313.

REVIEW QUESTIONS

1. Which of the following is *most* consistent with a diagnosis of diabetes insipidus in brain dead patients?

    A. Urine osmolality = 500 mOsm/kg

    B. Urine specific gravity = 1.001

C. Urine output = 0.5 mL/kg/hr for 6 hours
D. Random urine sodium concentration = 100 mEq/L

2. Which of the following confounding factors should be routinely excluded before clinical brain death testing?

A. Hyperkalemia
B. Oliguria
C. Hypoglycemia
D. Anemia

3. During clinical brain death testing, a 19-year-old female has nystagmus when cold water is installed into her right ear but not her left ear. Which of the following is the correct interpretation of this finding?

A. Brain death
B. Residual neuromuscular blocking (NMB) drug action
C. Intact central reflex
D. Hypermagnesemia

4. During clinical brain-death testing, a 45-year-old patient does not respond to visual or verbal stimuli but has flexion at the hip, knee, and ankle in response to painful stimulation of the lower extremity. Which of the following is the *most* appropriate next action?

A. Discontinue clinical brain death testing since the patient moved during examination
B. Administer NMB drug to abolish confounding movement
C. Repeat urine drug screen to exclude residual CNS depressant drug effect
D. Continue clinical brain death testing and consider additional or ancillary testing if confusion about cause of lower extremity movement persists

5. Which of the following is an essential component to the diagnosis of brain death?

A. Identification of reversible nature of brain injury
B. Involvement of cortical structures only
C. Loss of central reflexes
D. Determination by single clinical examination as early as possible after injury

6. Which of the following is the most appropriate patient for additional or ancillary brain death testing?

A. A 70-year-old patient who has cardiopulmonary arrest and does not have return of spontaneous circulation after 30 minutes of care according to ACLS protocols
B. A 19-year-old patient with severe traumatic brain injury and uncal herniation according to radiographic imaging and who has persistent loss of consciousness, loss of voluntary and involuntary responses, and loss of central reflexes and does not breath during an apnea test, according to clinical examination by 2 different clinicians.
C. A 45-year-old patient with Guillain-Barre syndrome who cannot move upper or lower extremities due

to increasing neuromotor weakness over the past several days
D. A 25-year-old patient with severe penetrating brain injury by radiographic imaging who has required emergent operation for irrigation and debridement of his wound, as well as enucleation of his left eye

7. Following the diagnosis of brain death, a 23-year-old male with severe traumatic brain injury and uncal herniation develops complications related to diabetes insipidus. Which of the following is the most appropriate therapy to restore appropriate hemodynamic and renal function?

A. Epinephrine
B. Vasopressin
C. Norepinephrine
D. Dopamine

8. A 35-year-old female becomes hypotensive despite fluid resuscitation and norepinephrine infusion following brain death following severe traumatic brain injury. Which of the following should be administered to restore normal hemodynamic status?

A. Estrogen
B. Hydrocortisone
C. Antidiuretic hormone
D. Growth hormone

9. A brain dead patient being worked up for organ harvest develops ventricular fibrillation. Which of the following is the *most* appropriate therapy for this patient?

A. Start chest compressions and prepare for defibrillation following ACLS protocols to establish return of spontaneous circulation
B. Inform the organ procurement organization that the patient has suffered cardiac arrest and that the patient can now no longer be an organ donor
C. Immediately institute ECLS to restore organ perfusion
D. Transport the patient to the operating room for emergency organ harvest procedures

10. Approximately 3 minutes after the start of apnea testing of a patient with severe traumatic brain injury, she develops cardiac arrhythmias and hypotension. She had previously demonstrated persistent loss of consciousness, loss of voluntary and involuntary response, and loss of central reflexes. After terminating the apnea test, which of the following is the *most* appropriate next therapy?

A. Pronounce the patient brain dead as she has demonstrated loss of all essential components of the clinical brain death examination
B. Discontinue brain death examination and continue care of this patient until cardiac death has occurred
C. Wait 5 minutes and attempt apnea test with lower fraction of inspired oxygen (FiO2)
D. Order additional or ancillary tests to confirm the diagnosis of brain death

ANSWERS

1. B. Diabetes insipidus is common following brain death due to the loss of ADH release from the posterior pituitary. DI is commonly diagnosed in patients with polyuria and laboratory assessment of low urine specific gravity, low urine osmolality, and low urine sodium concentration. The answer B is correct because urine specific gravity = 1.001 is very low. Answer A is not correct because urine osmolality = 500 mOsm/kg is not low enough to meet diagnostic criteria, typically < 350 mOsm/kg. Answer C is not correct because urine output = 0.5 mL/kg/hr for 6 hours is the definition of oliguria, not polyuria. Answer D is not correct because random urine sodium concentration = 100 mEq/L is not low and does not fulfill diagnostic criteria, typically < 20 mEq/L.

2. C. During brain death testing, confounding factors should be excluded prior to the start of clinical examination. Common confounding factors include hypothermia, hypotension, electrolyte and metabolic disturbances, residual CNS depressing drugs or NMB drugs. Answer C is therefore correct because hypoglycemia is a confounding endocrine or metabolic disturbance that should be excluded prior to clinical brain death examination. Answer A is not correct because hyperkalemia, while a metabolic disturbance, does not confound clinical brain death examination. Answer B is not correct because oliguria is not a confounder for clinical brain death examination. Likewise, Answer D is not correct because anemia is not a confounder of clinical brain death examination.

3. C. During clinical brain death testing, the vestibulo-ocular reflex should be tested by instillation of cold water into each ear. If brain dead, the patient will have no eye movement from this action; however, if eyes move (typically, by deviating to the ipsalateral side) with nystagmus to the opposite side, this is a sign of an intact vestibulo-ocular reflex (answer C). Answer A is not correct because the diagnosis of brain death requires loss of all central reflexes, including the vestibulo-ocular reflex. Answer B is not correct because residual NMB drug would cause loss of reflexes secondary to neuromuscular weakness, not nystagmus. Answer D is not correct because hypermagnesemia does not typically cause nystagmus.

4. D. During clinical brain death examination, painful stimuli should be applied to all 4 extremities. When painful stimuli is applied to the lower extremities, spinal reflexes, including the so-called triple flexion reflex, may occur. In this reflex, flexion occurs at the hip, knee, and ankle in response to spinal reflexes that do not involve brain responses. Patients with this triple flexion reflex may still be diagnosed with brain death according to clinical criteria; however, additional or ancillary testing may still be ordered if there is confusion about the cause of lower extremity movement. Answer A is not correct because this triple flexion reflex does not preclude the diagnosis of brain death by clinical examination. Answer B is not correct because NMB drugs should never be administered during clinical brain death examination. Answer C is not correct because CNS depressant drugs would not generally be present in the urine drug screen after initial negative testing.

5. C. Brain death is characterized by the irreversible cessation of all brain functions. The essential components of brain death in patients with known and severe neurologic injury are persistent loss of consciousness (coma); loss of voluntary and involuntary responses to visual, verbal, and painful stimuli; and loss of central reflexes, including respiratory drive in patients without confounding factors. Answer C is correct because loss of central reflexes is an essential component in the diagnosis of brain death. Answer A is incorrect because brain death patients must have an *irreversible* brain injury. Answer B is incorrect because all areas of the brain must have irreversible loss of function, including cortical, cerebral, and central nerves. Answer D is not correct because clinical examination should be performed by 2 clinicians and only after sufficient time has passed from the injury to demonstrate persistence of clinical examination findings..

6. D. Additional or ancillary brain death testing is indicated for patients with unclear clinical brain death examination findings or for patients who have confounding factors that cannot be excluded. Patients who are not able to demonstrate loss of bilateral central reflexes should also undergo additional or ancillary brain death testing once clinical examination has been shown to be consistent with brain death in all other tests. Answer D is most correct because surgical enucleation prevents testing of several bilateral central reflexes. Answer A is not correct because this patient has experienced cardiac death. Answer B is not correct because this patient has completed clinical examinations consistent with brain death. Answer C is not correct because this patient has a diagnosis of Guillain-Barre disease, a confounding disease that causes neuromuscular paralysis rather than brain death.

7. B. DI is a common clinical problem following brain death. DI occurs secondary to loss of ADH. Vasopressin is a synthetic analogue of ADH, and vasopressin infusion is used to treat DI in patients with brain death. For this reason, answer B is the correct answer. The other vasopressors, including epinephrine (answer A), norepinephrine (answer C), and dopamine (answer D), are not used to treat DI in brain dead patients.

8. B. Distributive shock occurs in brain dead patients due to loss of corticosteroid secretion from the adrenal glands secondary to loss of adrenocorticotropic hormone from the anterior pituitary gland. Following fluid resuscitation and norepinephrine infusion, hydrocortisone (answer B) should be administered to replace lost steroid secretion after brain death. The secretion of other hormones, including estrogen (answer A), antidiuretic hormone (answer C), and growth hormone (answer D) will also be lost; however, they are not routinely replaced to correct distributive shock.

9. A. Brain dead patients who develop cardiac arrest while awaiting organ harvest procedures should, unless otherwise requested by family order or organ procurement organization, be resuscitated using routine ACLS protocols. In this case, immediate chest compressions and preparation for early defibrillation (answer A) would be the most appropriate therapy for ventricular fibrillation. Answer B is not correct because patients who have cardiac arrest remain potential organ donors, provided that adequate organ function is maintained.

Answer C is not correct because ECLS is indicated only when return of spontaneous circulation (ROSC) has not been successful through traditional ACLS protocols. Similarly, answer D is not correct because transportation of the patient to the operating room for emergency organ harvest procedures is not indicated unless ROSC has not been successful through traditional ACLS protocols.

10. D. The apnea test is a critical care part of the clinical brain death examination. In this test, the patient is removed from mechanical ventilation and monitored for spontaneous respirations for a 10- to 15-minute period. If patients cannot tolerate apnea testing, additional or ancillary testing should be ordered. Answer D is most correct because additional testing would be most appropriate when apnea testing is aborted. Answer A is not correct because brain death cannot be determined clinically without apnea testing. Answer B is not correct because brain death can still be determined without apnea testing if additional or ancillary testing is consistent with brain death. Answer C is not correct because waiting 5 minutes and lowering FiO2 is likely to exacerbate the underlying arrhythmia and may make apnea testing more difficult.

35.

ETHICS IN CRITICAL CARE

Paul D. Weyker and Alessandro R. DeCamilli

STEM CASE AND KEY QUESTIONS

A 63-year-old man with a history of hypertension, chronic hepatitis C, and chronic kidney disease presents to a surgeon's clinic with his wife for evaluation of a 1.4 cm head of pancreas tumor suspected to be adenocarcinoma. Preoperative laboratory results are significant for a creatinine of 2.3 and a hemoglobin of 8.3 mg/dL. All other studies are within normal limits. An abdominal computed tomography (CT) scan shows no evidence of enlarged lymph nodes but shows the tumor may come in contact with the portal vein. The patient informs the surgeon that he is a practicing Jehovah's Witness and will not accept transfusion of blood products.

WHAT IS THE NEXT MOST APPROPRIATE STEP FOR THE SURGEON TO TAKE?

The surgeon proceeds with informed consent, discussing the high likelihood of blood loss during the procedure and the physiologic ramifications for not providing blood transfusions. Among other potential complications, the surgeon explains the risks of renal failure, myocardial ischemia, stroke, and death. In accordance with his religious beliefs, the patient is adamant that he would rather die than receive a blood transfusion. To clarify further, the surgeon goes through a complete list of blood products including red blood cells, fresh frozen plasma, platelets, and albumin, all of which are harvested from human donor sources. The refusal of these products is documented in detail in the surgeon's note.

At this point the surgeon politely asks the wife to leave the exam room to perform the physical exam. During the physical exam the surgeon again asks the patient in privacy to confirm his desire to abstain from blood transfusions. The patient once again reaffirms his strong refusal to accept human transfusion products.

WHY IS IT IMPORTANT FOR THE SURGEON TO ASK ABOUT BLOOD TRANSFUSION WITHOUT THE WIFE PRESENT?

Prior to scheduling a date for the surgery, the surgeon then consults a hematologist for optimization of blood counts and coagulation prior to surgery and schedules an appointment in the preanesthesiology clinic so the patient can meet with an anesthesiologist.

WHY ARE THESE APPROPRIATE CONSULTATIONS PRIOR TO SCHEDULING SURGERY FOR THIS PATIENT? WHY SHOULD THE ANESTHESIOLOGY DEPARTMENT BE MADE AWARE OF THIS CASE EARLY IN THE PROCESS?

On the day of surgery, an anesthesiologist who is comfortable with the patient's care limitations meets the patient for the first time and discusses informed consent for the anesthetic and supportive care during the procedure. The anesthesiologist again confirms and documents the list of human-derived, blood-related products that the patient will not accept. The patient also is unwilling to accept cell reclamation techniques (i.e., Cellsaver™) or acute, normovolemic hemodilution as his interpretation of his faith is that even his own blood cannot be separated from his body and then given back. The patient's starting hemoglobin is noted to be to 10 mg/dL on the morning of surgery as the patient was not compliant with the preoperative hematology recommendations. Anesthesia is induced without incident, and a right internal jugular central venous catheter and a radial arterial catheter are placed after intubation for the purpose of fluid administration and hemodynamic monitoring. During the surgery, the tumor is noted to be invading the porta hepatis structures and is firmly adherent to the portal vein. The surgeon decides he will need to perform a portal vein reconstruction. To do so, he harvests the patient's left internal jugular vein and proceeds with the resection. During the course of the surgery the patient loses about 3.5 L of blood, which is replaced with crystalloid solution to prevent hypotension but as judiciously as possible to prevent excessive dilution of the patient's cell counts and coagulation factors. The patient's blood pressure is supported with an infusion of norepinephrine, and at the end of the procedure the decision is made not to attempt mechanical liberation. Instead, he is transferred to the intensive care unit (ICU) sedated, intubated, and supported by vasoactive medications and a ventilator.

WOULD IT HAVE BEEN REASONABLE TO DENY THIS PATIENT SURGERY IF THE SURGEON FELT THERE WAS A HIGH POSSIBILITY OF BLOOD LOSS?

In the ICU, the patient requires moderately high doses of norepinephrine to maintain and adequate perfusion pressure. It is also noted that the patient is oliguric soon after arrival to the ICU. Initial lab tests in the ICU reveal the patient's hemoglobin is now 4.1 mg/dL and the arterial lactate is 8 mmol/L. The initial postoperative evening, patient becomes anuric, and over the course of postoperative day 1, the patient's creatinine doubles and the potassium level begins to rise aggressively. The hemoglobin continues to downtrend to 3.8 mg/dL, and the patient's family is updated about the grim prognosis.

SHOULD DIALYSIS BE OFFERED TO THIS PATIENT?

The intensivist and nephrologist both agree that the worsening acute kidney injury and resultant electrolyte imbalance can only be treated with emergent dialysis at this point. However, dialysis will further worsen the patient's already critical anemia to a level that is unsurvivable. The intensivist and nephrologist call in the family to update them again that his kidneys "have shut down" possibly due to the lack of oxygen delivery as a result of the patient's severe anemia. The family, like the patient preoperatively, agree to continue treatment without a blood transfusion but remain adamant that they want "everything else done."

The family requests that the patient be placed on dialysis, but the intensivist and consultant nephrologist do not offer dialysis as a treatment option as they deem it to be "futile" given his rapidly worsening anemia. At this point the intensivist discusses code status and recommends that they change his code status to "Do Not Resuscitate" (DNR). However, the family continues to request that everything be done.

DOES THE FAMILY HAVE THE RIGHT TO REFUSE THE CHANGE IN CODE STATUS IF THE TREATING PHYSICIANS AGREE THAT CARE IS FUTILE?

The following day that patient has a pulseless electrical activity arrest. Despite 20 minutes of high-quality advanced cardiac life support, the patient dies.

DISCUSSION

The Jehovah's Witness religion started in the late 1800s, after the realization of transfusions as a life-saving medical procedure but long before it was common proactive or blood blanking had begun. It was not in until the mid-twentieth century in 1945 that the Zion's Watch Tower Bible and Tract Society of Pennsylvania (often simply referred to as The Watch Tower Society), the governing body of the Jehovah's Witness religious organization, made rules banning members from receiving transfusion of blood products. While most observant Jehovah's Witness do not accept whole or component blood therapy, a growing number of individuals will accept laboratory-created or separated coagulation factors and colloid-based transfused products like albumin.

Prior to any medical procedure, it is important to ascertain if a patient demonstrates appropriate decision-making capacity and understanding of his or her choices. The surgeon must ensure a thorough informed consent, with all the risks, benefits, and alternatives discussed. As such, it would seem most appropriate the patient's surgeon should initiate this discussion as the patient has specifically had the opportunity to choose a practitioner to care for him or her. It is important that complete documentation of specific products that patient refuses to and, more importantly, is willing to accept be included in the preoperative notes.

Informed consent has essential components. The first is that the patient is able to comprehend medical information relevant to his or her care—this assessment must be made by the physician. In this case, the patient must have a general concept of the role of blood in supporting vital organ function and how severe anemia can result in organ dysfunction and death. The information should be conveyed sensitively but factually. Access to medical information has evolved over the last decade such that patients now have a wealth of access to informed medical sources. Each Kingdom Hall of Jehovah's Witnesses has a body of elders to help members with decisions regarding their faith. Additionally, The Watch Tower Society has a plethora of informational material available on its website and offers phone and in-person support for medical decisions. It is the role of the physician to help the patient navigate these sources and help provide meaningful perspective. It is important to ask which sources a patient has evaluated prior to any discussion so as to the vet the quality of the information on which the foundation learning has been built. For example, a patient who is well-read on the burgeoning field of robotic hernia repairs in minimizing postoperative pain and early ambulation may not realize that severe lung disease and a history of cerebral aneurysms conveys a massive increase in risk that can be ameliorated by simple doing a classic, open inguinal herniorrhaphy.

Next, the risks, benefits, and alternatives should be stated clearly and thoroughly, and while it is important not to unduly scare a patient, sugarcoating the situation will provide a false sense of security. In this case, the consequences of not receiving blood, including death, should be stated clearly and succinctly. Avoid euphemisms like "pass" or "not thrive," which can sow confusion when clarity is of the utmost importance. Patients should not be coerced, and physicians should also not use complex medical language to persuade the patient into agreement. A common scenario that may arise in the setting of serious, multiorgan illness is the "list of options" that are presented to a patient by the clinical team. Take the common example of a patient with metastatic cancer in the ICU facing the need for dialysis and a gastrostomy tube. While it is important for a physician to present options, it is also important to serve as a steward for navigating complex decision-making. Rather than sharing a list of options, a physician might instead discuss overall goals of care and recommend a pathway to achieve these goals and how each procedure would fit into such a scenario.

It is also important that the patient is free from coercion by others, including family members, friends, or spiritual advisors. While a patient may prefer to have a full discussion with family/friends/advisor present, it is incumbent upon the physician to reassess the patient's wishes while he or she is alone. It is true that some patients, including Jehovah's Witnesses, may be willing to accept transfusions if the family members are not present and will not be told about it. This in itself can add another layer of ethical cloudiness to these discussions, especially given the implications of what it could mean for the patient if his or her family, friends, or spiritual advisors find out. Again, respect for patient autonomy and nonmaleficence are brought to the forefront.

PREOPERATIVE MODIFICATION OF RISK

Optimization of the patient prior to undergoing a potentially high-risk surgery is of utmost importance. Preoperative hematologist consultation can recommend interventions to help optimize hemoglobin levels prior to the day of surgery utilizing iron supplementation and even erythropoietin derivatives, but these can take several weeks for full benefit. A simple adaptation to operating room setup, such as keeping a patient's blood "in continuity" with his or her body via tubing, is an option that Jehovah's Witnesses may accept and allows for the use of normovolemic hemodilution or red cell reclamation techniques. Intraoperative use of desmopressin and tranexamic acid may also be indicated, despite their intrinsic risks, to limit bleeding in patients where anemia could carry a risk of death. New technologies in bovine hemoglobin extracts can be administered to increase the oxygen-carrying capacity of blood; however, most of these products remain in the experimental phase and can be hard to obtain. A discussion between the surgeon, oncologist, and hematologist can weigh the risks of procedural delay and tumor progression against the benefits of preoperative optimization.

Additionally, the patient should be referred to the anesthesiology department for further discussion regarding intraoperative management. Reassurance is often needed that a patient's specific limitations to care will be followed. As a corollary to patient autonomy, it is not unreasonable for an anesthesiologist to refuse to participate in the care of a patient in which restrictions on transfusion might be seen as a "death sentence." Respecting the patient's sovereignty may contradict the physician's own guiding ethical principle of nonmaleficence, creating a personal moral impasse. This case has long been argued professionally by anesthesiologists, as well as legally in some states. In general, it is believed that a patient's choice is paramount and transfusion against the will of a person, even if life-saving, is in direct contradiction to that person's autonomy. However, if a provider does not feel ethically comfortable withholding potentially life-saving treatment, he or she should not be forced to provide such care. Therefore, careful planning ahead of time can ensure that an anesthesiologist who is comfortable caring for these patients is assigned to the procedure.

A situation may arise in which the patient does not wish to disclose his or her willingness to receive blood to his or her spouse, and patient privacy should be respected. This wish should be carried out, as it represents the patient's own will and respects autonomy. The more ethically challenging case is the case of a pediatric Jehovah's Witness who refuses blood

transfusion. In such situations, consent is left to the parent or legal guardian, as the minor may not legally consent for him- or herself. The parent or guardian, who may not consent for blood on similarly religious grounds, is putting the child in serious danger. In a situation where the physician feels that a parent is not deciding in a child's best interest, a court order can be sought. Parents and guardians, regardless of the motive, cannot make choices that result in direct harm to their children, and it would be unethical to carry out such choices. Currently, case law in regards to transfusion refusal for a minor by a guardian is a state-based decision and should be discussed prior to performing procedures.

CONCLUSION

This case illustrates a common conflict in medical ethics between patient autonomy and physician nonmaleficence. Patient autonomy is essential and relies on the ability of a patient to rationally comprehend medical information including risks, benefits, and alternatives. A patient's decision-making takes into consideration cultural, religious, and socioeconomic factors that are beyond the ethical scope of physicians to exert influence. The role of the physician is not to coerce a patient but to serve as a guide, melding the patient's goals with a reasonable course of action. If a physician feels the course of action takes on elevated risk, this risk should be clearly communicated, an appropriate discourse held, and final decisions documented so all providers are aware. If the physician feels it is not compatible with safe care, the physician may ethically recuse him- or herself and attempt to transition care to another provider. Such situations may arise in which a patient or a family requests a potentially futile treatment or refutes a life-saving treatment. In the case of refusal, if the patient is a minor or unable to make medical decisions, a surrogate should be sought. If the surrogate makes a decision that a physician feels to be unreasonably harmful, a court order may be sought, and each state's own legal precedence will guide the outcome.

As medicine becomes increasingly super-subspecialized, as scientific and medical information becomes more easily accessible to patients, and as novel medical care for critically ill patients pushes to new frontiers, the role of the physician is ever-changing. The paternalistic era of doctoring where physicians took charge of what was "best" for their patients with its potential for religious, gender, or behavioral bias has given way to one of autonomy. However, it is important to preserve the physician's role as an expert guide through this complex landscape and work hard to align a patient's goals with treatment options that are respectful, reasonable, and not futile.

REFERENCES

105th Congress Report, House of Representatives. Aviation Medical Assistance Act of 1998. House of Representatives; 1998.
American Medical Association Education. AMA principles of medical ethics. American Medical Association; 2016. https://www.ama-assn.org/sites/default/files/media-browser/principles-of-medical-ethics

American Medical Association Education. Sedation to unconsciousness in end-of-life care. American Medical Association; 2017. https://www.ama-assn.org/delivering-care/sedation-unconsciousness-end-life-care

Cho B, et al. Impact of preoperative erythropoietin on allogeneic blood transfusions in surgical patients: results from a systematic review and meta-analysis. *Anesthes Analges*. 2019 May;128(5):981–992.

Gabbay E, Meyer KB. Identifying critically ill patients with acute kidney injury for whom renal replacement therapy is inappropriate: an exercise in futility? *NDT Plus*. 2009;2(2):97–103.

Lin ES, Kaye AD, Baluch AR. Preanesthetic assessment of the Jehovah's Witness patient. *Ochsner J*. 2012;12(1):61–69.

Lawson T, Ralph C. Perioperative Jehovah's Witnesses: a review. *Brit J Anaesth*. 2015;115(5):676–687. https://doi.org/10.1093/bja/aev161

Quill TE, Brody H. Physician recommendations and patient autonomy: finding a balance between physician power and patient choice. *Ann Intern Med*. 1996;125(9):763.

West JM. Ethical issues in the care of Jehovah's Witnesses. *Curr Opin Anaesthesiol*. 2014;27(2):170–176.

REVIEW QUESTIONS

1. An anesthesiologist is called to assist with airway management for a patient who is currently undergoing chest compressions. Upon chart review, it is noted that the patient's code status is do not intubate. Which of the following ethical principles *most* supports the anesthesiologist's decision to not intubate the patient?

A. Autonomy
B. Beneficence
C. Nonmaleficence
D. Justice

Answer: A. Autonomy is the right of the patient to make decisions about his or her own treatment. Advanced directives allow patients to exert their autonomy even when they are not capable of making decisions at the time.

2. A 32-year-old female who is 36 hours status-post a pregnancy termination performed at 18 weeks gestation presents to the emergency room with fever, rigor, and hypotension. She is started on appropriate antibiotics and scheduled for an emergent dilation and curettage. The anesthesiologist on call has religious objections to abortion. It is 3 AM and there are no other anesthesiologists in house. What is the appropriate course of action?

A. Delay the procedure until another anesthesiologist who is comfortable with abortion procedures can staff the case
B. Arrange to have the case performed under nurse-administered sedation
C. Perform the case regardless of religious objection due to its emergent status
D. Arrange for emergent transfer to an outside facility that can provide the procedure without religious objection

Answer: C. According to the American Medical Association's Guideline for the Ethical Practice of Medicine, "A physician shall, in the provision of appropriate patient care except in emergencies, be free to choose whom to serve, with whom to associate and the environment in which to provide medical care." In this emergent case, delay of care or substandard care would harm the patient and thus not be ethical. It would only be ethical to change cases or assignments if there were appropriate and available staff to do so. Source: https://www.ama-assn.org/sites/default/files/media-browser/principles-of-medical-ethics.pdf

3. A patient presents for an open pancreatectomy. After a thorough discussion about the risks and benefits of a thoracic epidural, she declines to have it performed. She understands the explanation of multimodal analgesia and accepts the risk of higher postoperative opiate use. The attending anesthesiologist is accustomed to performing these procedures using epidurals and is concerned about difficult-to-manage postoperative pain. The surgeon reminds the anesthesiologist that there have been several recent studies showing that epidural use decreases the risk of postoperative ileus and decreases length of stay. The appropriate course of action is to

A. Return with the surgeon and relate her favorable experience with epidurals for postoperative pain management in an attempt to convince the patient this is her best option.
B. Restate that the risks of permanent nerve injury are almost nonexistent and that she should not be dissuaded by such concerns.
C. Relay several anecdotes of patients with favorable epidural experiences and state that "I would have an epidural done for myself in this situation."
D. Suggest to the patient that she will be heavily sedated for the procedure, so she won't feel any pain or discomfort, and that this is the standard protocol.
E. Respect the patient's wishes.

Answer: E. Physicians should respect patients' rights to self-determination. Provided the patient has decision-making capacity and has been given thorough and evidence-based risks, benefits, and alternatives, physicians should not use their medical expertise to coerce patients into a procedure.

4. An elderly patient with metastatic pancreatic cancer is in the ICU with a small bowel obstruction, pneumonia, and severe, intractable pain. After a multidisciplinary discussion with the patient and his surrogates, a decision is made to transition to comfort measures only. The patient is in severe, distressing pain. He is started on an infusion of fentanyl and midazolam, and his pain is only manageable on doses that make him minimally responsive. Which of the following does *not* apply to palliative sedation?

A. Consultation with a palliative care team should occur to ensure that appropriate symptom-specific pain control is being addressed and that palliative sedation to unconsciousness is the most appropriate course of treatment.
B. Sedation can be titrated to visceral and somatic pain.
C. Sedation can be increased if appropriate even in the setting of bradypnea.

D. Sedation can be provided to cope with existential despair and family distress.

E. Sedation titrated to unconsciousness should be restricted for the final stages of terminal illness.

Answer: D. It is the duty of the physician to relieve pain and suffering from terminal disease. In the appropriate clinical scenario, it may be necessary to treat refractory pain in the end stages of life with sedation titrated to unconsciousness. However, such sedation should be symptom guided and guided by physicians trained in palliative care. A multidisciplinary team consisting of personnel able to provide psychotherapy, emotional support, and spiritual guidance should be provided to cope with nonclinical sources of suffering such as existential despair, sense of loss of control, and family distress. Source: https://www.ama-assn.org/delivering-care/sedation-unconsciousness-end-life-care

5. A 32-year-old male who suffered a self-inflicted gunshot wound is in the ICU. Magnetic resonance imaging confirms diffuse cerebral edema, and a neurologist has deemed his degree of damage unrecoverable. A family is assembled to discuss end-of-life issues. When it comes to organ donation, which of the following is true?

A. Physicians who are involved in the organ donation process may be involved in end-of-life decision-making or the decision to withdraw care.

B. The primary medical team should broach the topic of organ donation.

C. It is acceptable to adhere to a "protocol" of organ support including intravenous fluids, blood pressure management, and electrolyte management to a patient on "comfort measures only" whose family has accepted organ donation.

D. The donation of organs should be discussed before the decision has been made to withdraw life-sustaining treatment, so that potential donor organ viability can be maximized.

Answer: C. There is an established set of physiologic parameters that the United Network for Organ Sharing has outlined for the preservation of deceased brain donors to preserve organ viability. It is ethical and optimal to enact these therapies in such patients, provided it does not conflict with other care goals and the patient's surrogates have accepted donation. It is important to ensure that healthcare professionals who are providing care at the end of life are not responsible for procuring organs. To prevent conflict of interest, these should be distinct from the primary medical team. The discussion of donation should be done after the decision to transition to comfort measures only, unless the patient's surrogates bring up the issue independently. It is important to balance the obligation to increase the supply of donor organs (justice) with the interests of the individual patient (beneficence). Source: https://www.unos.org/wp-content/uploads/unos/Critical_Pathway.pdf

6. To which of the following situations is a physician *not* ethically bound?

A. Reporting an elderly patient to the Department of Motor Vehicles (DMV) who has impaired vision and hearing who the physician feels to be unfit to drive and who has refused to stop driving

B. Reporting a patient with a new diagnosis of HIV to the Centers for Disease Control and Prevention

C. Reporting a case of suspected elder abuse to the police

D. Mandating the use of birth control in a female patient of child-bearing age with a severe congenital heart condition

Answer: D. The physician should have a thorough discussion concerning the risks of childbirth to her and her baby's health but is not mandated nor encouraged to mandate birth control methods. In a patient with decision-making capacity who is informed, this would be a violation of autonomy. Physicians should assess elderly patients on an individual, case-by-case basis for fitness to drive. The patient in answer choice A is clearly unfit and should be counseled and reported to the DMV. Using their best professional judgment, providers can anonymously report patients who are unable to drive to the DMV. However, the first step is to tactfully discuss this risk with the patient and his or her family and devise a fair plan. Most sexually transmitted infections (STIs) are reportable and vary on a state by state basis. The most common reportable STIs are HIV and syphilis. Elder abuse and child abuse are conditions under which physicians are legally required as well as ethically bound to report.

7. A 16-year-old patient and his mother are in the preoperative clinic discussing planned resection of a tibial tumor. According to the surgeon, there is a greater than 50% chance of requiring a blood transfusion, and, according to the oncologist, resection is the only viable option. The mother and son will not consent to a blood transfusion due to religious preferences. In this situation, the medical team should

A. Accept this preference, proceed with the surgery, and not transfuse the patient under any circumstances.

B. Deem the patient nonoperative due to refusal of a blood transfusion.

C. Attempt to obtain a court order before surgery to transfuse the child's blood if the situation becomes life-threatening.

D. Proceed with the surgery and transfuse the child if necessary, despite the preference, because the child is a minor and cannot consent for himself.

Answer: C. It is generally acceptable in this clinical scenario to seek a court order to transfuse blood. For obvious reasons, a life-saving blood transfusion is of benefit to the child. It poses minimal risk, is very efficacious, and has no viable alternative. What distinguishes this case from an adult case is that the child is a minor and cannot consent for himself. However, adults cannot choose to be responsible for the death of their children, regardless of religious beliefs. Source: https://adc.bmj.com/content/90/7/715

8. A 76-year-old female with metastatic ovarian cancer is admitted to the medical ICU with shortness of breath. CT

scan shows evidence of widely metastatic disease and innumerable pulmonary nodules. The oncology team states there are no chemotherapeutic or radiation options. The surgical team states she is not a candidate for surgery due to her widely metastatic disease. She is on high-flow oxygen and cannot lay flat. She has gone into renal failure now with indications for dialysis due to hyperkalemia. The nephrology team agrees with the ICU team that there is no utility to dialysis, and it would only carry discomfort and risk. The patient cannot tolerate the Trendelenburg position. The family would like all aggressive measures done and are adamantly requesting dialysis. They say that if dialysis is refused, they will transfer care to another facility. Which of the following is *not* a correct course of action for the intensivist?

A. Reassure the patient and surrogates that while all other medical therapies will be continued, dialysis will not be offered due to medical futility, risk, and pain.
B. Discuss transfer with another nearby institution that will perform dialysis.
C. Consult the ethics committee for further guidance.
D. Perform dialysis at the family's request and document disapproval and medical futility.

Answer: D. Patients and their surrogates often request interventions at the end-of-life that are deemed by the physician to be futile. These situations can be difficult to navigate because they require balancing respect for patient's autonomy and the desire to avoid unnecessary harm. They can also threaten the patient/family relationship. Physicians should only offer interventions that are felt to be medically appropriate. Dialysis was determined by the intensivist and nephrologist in this case to be medically inappropriate for a number of legitimate reasons—they should thus not proceed with it. However, it is reasonable to consult the ethics committee in such challenging cases. It is also acceptable and not uncommon practice to arrange for second opinions or transfers to outside hospitals, within clinical feasibility. There is no single definition for "futility" that applies to all patients and all providers.

9. A patient is interested in enrolling in a double-blind, placebo-controlled trial to test a new blood glucose lowering agent. Which of the following is *not* an ethical practice in research recruitment?

A. Offering small financial compensation to physicians for recruiting patients to studies
B. Explaining any conflicts of interest applicable to the physician performing the study
C. Engaging in randomized trials in emergency or life-threatening scenarios
D. Describing the likelihood of therapeutic benefit in the consent process
E. Administering a placebo labeled as a study drug

Answer: A. It is unethical to accept financial reward for recruitment of patients to clinical trials, as this would represent a conflict of financial interest. It is acceptable to be paid for involvement in research in other capacities, but payment should not exceed efforts or time spent on the projects. The consent process for enrolling a patient in a trial includes describing any potential benefit or harm of the study drug, the likelihood of therapeutic benefit, disclosing any conflict of interest, alternatives to the trial, and the exact nature of the drug and proposed mechanism of benefit. Physicians should make clear their role as researchers and how this differs from their role as clinicians. Randomized controlled trials may be conducted in life-threatening scenarios without informed consent, provided a set of ethical guidelines are upheld and there are not major deviations from standards of care.

10. A 46-year-old male suffers a prolonged seizure while aboard a domestic flight. A physician on board is called to the scene, and a nurse begins to provide jaw thrust support and calls for the first-aid kit, which contains anti-epileptic drugs. A physician is called to the scene and told that the first-aid kit contains an intubation kit and anti-epileptic drugs. Which of the following is *not* an appropriate course of action?

A. The physician refuses to administer the anti-epileptic because she is not readily familiar with the dosing regimen.
B. The physician refuses to provide care because she has had a glass of wine.
C. The physician assists with airway support but states that an emergency landing is necessary for further care.
D. The physician refuses to help, stating that she is not credentialed to provide flight medicine and legal action may be taken against her.

Answer: D. According to the Aviation Medical Assistance Act of 1998, as long a physician is not conducting "willful misconduct" or "gross negligence," he or she is protected under law in this situation. Physicians are not, however, required to provide assistance and may decline. Physicians should not act beyond the bounds of their clinical expertise or if they are under the influence of sedative substances. Source: https://www.gpo.gov/fdsys/pkg/CRPT-105hrpt456/pdf/CRPT-105hrpt456.pdf

11. A 76-year-old male with a debilitating stroke is in the ICU with persistent bacteremia, vasopressor requirement, and dependence upon continuous hemodialysis. The patient's family becomes irate during a family meeting, and an altercation occurs between them and the nephrologist consultant. They firmly refuse this nephrologist's further involvement on the case. Which of the following scenarios is an appropriate course of action?

A. The neurologist arranges for transition of care to another nephrologist.
B. The intensivist refuses to continue dialysis on the patient due to the family's inability to cooperate with the nephrology team.
C. The nephrologist stops seeing the patient but continues to write dialysis orders and has his fellow examine the patient on rounds.

D. A nephrologist refuses to leave the care team and continues to round on the patient.

Answer: A. Physicians can fire patients as long as they arrange for transition of care to another physician. In this case the family has fired the physician but they cannot easily seek out another nephrologist. It is therefore the obligation of the primary physician to find a replacement nephrologist to assume care of this patient. Source: https://www.ama-assn.org/delivering-care/frequently-asked-questions-ethics

INDEX

Tables, figures, and boxes are indicated by *t, f,* and *b* following the page number

anaphylaxis, 125–129. *See also* anaphylactic
reactions
causes of, 126
conclusions, 128
defined, 125
diagnosis of, 125, 127
differential diagnosis of, 125
discussion, 126–128
food allergies–related, 125–126
incidence of, 126
management of, 125–128
follow-up care, 128
pathogenesis of, 126
prevention of
counseling in, 126
review questions, 128–129
risk factors for, 126–127
signs and symptoms of, 126
stem case and key questions, 125–126
triggers for, 125–127
WAO guidelines for, 125
anemia
differential diagnosis of, 94
anesthesia/anesthetics
in AIS/LVO management, 81–82
general
in PEC management, 151–152
inhaled-halogenated
in status asthmaticus management, 4
aneurysm(s)
clipping of
after SAH, 59
hemorrhagic CVA, 55–62. hemorrhagic
CVA/aneurysm, with cerebral arterial
vasospasm; (*see also* acute subarachnoid
hemorrhage (aSAH); subarachnoid
hemorrhage [SAH])
angina
atypical
defined, 102
typical
defined, 102
unstable
defined, 102
risk factors for, 103, 103b
angioedema
airway management for, 125
angiography
in AIS/LVO diagnosis, 80, 81t
CT
in AIS/LVO diagnosis, 79
in LVAD–associated intracranial hemorrhage, 245f, 248
magnetic resonance
in mesenteric ischemia diagnosis, 183
Ankola, A.A., 15
Annals of Thoracic Surgery, 261–262
antiarrhythmics
in ventricular arrhythmias after CABG
management, 230, 231t–232t

anticholinergics
in status asthmaticus management, 2
anticoagulation
in AF management, 222–223
in AF with rapid ventricular response post
mitral valve repair management, 220
in LVAD–associated intracranial hemorrhage management, 246, 249
after bleeding complication, 250
emergent reversal of, 249
parenteral
in POMI management, 96
antihistamine(s)
H1
in anaphylaxis management, 127
H2
in anaphylaxis management, 127
anti-NMDA receptor (anti-NMDAR) encephalitis. *See* anti-NMDAR encephalitis
anti-NMDAR encephalitis, 71–76
conclusion, 75
diagnosis of, 71, 73
differential diagnosis of, 73
discussion, 72–75
mechanism of, 73–74
neurologic symptoms of, 72
presentation of, 72
prodrome of, 72
prognosis of, 74–75
psychiatric symptoms of, 72
recovery following, 74–75
relapses following, 75
review questions, 76
seizures in
differential diagnosis of, 71
sequelae, 75
stem case and key questions, 71–72
supplemental charts and images, 76
treatment of, 71–72, 74
future directions in, 75
antithrombotic therapy
in POMI management, 96
APAP devices. *See* autotitrating positive
airway pressure (APAP) devices
apnea
obstructive sleep. *See* obstructive sleep
apnea (OSA)
apnea-hypopnea index (AHI), 175
apoplexy
pituitary, 87–92. (*see also* pituitary
apoplexy)
ARDS. *See* acute respiratory distress syndrome (ARDS)
ARDSnet protocol, 50
arrhythmia(s)
ventricular. (*see* ventricular arrhythmias)
arterial embolization
in PPH management, 160
arterial ligation
in PPH management, 160

ASA. *See* alcohol septal ablation (ASA)
aSAH. *See* acute subarachnoid hemorrhage
(aSAH)
Ashbaugh, D.G., 25
ASPECTS. *See* Alberta Stroke Program
Early CT Score (ASPECTS)
asthma. *See also specific types and* status
asthmaticus
acute
hallmarks of, 2
airway response in, 2
causes of, 2
conclusions, 5
costs related to, 2
defined, 2
discussion, 2–5, 3t
pathogenesis of, 2
pathology of, 2
prevalence of, 2
refractory
in pediatric patient, 1–8. (*see also* refractory asthma, in pediatric patient)
review questions, 6–8
severe
medical management of, 2–4, 3t. (*see
also* status asthmaticus)
atrial fibrillation (AF)
causes of, 220
HCM–related, 111–112
OSA and, 174
pathophysiology of, 220
postoperative. (*see* postoperative atrial
fibrillation [POAF])
with rapid ventricular response post mitral
valve repair, 219–226. (*see also* postoperative atrial fibrillation [POAF])
anticoagulation for, 220
conclusions, 223
diagnosis of, 219
discussion, 220–223
implications of, 221
incidence of, 220
management of, 219–223
preventive measures, 222
review questions, 224–226
risk factors for, 219, 221
stem case and key questions, 219–220
atypical angina
defined, 102
automatic internal cardiac defibrillator (AICD)
American College of Cardiology guidelines for, 233
in ventricular arrhythmias after CABG
management, 233
auto-PEEP, 5
autotitrating positive airway pressure
(APAP) devices
in OSA management, 175
AVWS. *See* acquired von Willebrand syndrome (AVWS)

hypertrophic cardiomyopathy
(HCM) (*cont.*)
management of, 110–111
ASA in, 108, 111
future interventions, 112
ICD in, 108, 111, 111*b*
invasive, 111
medications in, 107
noninvasive, 110–111
surgical myectomy in, 108, 111
murmurs associated with, 107
natural history of, 108
obstructive, 109–110
conclusions, 112
management of, 108, 110–111
review questions, 113–115
with SAM, 107–115
stem case and key questions, 107–108
pathophysiology of, 109–110, 110*f*
review questions, 113–115
SAM with, 109–111, 110*f*
SCD in
prevention of, 111, 111*b*
risk factors for, 108, 111
sequelae, 108
stem case and key questions, 107–108
hypertrophy
HCM–related, 109–110
hypocalcemia
massive blood transfusion–related, 48, 49
hypoplastic left heart syndrome (HLHS),
15–17, 16*f*, 17*f*
hypotension
maternal
during labor induction, 165
hypothermia
massive blood transfusion–related, 48, 49
hypovolemia
LVAD–associated, 247*t*, 248
hypoxia
causes of, 39
hysterectomy
caesarean
in PPH management, 160–161

I

IABP. *See* intra-aortic balloon pump
(IABP)
IAH. *See* intra-abdominal hypertension
(IAH)
ICD. *See* implantable cardioverter-defibrillator (ICD)
immunotherapy
second-line
in anti-NMDAR encephalitis management, 74
implantable cardioverter-defibrillator (ICD)
in HCM management, 108, 111, 111*b*
inhaled bronchodilators
in status asthmaticus management, 2

inhaled-halogenated anesthetics
in status asthmaticus management, 4
in-hospital acute coronary syndrome,
101–106. *See also* acute coronary
syndrome, in-hospital
in-stent stenosis
with ACS
treatment of, 104
*Interactive Cardiovascular and Thoracic
Surgery,* 260
Interagency Registry for Mechanically
Assisted Circulatory Support
(INTERMACS), 238
database report, 250
INTERMACS. *See* Interagency Registry for
Mechanically Assisted Circulatory
Support (INTERMACS)
internal cardiac defibrillator
in VT/VF management, 227
International Society for Heart and Lung
Transplantation Guidelines for
Mechanical Circulatory Support, 249
International Society of Thrombosis and
Hemostasis, 198
intra-abdominal hypertension (IAH),
203–211
becoming ACS, 203–204
causes of, 203, 204, 205*b*
concerns related to, 203
conclusions, 208
described, 203
diagnosis of, 203, 205, 205*f*, 205*b*
discussion, 204–208, 205*b*, 204*b*, 205*f*–
208*f*, 208*b*
grades of, 204, 204*b*
management of, 204–208, 206*f*–208*f*,
208*b*
outcomes of, 208
pathogenesis of, 204
review questions, 209–211
stem case and key questions, 203–204
intra-abdominal pressure
measurement of, 205, 205*b*
intra-aortic balloon pump (IABP)
advantages/disadvantages of, 94
CABG vs., 94
in cardiogenic shock management, 97–98,
97*f*
counterpulsation associated with
complications of, 94
hemodynamic effects of, 94
for refractory shock, 93–94
in VT management, 119
intracranial hemorrhage
LVAD patient presenting with, 245–253.
(*see also* left ventricular assist
device (LVAD), intracranial hemorrhage in patient with)
intracranial hypertension
assessment of, 65–66

conclusions, 66–67
defined, 65
discussion, 65–67, 66*f*
management of, 66
review questions, 67–69
stem case and key questions, 63–64
TBI related to, 66. (*see also* traumatic
brain injury [TBI])
intubation
in status asthmaticus management, 5
ischemia
cerebral
delayed. (*see* delayed cerebral ischemia)
mesenteric, 181–187. (*see also* mesenteric
ischemia)
myocardial. (*see* myocardial ischemia)

J

Jehovah's Witness religion
ethics in critical care factors related to,
275–281
conclusion, 277
discussion, 276–277
preoperative modification of risk, 277
review questions, 278–281
stem case and key questions, 275–276
Johnson, S.B., II, 9
*Journal of Cardiothoracic and Vascular
Anesthesia,* 262
J-waves, 48*f*, 49

K

ketamine
in status asthmaticus management, 3*t*, 4
Ketzler, J., 139
kidney injuries, 144, 145*t*
grading of, 144, 145*t*

L

LABAs. *See* long-acting beta-2 agonists
(LABAs)
labor induction
maternal hypotension during
differential diagnosis of, 165
Lancet, 261
Landry, D.W, 258
laparoscopic bowel surgery
sepsis following, 197–202. (*see also*
sepsis, laparoscopic bowel
surgery–related)
laparoscopic gastric bypass surgery
OSA after, 173–179. (*see also* obstructive
sleep apnea (OSA), after laparoscopic gastric bypass surgery)
large vessel occlusion (LVO). *See also* acute
ischemic stroke/large vessel occlusion (AIS/LVO)
described, 79
left middle cerebral artery (MCA) acute
stroke syndrome